Paramedic Exam Review

Third Edition

Bob Elling, MPA, EMT-P
Kirsten M. Elling, BS, EMT-P

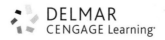
DELMAR
CENGAGE Learning·

Australia • Brazil • Japan • Korea • Mexico • Singapore • Spain • United Kingdom • United States

DELMAR
CENGAGE Learning

Paramedic Exam Review, Third Edition
Bob Elling and Kirsten M. Elling

Vice President, Careers & Computing:
    Dave Garza

Director of Learning Solutions: Sandy Clark

Senior Acquisitions Editor: Janet E. Maker

Managing Editor: Larry Main

Senior Product Manager: Jennifer Starr

Editorial Assistant: Leah Costakis

Vice President, Marketing: Jennifer Baker

Marketing Director: Deborah Yarnell

Associate Marketing Manager: Erica Glisson

Senior Production Director: Wendy Troeger

Production Manager: Mark Bernard

Content Project Management: PreMediaGlobal

Cover Design: PreMediaGlobal

For product information and technology assistance, contact us at
Cengage Learning Customer & Sales Support, 1-800-354-9706

For permission to use material from this text or product,
submit all requests online at **cengage.com/permissions.**
Further permissions questions can be e-mailed to
permissionrequest@cengage.com

Library of Congress Control Number: 2012933139

ISBN-13: 978-1-133-13129-8

ISBN-10: 1-133-13129-8

Delmar
5 Maxwell Drive
Clifton Park, NY 12065-2919
USA

Cengage Learning is a leading provider of customized learning solutions with office locations around the globe, including Singapore, the United Kingdom, Australia, Mexico, Brazil, and Japan. Locate your local office at:
international.cengage.com/region

Cengage Learning products are represented in Canada by Nelson Education, Ltd.

To learn more about Delmar, visit **www.cengage.com/delmar**

Purchase any of our products at your local college store or at our preferred online store **www.cengagebrain.com**

Notice to the Reader
Publisher does not warrant or guarantee any of the products described herein or perform any independent analysis in connection with any of the product information contained herein. Publisher does not assume, and expressly disclaims, any obligation to obtain and include information other than that provided to it by the manufacturer. The reader is expressly warned to consider and adopt all safety precautions that might be indicated by the activities described herein and to avoid all potential hazards. By following the instructions contained herein, the reader willingly assumes all risks in connection with such instructions. The publisher makes no representations or warranties of any kind, including but not limited to, the warranties of fitness for particular purpose or merchantability, nor are any such representations implied with respect to the material set forth herein, and the publisher takes no responsibility with respect to such material. The publisher shall not be liable for any special, consequential, or exemplary damages resulting, in whole or part, from the readers' use of, or reliance upon, this material.

Printed in the United States of America
1 2 3 4 5 6 7 16 15 14 13 12

Dedication

This work is dedicated to Kirsten and my daughters Laura and Caitlin.
May you always maintain humility as your accomplishments meet the stars.

—BOB ELLING

In memory of my mother Inge Nicholson, 1940–2000, whose love and support I miss very much.
To my husband Bob, whose support and inspiration continue to drive me to
continuously improve patient care in the field.

—KIRSTEN M. ELLING

Contents

Preface

Intent of This Book

Paramedic Exam Review, third edition, is an excellent resource for preparing for your State or National Registry written exams. This book is a valuable tool to help review your knowledge, and practice the content requirements in order to build confidence for the actual exam. Intended as a review for both state and national paramedic examinations, the book is designed to follow the organizational chapter format of the 2009 National Emergency Medical Services Education Standards: Paramedic Instructional Guidelines as well as the 2010 American Heart Association Guidelines for Emergency Cardiovascular Care and CPR.

Why We Wrote This Book

Paramedic training has evolved quite a bit since I first completed the program at the Institute of Albert Einstein Medical School in "da-Bronx" back in 1978. I remember the first day of class when Dr. Jacobson and the instructor coordinators (Ronnie & Kevin) wheeled in a hand truck piled high with papers that we used as our textbook. Most of the materials consisted of the yet-unpublished draft of the paramedic book that Nancy Caroline, M.D., had just completed for the U.S. DOT and lots of interesting articles from the medical journals. These days, it is hard to find a "15-module trained" medic still working in the field. Both Kirsten, my co-author and partner, and I have seen the curriculum become more enriched and sophisticated in 1985 with the six-division program and then again in 1998 and once again in 2009 with the latest revision. Working as paramedics and EMS educators for the past three decades, both Kirsten and I have seen medic training evolve firsthand. Today there are many choices of books, magazines, video, workbooks, and Web sites for instructors to use to prepare their students for the streets.

We sincerely hope you will enjoy *Paramedic Exam Review*, third edition, and benefit from the test-taking review to expand your knowledge base. After all, when the real test occurs, in the field, our patients rely on us to be prepared. See you in the streets!

—*Bob & Kirsten Elling*

Features of This Book

- *Accessible for Both Certification and Refresher Exams* These questions allow you to study for the exam whether you are a candidate for paramedic certification, or a current paramedic working to renew certification.
- *Aligns with the National Instructional Guidelines* The chapter order follows that of the curriculum for ease of reference and use. Early in this project we also made a decision that the questions would only be the multiple choice style with the standard format of three distractors and one correct answer to each question. Because this book will be used to prepare for both state and national paramedic examinations, it makes the most sense to use the format and style of questions used on these types of exams, in order to provide the best possible practice and build confidence for the actual exam.
- *Literally thousands of questions* We suggest you tackle a chapter at a time and, after taking each exam, check the answer key and mark the ones you need to review. The more time you spend using the practice questions, the better your chances for success on the exam.
- *Answers and Rationale* The rationale for correct answers provides you with the necessary feedback for understanding the context of the question, and, if applicable, a point of reference for review.
- *NREMT Skill Sheets* are provided in the Appendices, offering the necessary knowledge of the requirements for those preparing for the National Registry Paramedic certification exam.
- *An Interactive CD* offers further practice and review including two full-length simulated practice exams.

New to This Edition

- *Covers New Content Areas in the Instructional Guidelines* Additional chapters have been added to cover all the additional content areas of the new curriculum.

- *New Scenario-Based Questions* Practice crucial critical-thinking skills that will be required on the job as a paramedic.

- *10% New Questions* A fresh approach to the content ensures that the questions remain up to date with the latest information required on the state and national paramedic exams.

- *Updated to the 2010 AHA Guidelines* The questions provide technical information that remains updated to the latest procedures outlined by the 2010 edition of the American Heart Association Guidelines for Emergency Cardiovascular Care and CPR.

- *Accompanying CD Includes Interactive Practice Exams, Games, and More* reflecting current information of the National EMS Educational Standards and the 2010 AHA Guidelines and offering additional review for the exam.

About the Authors

Bob Elling, MPA, EMT-P

Bob has been involved in EMS since 1975. He is an active paramedic with Colonie EMS Department, the Times Union Center, and Whiteface Mountain Medical Services, all in upstate New York. He is a passionate volunteer for the American Heart Association and has served as national faculty as well as a board member and advocate for strengthening the links in the chain of survival. He is also regional faculty for the NYS Bureau of EMS. Bob is a clinical instructor for Albany Medical Center assigned to teach in the paramedic program at Hudson Valley Community College. He has also served as a paramedic and lieutenant for NYC EMS, program director for the Institute of Prehospital Emergency Medicine of HVCC, associate director of the NYS EMS Program, and the education coordinator for PULSE: Emergency Medical Update. Bob is an author/coauthor of many CengageLearning titles in addition to *Paramedic Exam Review*, 3e, including: *Principles of Assessment in EMS*, *Why-Driven EMS Review*, 2e, and *Advanced EMT Exam Review, 2e.*

Kirsten M. Elling, BS, EMT-P

Kirsten (Kirt) Elling is a career paramedic who works in the Town of Colonie in upstate New York. She began work in EMS in 1988 as an EMT/firefighter and has been a National Registered paramedic since 1991. She has been an EMS educator since 1990 and teaches basic and advanced EMS programs at the Institute of Prehospital Emergency Medicine in Troy, New York. Kirsten serves as regional faculty NYS DOH, Bureau of EMS and regional faculty American Heart Association, Northeast region. In addition to *Paramedic Exam Review*, 3e, Kirsten is the author/coauthor of the following: Numerous scripts for the EMS training video series PULSE: Emergency Medical Update; *EMT Exam Review*, 2e; *Emergency Medical Responder Exam Review*; *Advanced EMT Exam Review,*; *Why-Driven EMS Review*, 2e; *Principles of Assessment for the EMS Provider*; contributing author of the Paramedic Lab Manual for the IPEM, and an adjunct writer for the 1998 and 2009 revisions of the National Highway Traffic Safety Administration, EMT-Paramedic and EMT-Intermediate: National Standard Curricula.

Also Available

Elling, Elling & Rothenburg/*Why-Driven EMS Review*, Second Edition
(978-1-4180-3817-5)

Elling, Kirsten/*Emergency Medical Responder Exam Review*
(978-1-4180-7286-5)

Elling, Kristen/*Emergency Medical Technician Exam Review*, Second Edition
(978-1-1133131281)

Elling, Elling/*Advanced EMT Exam Review* (978-1-1336-8702-3)

Acknowledgments

Thank you to the editorial and production team at Delmar Cengage Learning who contributed to this new edition, especially Janet Maker, Jennifer Starr, Jim Zayicek, and Jennifer Hanley, as well as the project team at PreMedia Global.

Also, special thanks to our reviewers:

Linda Anderson
Director, Paramedic Education
Santa Rosa Junior College
Windsor, CA

Mike McLaughlin
Director of Health Occupations
Kirkwood Community College
Cedar Rapids, IA

David McDonald
Program Faculty
Greenville Technical College
Greenville, SC

Gordon Kokx
Associate Professor
College of Southern Idaho
Twin Falls, ID

Workforce Safety and Wellness

1. _____ is defined as a state of complete physical, mental, and social well-being.
   a. Health
   b. Wellness
   c. Fitness
   d. Nutrition

2. The components of wellness include physical well-being, proper nutrition, and:
   a. vaccinations.
   b. past medical history.
   c. mental and emotional health.
   d. compliance with prescribed medications.

3. Proper nutrition involves an understanding of nutrients the body needs, as well as the principles of:
   a. mental health.
   b. emotional well-being.
   c. exercise.
   d. weight control.

4. According to the Surgeon General's Report on Nutrition and Health, diet-related diseases account for over _____ of all deaths in the United States.
   a. one-quarter
   b. one-third
   c. one-half
   d. two-thirds

5. Poor diet and nutrition can be attributed to the development of degenerative diseases such as:
   a. gout.
   b. anxiety.
   c. diabetes.
   d. chronic lung disease.

6. The diets of paramedics are often complicated by meals that are rushed, interrupted, and:
   a. provide limited access to choices of food types.
   b. provide increased susceptibility to lactose intolerance.
   c. low in cholesterol.
   d. high in vitamins and complex carbohydrates.

7. For the paramedic who is making a conscious effort to eat better at work, which of the following activities should be avoided?
   a. preparing meals at home in advance
   b. expanding the range of foods from your normal choices
   c. stopping for fast food when you are hungry and did not bring a meal
   d. bringing along a small cooler with fresh fruits or vegetable snacks

8. Which of the following modifications to a diet is considered to be a reasonable and healthy change?
   a. watching the fat content, not the calories
   b. making small changes with a slow transition
   c. drinking less fluid before and during meals
   d. watching only the calories, not the fat content

9. Which of the following tips about snacking is most accurate?
   a. Low-fiber snacks are better for dental health.
   b. Snacking will make you fat and should be avoided.
   c. Waiting until you are starving before you eat a snack will better satisfy your hunger.
   d. Snacks can fill the voids between meals and should be a part of your food plan.

10. Being physically fit involves a combination of elements, including aerobic conditioning, strength, endurance, and:
    a. attitude.
    b. monitoring your heart rate.
    c. having a personal trainer.
    d. being able to run several miles a week.

11. Before starting a fitness program, it is a good idea to get a physical examination by a physician because:
    a. a physician will identify any specific limitations to consider.
    b. most gyms require medical clearance before joining.
    c. athletic trainers require medical clearance before working with new clients.
    d. your physician will prescribe steroids to help you increase muscle mass.

12. Which of the following immunizations may be recommended rather than required for some paramedics?
    a. rubella
    b. hepatitis B
    c. Lyme disease
    d. tetanus and diphtheria

13. Being physically fit has many benefits, including:
    a. decreased metabolism.
    b. decreased resistance to injury and illness.
    c. improved personal appearance and self-image.
    d. increased blood pressure and resting heart rate.

14. Routine aerobic exercise lasting at least 20 minutes, three times a week, improves the cardiac stroke volume of the heart while increasing:
    a. the resting heart rate.
    b. wear and tear on the heart.
    c. nutritional fortitude.
    d. physical endurance.

15. _____ are regular changes in mental and physical characteristics that occur in the course of a day.
    a. Anxieties
    b. Circadian rhythms
    c. Addictions
    d. Stimulants

16. Major industrial accidents, such as the Exxon Valdez oil spill, have been attributed partly to errors made by:
    a. fatigued night-shift workers.
    b. smokers who suffered a stroke.
    c. stressed, obese shift workers.
    d. overdose on NoDoz®.

17. When considering the risk assessment for cardiovascular disease, the paramedic should take into account:
    a. blood pressure.
    b. personal hygiene.
    c. exposure to the sun.
    d. proper lifting techniques.

18. To avoid contact with a potentially infectious body fluid found on a piece of your equipment, you remove the substance. You use a product that is designed to kill all forms of microbial life, except high numbers of bacterial spores. This level of cleaning is called:
    a. low-level disinfection.
    b. intermediate-level disinfection.
    c. high-level disinfection.
    d. sterilization.

19. Which of the following is considered an unsafe practice rather than a proper lifting technique?
    a. bending at the hips
    b. avoiding any twisting when lifting
    c. using caution and knowing your limits
    d. keeping the load close to your body

20. A low-priority call at a two-story apartment building for an elderly woman who fell has suddenly turned into a hostile scene. The patient is conscious and confused, with an obvious fracture to the left ankle. She is refusing transport, throwing objects, and spitting. Which of the following actions is most appropriate for this scenario?
    a. Stand your ground while waiting for the police.
    b. Retreat to your ambulance until the police arrive.
    c. Leave yourself an exit and be prepared to retreat.
    d. Force a mask onto the patient's face, and then physically restrain her.

21. A frequent and typical profile of an ambulance collision is one that occurs in the:
    a. daytime, on clear, dry roads.
    b. night, involving intoxicated drivers.
    c. winter, while driving on snow and ice.
    d. fall, when the roads are covered with wet leaves.

22. Knowledge of the proper use of lights and sirens, as well as the public's typical reactions, includes the understanding that:
    a. these devices guarantee you the right of way.
    b. there are limitations with the use of lights and sirens.
    c. the public has to yield the right of way.
    d. driving an emergency vehicle requires a special course.

23. Which of the following actions can a paramedic employ to reduce the risks associated with driving an emergency vehicle?
    a. using lights and sirens on training drills
    b. using a police escort whenever possible
    c. avoiding the use of flashing lights at night and in fog
    d. driving with due regard for the safety of other drivers

24. When developing strategies to help reduce or eliminate ambulance collisions, you should consider which of the following?
    a. Provide instruction on the use of global positioning systems (GPS).
    b. Ensure that vehicle operators know the proper way to change a tire.
    c. Test all drivers on their knowledge of standard operating procedures (SOPs).
    d. Ensure that only the most senior operators drive with the siren and lights on.

25. For which emergency vehicle operation topic should each emergency service have an SOP?
    a. What to do when a collision occurs?
    b. How to load and unload a stretcher?
    c. How to deal with uncooperative drivers?
    d. How to avoid inclement weather conditions?

26. Safety equipment that paramedics use at the scene of a collision may include:
    a. head protection, such as a helmet.
    b. eye protection, such as safety goggles or shields.
    c. a turnout coat to protect from sharp objects.
    d. all of the above.

27. Twenty minutes after the cessation of smoking a cigarette, which of the following physical changes occurs?
    a. The pulse rate increases.
    b. The blood pressure increases.
    c. The blood pressure decreases.
    d. The body temperature of the hands and feet decreases.

28. At 1 year after the cessation of cigarette smoking, the excess risk of coronary heart diseases is decreased to _____ of a smoker.
    a. one-fourth
    b. one-third
    c. one-half
    d. two-thirds

29. Which of the following is inaccurate about the cessation of cigarette smoking?
    a. Even heavy smokers can benefit significantly by stopping.
    b. For longtime smokers, stopping is not of any benefit.
    c. At 5–10 years after quitting, the stroke risk is reduced to that of nonsmokers.
    d. Nicotine is a drug that causes addiction.

30. All of the following are accurate about the effects of nicotine, *except*:
    a. nicotine has no effect on nerve cells.
    b. withdrawal is difficult with nicotine.
    c. nicotine can act as a stimulant.
    d. nicotine can act as a sedative.

31. A(n) _____ is a compulsive need for, and use of, a habit-forming substance.
    a. anxiety
    b. addiction
    c. agonist
    d. stimulant

32. Which of the following statements is most correct in reference to stress?
    a. Stress is associated with positive events.
    b. Stress is only associated with negative events.
    c. Stress is an unnatural and unnecessary emotion.
    d. Stress is a harmful emotion that should be avoided.

33. The three distinct phases of a stress response include:
    a. anxiety, panic, and relief.
    b. alarm, denial, and acceptance.
    c. alarm, resistance, and exhaustion.
    d. physical, emotional, and behavioral.

34. A person can become desensitized or adapted to extreme stressors. This is a result of an increase in the:
    a. level of resistance in the resistance phase of the stress reaction.
    b. production of epinephrine in the alarm reaction phase.
    c. norepinephrine released during the denial phase.
    d. glucose production from a pituitary response.

35. As stress continues, and coping mechanisms are exhausted, the body will have an increased:
    a. release of adrenocorticotropic hormones.
    b. pulse rate and blood pressure.
    c. resistance to stressors.
    d. susceptibility to physical and psychological ailments.

36. You are treating a patient who is having a lot of stress in his life. Which of the following is a cognitive sign or symptom of stress?
    a. anger
    b. disorientation
    c. chest tightness
    d. aching muscles and joints

37. An emotional sign or symptom of stress may include:
    a. depression.
    b. panic reaction.
    c. poor concentration.
    d. increased smoking.

38. Which of the following is a physical sign or symptom of stress?
    a. nausea and vomiting
    b. feeling overwhelmed
    c. fighting with coworkers
    d. increased alcohol consumption

39. You are evaluating a patient with multiple general complaints. During your interview and physical assessment, you have learned that this patient is experiencing withdrawal, is smoking more than usual, and displays hyperactivity. These are all _____ signs and symptoms of stress.
    a. cognitive
    b. physical
    c. emotional
    d. behavioral

40. _____ is an example of an environmental stress trigger.
    a. Siren noise
    b. Inclement weather
    c. Confined workspace
    d. All of the above

41. An example of a psychosocial stress trigger is:
    a. a conflict with a supervisor or coworker.
    b. a rapid scene response.
    c. life and death decision making.
    d. hyperventilation syndrome.

42. Personality and emotional stress in paramedics is often caused by a trigger such as:
    a. feelings of guilt.
    b. changes in eating habits.
    c. changes in sleep patterns.
    d. cardiac rhythm disturbances.

43. _____ is an active process of confronting the stress or the cause of the stress.
    a. Putting up defenses
    b. Coping
    c. Exposure
    d. Gaining experience

44. _____ is a technique used to manage stress.
    a. Circadian rhythms
    b. Controlled breathing
    c. Guided hyperactivity
    d. Sleep deprivation

45. _____ is an organized process that enables emergency personnel to vent feelings and facilitates understanding of stressful situations.
    a. Coping for EMS providers (CEMSP)
    b. EMS problem solving (EMSPS)
    c. Emergency EMS distress (EEMSD)
    d. Critical incident stress management (CISM)

46. You are concerned about your partner since the fire where the two of you pulled out an entire family with critical burns. One of the indications that a coworker may be experiencing a crisis-induced stress reaction would be:
    a. getting plenty of rest.
    b. focusing on the positives.
    c. signs of gastrointestinal distress.
    d. maintaining a good sense of humor.

47. A characteristic example of an incident that might provoke a crisis-induced stress reaction in a paramedic would be:
    a. a prolonged incident.
    b. defusing a large-scale incident.
    c. line-of-duty death or serious injury.
    d. successful reversal of a cardiac arrest.

48. A practice for paramedics to avoid when trying to reduce crisis-induced stress would be:
    a. getting plenty of rest.
    b. replacing fluids and food.
    c. increased cigarette smoking.
    d. limiting exposure to the provoking incident.

49. During the grieving process, it is not unusual for families to vent their anger on the paramedic. As long as there is no perceived physical harm to you, it is best to:
    a. allow them to express their feelings as best as you can.
    b. walk away, as it could get personal.
    c. give them your opinion based on your experience.
    d. let them argue with the police instead.

50. In which developmental age group do children begin to understand the finality of death?
    a. 3–6 years old
    b. 6–9 years old
    c. 9–12 years old
    d. adolescence

51. Which of the following statements about helping children deal with grief is most accurate?
    a. It is less distressing for the child to see that "everything is normal."
    b. Tell the truth and be straightforward when talking about the death of a loved one.
    c. Shielding a child from grief may protect her in the long run.
    d. A child seeing his father cry over the mother's death is an unnecessary burden on the child.

52. You are treating a family who is upset due to the recent loss of their 12-year-old son in a skiing accident. The stages of the grieving process will vary for any given individual; however, most will experience all of the stages, beginning with:
    a. anger.
    b. shock.
    c. denial.
    d. bargaining.

53. Prevention of disease transmission by the paramedic includes all the following, *except*:
    a. protection against airborne pathogens.
    b. protection against blood-borne pathogens.
    c. following recommended guidelines for proper cleaning and disinfection.
    d. sterilizing all ambulance equipments on a regular basis.

54. A(n) _____ is contact with a potentially infectious body fluid substance that may be carrying a pathogen.
    a. exposure
    b. removal
    c. reaction
    d. preventive measure

55. The procedure used to manage an exposure includes:
    a. conducting the incident investigation.
    b. conducting a period risk assessment.
    c. completing the required medical follow-up.
    d. safeguarding against potential disciplinary action.

56. When documenting an exposure, the paramedic should include:
    a. periodic risk assessment.
    b. ongoing exposure-control training.
    c. actions taken to reduce chances of infection.
    d. obtaining proper immunization boosters.

57. _____ is cleaning the surface of objects with a specific agent designed to kill pathogens that may have come in contact with the object.
    a. Cleaning
    b. Disinfection
    c. Sterilization
    d. Isolation precaution

58. Your agency's SOPs require that you follow standard precautions. Standard precautions are a series of practices designed to:
    a. prevent lapses in immunizations.
    b. improve screening for exposures.
    c. improve personal hygiene habits.
    d. prevent contact with body substances such as blood and urine.

59. There are a number of effective ways paramedics can positively deal with excessive stress, such as:
    a. alcohol.
    b. biofeedback.
    c. decreasing exercise.
    d. overeating.

60. You are treating a patient who is under a doctor's care for a stress disorder. All of the following are used to treat stress, *except*:
    a. vaccination.
    b. patient education.
    c. medication.
    d. psychotherapy.

Exam #1 Answer Form

	A	B	C	D			A	B	C	D
1.	❏	❏	❏	❏		31.	❏	❏	❏	❏
2.	❏	❏	❏	❏		32.	❏	❏	❏	❏
3.	❏	❏	❏	❏		33.	❏	❏	❏	❏
4.	❏	❏	❏	❏		34.	❏	❏	❏	❏
5.	❏	❏	❏	❏		35.	❏	❏	❏	❏
6.	❏	❏	❏	❏		36.	❏	❏	❏	❏
7.	❏	❏	❏	❏		37.	❏	❏	❏	❏
8.	❏	❏	❏	❏		38.	❏	❏	❏	❏
9.	❏	❏	❏	❏		39.	❏	❏	❏	❏
10.	❏	❏	❏	❏		40.	❏	❏	❏	❏
11.	❏	❏	❏	❏		41.	❏	❏	❏	❏
12.	❏	❏	❏	❏		42.	❏	❏	❏	❏
13.	❏	❏	❏	❏		43.	❏	❏	❏	❏
14.	❏	❏	❏	❏		44.	❏	❏	❏	❏
15.	❏	❏	❏	❏		45.	❏	❏	❏	❏
16.	❏	❏	❏	❏		46.	❏	❏	❏	❏
17.	❏	❏	❏	❏		47.	❏	❏	❏	❏
18.	❏	❏	❏	❏		48.	❏	❏	❏	❏
19.	❏	❏	❏	❏		49.	❏	❏	❏	❏
20.	❏	❏	❏	❏		50.	❏	❏	❏	❏
21.	❏	❏	❏	❏		51.	❏	❏	❏	❏
22.	❏	❏	❏	❏		52.	❏	❏	❏	❏
23.	❏	❏	❏	❏		53.	❏	❏	❏	❏
24.	❏	❏	❏	❏		54.	❏	❏	❏	❏
25.	❏	❏	❏	❏		55.	❏	❏	❏	❏
26.	❏	❏	❏	❏		56.	❏	❏	❏	❏
27.	❏	❏	❏	❏		57.	❏	❏	❏	❏
28.	❏	❏	❏	❏		58.	❏	❏	❏	❏
29.	❏	❏	❏	❏		59.	❏	❏	❏	❏
30.	❏	❏	❏	❏		60.	❏	❏	❏	❏

CHAPTER 2

EMS Systems, Roles and Responsibilities of the Paramedic

1. The first civilian ambulance service was started in _____ in 1865.
   a. New York City
   b. Cincinnati
   c. Philadelphia
   d. Chicago

2. In _____ the first rescue squad was launched by Julien Stanley Wise in Roanoke, VA.
   a. 1903
   b. 1928
   c. 1955
   d. 1962

3. In 1956, Dr. Safar and Dr. Elan demonstrated the effectiveness of:
   a. public access defibrillation.
   b. mouth-to-mouth resuscitation.
   c. seat belts to save lives in motor vehicle collisions.
   d. electricity to convert ventricular fibrillation to an organized rhythm.

4. In 1959, the first _____ was developed at Johns Hopkins Hospital for the treatment of cardiac arrest.
   a. intubation
   b. epinephrine administration
   c. sodium bicarbonate
   d. portable defibrillator

5. In 1966, landmark legislation called the _____ created the U.S. Department of Transportation (DOT) as a cabinet-level department.
   a. White Paper
   b. Highway Safety Act
   c. Committee on Traffic Safety report
   d. EMT-ambulance curriculum

6. In 1972, the _____ was developed to portray the role of rescue workers and paramedics working in the streets.
   a. television show *EMERGENCY!*
   b. Board of Directors of the National Registry of EMTs
   c. Emergency Medical Services Systems Act
   d. National Highway Traffic Safety Administration

7. In 1974, DOT published the "KKK-A-1822" Federal:
   a. educational standards.
   b. Emergency Medical Dispatch system.
   c. Ambulance Specifications.
   d. Standards for CPR.

8. In 1975, the development of the first EMT-Paramedic National Standard Curriculum was contracted to:
   a. the American Academy of Orthopedic Surgeons in Chicago, IL.
   b. Nancy Caroline, MD, and the University of Pittsburgh, PA.
   c. Eugene Nagel, MD, in Jacksonville, FL.
   d. Frank Pantridge, MD, in Belfast Ireland.

9. The _____ EMT-basic curriculum included the use of the automated external defibrillator as a skill taught to the EMT, rather than reserved for only the advanced levels of EMTs.
   a. 1985
   b. 1990
   c. 1995
   d. 1998

10. A(n) _____ is a coordinated effort to bring together a minimum of ten key components to reduce out-of-hospital morbidity and mortality.
    a. EMS curriculum
    b. NHTSA Act
    c. EMS system
    d. emergency medical dispatch flowchart

11. Permission that is granted by a government authority to practice in a profession, business, or activity is called:

a. certification.

b. licensure.

c. public access.

d. registration.

12. A _____ is a document testifying to the fulfillment of the requirements for practice in the field.

a. certification

b. licensure

c. public access

d. registration

13. Which of the following is not one of the four national levels of out-of-hospital training that is recognized by the National Registry of Emergency Medical Technicians?

a. emergency medical responder

b. EMT

c. critical care technician

d. paramedic

14. The level of provider that is not intended to be utilized as the minimum staffing for an ambulance is the:

a. emergency medical responder.

b. critical care technician.

c. EMT.

d. advanced EMT.

15. The roles and responsibilities of the _____ include: providing safety, primary assessment and treatment, including immediate resuscitative measures, and portraying a professional and positive appearance.

a. emergency medical responder

b. advanced EMT

c. paramedic

d. all the above

16. One of the roles of the National Registry of Emergency Medical Technicians (NREMT) is:

a. eradicating the process of state-to-state reciprocity.

b. contributing to the development of professional standards.

c. issuing licensure to the EMS provider once competency has been verified.

d. providing constructive feedback in association with verifying competency.

17. Select the statement that is most accurate regarding paramedic recertification.

a. All states require recertification through the same process.

b. The current paramedic curriculum contains recertification curricula.

c. The current paramedic curriculum does not contain recertification curricula.

d. The medical director of an EMS agency can determine how recertification is to be accomplished.

18. _____ is the legal recognition of training obtained in another state.

a. Recertification

b. Challenging

c. Reciprocity

d. National registration

19. One of the benefits of participating in continuing education is that it:

a. provides positive feedback.

b. guarantees reciprocity to other states.

c. improves your image in the public's eyes.

d. refreshes knowledge and skills, and introduces new material.

20. What is the single most important attribute of a paramedic?

a. integrity

b. indifference

c. good personal hygiene

d. good time management

21. Select the most accurate statement about health care professionals.

a. Smoking in public is viewed as a positive attribute by society.

b. Society's expectations of health care professionals are high, both on and off duty.

c. Working as part of a team is not an essential attribute for the health care profession.

d. When the public sees you without your seat belt on while driving the ambulance, your public image is unaffected.

22. _____ are moral principles of one's practice in his or her profession.

a. Standards of care

b. Ethics

c. Peer review

d. Professional conduct

23. Constructive feedback by other EMS providers in a genuine effort to improve future performance is called:
    a. quality control.
    b. quality improvement.
    c. peer review.
    d. the standard of care.

24. After turning a patient over to the emergency department (ED) staff and giving a verbal report, you complete your documentation for the call. As usual, you are conscientious about providing accurate documentation and completing all necessary paperwork. This attribute is an example of:
    a. integrity.
    b. empathy.
    c. good time management.
    d. working well with others.

25. You are on the scene with an elderly female patient who had a syncopal event, but is now awake and alert. She denies dyspnea and chest pain, and admits to having recent fainting spells. She lives alone and is worried about leaving her home and not being able to return. Your assessment findings are that she is hypotensive and has a third-degree heart block. As you begin treatment, you also address the patient's concern and provide an understanding of her feelings. This is an example of behavior demonstrating:
    a. ethics.
    b. empathy.
    c. sympathy.
    d. self-motivation.

26. _____ acknowledges the patient's circumstances and how serious they must be without the provider becoming emotionally involved.
    a. Empathy
    b. Sympathy
    c. Pity
    d. Kindness

27. Examples of demonstrating self-confidence include:
    a. consulting with medical direction after the patient's condition deteriorates.
    b. having a good understanding of your limitations.
    c. calling for backup after realizing the patient you are lifting is too heavy.
    d. being able to call for help once you are overwhelmed.

28. A neat and professional appearance and being well groomed and clean are important and:
    a. very subjective qualities of an EMT.
    b. an indication of your competency and skills.
    c. show diplomacy to the patient and his family.
    d. help to instill confidence in the patient and his family.

29. An example of the paramedic who demonstrates good time management skills is one who:
    a. is accepting of all learning opportunities.
    b. attends a required continuing education class.
    c. shows enthusiasm for learning and continuous improvement.
    d. is dressed appropriately and prepared to work when the shift begins.

30. Each of the following is an example of a type of way in which errors happen, *except*:
    a. careful documentation of care administered.
    b. skills-based failures.
    c. rules-based failures.
    d. knowledge-based failures.

31. _____ is defined as tact and skill in dealing with people.
    a. Respect
    b. Diplomacy
    c. Teamwork
    d. Communication

32. Which of the following examples of behavior demonstrates unprofessional conduct rather than a teamwork effort?
    a. Disagreeing with a coworker in private
    b. Disagreeing with a coworker in public
    c. Remaining flexible and open to changes
    d. Communicating in an effort to solve problems

33. Patients are at a disadvantage when thrust into the health care system because of a sudden illness or injury; this is why part of the responsibility of the paramedic is to:
    a. let their neighbors know which hospital you took them to.
    b. let them use your cell phone to call a friend.
    c. take their wallet or purse for safekeeping.
    d. be an advocate for your patient.

34. For the paramedic who is making an effort to be conscientious about patient advocacy activities, which of the following should be avoided?
    a. placing the patient's needs ahead of your own
    b. telling a patient who smokes that he is really stupid for doing so
    c. placing your safety and the safety of the crew ahead of your patient's
    d. explaining to an unrestrained patient injured in a motor vehicle collision that being belted during a collision is a safer practice

35. Examples of behavior demonstrating patient advocacy include:
    a. placing the patient's safety above your own.
    b. protecting the patient's confidentiality.
    c. rushing a patient report to get out of work on time.
    d. allowing personal bias to influence patient care.

36. An important attribute for the paramedic is being careful in the delivery of services to the patient. An example of this would be:
    a. consistently adhering to a nutritional diet.
    b. getting to know all the residents in your district.
    c. protecting the patient's furniture while moving your stretcher through the living room.
    d. helping to implement legislation that provides protection from liability for EMS providers when dealing with unusual situations.

37. The primary role of the medical director of an EMS agency is to:
    a. ensure quality patient care.
    b. oversee all continuing education.
    c. delineate the quality control process.
    d. evaluate and revise patient access to definitive care.

38. _____ are guidelines for the management of specific patient-presenting problems.
    a. Diagnoses
    b. Algorithms
    c. Protocols
    d. Definitive care standards

39. The role of the medical director has expanded over the past decade and now typically includes:
    a. participating in the development of continuing education.
    b. developing policies and procedures for billing patient services.
    c. providing interface between EMS systems and the families of patients.
    d. ensuring the proper utilization of safety equipment by EMS personnel.

40. Potential benefits of online (direct) medical control include:
    a. the ability to obtain real-time direction and orders.
    b. interfacing with a physician for more effective treatment.
    c. treatment orders that are more efficient.
    d. quicker access to definitive care.

41. Off-line (indirect) medical control primarily relies on:
    a. judgment.
    b. protocols.
    c. ACLS algorithms.
    d. advanced directives.

42. You are at the scene of a motor vehicle collision treating a head injured patient. If a physician stops at the scene of your call and offers assistance, which of the following should you do before consenting to allow his assistance?
    a. Confirm that the person is actually a medical doctor and not a Ph.D.
    b. Confirm that the physician is willing to come to the hospital with you and the patient.
    c. Let the physician speak to your medical control so they can work together.
    d. All of the above.

43. EMS providers are responsible for being prepared to work in the field as a paramedic in which of the following ways?
    a. by getting a college education
    b. by having a lawyer on retainer for potential lawsuits
    c. by personally knowing many residents in the area where you work
    d. by conforming to the standards of a health care professional providing quality patient care

44. After assessing and managing your patient at the scene, you will need to determine the most appropriate hospital destination. When making the determination about the appropriate destination for your patient, which of the following factors regarding the hospitals in your area should be considered?
    a. clinical capabilities
    b. discharge capacity
    c. rehabilitation resources
    d. availability of critical care beds

45. When returning the ambulance to service after a serious trauma call, one of the primary responsibilities of the paramedic and crew is:
    a. filling any oxygen tanks used on the call.
    b. disinfecting all items used on the call.
    c. performing a complete equipment checklist.
    d. replacing disposable items available from the hospital.

46. Which of the following is the most practical benefit of having paramedics teach in the community?
    a. It enhances the visibility and positive image of paramedics and their agencies.
    b. It ensures the safety of all the children in the community.
    c. It ensures proper utilization of safety helmets.
    d. It helps to get the elderly compliant with medication use.

47. Examples of citizen involvement in EMS systems include all of the following, *except*:
    a. learning how to access EMS.
    b. training and being willing to do bystander CPR.
    c. training to be a career paramedic/firefighter.
    d. fund-raising and lobbying for EMS improvements.

48. As the "scope of practice" evolves, the paramedic may be utilized in nontraditional activities such as:
    a. patient well-care visits.
    b. assisting with daily living activities.
    c. assisting with physical therapy.
    d. minor surgical procedures.

49. The expanded scope pilots have been utilized to bring medically trained health care professionals to the patients when they are underserved or:
    a. in a hospice program.
    b. the transportation alternatives are very costly.
    c. dental or chiropractic services are not affordable.
    d. they cannot prepare their own meals.

50. In the document EMS Agenda for the Future, integration of health services specifically refers to the:
    a. allocation of funding for HMOs.
    b. development of paramedic jobs in private home care.
    c. integration of EMS with other health care providers to deliver quality care.
    d. implementation of laws that provide protection from liability for EMS providers.

51. In the document EMS Agenda for the Future, EMS research is developing strategies to:
    a. address the portion of the population with special needs.
    b. develop a system of reciprocity for EMS provider credentials.
    c. develop information systems that provide linkage between various health care services.
    d. expand the EMS role in public health and involve EMS in community health monitoring activities.

52. Legislation and regulation recommendations for the future of EMS are focused on:
    a. authorizing and funding a leading federal EMS agency.
    b. ensuring the adequacy of EMS education programs.
    c. developing laws for the accreditation of EMS education programs.
    d. developing laws that provide liability insurance for all career and volunteer EMS providers.

53. System finance in EMS is striving for which of the following?
    a. to commission the development of government-funded health care
    b. collaboration with other health care providers and insurers to enhance patient care efficiency
    c. to compensate EMS on the basis of volume
    d. to provide immediate access to the Medicare approval process

54. In the document EMS Agenda for the Future, strategies for human resources include:
    a. conducting EMS occupation health research.
    b. formalizing paramedicine as a subspecialty of home health care.
    c. requiring appropriate credentials for all physicians who provide online medical direction.
    d. enhancing the ability of EMS systems to triage calls and providing resource allocation that is tailored to patients' needs.

55. A key proposal for medical direction in the future is to:
    a. require appropriate credentials for all those who provide online medical direction.
    b. develop a system for reciprocity of EMS physician credentials.
    c. ensure that medical directors are allocated federal funding for participating in an EMS system.
    d. appoint national EMS medical directors.

56. In the document EMS Agenda for the Future, strategies for educational systems include:
    a. accrediting only college-based EMS education.
    b. promulgating and updating standards for EMS dispatch.
    c. acknowledging that public education is a critical EMS activity.
    d. developing, bridging, and transitioning EMS programs with all health professions' education.

57. Goals for EMS public education for the future include:
    a. relying on HMOs to get the message out.
    b. collaborating efforts with federally funded programs.
    c. exploring and evaluating public education alternatives.
    d. supporting legislation that results in injury prevention.

58. A major goal for the future in EMS communications systems is to:
    a. acknowledge that public education is a critical EMS activity.
    b. assess the effectiveness of resource attributes for EMS dispatching.
    c. provide the 9-1-1 emergency telephone service to all global positioning system (GPS) monitors.
    d. develop models for EMS evaluations that incorporate consumer input.

59. One of the major goals for the future in the clinical care aspect of EMS is to:
    a. evaluate EMS effects on various medical conditions.
    b. evaluate EMS standards for higher earning potentials.
    c. obtain legal advice on how to obtain informed consent.
    d. commit to a common definition of what constitutes baseline community EMS care.

60. One of the goals that EMS information systems is striving for in the future is to:
    a. incorporate task analyses to configure staffing of patient transfers.
    b. employ new care techniques and technology after they are shown to be effective.
    c. develop a mechanism to generate and transmit data that are valid, reliable, and accurate.
    d. facilitate the exploration of potential uses of advancing communication technology.

61. In the document EMS Agenda for the Future, one of the elements of the evaluation components is to:
    a. value peer review and publishing research.
    b. establish proactive relationships between EMS and other health care providers.
    c. determine EMS effects for multiple outcome categories and cost-effectiveness.
    d. update geographically integrated and function-based EMS communications networks.

62. Continuous quality improvement (CQI) is a process that is designed to:
    a. focus on specific problem individuals within an organization.
    b. uncover problems and provide solutions.
    c. correct life-threatening patient conditions.
    d. monitor the work performance of field paramedics.

63. The education that a paramedic should receive to become a competent entry-level provider is outlined in the:
    a. National Registry guidelines.
    b. AHA guidelines.
    c. National EMS Education Standards.
    d. state medical practice act.

64. _____ is unrecognized in the National EMS Educational Standards as an EMS provider level.
    a. EMT
    b. Cardiac rescue technician (CRT)
    c. Advanced EMT
    d. Paramedic

65. A _____ is a "calling" requiring specialized preparation and specific academic preparation.
    a. validation
    b. credential
    c. profession
    d. business

66. Which of the following is inaccurate about the public image of health care workers?
    a. Your image and behavior in the public's eye are insignificant.
    b. EMS providers are very visible role models whose behaviors are closely observed.
    c. Your actions in public represent the image of your peers as well as your own.
    d. If people see you not wearing your seat belt, they may think that seat belts are really unnecessary.

67. Empathy is an attribute the paramedic would typically demonstrate to:
    a. him- or herself.
    b. the general public.
    c. the EMS profession.
    d. patients and their families.

68. Which of the following is an example of behavior that demonstrates self-motivation by the paramedic?

    a. not accepting constructive feedback, because there is no such thing

    b. taking advantage of all learning opportunities

    c. taking on selective tasks as recommended by supervision

    d. making corrections to improve work performance when advised

69. At times the paramedic must be the diplomat, which means saying and doing things that are considered by some to be:

    a. status quo.

    b. newsworthy.

    c. political suicide.

    d. politically correct.

70. Why is it necessary for paramedics to be good communicators?

    a. It is a prerequisite for an EMS provider.

    b. It is because many patients cannot communicate verbally.

    c. Most of what paramedics do involves communication skills.

    d. Good communication skills keep the paramedic from being overbearing.

Exam #2 Answer Form

	A	B	C	D			A	B	C	D
1.	❏	❏	❏	❏		31.	❏	❏	❏	❏
2.	❏	❏	❏	❏		32.	❏	❏	❏	❏
3.	❏	❏	❏	❏		33.	❏	❏	❏	❏
4.	❏	❏	❏	❏		34.	❏	❏	❏	❏
5.	❏	❏	❏	❏		35.	❏	❏	❏	❏
6.	❏	❏	❏	❏		36.	❏	❏	❏	❏
7.	❏	❏	❏	❏		37.	❏	❏	❏	❏
8.	❏	❏	❏	❏		38.	❏	❏	❏	❏
9.	❏	❏	❏	❏		39.	❏	❏	❏	❏
10.	❏	❏	❏	❏		40.	❏	❏	❏	❏
11.	❏	❏	❏	❏		41.	❏	❏	❏	❏
12.	❏	❏	❏	❏		42.	❏	❏	❏	❏
13.	❏	❏	❏	❏		43.	❏	❏	❏	❏
14.	❏	❏	❏	❏		44.	❏	❏	❏	❏
15.	❏	❏	❏	❏		45.	❏	❏	❏	❏
16.	❏	❏	❏	❏		46.	❏	❏	❏	❏
17.	❏	❏	❏	❏		47.	❏	❏	❏	❏
18.	❏	❏	❏	❏		48.	❏	❏	❏	❏
19.	❏	❏	❏	❏		49.	❏	❏	❏	❏
20.	❏	❏	❏	❏		50.	❏	❏	❏	❏
21.	❏	❏	❏	❏		51.	❏	❏	❏	❏
22.	❏	❏	❏	❏		52.	❏	❏	❏	❏
23.	❏	❏	❏	❏		53.	❏	❏	❏	❏
24.	❏	❏	❏	❏		54.	❏	❏	❏	❏
25.	❏	❏	❏	❏		55.	❏	❏	❏	❏
26.	❏	❏	❏	❏		56.	❏	❏	❏	❏
27.	❏	❏	❏	❏		57.	❏	❏	❏	❏
28.	❏	❏	❏	❏		58.	❏	❏	❏	❏
29.	❏	❏	❏	❏		59.	❏	❏	❏	❏
30.	❏	❏	❏	❏		60.	❏	❏	❏	❏

Exam #2 Answer Form

	A	B	C	D			A	B	C	D
61.	❏	❏	❏	❏		66.	❏	❏	❏	❏
62.	❏	❏	❏	❏		67.	❏	❏	❏	❏
63.	❏	❏	❏	❏		68.	❏	❏	❏	❏
64.	❏	❏	❏	❏		69.	❏	❏	❏	❏
65.	❏	❏	❏	❏		70.	❏	❏	❏	❏

CHAPTER 3

Public Health and Research

1. _____ is the study of occurrence of disease.
   a. Morbidity
   b. Mortality
   c. Incidence
   d. Epidemiology

2. The extent of an injury or illness is called:
   a. morbidity.
   b. mortality.
   c. incidence.
   d. epidemiology.

3. What is the leading cause of overall deaths in the United States?
   a. heart disease
   b. malignant tumors
   c. cerebrovascular diseases
   d. COPD

4. Which of the following is most accurate about causes of death when broken down by gender, age, and race?
   a. Accidents are the leading cause of death for ages 1–44.
   b. Those who marry have a higher mortality rate than those who do not.
   c. Life expectancy for males has recently surpassed that of females.
   d. Cerebrovascular disease is the leading cause of death for those over 60 years of age.

5. Which of the following is an effect that has occurred as a result of early release/discharge of patients from the hospital?
   a. Home health care will reduce the overall lifetime cost of injuries.
   b. There are more expectations for EMS services to provide care for patients being managed in the home setting.
   c. This cost-cutting trend is going to decrease the reliance on EMS.
   d. More hospitals will rely on EMS to care for and transport patients that have had outpatient procedures.

6. The leading cause of death for white males aged 15–24 is:
   a. accidents.
   b. homicide.
   c. HIV infection.
   d. suicide.

7. _____ is defined as a real or potentially hazardous situation that puts individuals at risk for sustaining an injury.
   a. Harm's way
   b. Injury surveillance
   c. Injury prevention
   d. Injury risk

8. An important part of any injury surveillance program is the timely dissemination of the data to those who need to use it for:
   a. prevention and control efforts.
   b. obtaining funding through grants.
   c. treatment of patients.
   d. reversal of management plans.

9. _____ injury preventions are activities involved in the care of an injury that has already occurred to prevent it from getting worse.
   a. Primary
   b. Secondary
   c. Tertiary
   d. Productive

10. Activities that are involved in the rehabilitation of an injured person, such as preventing infections, are known as:
    a. a teachable moment.
    b. tertiary injury prevention.
    c. sensible ongoing care.
    d. productive quality care.

11. You have decided that it is sensible to be involved in injury and illness prevention efforts in the community where you live and work. One of the ways to act on this decision is to:
    a. visit each school in the community.
    b. pick a cause that best suits your interests.
    c. visit each nursing home in the community.
    d. always wear your seat belt, on and off duty.

12. Which of the following statements about bicycle-related head injuries is most accurate?
    a. The solution to preventing these injuries is to make better helmets.
    b. The lack of parental supervision is the primary contributing factor to these injuries.
    c. Over 95% of victims of bicycle-related head injuries were not wearing helmets when injured.
    d. Reducing speed limits in residential communities is the solution to preventing these types of injuries.

13. In addition to public education in the prevention of drowning, which of the following is a recommended solution for prevention?
    a. assuring adequate supervision of adults who drink while boating
    b. legislation banning any alcohol consumption while in or near water
    c. requiring that personal flotation devices (PFDs) be worn whenever children or adults who cannot swim are in or near water
    d. legislation requiring that all school-age students receive swimming lessons for 2 years

14. The key strategy for reducing deaths from motor vehicles is:
    a. reducing speed limits in school zones.
    b. mandating lower speed limits on the highways.
    c. advocating for more vehicles to include airbags.
    d. getting everyone in the vehicle to wear seat belts.

15. In 1970, the Poison Prevention Act required the U.S. Consumer Product Safety Commission to require the:
    a. use of residential smoke detectors.
    b. use of carbon monoxide detectors in commercial properties.
    c. installation of locks for the storage of toxic substances in schools.
    d. use of child-resistant packaging of toxic substances for in-home use.

16. According to the U.S. Poison Control Centers, more than 90% of poison exposures occur in:
    a. schools.
    b. hospitals.
    c. homes.
    d. work facilities.

17. A strategy for fire prevention safety that you can use at home is to:
    a. practice family fire escape plans every 6 months.
    b. get everyone in your family to stop smoking as soon as possible.
    c. change the batteries on carbon monoxide and smoke alarms every 5 years.
    d. increase the amount of coverage on your homeowner's or renter's insurance.

18. A key strategy to reduce injury and death that occur from motorcycle collisions is to:
    a. educate riders to always wear a helmet and protective gear.
    b. educate motor vehicle drivers to give way to riders.
    c. increase insurance rates for riders who drink and drive.
    d. offer insurance discounts for riders who drive slower.

19. Two key strategies for playground safety are adult supervision and:
    a. making hourly inspections for equipment in need of repair.
    b. making sure that any surface that children may fall onto is soft and padded.
    c. ensuring that all playground surfaces have shredded rubber to cushion a fall.
    d. ensuring that all playground surfaces use fine sand or pea gravel to cushion a fall.

20. Select the most accurate statement about common injuries related to falls.
    a. Toddlers should not be allowed to sit in shopping carts.
    b. Every adult aged 65 or older will fall at least once each year.
    c. Injuries from falls affect the very young and the elderly more severely.
    d. The use of handrails when walking on stairs will eliminate any chance of falling.

21. Which of the following practices should be avoided as a strategy for prevention of falls among the elderly?
    a. installing metal grates on windows in high-rise buildings
    b. installing tiles in kitchens and baths
    c. eliminating throw rugs and other trip hazards
    d. using shopping carts with straps for holding toddlers

22. Which of the following is often a frequent cause of strangulation among infants and children?
    a. locks on bathroom doors
    b. unattended child in a vehicle
    c. drawstrings on curtains or blinds
    d. shopping carts with straps for holding infants

23. Key strategies for the prevention of firearm injuries and fatalities include all the following, *except*:
    a. disassembling the National Rifle Association.
    b. gun control and proper storage.
    c. training and licensing of handgun owners.
    d. mandates for trigger locks and loading indicators.

24. Of the approximately 82,000 auto–pedestrian injuries that occur annually, over _____ of those include children who often receive serious brain injury.
    a. 10,000
    b. 20,000
    c. 35,000
    d. 50,000

25. A key strategy for injury prevention and pedestrian safety is to:
    a. avoid drinking and walking.
    b. have a good sense of timing.
    c. avoid crossing the road with small children.
    d. wear reflective clothing both day and night.

26. One of the most effective ways EMS providers can provide leadership in the area of illness and injury prevention is to:
    a. say they are in support of prevention programs.
    b. set examples in all activities of the organization.
    c. give an in-service training program on injury prevention.
    d. advocate for state laws requiring helmet use.

27. An EMS leader has the responsibility to protect individual EMS providers from injury while on duty. One of the things that a leader is expected to do is:
    a. seek out financial resources to sponsor injury prevention programs.
    b. develop sensible policies and procedures promoting safety in all work activities.
    c. mandate each employee to teach injury prevention in one of the local schools or nursing homes.
    d. participate in a wellness program for EMS providers, but not for management and office staff.

28. An example of an exposure to a potential injury for the paramedic at the scene of a call is:
    a. day care centers.
    b. unconscious patients.
    c. extremely ambient temperatures.
    d. a broken or faulty blood pressure cuff.

29. An example of a resource that the paramedic should be aware of as part of an injury prevention program is:
    a. retirement options.
    b. child protective services.
    c. utility reimbursement resources.
    d. recreation options for the elderly.

30. One concept of effective communication that the paramedic can use as part of the on-scene education strategy for injury prevention is:
    a. to avoid being objective.
    b. recognizing the teachable moments.
    c. being judgmental about safety issues.
    d. to avoid consideration of ethnic, religious, or social diversity.

31. When a paramedic documents a safety hazard, which of the following should be included?
    a. primary care provided
    b. primary injury data
    c. information required by the EMS agency
    d. all of the above

32. _____ is(are) example(s) of primary injury data.
    a. Scene conditions
    b. Time of response
    c. Past medical history
    d. Medications and allergies

33. Which of the following is associated with an overall lower risk of death?
    a. higher education attainment
    b. residing in warm climates
    c. residing in cold climates
    d. occupation in health care

34. Paramedics are in an ideal position to be frontline advocates for injury and disease prevention because:
    a. of the support provided by private sector groups.
    b. of their perspective offered in out-of-hospital care.
    c. of their knowledge of communicable diseases.
    d. all EMS leaders are progressive with injury prevention.

35. _____ is an effort to keep an injury from ever occurring.
    a. Incidence prevention
    b. Injury surveillance
    c. Primary injury prevention
    d. Accident Watch®

36. Research in EMS is important for all the following reasons, *except*:
    a. research helps to enhance recognition and respect for EMS professionals.
    b. outcome studies are needed to assure the continued funding for EMS system grants.
    c. changes in professional standards, training, and equipment need to be based on empirical data.
    d. research can be influenced by biases.

37. The role of EMS providers in data collection is to enthusiastically participate and honestly comply with the study requirements without:
    a. changing the sample size.
    b. obtaining informed consent.
    c. changing the initial hypothesis.
    d. negatively affecting patient care.

38. One of the basic principles of research is understanding:
    a. what a randomized and controlled group is.
    b. how to change patient care standards.
    c. those populations that are to be researched.
    d. that there are no limitations within a study.

39. Which of the following is not one of the typical steps in the procedure for conducting research in EMS?
    a. Collect the funding needs for the hypothesis development.
    b. Prepare the question to be studied.
    c. Describe who the populations to be studied will be.
    d. Obtain legal advice on how to obtain informed consent.

40. The general areas of prehospital research include: answering clinically important questions, arriving at conclusions based on scientifically sound procedures, and:
    a. obtaining informed consent.
    b. making decisions based on traditions or opinions.
    c. providing results that lead to system improvements.
    d. arriving at conclusions based on questionable ethical procedures.

Exam #3 Answer Form

	A	B	C	D			A	B	C	D
1.	❏	❏	❏	❏		21.	❏	❏	❏	❏
2.	❏	❏	❏	❏		22.	❏	❏	❏	❏
3.	❏	❏	❏	❏		23.	❏	❏	❏	❏
4.	❏	❏	❏	❏		24.	❏	❏	❏	❏
5.	❏	❏	❏	❏		25.	❏	❏	❏	❏
6.	❏	❏	❏	❏		26.	❏	❏	❏	❏
7.	❏	❏	❏	❏		27.	❏	❏	❏	❏
8.	❏	❏	❏	❏		28.	❏	❏	❏	❏
9.	❏	❏	❏	❏		29.	❏	❏	❏	❏
10.	❏	❏	❏	❏		30.	❏	❏	❏	❏
11.	❏	❏	❏	❏		31.	❏	❏	❏	❏
12.	❏	❏	❏	❏		32.	❏	❏	❏	❏
13.	❏	❏	❏	❏		33.	❏	❏	❏	❏
14.	❏	❏	❏	❏		34.	❏	❏	❏	❏
15.	❏	❏	❏	❏		35.	❏	❏	❏	❏
16.	❏	❏	❏	❏		36.	❏	❏	❏	❏
17.	❏	❏	❏	❏		37.	❏	❏	❏	❏
18.	❏	❏	❏	❏		38.	❏	❏	❏	❏
19.	❏	❏	❏	❏		39.	❏	❏	❏	❏
20.	❏	❏	❏	❏		40.	❏	❏	❏	❏

CHAPTER

Communications: EMS Systems & Therapeutic

1. An example of electronic communication that is used by paramedics on many ALS calls is:
   a. triage.
   b. 10 codes.
   c. telephone interrogation.
   d. the code summary on a monitor-defibrillator unit.

2. When a citizen driving by a collision notices the patient and calls 9-1-1, this is called:
   a. notification.
   b. response.
   c. detection.
   d. occurrence.

3. When the paramedic confers with medical control over the field treatment of the patient, this is referred to as the _____ phase of communication.
   a. notification
   b. treatment
   c. preparation for the next call
   d. response

4. The basic model of communication includes which of the following steps?
   a. Receiver has a message.
   b. Receiver gives feedback.
   c. Sender decodes the message.
   d. Receiver sends the message.

5. On an EMS call the paramedic is required to interact with each of the following, *except*:
   a. emergency service personnel at the scene.
   b. the crew members and bystanders.
   c. the patient's family physician.
   d. the ED staff who will be taking over management of the patient.

6. Special radio codes:
   a. lead to a clearer understanding of the message.
   b. are necessary to avoid listeners.
   c. add an unnecessary level of complexity.
   d. should be used in public.

7. Newer cell phones are required to have a(n) _____, which can help identify the location of a caller in an emergency.
   a. caller identification
   b. amplitude modulator
   c. global positioning device
   d. enhanced caller identification

8. The study of the meaning in language is called:
   a. diction.
   b. semantics.
   c. linguistics.
   d. context.

9. When talking with a child on an EMS call, it is important to:
   a. avoid technical terms.
   b. stretch the truth so it sounds better.
   c. use buzzwords.
   d. use only short words.

10. When speaking on a portable radio, you should depress the microphone for a moment prior to beginning to speak because:
    a. it will get everyone's attention.
    b. it helps to avoid cutting off the first few words.
    c. the radio will transmit louder.
    d. the receivers will be ready to hear you.

11. You are caring for a patient who is very angry and is taking his anger out on you. Which of the following should you avoid doing?

   a. getting angry in return

   b. doing a quick pat down for weapons

   c. keeping the situation calm

   d. requesting police

12. You are inside an office building taking care of a patient with severe respiratory distress. When you attempt to use your portable radio to call out, you get a buzzing noise and suspect that it is 60-cycle interference. Which of the following factors is most likely causing the radio interference?

   a. close proximity to computers

   b. thickness of the walls of the building

   c. metal skeletal structure of the building

   d. the cell phone the patient is using to call his family

13. When the EMD gives instructions on CPR compressions to the family member who called, this is known as:

   a. interrogation.

   b. pre-arrival instructions.

   c. radio dispatch.

   d. logistics coordination.

14. During an interview with a patient in severe respiratory distress, you ask the patient to "nod yes or shake no" to answer your questions. This is an example of asking questions that are:

   a. direct.

   b. leading.

   c. patronizing.

   d. open-ended.

15. The time between the receipt of the call and the time the call is given to the emergency unit to respond is called _____ time.

   a. response

   b. alerting

   c. dispatch

   d. queue

16. When analyzing the time segments of a call, it is important to remember that:

   a. scene time begins upon arrival at the patient's side.

   b. the scene time may be inaccurately lengthened.

   c. scene time ends once you load the patient on the stretcher.

   d. most times are usually inaccurate.

17. An example of a factor that may lengthen the actual scene time is:

   a. heavy traffic conditions.

   b. a lengthy extrication.

   c. the dispatch priority.

   d. a change in transport destination.

18. _____ is part of the communication process rather than a communication technique.

   a. Silence

   b. Encoding

   c. Listening

   d. Explanation

19. When called by someone who is in direct contact with the patient, this is referred to as a:

   a. first-party caller.

   b. second-party caller.

   c. third-party caller.

   d. fourth-party caller.

20. The new roles of the Federal Communication Commission include:

   a. creating a model agency for the digital age.

   b. managing the electromagnetic spectrum.

   c. promoting competition in all communication markets.

   d. all of the above.

21. What medical breakthrough is referred to as zero-minute response time?

   a. Public Access Defibrillation

   b. pre-arrival instructions

   c. system status management

   d. rapid response vehicles

22. Why should the paramedic avoid providing false reassurance when the situation is serious?

   a. The patient will sue if she finds out the truth.

   b. The patient will suffer harm.

   c. The paramedic could lose her certification.

   d. The paramedic could lose the patient's trust.

23. The main purpose of a verbal report over the radio to the hospital is to:

   a. document on tape the patient's problem.

   b. document the run on tape for QI purposes.

   c. give them time to prepare for the patient.

   d. assess the need for diversion.

24. Which of the following pieces of information should the paramedic avoid giving over the radio as part of the report to the hospital?
    a. patient's name
    b. chief complaint
    c. baseline vital signs
    d. response to emergency interventions

25. In addition to the standard radio report, the paramedic report to medical control should also include:
    a. drugs administered on standing orders.
    b. a second set of vital signs.
    c. the patient's ETA.
    d. the patient's age.

26. In the communication process, the message moves through various forms, including: verbal, nonverbal, encoding, and:
    a. receiver.
    b. translator.
    c. interpreter.
    d. forecaster.

27. When speaking on a portable radio you should:
    a. only use the last names of patients.
    b. be courteous and say please and thank you.
    c. say each digit for clarity when transmitting a number.
    d. speak quickly with your lips about an inch from the microphone.

28. One major advantage of digital technology in communication for emergency responders is that:
    a. digital transmitters are not affected by typical sources of interference.
    b. digital transmitters do not require voice transmission time over the radio.
    c. technology makes it impossible for people with scanners to listen in on transmissions.
    d. technology reduces scene time by eliminating the need to talk to dispatch on the radio.

29. The number of repetitive cycles per second completed by a radio wave is called the:
    a. telemetry.
    b. frequency.
    c. amplitude modulation.
    d. call simplex.

30. When a radio transmits and receives on the same frequency, this is called:
    a. simplex.
    b. duplex communications.
    c. telemetry.
    d. ultra-high frequency.

31. When the radio power of a portable is not strong enough to reach a base station, this system can be improved by the use of a(n):
    a. amplitude modulator.
    b. frequency modulator.
    c. duplex system.
    d. repeater.

32. Like many professions, _____ is an integral component of the EMS profession.
    a. encoding
    b. communication
    c. sign language
    d. diet

33. The _____ band is less susceptible to interference than _____, so it is more frequently used in EMS communications.
    a. cellular; AM
    b. FM; AM
    c. AM; FM
    d. UHF; FM

34. Voice transmission is also referred to as:
    a. simplex.
    b. analog transmission.
    c. digital transmission.
    d. duplex.

35. Which of the following is an example of a condescending question to be avoided during an interview?
    a. How much did you have to drink tonight?
    b. You don't smoke, do you?
    c. Do you take your medications every day?
    d. When was your last menstrual period?

36. In an effort to keep a patient from becoming more anxious during a patient interview, the paramedic should:
    a. shun nonverbal communication.
    b. avoid facilitation whenever possible.
    c. stay away from silence as an interview technique.
    d. avoid the use of complicated medical terminology.

37. An example of a negative communication technique that the paramedic should avoid with patients and their families is:
    a. reflection.
    b. inattentiveness.
    c. asking for clarification when a patient's response is ambiguous.
    d. being conscious of the amount of physical space between you and the patient.

38. _____ is the way you speak, and how your posture and your actions are used to encourage the patient to say more.
    a. Empathy
    b. Confrontation
    c. Facilitation
    d. Reflection

39. To repeat or echo the patient's own words as a way of encouraging the flow of conversation without interrupting the patient's concentration is referred to as:
    a. interpretation.
    b. clarification.
    c. facilitation.
    d. reflection.

40. _____ is reasoning based not on what you observed from the patient, but on what you have concluded from the information you have compiled.
    a. Interpretation
    b. Clarification
    c. Empathy
    d. Silence

41. Which of the following conditions is least likely to be an obstacle during a patient interview?
    a. a patient who is blind
    b. a patient who is overtalkative
    c. a patient who is symptomatic
    d. a patient who is developmentally disabled

42. A rolled piece of paper in a plastic container, which contains medical information about a patient, is a(n):
    a. MedicAlert tag®.
    b. prescription bottle.
    c. Vial of Life®.
    d. Emergency Lifeline®.

43. When treating a patient who only speaks a foreign language that you do not, and no interpreter is immediately available, which of the following can you do to best facilitate care?
    a. Use positive body language while you begin care.
    b. Wait for a translator before initiating care.
    c. Ask police for assistance.
    d. Call the paramedic supervisor.

44. While caring for a blind patient, it is appropriate to announce yourself, to explain as much as possible, and to:
    a. secure the seeing eye dog for your protection.
    b. speak while facing the patient.
    c. interact with the patient the same as with a seeing patient.
    d. ask permission to touch the patient before actually touching him.

45. Sleep disorders, appetite disturbances, the inability to concentrate, and lack of energy are all signs of:
    a. fear.
    b. confusion.
    c. depression.
    d. abuse.

46. When interviewing a patient who is extremely talkative, but is not providing you with the information you need, which of the following techniques might be useful in obtaining what you need?
    a. Ignore the patient.
    b. Ask the patient to stop talking and listen.
    c. Try using diversion tactics.
    d. Try using direct "yes" or "no" questions.

47. _____ and history taking are significant portions of the patient interview.
    a. Dispatch information
    b. A rapid response time
    c. Establishing a rapport with the patient
    d. Professional appearance

48. _____ may be found on necklaces, bracelets, and anklets, and provide vital medical information such as a medical condition or reaction.
    a. Dog tags®
    b. Lucky charms®
    c. MedicAlert tags®
    d. Coils

49. Once you have arrived at the ED with a hearing-impaired patient, the _____ requires that the hospital provide a sign interpreter within 30 minutes of the patient's arrival.
    a. American's with Disabilities Act (ADA)
    b. Veteran's Administration (VA)
    c. Centers for Disease Control (CDC)
    d. American Sign Language (ASL) bill

50. When caring for a hearing-impaired patient, be sure to face the patient when you are speaking and to:
    a. speak very slowly.
    b. use a family member to communicate.
    c. exaggerate your speech.
    d. look to see if his hearing aid is on.

Exam #4 Answer Form

	A	B	C	D		A	B	C	D
1.	❏	❏	❏	❏	26.	❏	❏	❏	❏
2.	❏	❏	❏	❏	27.	❏	❏	❏	❏
3.	❏	❏	❏	❏	28.	❏	❏	❏	❏
4.	❏	❏	❏	❏	29.	❏	❏	❏	❏
5.	❏	❏	❏	❏	30.	❏	❏	❏	❏
6.	❏	❏	❏	❏	31.	❏	❏	❏	❏
7.	❏	❏	❏	❏	32.	❏	❏	❏	❏
8.	❏	❏	❏	❏	33.	❏	❏	❏	❏
9.	❏	❏	❏	❏	34.	❏	❏	❏	❏
10.	❏	❏	❏	❏	35.	❏	❏	❏	❏
11.	❏	❏	❏	❏	36.	❏	❏	❏	❏
12.	❏	❏	❏	❏	37.	❏	❏	❏	❏
13.	❏	❏	❏	❏	38.	❏	❏	❏	❏
14.	❏	❏	❏	❏	39.	❏	❏	❏	❏
15.	❏	❏	❏	❏	40.	❏	❏	❏	❏
16.	❏	❏	❏	❏	41.	❏	❏	❏	❏
17.	❏	❏	❏	❏	42.	❏	❏	❏	❏
18.	❏	❏	❏	❏	43.	❏	❏	❏	❏
19.	❏	❏	❏	❏	44.	❏	❏	❏	❏
20.	❏	❏	❏	❏	45.	❏	❏	❏	❏
21.	❏	❏	❏	❏	46.	❏	❏	❏	❏
22.	❏	❏	❏	❏	47.	❏	❏	❏	❏
23.	❏	❏	❏	❏	48.	❏	❏	❏	❏
24.	❏	❏	❏	❏	49.	❏	❏	❏	❏
25.	❏	❏	❏	❏	50.	❏	❏	❏	❏

CHAPTER

Documentation

1. In a medicolegal case review, poor documentation is:
   a. only a problem with new EMS personnel.
   b. an indication of poor assessment.
   c. usually caused by lack of training or supervision.
   d. a sign of laziness.

2. Which of the following statements about the documentation of patient care is most correct?
   a. Documentation serves as a legal record of the incident.
   b. A well-written prehospital care report (PCR) needs only the baseline set of vital signs.
   c. There is no standardization of data between different agencies and systems.
   d. Administrative data is listed on only the original copy of the PCR.

3. _____ has defined a minimum data set to be included in all prehospital care reports.
   a. NHTSA
   b. DOT
   c. State EMS
   d. DOH

4. Which of the items listed is an example of patient data?
   a. run times
   b. name of the service
   c. disposition of the call
   d. name of the crew members

5. Which of the items listed is an example of run data?
   a. nature of illness
   b. mechanism of injury
   c. location of the patient
   d. level of training of the crew members

6. All of the following are names for the out-of-hospital patient care documentation prepared by paramedics, *except* the:
   a. PCR.
   b. run sheet.
   c. ambulance call report.
   d. DNAR.

7. Which of the items listed is an example of patient demographic data?
   a. past medical history
   b. the patient's address
   c. time en route to the patient
   d. treatment self-administered prior to EMS arrival

8. Before a PCR can be used for quality improvement or educational purposes, what action must be taken?
   a. Obtain verbal consent from patient.
   b. Obtain written consent from patient.
   c. Remove patient's name from documentation.
   d. Remove paramedic's name from documentation.

9. Which of the following is most accurate about documentation of vital signs?
   a. Vital signs should be documented before and after a medication administration.
   b. Three sets of vital signs should be documented for every patient.
   c. Vital signs should be documented at least every 10 minutes for critical patients.
   d. It is not difficult to make treatment decisions based on one set of vital signs.

10. Standard guidelines for documentation of out-of-hospital assessment and management include:
    a. always using print on the PCR.
    b. being objective, specific, and concrete.
    c. minimizing the use of abbreviations.
    d. avoiding the use of quotations.

11. The prefix *ambi–* means:
    a. around.
    b. both sides.
    c. dim, dull, or lazy.
    d. against, opposed to.

12. The suffix *–plasia* means:
    a. paralysis.
    b. surgical repair.
    c. painful condition.
    d. development, formation.

13. Because the paramedic will not be present to explain his findings to all who ultimately read the PCR, the form should be so complete that it:
    a. leaves no doubt about the patient's diagnosis.
    b. contains the patient's entire past medical history.
    c. includes only objective findings by the paramedic.
    d. "speaks for itself."

14. The presence of a complete and accurate record is helpful in:
    a. keeping the patient from harm or embarrassment.
    b. ensuring and maintaining patient confidentiality.
    c. averting further legal action during the "discovery phase" of a lawsuit.
    d. developing a plan for definitive treatment.

15. A statement like _____ is an example of a professional statement the paramedic should include in documenting the PCR.
    a. "The patient had the beating coming to him."
    b. "The skell just wanted another ride across town."
    c. "She is lonely and is just looking for a little attention."
    d. "The patient stated she vomited four times last night."

16. You are charting a PCR for your last patient and are documenting the intubation you performed. Which of the following aspects of this skill is extraneous information that you need not chart?
    a. the correction of a misplaced tube
    b. the depth of the tube and the method of securing
    c. at least three methods of ensuring correct tube placement
    d. the length and design of stylet used to facilitate the intubation

17. Select the statement that is an example of a pertinent negative that the paramedic would document about a patient.
    a. A patient struck his head in an MVC and denies a loss of consciousness.
    b. A patient with dyspnea denies a smoking history of more than 10 years.
    c. A patient with a lengthy medical list denies any allergies to medications.
    d. A patient in an MVC has never been involved in a collision until now.

18. _____ findings are information the patient or bystanders tell the paramedic.
    a. Subjective
    b. Neutral
    c. Objective
    d. Biased

19. _____ findings are information the paramedic can measure, such as vital signs.
    a. Subjective
    b. Neutral
    c. Objective
    d. Lawful

20. Patients have a right to have their medical records be:
    a. held from third-party billing agencies.
    b. withheld from medical students.
    c. partially restricted from their HMOs.
    d. held in confidence.

21. You are caring for a 48-year-old male patient with acute abdominal pain. He is pale and diaphoretic. During your examination of his abdomen, he tells you he is feeling dizzy and is nauseated. Which of the following will you document as an *objective* finding on the PCR?
    a. nausea
    b. dizziness
    c. pale, diaphoretic skin
    d. acute abdominal pain

22. It is necessary to document multiple sets of vital signs on the PCR:
    a. only when the patient is unstable.
    b. to show trends in the patient's condition.
    c. only when interventions have been applied.
    d. only when the baseline vital signs are abnormal.

23. When documentation is anything less than complete or accurate, the presumption is that the paramedic either did not do the proper care or:
    a. had a bad day.
    b. forgot to include something.
    c. had something to hide.
    d. was not trained properly.

24. You are evaluating a 20-year-old male with a traumatic injury to the hand and wrist. While at work, his right hand became entangled in equipment, causing it to bend backward in hyperextension. When you document the MOI, which of the following standard terms or planes can you use to describe the injury?

    a. protraction
    b. dorsiflexion
    c. lateral rotation
    d. cephalad extension

25. The documentation for starting IVs in the field should include all the following information, *except*:

    a. the size of the angiocath used.
    b. who started the IV.
    c. who adjusted the drip rate.
    d. the number of attempts if the first was not successful.

26. Most often there is additional documentation associated with the administration of drugs such as morphine of valium. Which of the following is not included in that information?

    a. the patient's name
    b. the patient's medical insurance information
    c. the physician who authorized the administration
    d. what effect the medication had on the patient

27. Which of the following is often used as the first line of documentation at an MCI?

    a. donning identification vests
    b. triage tags
    c. labeling sectors
    d. recording transportation destinations

28. You have arrived at the ED with a 7-year-old male patient who you suspect is a victim of child abuse. As this type of call requires mandatory reporting in every state, you will:

    a. complete a special incident form.
    b. follow your state and local guidelines.
    c. document your suspicions on the PCR.
    d. provide a written statement to the state police.

29. When making corrections of a recorded error on a PCR, which of the following is the incorrect way to make the change?

    a. Initial and date the mistaken entry.
    b. Draw a single line through the entry.
    c. Write "error" above or next to the entry.
    d. Erase the entry.

30. Which of the following is an example of an unusual situation that the paramedic should record on a PCR?

    a. During the transport, your ambulance passed by a serious MVC.
    b. While immobilizing an extremity that was swollen and deformed, the patient cried out in pain.
    c. Radio failure delayed contact with medical control and subsequent medical orders.
    d. After transferring the patient to a bed in the ED and giving the report, the patient became unresponsive.

31. Documentation of which of the following findings is vital in defending your care of a patient with a suspected fracture or dislocation?

    a. adequacy of the neurovascular supply before and after immobilization
    b. the manner in which the fracture/dislocation was immobilized
    c. the type of splint used
    d. the use of analgesia for pain management

32. If a patient makes statements to questions that do not appear in a check box on the PCR, the paramedic should:

    a. paraphrase the patient's statement into the narrative.
    b. document the statement in "quotes."
    c. use a special incident form for complete accuracy.
    d. write in additional check boxes.

33. The PCR is a legal document in which the paramedic should assure that the expressions and terms used are:

    a. derogatory.
    b. approved by the DOH.
    c. standardized and professional.
    d. judgment biased.

34. When a paramedic documents information about a patient's medication that is being taken "four times a day," which of the following would she use?

    a. q. d.
    b. q. i. d.
    c. t. i. d.
    d. p. r. n.

35. An example of a situation that is not typically documented on a PCR is the:

    a. restraining of the patient.
    b. hostile or abusive behavior of the patient.
    c. patient's marital status.
    d. patient's date of birth.

36. Standardization of the data elements to be included in all PCRs or on electronic call reports helps to make it easier to:
    a. facilitate corroborating testimony in court.
    b. avoid litigation in the future.
    c. compare data from different agencies.
    d. document the disposition of the call.

37. Which of the following is meant by the legal expression that the document should "stand on its own"?
    a. The record contains everything it should in a clear, legible, and concise fashion.
    b. The record does not contain unprofessional language.
    c. The record does not contain any pertinent negatives.
    d. There are no documented errors.

38. Acronyms used for two types of narrative formats used in documentation of PCRs are:
    a. SOAP and CHART.
    b. CUPS and AVPU.
    c. PMHx and OPQRST.
    d. SAMPLE and APGAR.

39. Ensuring that your documentation is complete, accurate, and legible is one of the _____ of the paramedic.
    a. standing orders
    b. local protocols
    c. professional responsibilities
    d. state DOH regulations

40. Legally, with whom are you not allowed to share a patient's medical information?
    a. the health-care provider continuing care
    b. a lawyer with a subpoena
    c. a police officer who is a friend of the patient
    d. third-party billing companies

41. Which of the following situations requires extra attention to detail when documenting a PCR?
    a. MCI
    b. refusal of medical assistance (RMA)
    c. correcting an error
    d. all of the above

42. When the paramedic documents a call where the patient is refusing care or transport, yet strongly feels that the patient needs medical attention, which of the following should be recorded?
    a. the specific recommendation for care and transport, and the consequences of refusing care
    b. a statement that describes your opinion of how difficult and obnoxious the patient was
    c. a subjective reference to how ignorant and indifferent the patient was to your efforts to take care of him
    d. the patient's Social Security number, driver's license number, and insurance information, if possible

43. Ideally, the best time for the paramedic to complete a PCR on a patient is:
    a. en route to the hospital.
    b. while waiting to transfer the patient to a bed.
    c. at the ED, after transfer of the patient to a bed.
    d. after returning to your station from the ED.

44. The part of a PCR that contains the written report that depicts the call is the:
    a. narrative.
    b. addendum.
    c. administrative section.
    d. demographic section.

45. When documenting assessment findings, which of the following is not necessary to record?
    a. pertinent positives
    b. pertinent negatives
    c. normal findings
    d. all findings should be recorded

46. _____ is the writing of false and malicious statements intended to damage a person's character.
    a. Bias
    b. Jargon
    c. Slander
    d. Libel

47. Which of the following statements about documenting PCRs is most correct?
    a. All personnel and resources involved in the call should be recorded.
    b. Using various formats when documenting helps the paramedic to become a proficient narrator.
    c. When documentation is complete, accurate, and legible, there is no chance of becoming involved in litigation.
    d. The discovery phase is the only time a lawyer will be able to gain access to your documentation.

48. Which of the following is a standard term used by the paramedic in documenting something that is situated near the surface of the body?
    a. superior
    b. sagittal
    c. efferent
    d. superficial

49. _____ is a common medical suffix that means stopping or controlling.
    a. Stasis
    b. Stomy
    c. Scopy
    d. Plasty

50. When a paramedic sees the prefix _____, he can recognize that the term is referring to the kidney.
    a. nephr/o–
    b. hepat/o–
    c. gangli/o–
    d. dacry/o–

Exam #5 Answer Form

	A	B	C	D			A	B	C	D
1.	❏	❏	❏	❏		26.	❏	❏	❏	❏
2.	❏	❏	❏	❏		27.	❏	❏	❏	❏
3.	❏	❏	❏	❏		28.	❏	❏	❏	❏
4.	❏	❏	❏	❏		29.	❏	❏	❏	❏
5.	❏	❏	❏	❏		30.	❏	❏	❏	❏
6.	❏	❏	❏	❏		31.	❏	❏	❏	❏
7.	❏	❏	❏	❏		32.	❏	❏	❏	❏
8.	❏	❏	❏	❏		33.	❏	❏	❏	❏
9.	❏	❏	❏	❏		34.	❏	❏	❏	❏
10.	❏	❏	❏	❏		35.	❏	❏	❏	❏
11.	❏	❏	❏	❏		36.	❏	❏	❏	❏
12.	❏	❏	❏	❏		37.	❏	❏	❏	❏
13.	❏	❏	❏	❏		38.	❏	❏	❏	❏
14.	❏	❏	❏	❏		39.	❏	❏	❏	❏
15.	❏	❏	❏	❏		40.	❏	❏	❏	❏
16.	❏	❏	❏	❏		41.	❏	❏	❏	❏
17.	❏	❏	❏	❏		42.	❏	❏	❏	❏
18.	❏	❏	❏	❏		43.	❏	❏	❏	❏
19.	❏	❏	❏	❏		44.	❏	❏	❏	❏
20.	❏	❏	❏	❏		45.	❏	❏	❏	❏
21.	❏	❏	❏	❏		46.	❏	❏	❏	❏
22.	❏	❏	❏	❏		47.	❏	❏	❏	❏
23.	❏	❏	❏	❏		48.	❏	❏	❏	❏
24.	❏	❏	❏	❏		49.	❏	❏	❏	❏
25.	❏	❏	❏	❏		50.	❏	❏	❏	❏

CHAPTER

6

Medical/Legal Issues

1. A state's EMS Act, which defines the governmental agency taking the lead in supervising the EMS and issuing certifications, is an example of _____ law.
   a. civil
   b. common
   c. legislative
   d. administrative

2. The statutes that are voted on and passed by the city council, county board, state legislature, or U.S. Congress are called _____ law.
   a. legislative
   b. civil
   c. tort
   d. common

3. A jury panel composed of a selection of people from the community is often referred to as a(n):
   a. appellate jury.
   b. legislative body.
   c. "jury of your peers."
   d. party of legal action.

4. The rules and regulations that outline the specifics of the enacting EMS law in each state are called the:
   a. standard operating procedure (SOP).
   b. EMS code.
   c. state protocols.
   d. Practice Act.

5. Precedents are often decided in a court of law based upon _____ law.
   a. criminal
   b. tort
   c. case
   d. administrative

6. A paramedic found purposely hurting patients by withholding essential medications would be charged in a(n) _____ court.
   a. small claims
   b. criminal
   c. civil
   d. administrative

7. When a plaintiff sues a paramedic for a breach of confidentiality in which she felt harm was caused to her reputation in the community, this action would take place in _____ court.
   a. criminal
   b. administrative
   c. civil
   d. case law

8. The person or institution (corporation) being sued is called the:
   a. plaintiff.
   b. responder.
   c. claimant.
   d. defendant.

9. A less formal legal process, which involves a judge and attorneys but no jury, is called a(n):
   a. civil trial.
   b. hearing.
   c. common law action.
   d. appellate court.

10. In a trial court, the _____ is responsible for deciding the facts of the case as presented by the competing attorneys.
    a. judge
    b. jury
    c. hearing officer
    d. respondent's attorney

11. If a party to a legal action is not satisfied with the results of the case in a trial court, the decision:
    a. is conclusive and final.
    b. may be appealed to a higher court.
    c. cannot be overruled by another court.
    d. is automatically remanded to a higher court.

12. A(n) _____ is convened to help decide if the district attorney or prosecutor has enough evidence to indict an individual to stand trial for a crime.
    a. appellate court
    b. civil court
    c. grand jury
    d. higher court

13. Deviation from the accepted standard of care is called:
    a. abandonment.
    b. negligence.
    c. confidentiality.
    d. a civil tort.

14. When a plaintiff's objective is to receive a financial award for damages that were allegedly caused by the paramedic, this is conducted in a(n):
    a. grand jury.
    b. criminal court.
    c. civil court.
    d. administrative hearing.

15. If the paramedic has an established duty to act and does not comply with that duty, this is referred to as a(n):
    a. error of commission.
    b. breach of duty.
    c. error of omission.
    d. infraction of decorum.

16. The failure to do a required act or duty, such as CPR on a patient who has been down for 5 minutes prior to your arrival, is called:
    a. nonfeasance.
    b. breach.
    c. malfeasance.
    d. non-reliance.

17. In a malpractice case against a paramedic, the plaintiff's lawyer must prove the:
    a. proximate cause.
    b. presence of an advanced directive.
    c. absence of an advanced directive.
    d. lack of moral judgment related to societal standards.

18. When an expert witness is called to testify in a malpractice case, it is usually to establish:
    a. proximate cause.
    b. that a duty was present.
    c. that there was a breach of duty.
    d. that commission incurred.

19. If a paramedic was found to have administered an excessive dose of Lasix to a drug addict in order to get "pleasure" out of watching the patient urinate all over himself, this is an example of:
    a. proximate cause.
    b. gross negligence.
    c. abandonment.
    d. commission of duty.

20. The termination of a paramedic-patient relationship before assuring that a health-care provider of equal or higher training will continue care is called:
    a. false imprisonment.
    b. confidentiality.
    c. malpractice.
    d. abandonment.

21. Detaining a patient without her consent or legal authority is considered:
    a. abandonment.
    b. false imprisonment.
    c. slander.
    d. kidnapping.

22. A crime in which a patient, her character, or her reputation is injured by false statements of another person is called:
    a. false imprisonment.
    b. libel.
    c. slander.
    d. abandonment.

23. A crime in which a person, her character, or her reputation is injured by the false written statements of another person is called:
    a. libel.
    b. slander.
    c. graffiti.
    d. confidentiality.

24. The granting of medical privileges by a physician either online or off-line is called:
    a. libel.
    b. delegation.
    c. confiscation.
    d. scope of practice.

25. The range of duties and skills a paramedic is expected to perform when necessary is called the:
    a. scope of practice.
    b. delegated authority.
    c. protocol.
    d. negligence per se.

26. The Latin term _____ means "the thing speaks for itself."
    a. veni, vidi, vici
    b. semper fi
    c. res ipsa loquitor
    d. negligence per se

27. Negligence shown because the law was violated and an injury occurred is called:
    a. res ipsa locquitor.
    b. causation implied.
    c. negligence per se.
    d. contributory negligence.

28. In a rear-end collision, the driver sustained a neck injury. Despite wearing a seat belt, the headrest was improperly positioned, which most likely contributed to the injury. At sentencing, the judge reduces the award to the injured party; this may be because of:
    a. negligence per se.
    b. government immunity.
    c. abandonment.
    d. contributory negligence.

29. One of the first steps taken in the most basic process of civil litigation is:
    a. the trial.
    b. an investigation.
    c. the discovery phase.
    d. the serving of the defendant.

30. The period during the pretrial phase when opposing sides get the opportunity to obtain the facts and information from the other side in preparation for the trial is called:
    a. interrogations.
    b. discovery.
    c. settlement.
    d. deposition.

31. The damages and awards that are given to the plaintiff is(are) called the:
    a. settlements.
    b. interrogatories.
    c. sentencing.
    d. depositions.

32. Written answers to a list of questions about charges are called:
    a. interrogatories.
    b. settlements.
    c. depositions.
    d. discoveries.

33. The responsibility for one's own actions is also called:
    a. immunity.
    b. per se negligence.
    c. liability.
    d. malpractice.

34. The time limit within which a lawsuit may be filed is called the:
    a. penalty clause.
    b. statute of limitations.
    c. maximum penalty.
    d. government immunity option.

35. When we discuss and study ethical principles, this practice serves to:
    a. maintain a high degree of integrity.
    b. strengthen and validate our own inner value system.
    c. define a futile situation and who makes the decision.
    d. prevent incorrect documentation or record tampering.

36. When an adult patient agrees to your care, this is called _____ consent.
    a. expressed
    b. informed
    c. implied
    d. detailed

37. After full disclosure or explanation, the patient is said to have given _____ consent.
    a. expressed
    b. implied
    c. involuntary
    d. informed

38. Another name for implied consent is the:
    a. writ of Hypheas.
    b. emergency doctrine.
    c. mental health law.
    d. nolo de solvo.

39. Can an unemancipated minor refuse care?
    a. No.
    b. Yes.
    c. Sometimes.
    d. Yes, but only when a parent cannot be contacted.

40. When a patient wants to refuse treatment or transport, but the paramedic believes the patient needs immediate care, the paramedic can avoid an ethical dilemma by:
    a. using value judgment.
    b. acting in the patient's best interest.
    c. letting the patient sign a waiver of care.
    d. preemptively calling a personal lawyer after the call.

41. A refusal of medical care is considered legal when:
    a. the patient signs a release.
    b. the Medical Director was contacted.
    c. a parent or family member was contacted.
    d. full disclosure was provided to an alert patient.

42. When a patient refuses any part of medical care or transport for evaluation that you deem necessary, despite all of your efforts to convince the patient otherwise, it may be helpful to:
    a. ask the police to threaten the patient with arrest.
    b. get the patient to sign a release.
    c. consult medical control.
    d. avoid a conflict and return to service.

43. Can intoxicated patients refuse care?
    a. Yes; if they do not want transport, just leave them.
    b. Yes, unless they are minors.
    c. No; persons with altered mental status are not considered able to make a competent decision.
    d. No; they can only make decisions of implied consent.

44. Can the paramedic determine how intoxicated a patient may be?
    a. yes
    b. not without additional training
    c. only if the Medical Director is involved
    d. yes, after ruling out medical causes of the altered behaviors

45. If a patient who is refusing care becomes unconscious, can the paramedic treat him?
    a. yes, under the informed consent provision
    b. yes, under the emergency doctrine
    c. not without the police present
    d. not without permission of medical control

46. Who can take a patient away against his will for evaluation in a hospital?
    a. a spouse
    b. a mental health officer
    c. the paramedic
    d. the medical control physician

47. When a police officer agrees that a patient who is refusing your care may be harmful to himself, he/she can order the patient to the hospital under:
    a. executive powers.
    b. protective custody.
    c. mental health laws.
    d. offensive consent.

48. You are called to the scene of a private residence. The patient is an elderly man whose two daughters meet you at the door and proceed to tell you how he is acting crazy and is so much trouble to care for. They would like you to take him to the hospital. If the patient refuses to go and is alert with no life threats, what should you do?
    a. Just take him in restraints.
    b. Involve the police for some assistance.
    c. Call medical control to get an order to take him in.
    d. Call a mental health officer.

49. The federal rules on sexual harassment are found in the:
    a. state harassment code.
    b. Civil Rights Act.
    c. OSHA regulations.
    d. NFPA guidelines.

50. A living will is a document that states the type of life-saving medical treatment a patient wants or does not want to be employed in case of:
    a. terminal illness.
    b. coma.
    c. persistent vegetative state.
    d. all of the above.

51. A _____ allows a person to designate an agent in cases where the person is unable to make decisions for himself.
    a. living will
    b. health-care proxy
    c. patient self-determination act
    d. release

52. In which of the following cases it is legal for the paramedic or an EMS agency to release confidential information about a patient to others?
    a. when a third party requires the information for billing
    b. when the receiving hospital requests the patient's name over the radio
    c. when the patient's lawyer goes to the EMS office and verbally requests it
    d. when a spouse calls on the phone asking for a fax of the billing information

53. _____ is(are) the use of sheets, tape, or leather-padded restraints to reduce the potential harm to a patient who is unruly or violent.
    a. Humane restraints
    b. Hog tying
    c. Proven binding
    d. Mummy wrapping

54. The paramedic has a(n) _____ responsibility to resuscitate all potential organ donors so that others may benefit from the organs.
    a. legal
    b. ethical
    c. moral
    d. religious

55. It is important for the paramedic to write the patient care report (PCR) "in the course of business" for all of the following reasons, *except* when:
    a. completing the paperwork at a later time looks suspicious.
    b. the information is fresh in the paramedic's mind.
    c. the information has to be quickly available for billing.
    d. a copy needs to go to the ED to be placed in the patient's record.

56. Punitive damages are designed to punish the defendant for:
    a. her harmful actions.
    b. the extended response time.
    c. the delay in responding to the patient's needs.
    d. discourteous language used.

57. Which of the following is an example of an ethical dilemma the paramedic may experience as a physician extender?
    a. an indirect (off-line) protocol is not in the patient's best interest
    b. an indirect (off-line) protocol is contraindicated but morally right
    c. receiving a direct (online) order that is not part of standing orders
    d. receiving a direct (online) order that is medically acceptable but morally wrong

58. Who has the burden of proof in a lawsuit?
    a. defendant
    b. plaintiff
    c. responder
    d. hearing officer

59. _____ is the range of skills and knowledge the paramedic is trained in.
    a. Scope of practice
    b. Standard of care
    c. Protocol
    d. Code of ethics

60. The _____ makes certain types of information collected by public agencies available to the media, legal council, or the public upon demand.
    a. "standards of care"
    b. Burden of Proof Act
    c. Freedom of Information Act
    d. innocent until proven guilty pretext

61. The paramedic is responsible for the actions of the intern under the _____ concept.
    a. "cloak of secrecy"
    b. medical extender
    c. Good Samaritan
    d. "borrowed servant"

62. Except for the unconscious patient, all EMS providers must get the patient's consent for treatment or they could be charged with:
    a. battery and assault.
    b. sexual harassment.
    c. false imprisonment.
    d. nothing.

63. In determining whether or not an ambulance operator was exercising due regard in the use of signaling equipment, the courts will consider which of the following?
    a. Was the given signal audible and/or visible to motorist and pedestrians?
    b. Does the insurance company require the use of lights and sirens for all calls?
    c. Does the insurance company require the use of lights and sirens for emergency calls?
    d. Does the insurance company require the use of lights and sirens for all nonemergency calls?

64. Society attempts to resolve global ethical conflicts by using preplans such as wills and advanced directives to make a patient's wishes known, and by:
    a. preprogramming the phone to dial 9-1-1.
    b. using enhanced 9-1-1 and emergency medical dispatch.
    c. creating laws protecting patient's rights.
    d. researching prospective medical decisions.

65. A _____ is a document testifying that one has fulfilled certain requirements, such as a course of instruction.
    a. certificate
    b. license
    c. permit
    d. regents insignia

66. Select the most accurate statement regarding the use of lights and sirens during an emergency response.
    a. The use of lights and sirens during an emergency response gives the operator complete immunity.
    b. The operator of the emergency vehicle assumes the extra burden of driving with due regard for others.
    c. The emergency vehicle operator will be held to a lower standard than the average driver in the eyes of the law.
    d. The use of lights and sirens during an emergency response gives the operator and EMS agency complete immunity.

67. The Americans with Disabilities Act (ADA) is a federal law designed to protect qualified persons with disabilities, such as one who _____, from discrimination in employment.
    a. is pregnant
    b. uses illegal drugs
    c. has hearing impairment
    d. fractured an ankle on the job

68. An example of unethical behavior would be:
    a. treating and transporting a patient with no health insurance.
    b. witnessing a coworker do something unethical and saying nothing.
    c. transporting a trauma arrest patient to the nearest hospital instead of a trauma center.
    d. transporting a patient to a hospital that is not the closest because it has more appropriate resources for the patient.

69. The _____ is the federal law that has an impact on issues such as on-call pay, comp time, and long-shift and overtime pay.
    a. Family and Medical Leave Act (FMLA)
    b. Fair Labor Standards Act (FLSA)
    c. Federal Insurance Contributions Act (FICA)
    d. Occupational Safety and Health Administration (OSHA)

70. One of the major roles of the Occupational Safety and Health Administration (OSHA) is to:
    a. enforce regulations within employment by federal agencies.
    b. encourage the improvement of existing safety and health programs.
    c. assure that self-employed workers are covered by OSHA regulations.
    d. enforce safety regulations and fine noncompliant farmers where only family members are employed.

71. It is good practice to wear an ID tag and introduce yourself to your patient by name and level of training because:
    a. it is the polite thing to do.
    b. she will know who to sue if she feels treatment was inappropriate.
    c. she will know to send a tip and thank-you letter.
    d. patients have a right to know who you are and your level of training.

72. The Medical Director's liability for prehospital care falls into the two categories of:
    a. training and continuing education.
    b. online and off-line supervision.
    c. quality improvement and quality assurance.
    d. omission and commission.

73. The best way for a paramedic to avoid a lawsuit is to:
    a. always be respectful and pleasant to patients, their families, and their property.
    b. practice good medicine and be a competent caregiver.
    c. accurately document the assessment and management of the patient clearly on the PCR.
    d. All of the above.

74. The first responsibility the paramedic has at a crime scene is to:
    a. protect potential evidence.
    b. provide care for the patient.
    c. protect herself and the crew.
    d. notify law enforcement if not already done.

75. In an effort to maintain the paramedic–patient relationship, which of the following pieces of information must be kept confidential?
    a. gunshot and stab wounds
    b. signs of suspected abuse
    c. signs of a communicable disease
    d. observations made of the patient's residence

76. In the EMS community, global ethical conflicts are typically resolved by utilizing standards of care and:
    a. treatment protocols.
    b. maintaining a high degree of suspicion.
    c. involving a family member whenever possible.
    d. avoiding having family involved whenever possible.

77. Ethics are defined as:
    a. a system of principles governing moral conduct.
    b. not acting in a rude or crude manner.
    c. never cheating on your taxes.
    d. a true measure of honesty.

78. Morals relate to _____ standards and ethics relate to _____ standards.
    a. high; objective
    b. subjective; high
    c. personal; societal
    d. societal; personal

79. Which of the following questions should the paramedic consider when confronted with an ethical dilemma?
    a. "What is in the EMS agency's best interest?"
    b. "How will I keep from getting sued?"
    c. "How can my interest best be preserved?"
    d. "What is in the patient's best interest?"

80. How can a refusal of medical assistance involve ethical decisions?
    a. Once the standard of care has been applied, there are no ethical issues.
    b. Ethics are not really a factor when the patient has given informed consent.
    c. Ethics can affect the extent to which you should persuade a patient to receive treatment.
    d. Ethics can affect how much your agency will bill a patient for services after the patient refuses transport.

81. Some states have laws to provide immunity from _____ for the paramedic who begins CPR on a patient with a DNAR order.
    a. liability
    b. willful disregard
    c. wanton disregard
    d. malicious disregard

82. For the patient to be able to be well informed in his decisions regarding care, the paramedic, as a rule, should be honest and:
    a. have a family member involved when possible.
    b. use language/terms the patient can understand.
    c. ask the patient to sign for consent for treatment.
    d. avoid having family involved whenever possible.

83. When the paramedic is faced with a global ethical conflict, which of the following should he avoid using to help resolve the conflict?
    a. standards of care
    b. treatment protocols
    c. retrospective reviews of medical decisions
    d. preplanned wills

84. The American Medical Association's (AMA) Code of Medical Ethics states that patients have the right to:
    a. refuse payment when they are dissatisfied with care rendered.
    b. name the physician who will not do their surgery.
    c. waive their ethical options.
    d. make decisions on health care.

85. In which of the following areas might a paramedic have to make an ethical decision?
    a. implied consent
    b. billing
    c. privacy disclosure
    d. reporting suspected child abuse

86. In EMS systems with multiple hospitals and ill-defined transport protocols, the paramedic should use which of the following to influence the patient's decision on where to be transported?
    a. capabilities of the hospital
    b. the closest hospital to the patient's residence
    c. the fastest trip to the hospital
    d. the hospital that accepts the patient's insurance

87. Which of the following is an example of a prehospital ethical decision the paramedic may be confronted with?
    a. deciding to stay home from work when injured
    b. dealing with a patient who is experiencing a behavioral emergency
    c. deciding whether or not to stop to render assistance when not on duty
    d. receiving and confirming a physician order that seems medically acceptable

88. Select the most accurate statement about ethics in the EMS profession.
    a. There is really no difference between ethics and morals.
    b. Ethics involve larger issues than a paramedic's practice.
    c. Every treatment decision the paramedic makes is based on ethics.
    d. Making a medication error and reporting it is an example of unethical behavior.

89. Criteria that are used for allocating scarce EMS resources include: need based upon established criteria, value earned based upon an established criteria awarding points or value, and:
    a. true parity.
    b. hardship.
    c. distribution.
    d. prerequisite.

90. _____ is an attempt to make a comparison of all variables in an effort to arrive at a similarity.
    a. True parity
    b. Objective standard
    c. Subjective parity
    d. True standard

91. The paramedic is ethically accountable to all of the following, *except*:
    a. the patient.
    b. the patient's advanced directives.
    c. the Medical Director.
    d. fulfilling the standard of care.

92. When answering an ethical question regarding a patient, which of the following should be considered?
    a. passion
    b. good faith
    c. sentiment
    d. sympathy

93. When the paramedic is making a determination of "what is in the patient's best interest," which of the following should be considered first?
    a. the patient's statements
    b. input from the patient's lawyer
    c. unsigned advanced directives
    d. input from the patient's physician

94. A husband called 9-1-1 when he found his wife unresponsive. You arrived and began resuscitation efforts, but shortly thereafter the patient's son arrives and tells you that the patient did not want any type of resuscitation. There is no Do Not Attempt Resuscitation (DNAR) order for the patient. What should you do next?
    a. Stop CPR and call the coroner.
    b. Call the patient's physician for his advice.
    c. Ask the police to keep the son away.
    d. When in doubt, resuscitate.

95. _____, as we know it today, stands for soundness of moral principle and character, uprightness, and honesty.
    a. Ethics
    b. Integrity
    c. Candor
    d. Sincerity

Exam #6 Answer Form

	A	B	C	D			A	B	C	D
1.	❏	❏	❏	❏		33.	❏	❏	❏	❏
2.	❏	❏	❏	❏		34.	❏	❏	❏	❏
3.	❏	❏	❏	❏		35.	❏	❏	❏	❏
4.	❏	❏	❏	❏		36.	❏	❏	❏	❏
5.	❏	❏	❏	❏		37.	❏	❏	❏	❏
6.	❏	❏	❏	❏		38.	❏	❏	❏	❏
7.	❏	❏	❏	❏		39.	❏	❏	❏	❏
8.	❏	❏	❏	❏		40.	❏	❏	❏	❏
9.	❏	❏	❏	❏		41.	❏	❏	❏	❏
10.	❏	❏	❏	❏		42.	❏	❏	❏	❏
11.	❏	❏	❏	❏		43.	❏	❏	❏	❏
12.	❏	❏	❏	❏		44.	❏	❏	❏	❏
13.	❏	❏	❏	❏		45.	❏	❏	❏	❏
14.	❏	❏	❏	❏		46.	❏	❏	❏	❏
15.	❏	❏	❏	❏		47.	❏	❏	❏	❏
16.	❏	❏	❏	❏		48.	❏	❏	❏	❏
17.	❏	❏	❏	❏		49.	❏	❏	❏	❏
18.	❏	❏	❏	❏		50.	❏	❏	❏	❏
19.	❏	❏	❏	❏		51.	❏	❏	❏	❏
20.	❏	❏	❏	❏		52.	❏	❏	❏	❏
21.	❏	❏	❏	❏		53.	❏	❏	❏	❏
22.	❏	❏	❏	❏		54.	❏	❏	❏	❏
23.	❏	❏	❏	❏		55.	❏	❏	❏	❏
24.	❏	❏	❏	❏		56.	❏	❏	❏	❏
25.	❏	❏	❏	❏		57.	❏	❏	❏	❏
26.	❏	❏	❏	❏		58.	❏	❏	❏	❏
27.	❏	❏	❏	❏		59.	❏	❏	❏	❏
28.	❏	❏	❏	❏		60.	❏	❏	❏	❏
29.	❏	❏	❏	❏		61.	❏	❏	❏	❏
30.	❏	❏	❏	❏		62.	❏	❏	❏	❏
31.	❏	❏	❏	❏		63.	❏	❏	❏	❏
32.	❏	❏	❏	❏		64.	❏	❏	❏	❏

Exam #6 Answer Form

	A	B	C	D			A	B	C	D
65.	❏	❏	❏	❏		81.	❏	❏	❏	❏
66.	❏	❏	❏	❏		82.	❏	❏	❏	❏
67.	❏	❏	❏	❏		83.	❏	❏	❏	❏
68.	❏	❏	❏	❏		84.	❏	❏	❏	❏
69.	❏	❏	❏	❏		85.	❏	❏	❏	❏
70.	❏	❏	❏	❏		86.	❏	❏	❏	❏
71.	❏	❏	❏	❏		87.	❏	❏	❏	❏
72.	❏	❏	❏	❏		88.	❏	❏	❏	❏
73.	❏	❏	❏	❏		89.	❏	❏	❏	❏
74.	❏	❏	❏	❏		90.	❏	❏	❏	❏
75.	❏	❏	❏	❏		91.	❏	❏	❏	❏
76.	❏	❏	❏	❏		92.	❏	❏	❏	❏
77.	❏	❏	❏	❏		93.	❏	❏	❏	❏
78.	❏	❏	❏	❏		94.	❏	❏	❏	❏
79.	❏	❏	❏	❏		95.	❏	❏	❏	❏
80.	❏	❏	❏	❏						

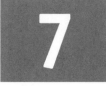

Anatomy, Physiology, and Medical Terminology

1. The study of the function of the body is called:
   a. anatomy.
   b. physiology.
   c. pathophysiology.
   d. functionality.

2. The study of the components of the body is called the:
   a. anatomy.
   b. physiology.
   c. pathology.
   d. pathophysiology.

3. The study of how a disease develops and progresses is covered best in:
   a. anatomy.
   b. microbiology.
   c. pathophysiology.
   d. prognosis.

4. The functions of the body which attempt to keep metabolism functioning within normal ranges of temperature and pH is referred to as:
   a. heredity.
   b. immunity.
   c. nutritional balance.
   d. homeostasis.

5. When preparing a report and giving a report, a paramedic should refer to the patient's "armpit" as their:
   a. brachial.
   b. axillary.
   c. cervical.
   d. perineal.

6. An artery found in the upper arm which is used for obtaining a blood pressure is called the:
   a. femoral.
   b. brachial.
   c. pectoral.
   d. deltoid.

7. The area of the spine which is posterior to the abdomen is most likely the _____ spine.
   a. plantar
   b. cervical
   c. lumbar
   d. thoracic

8. How is the term "buccal" typically used by the paramedic?
   a. in describing a route of medication administration
   b. in describing the location of an artery
   c. in describing the degree of severity of pain
   d. in describing a location on the top of the foot

9. A condition that affects the heart of the patient is referred to as a _____ condition.
   a. cerebral
   b. gastric
   c. cardiac
   d. occipital

10. The muscles on the anterior surface of the patient's chest wall are referred to as:
    a. inguinal.
    b. hyperplasia.
    c. parietal.
    d. pectoral.

11. Of the following terms, which is not referring to an area of the patient's head?
    a. parietal
    b. temporal
    c. plantar
    d. occipital

12. What is the term for the major artery in the kidneys?
    a. volar
    b. renal
    c. hepatic
    d. inguinal

13. What is the term for the artery that supplies oxygen to a growing fetus?
    a. mammary
    b. umbilical
    c. perineal
    d. volar

14. Of the following terms, which one is a name of a location for an artery in the extremity?
    a. hepatic
    b. mammary
    c. popliteal
    d. cutaneous

15. Pain caused by an injury to the ligament between the abdomen and the pelvis is said to be:
    a. inguinal.
    b. gluteal.
    c. plantar.
    d. patellar.

16. The larger quantities of IM injections are given in the:
    a. deltoid.
    b. brachial.
    c. gluteal.
    d. pectoral.

17. A baseball batter's helmet is designed to protect the _____ region of the brain.
    a. occipital.
    b. temporal.
    c. frontal.
    d. sacral.

18. Which plane or view shows the bone in the middle and the nerves, artery, veins, and lymphatic vessel surrounding the bone?
    a. longitudinal section
    b. midsaggital plane
    c. cross-section
    d. sagittal plane

19. The bones are a component of the _____ system.
    a. nervous
    b. skeletal
    c. endocrine
    d. circulatory

20. Which organ system takes up the largest space?
    a. endocrine system
    b. renal system
    c. integumentary system
    d. respiratory system

21. The alveoli are a component of the _____ organ system.
    a. digestive
    b. muscular
    c. endocrine
    d. respiratory

22. The alimentary canal is a part of the _____ organ system.
    a. endocrine
    b. renal
    c. digestive
    d. lymphatic

23. Of the following, which is considered in a dorsal cavity?
    a. spinal
    b. pelvic
    c. abdominal
    d. thoracic

24. Immune cells are found in the _____ organ system.
    a. skeletal
    b. lymphatic
    c. endocrine
    d. respiratory

25. Each of the following is considered carbohydrates, *except*:
    a. starches.
    b. oligosaccharides.
    c. triglycerides.
    d. glycogen.

26. Steroids are a chemical form of a(n):
    a. carbohydrate.
    b. protein.
    c. lipid.
    d. enzyme.

27. Which of the following is not considered a nucleic acid?
    a. DNA
    b. polypeptide
    c. ATP
    d. RNA

28. The specialized extracellular fluid found in the joints is called _____ fluid.
    a. cerebrospinal
    b. synovial
    c. aqueous humor
    d. lymph

29. When cells surround and engulf a foreign substance, this is referred to as:
    a. filtration.
    b. active transport.
    c. phagocytosis.
    d. facilitated diffusion.

30. Areola is a form of _____ tissue.
    a. muscular
    b. epithelial
    c. connective
    d. neural

31. Which of the following is not considered a specialized connective tissue?
    a. simple cuboidal
    b. fibrous pericardium
    c. meninges
    d. perichondrium

32. Simple cuboidal, simple columnar, and transitional are types of _____ tissue.
    a. connective
    b. epithelial
    c. muscle
    d. neural

33. Each of the following is a type of muscle tissue, *except*:
    a. elastic.
    b. smooth.
    c. skeletal.
    d. cardiac.

34. Each of the following is a type of membrane, *except*:
    a. synovial.
    b. pleura.
    c. pericardial.
    d. peritoneum.

35. The connective tissue that the tip of your nose and ears are made of is called:
    a. periosteum.
    b. perichondrium.
    c. cartilage.
    d. adipose.

36. The skeleton has two major subdivisions, the axial and the:
    a. posterior.
    b. anterior.
    c. sphenoid.
    d. appendicular.

37. The rib cage consists of 12 pairs of ribs and the:
    a. manubrium and xiphoid process.
    b. coccyx and sacrum.
    c. floating ribs and ischium.
    d. scapula and clavicle.

38. When a patient falls on an outstretched arm, he may injure any of the following bones, *except* the:
    a. radius.
    b. ulna.
    c. metatarsals.
    d. humerus.

39. When a patient falls onto his knees, it is likely he may injure his:
    a. calcaneus.
    b. patella.
    c. phalanges.
    d. myofibrils.

40. What type of joint is the knee?
    a. gliding joint
    b. hinge joint
    c. saddle joint
    d. pivot joint

41. The sources for muscle contraction include creatinine phosphate and each of the following, *except*:
    a. cholinesterase.
    b. ATP.
    c. glycogen.
    d. glucose.

42. The membrane that surrounds the lung is called the:
    a. serious membrane.
    b. visceral pleura.
    c. intrapleural membrane.
    d. perineum.

43. Each of the following is a type of leukocyte, *except*:
    a. basophil.
    b. monocyte.
    c. eosinophil.
    d. prothrombin.

44. The inner ear contains the bony labyrinth, perilymph, and the:
    a. incus.
    b. stapes.
    c. cochlea.
    d. Eustachian tube.

45. The sebaceous, ceruminous, and eccrine glands are all found in the:
    a. ears.
    b. eyes.
    c. nose.
    d. skin.

46. Of the following hormones, which is not found in the anterior pituitary gland?
    a. calcitonin
    b. thyroid-stimulating hormone
    c. prolactin
    d. follicle-stimulating hormone

47. Diseases of the adrenal cortex include Cushing's syndrome and:
    a. diabetes.
    b. hypertension.
    c. Addison's disease.
    d. cystic fibrosis.

48. In addition to the parathyroid hormone, each of the following is a hormone that affects kidney function, *except*:
    a. atrial natriuretic peptide.
    b. cortisol.
    c. antidiuretic hormone.
    d. aldosterone.

49. Angiotensin II is responsible for stimulating the secretion of the hormone _____, which acts on the kidney to increase the reabsorption of sodium into the blood.
    a. adenosine
    b. aldosterone
    c. epinephrine
    d. norepinephrine

50. The term "cephalad" means:
    a. toward the top.
    b. toward the bottom.
    c. toward the tail.
    d. toward the head.

51. The imaginary plane that passes through the body and divides it into the upper and lower sections is called the:
    a. transverse plane.
    b. coronal plane.
    c. sagittal plane.
    d. frontal plane.

52. Which prefix means "with both sides?"
    a. adip–
    b. acou–
    c. ambi–
    d. brachi–

53. Which prefix means "within?"
    a. dexto–
    b. endo–
    c. extra–
    d. anterio–

54. The prefix that means "slow" is:
    a. end–.
    b. ana–.
    c. brady–.
    d. meta–.

55. The prefix that means "thicken" is:
    a. pachy–.
    b. trans–.
    c. tacky–.
    d. circum–.

56. The suffix that means "giving rise to" is:
    a. –genesis.
    b. –genic.
    c. –form.
    d. –cis.

57. The suffix that means "a viewing" is:
    a. –oma.
    b. –oid.
    c. –opsy.
    d. –ismus.

58. The term used for blood pressure that is excessive or beyond normal is:
    a. distension.
    b. hypotension.
    c. megatension.
    d. hypertension.

59. The term for the destruction by passage of an electric current is:
    a. hydrolysis.
    b. orthopnea.
    c. electrolysis.
    d. lithotripter.

60. What term is used to describe an inflammation of the tube where urine exits the body?
    a. urethritis
    b. urinalysis
    c. hypertrophic
    d. urinary

Exam #7 Answer Form

	A	B	C	D		A	B	C	D
1.	❏	❏	❏	❏	31.	❏	❏	❏	❏
2.	❏	❏	❏	❏	32.	❏	❏	❏	❏
3.	❏	❏	❏	❏	33.	❏	❏	❏	❏
4.	❏	❏	❏	❏	34.	❏	❏	❏	❏
5.	❏	❏	❏	❏	35.	❏	❏	❏	❏
6.	❏	❏	❏	❏	36.	❏	❏	❏	❏
7.	❏	❏	❏	❏	37.	❏	❏	❏	❏
8.	❏	❏	❏	❏	38.	❏	❏	❏	❏
9.	❏	❏	❏	❏	39.	❏	❏	❏	❏
10.	❏	❏	❏	❏	40.	❏	❏	❏	❏
11.	❏	❏	❏	❏	41.	❏	❏	❏	❏
12.	❏	❏	❏	❏	42.	❏	❏	❏	❏
13.	❏	❏	❏	❏	43.	❏	❏	❏	❏
14.	❏	❏	❏	❏	44.	❏	❏	❏	❏
15.	❏	❏	❏	❏	45.	❏	❏	❏	❏
16.	❏	❏	❏	❏	46.	❏	❏	❏	❏
17.	❏	❏	❏	❏	47.	❏	❏	❏	❏
18.	❏	❏	❏	❏	48.	❏	❏	❏	❏
19.	❏	❏	❏	❏	49.	❏	❏	❏	❏
20.	❏	❏	❏	❏	50.	❏	❏	❏	❏
21.	❏	❏	❏	❏	51.	❏	❏	❏	❏
22.	❏	❏	❏	❏	52.	❏	❏	❏	❏
23.	❏	❏	❏	❏	53.	❏	❏	❏	❏
24.	❏	❏	❏	❏	54.	❏	❏	❏	❏
25.	❏	❏	❏	❏	55.	❏	❏	❏	❏
26.	❏	❏	❏	❏	56.	❏	❏	❏	❏
27.	❏	❏	❏	❏	57.	❏	❏	❏	❏
28.	❏	❏	❏	❏	58.	❏	❏	❏	❏
29.	❏	❏	❏	❏	59.	❏	❏	❏	❏
30.	❏	❏	❏	❏	60.	❏	❏	❏	❏

CHAPTER

Pathophysiology

1. Pathophysiology is defined as:
   a. the study of disease.
   b. an abnormality of function or a structural problem.
   c. a description of how a disease develops from its onset.
   d. the study of how normal physiological processes are altered by disease.

2. The cause of a disease is referred to as the:
   a. pathogenesis.
   b. etiology.
   c. pathology.
   d. prognosis.

3. When the symptoms of a disease rapidly worsen, this is referred to as:
   a. remission.
   b. iatrogenic.
   c. exacerbation.
   d. prognosis.

4. Iatrogenic causes of injury or illness indicate that the cause, or the significant contribution to the cause, is:
   a. heredity.
   b. impaired immunity.
   c. nutritional imbalance.
   d. the actions of a heath care provider.

5. A group of symptoms or conditions that may be caused by a disease or various related medical problems is called a(n):
   a. toxidrome.
   b. infection.
   c. syndrome.
   d. malignancy.

6. A decreased size in the cell leading to a decrease in the size of the tissue and organ is called:
   a. atrophy.
   b. hypertrophy.
   c. acceleration.
   d. cellular adaptation.

7. Atrophy, hyperplasia, and neoplasia are forms of:
   a. muscular dysfunction.
   b. dysplasia.
   c. cellular adaptation.
   d. dysfunction syndrome.

8. An increase in the actual number of cells by hormonal stimulation is called:
   a. hypertrophy.
   b. dysplasia.
   c. metaplasia.
   d. hyperplasia.

9. An alteration in the size and shape of cells, as in a developing tumor, is called:
   a. dysplasia.
   b. hyperplasia.
   c. metaplasia.
   d. hypertrophy.

10. The development of a new type of cell with an uncontrolled growth pattern is called:
    a. neoplasia.
    b. hyperplasia.
    c. metaplasia.
    d. hypertrophy.

11. The ability of microorganisms to cause disease is called:
    a. toxicity.
    b. infectability.
    c. carcinogenesis.
    d. virulence.

12. Your patient was diagnosed with a bacterial disease. Many bacteria have a capsule that is designed to:
    a. hide the microorganism from its host.
    b. make it easier to infect the organism.
    c. protect it from ingestion and destruction by phagocytes.
    d. prevent destruction by a virus.

13. When large amounts of endotoxins are present in the body, the patient may develop:
    a. renal failure.
    b. septic shock.
    c. hypovolemic shock.
    d. liver dysfunction.

14. Your patient has a high white blood cell count. When white blood cells release endogenous pyrogens, it causes:
    a. the production of additional white blood cells.
    b. septic shock.
    c. the body to lower its temperature.
    d. fever to develop.

15. One major difference between viruses and bacteria is that:
    a. viruses are not encapsulated, unlike bacteria.
    b. viruses do not produce exotoxins or endotoxins.
    c. there is a symbiotic relation between viruses and bacteria.
    d. bacteria cause a decreased synthesis of macro-molecules, and viruses do not.

16. The body's most common reaction to the presence of bacteria is:
    a. inflammation.
    b. hemorrhage.
    c. hyperplasia.
    d. increased capillary pressure.

17. An example of an injurious genetic factor affecting the cell is:
    a. sepsis.
    b. hepatitis C.
    c. Down syndrome.
    d. mineral deficiency.

18. Why is good nutrition required by the cells?
    a. It helps the nerve cells to rejuvenate.
    b. It helps the cells fight off diseases.
    c. It helps the muscle cells multiply.
    d. It decreases the production of energy in the cells.

19. The cellular environment is associated with the:
    a. ability of the bladder to store urine.
    b. changes in cell distribution with aging.
    c. movement of potassium into the cells.
    d. movement of potassium out of the cells.

20. How much of the body's weight is fluid?
    a. 10–12%
    b. 30–40%
    c. 50–70%
    d. 70–90%

21. It has been said that humans are mostly fluid. Where, in the body, can most of the fluid be found?
    a. in the fluid between the cells
    b. intracellular fluids
    c. extracellular fluids
    d. in the bladder

22. How much fluid does the average adult take in each day?
    a. 1,500 ml
    b. 2,500 ml
    c. 3,500 ml
    d. 4,500 ml

23. When a person loses large quantities of water, he also loses the major extracellular cation:
    a. sodium.
    b. calcium.
    c. potassium.
    d. chloride.

24. Lymph fluid is a part of _____ fluid.
    a. interstitial
    b. intracellular
    c. extracellular
    d. transcellular

25. The movement of a substance from an area of higher concentration to an area of lower concentration is called:
    a. osmosis.
    b. filtration.
    c. active transport.
    d. diffusion.

26. When a cell membrane ingests a substance, this is called:
    a. exocytosis.
    b. pinocytosis.
    c. endocytosis.
    d. phagocytosis.

27. The engulfing of solid particles by a cell membrane is called:
    a. exocytosis.
    b. pinocytosis.
    c. endocytosis.
    d. phagocytosis.

28. The pressure that develops when two solutions of different concentrations are separated by a semipermeable membrane is called _____ pressure.
    a. intracranial
    b. osmotic
    c. colloid
    d. oncotic

29. Of the following male age groups, which patients have the greatest percentage of total body water?
    a. 10–18 years
    b. 18–40 years
    c. 40–60 years
    d. over 60 years

30. A solution with a lower solute concentration than the blood is referred to as a(n) _____ solution.
    a. hypertonic
    b. hypotonic
    c. isotonic
    d. neotonic

31. When a helper molecule, found within the membrane, helps the movement of a substance from areas of higher concentration to areas of lower concentration, this is called:
    a. facilitated diffusion.
    b. active transport.
    c. osmosis.
    d. filtration.

32. Which of the following plasma proteins is responsible for maintaining osmotic pressure?
    a. albumin
    b. globulin
    c. fibrinogen
    d. prothrombin

33. The pressure generated by dissolved proteins in the plasma that are too large to penetrate the capillary membrane is called:
    a. tissue colloidal osmotic pressure.
    b. capillary hydrostatic pressure.
    c. tissue hydrostatic pressure.
    d. capillary colloidal osmotic pressure.

34. The pressure that pushes water out of the capillary into the interstitial space is referred to as the:
    a. tissue colloidal osmotic pressure.
    b. capillary colloidal osmotic pressure.
    c. capillary hydrostatic pressure.
    d. tissue hydrostatic pressure.

35. Your patient has developed an accumulation of excess fluids in the interstitial space. This condition is called:
    a. edema.
    b. lymph.
    c. cellular swelling.
    d. engorgement.

36. Your patient has accumulated fluid in his peritoneal cavity. This condition is referred to as:
    a. ascites.
    b. sacral edema.
    c. intestinal swelling.
    d. pitting edema.

37. Edema can be caused by:
    a. increased capillary pressure.
    b. decreased colloidal osmotic pressure.
    c. lymphatic vessel obstruction.
    d. All of the above.

38. When a patient sustains an extensive full thickness burn injury, the swelling that develops is caused by:
    a. increased capillary pressure.
    b. decreased colloidal osmotic pressure.
    c. dehydration.
    d. lymphatic vessel obstruction.

39. When edematous tissue, such as in the ankles, is compressed with a finger, the fluid is pushed aside causing a temporary impression. This is referred to as:
    a. lymphatic edema.
    b. pitting edema.
    c. ascites.
    d. acute pulmonary edema (APE)

40. What is the main function of the sodium–potassium pump?
    a. pump sodium into the cells
    b. move potassium out of the cells
    c. exchange three sodium ions for every two potassium ions
    d. exchange two sodium ions for every three potassium ions

41. The tension exerted on cell size caused by water movement across the cell membrane is referred to as:
    a. tonicity.
    b. oncotic pressure.
    c. osmotic pressure.
    d. colloid pressure.

42. Cells with an osmolarity of 280 mOsm/L will neither shrink nor swell. This is because they:
    a. are considered hypotonic solutions.
    b. are high in both sodium and potassium.
    c. have the same osmolarity as intracellular fluid.
    d. are considered hypertonic solutions.

43. When a cell is placed in a _____ solution, it will shrink as the water is _____ the cell.
    a. hypotonic; pushed into
    b. hypotonic; pulled out of
    c. hypertonic; pushed into
    d. hypertonic; pulled out of

44. When a cell is placed in a hypotonic solution that has a _____ osmolarity than ICF, it will _____.
    a. lower; shrink
    b. lower; swell
    c. higher; shrink
    d. higher; swell

45. The most common cation in the body is:
    a. calcium.
    b. potassium.
    c. sodium.
    d. chloride.

46. Although the average adult ingests between 6 and 15 grams of sodium per day, the required amount is:
    a. 100 mg.
    b. 500 mg.
    c. 1,000 mg.
    d. 4 mg.

47. Angiotensin II is responsible for:
    a. dilating the renal blood vessels.
    b. increasing kidney blood flow.
    c. stimulating sodium reabsorption.
    d. increasing the glomerular filtration rate.

48. The protein enzyme that is released by the kidney into the blood stream in response to changes in blood pressure is called:
    a. renin.
    b. epinephrine.
    c. tensin.
    d. aldosterone.

49. Angiotensin II is responsible for stimulating the secretion of the hormone _____, which acts on the kidney to increase the reabsorption of sodium into the blood.
    a. adenosine
    b. aldosterone
    c. epinephrine
    d. norepinephrine

50. When a patient has excess body water loss without a proportionate sodium loss, she is said to be:
    a. hyponatremic.
    b. hypernatremic.
    c. dehydrated.
    d. edematous.

51. You suspect that your patient, who is an elderly male, has sustained hypernatremia. One of the most severe manifestations of hypernatremia is:
    a. oliguria.
    b. seizures and coma.
    c. decreased salivation.
    d. dry and flushed skin.

52. Which of the following is a classic cause of hyponatremia?
    a. sepsis
    b. esophageal varices
    c. vomiting and diarrhea
    d. intra-abdominal hemorrhage

53. An athlete who has had excessive sweating for a 3-hour period and has only been drinking water to rehydrate may suffer the symptoms of:
    a. hypovolemia.
    b. hypertension.
    c. hyponatremia.
    d. hypernatremia.

54. The major intracellular cation, which is critical to many of the functions of the cell, is:
    a. sodium.
    b. potassium.
    c. chloride.
    d. calcium.

55. A patient may become hypokalemic from:
    a. excessive vomiting or diarrhea.
    b. a diet deficient in sodium.
    c. excessive eating.
    d. decreased sweating.

56. ECG changes associated with a deficiency in potassium may include:
    a. depressed P wave.
    b. widening QRS complex.
    c. low T wave and sagging ST segment.
    d. peaked T waves and depressed ST segment.

57. When a patient has an elevated serum potassium level, this can be caused by:
    a. decreased potassium intake.
    b. excess use of diuretics.
    c. renal failure.
    d. treatment with angiotensin.

58. The clinical manifestations of hyperkalemia include:
    a. paresthesia and intestinal colic.
    b. a feeling of euphoria.
    c. excessive urination.
    d. muscle overactivity.

59. A hyperkalemic patient may exhibit ECG changes such as:
    a. peaked ST segments.
    b. depressed T waves.
    c. widened QRS.
    d. peaked P waves.

60. Where is the vast majority of the body's calcium found?
    a. kidneys
    b. teeth
    c. liver
    d. bones

61. The purpose of calcium is to provide:
    a. strength and stability to bones.
    b. increased conduction through muscles.
    c. enhanced renal effectiveness.
    d. maintenance of the blood pressure.

62. How does calcium enter the body?
    a. through the lungs
    b. by way of the bones
    c. through the GI tract
    d. through the skin

63. Hypocalcemia can be caused by:
    a. renal failure.
    b. decreased pH.
    c. decreased fatty acids.
    d. vomiting and diarrhea.

64. Other causes of hypocalcemia include:
    a. hypermagnesemia.
    b. rapid transfusion of citrated blood.
    c. decreased pH.
    d. excess vitamin D.

65. A patient with hypocalcemia often presents with:
    a. skeletal muscle cramps.
    b. absence of tetany.
    c. hypertension.
    d. hypoactive reflexes.

66. A patient who has frequent skeletal muscle cramps, abdominal spasms, and cramps, as well as frequent fractures, may benefit by supplementing his diet intake of:
    a. sodium.
    b. calcium.
    c. zinc.
    d. potassium.

67. Osteomalacia and carpopedal spasms have been found to be manifestations of:
    a. hyponatremia.
    b. hyperkalemia.
    c. hypophosphatemia.
    d. hypocalcemia.

68. Hypercalcemia can be caused by:
    a. increased pH.
    b. excess calcium in the diet.
    c. insufficient calcium in the diet.
    d. decreased levels of parathyroid hormone.

69. Kidney stones, constipation, and polyuria are sometimes a manifestation of:
    a. hypocalcemia.
    b. hyponatremia.
    c. hypercalcemia.
    d. hypokalemia.

70. A shortening QT interval and AV block on the ECG sometimes is found with which condition?
    a. hypercalcemia
    b. hyponatremia
    c. hypokalemia
    d. hyperkalemia

71. Hypophosphatemia is an abnormally low level of phosphate in the body and can be caused by:
    a. seizures.
    b. heat stroke.
    c. potassium deficiency.
    d. diabetic ketoacidosis.

72. The clinical manifestation of hypophosphatemia includes:
    a. impaired red blood cell function.
    b. hyperreflexia.
    c. hemolytic anemia.
    d. excessive hunger.

73. Often patients who experience trauma and have kidney failure are at risk to develop:
    a. hypokalemia.
    b. hyperphosphatemia.
    c. hypocalcemia.
    d. hyponatremia.

74. Malnutrition or starvation can be caused by which of the following conditions?
    a. hypocalcemia
    b. hypomagnesemia
    c. hypercalcemia
    d. hyponatremia

75. Positive Babinski's sign, positive Chvostek's sign, and positive Trousseau's sign may be found in the patient who has:
   a. hypomagnesemia.
   b. hypercalcemia.
   c. hypernatremia.
   d. hyponatremia.

76. A muscular spasm resulting from pressure applied to nerves and vessels of the upper arm is called _____ sign.
   a. Babinski's
   b. Chvostek's
   c. Trousseau's
   d. Cushing's

77. What is the normal pH range of the body?
   a. 7.15–7.25
   b. 7.25–7.35
   c. 7.35–7.45
   d. 7.45–7.55

78. A blood pH _____ than 7.45 is called _____.
   a. greater; acidosis
   b. greater; alkalosis
   c. greater; neutral
   d. less; alkalosis

79. Sepsis, diabetic ketoacidosis, and salicylate poisoning may cause:
   a. respiratory acidosis.
   b. metabolic acidosis.
   c. metabolic alkalosis.
   d. respiratory alkalosis.

80. When CO_2 retention leads to increased levels of pCO_2, the patient develops:
   a. respiratory acidosis.
   b. respiratory alkalosis.
   c. metabolic acidosis.
   d. metabolic alkalosis.

81. Patients who experience a medical condition causing hypoventilation may develop:
   a. metabolic acidosis.
   b. metabolic alkalosis.
   c. respiratory acidosis.
   d. respiratory alkalosis.

82. When a 24-year-old female patient has been hyperventilating from an anxiety attack, she may ultimately develop:
   a. metabolic acidosis.
   b. metabolic alkalosis.
   c. respiratory acidosis.
   d. respiratory alkalosis.

83. Analyzing disease risk involves reviewing all of the following, *except*:
   a. genetic histories of populations.
   b. rates of incidence.
   c. prevalence.
   d. mortality.

84. An example of a disease that is more prevalent in males is:
   a. osteoporosis.
   b. Parkinson's disease.
   c. breast cancer.
   d. rheumatoid arthritis.

85. Acquired hypersensitivity is called a(n):
   a. rheumatic fever.
   b. cancer.
   c. asthma.
   d. allergy.

86. You are treating a 45-year-old male patient who tells you he had a recent strep throat, and he has a history of myocarditis and arthritis. Which of the following conditions could he most likely have?
   a. Parkinson's disease
   b. rheumatic fever
   c. lung cancer
   d. diabetes

87. Which of the following signs or symptoms is an atypical finding associated with cancer?
   a. recent weight gain
   b. difficulty swallowing
   c. nagging cough or hoarseness
   d. change in bowel or bladder habits

88. A hypersensitivity reaction causing constriction of the bronchi, wheezing, and dyspnea is a chronic illness called:
   a. diabetes.
   b. anemia.
   c. asthma.
   d. cardiomyopathy.

89. The leading cause of chronic illness in children is:
    a. diabetes.
    b. chicken pox.
    c. cancer.
    d. asthma.

90. The leading cause of cancer deaths in both males and females combined is from _____ cancer.
    a. rectal
    b. brain
    c. lung
    d. breast

91. The difference between Type I and Type II diabetes is:
    a. Type I develops as a disease in adults.
    b. Type II does not become hypoglycemic.
    c. Type I requires exogenous insulin.
    d. Type II requires injected insulin.

92. Why do diabetic patients need to *inject* insulin?
    a. so they can take an entire day's dose at once
    b. their digestive juices would destroy oral forms
    c. pills do not counteract low blood pressure
    d. it is cheapest in this form

93. What organ is responsible for the production of insulin?
    a. kidney
    b. liver
    c. spleen
    d. pancreas

94. Exposure to benzene and bacterial toxins can cause the patient to develop:
    a. hemophilia.
    b. hematochromatosis.
    c. drug-induced anemia.
    d. septal hypertrophy.

95. Select the statement that is most correct about mitral valve prolapse condition.
    a. The cause is unknown.
    b. The condition is more prevalent in men.
    c. Management of this condition is focused on surgical repair.
    d. The mitral valve leaflets balloon into the right atrium during systole.

96. Long QT syndrome is a cardiac conduction system abnormality that:
    a. is inherited.
    b. cannot be treated.
    c. is not associated with other diseases.
    d. occurs as a result of abnormal iron retention by the liver.

97. A sex-linked hereditary disorder most commonly passed on from an asymptomatic mother to a male child is:
    a. anemia.
    b. hemophilia.
    c. ALS.
    d. hematochromatosis.

98. Incurable diseases of the heart, which ultimately lead to congestive heart failure or acute coronary syndrome (ACS), include:
    a. stroke.
    b. cardiomyopathies.
    c. mitral valve prolapse.
    d. hematochromatosis.

99. The disease mortality rate for _____ is significantly higher than that of other diseases.
    a. cancer
    b. accidents
    c. HIV/AIDS
    d. cardiovascular disease

100. What is the leading cause of stroke in the prehospital setting?
    a. brain aneurysm
    b. diabetes
    c. cigarette smoking
    d. hypertension

101. A disorder of protein metabolism that primarily affects males, leading to inflammation of the joints, is called:
    a. arthritis.
    b. lactose intolerance.
    c. gout.
    d. ulcerative colitis.

102. Chronic hypertension is a devastating disease that affects the cardiovascular system by:
    a. increasing the blood supply.
    b. changing the size and shape of the heart.
    c. causing the right ventricle to work harder than the left.
    d. increasing the blood volume pumped through the body.

103. Why is smoking a risk factor for stroke?
    a. The carbon dioxide levels run higher.
    b. It damages the lung cells.
    c. Nicotine causes vasoconstriction.
    d. It paralyzes the brain tissues.

104. The medical term for kidney stones is:
    a. uric acid crystals.
    b. renal calculi.
    c. hematuria.
    d. renal calcium.

105. Kidney stones are most common in _____ between the ages of _____.
    a. males; 50 and 70
    b. females; 30 and 70
    c. males; 30 and 50
    d. females; 50 and 70

106. A disorder affecting the rectum and colon, causing inflammation, lesions, and ulcerations of the mucosal layer, is called:
    a. lactose intolerance.
    b. irritable bowel syndrome.
    c. ulcerative colitis.
    d. Crohn's disease.

107. Patients who are unable to break down the complex carbohydrates found in ice cream have:
    a. renal calculi.
    b. lactose intolerance.
    c. ulcerative colitis.
    d. irritable bowel syndrome.

108. A group of disorders that occurs in areas of the upper GI tract that are normally exposed to acid pepsin secretions is referred to as:
    a. peptic ulcers.
    b. muscular dystrophy.
    c. Crohn's disease.
    d. Huntington's disease.

109. Cholelithiasis is the medical term for:
    a. kidney stones.
    b. peptic ulcers.
    c. gallstones.
    d. Crohn's disease.

110. When the flow of bile is obstructed, the patient may be suffering from:
    a. renal calculi.
    b. lactose intolerance.
    c. gallstones.
    d. Huntington's disease.

111. Each of the following is considered a health risk associated with obesity, *except*:
    a. hyperlipidemia.
    b. hypotension.
    c. gallbladder disease.
    d. insulin resistance.

112. Morbidly obese patients often have sleep apnea and:
    a. lactose intolerance.
    b. hypolipidemia.
    c. multiple sclerosis.
    d. respiratory function impairment.

113. A rare hereditary disorder involving chronic progressive chorea, psychologic changes, and dementia is called:
    a. Crohn's disease.
    b. Huntington's disease.
    c. multiple sclerosis.
    d. muscular dystrophy.

114. You are treating a patient who has a disease that manifests itself with acute episodes of paresthesia, optic neuritis, diplopia, or gaze paralysis. You suspect he may have a history of:
    a. multiple sclerosis.
    b. Huntington's disease.
    c. muscular dystrophy.
    d. Alzheimer's.

115. A patient who has stage 2 Alzheimer's disease may exhibit:
    a. indifference to food and inability to communicate.
    b. memory loss and lack of spontaneity.
    c. impaired cognition and abstract thinking.
    d. inability to taste spicy food and disorientation to time and date.

116. The most common cause of cardiogenic shock is:
    a. anaphylaxis.
    b. a ventricular septal defect.
    c. an extensive acute myocardial infarction.
    d. multiple organ dysfunction syndrome following a severe traumatic injury.

117. _____ is an example of a condition that can cause obstructive shock.
    a. Anaphylaxis
    b. Heart failure
    c. Pericardial tamponade
    d. Ventricular septal defect

118. Causes of hypovolemic shock include:
    a. heart failure.
    b. ventricular septal defect.
    c. electrolyte loss from dehydration.
    d. pericardial tamponade.

119. What is MODS?
    a. a disease of the brain
    b. advice for managing shock
    c. multiple organ dysfunction syndrome
    d. mutation of disease syndrome

120. When a patient who receives a blood transfusion from another person has a reaction to the red blood cells, this is called an _____ reaction.
    a. allergic
    b. isoimmune
    c. autoimmune
    d. inflammation

121. _____ is one of the local effects of an inflammation response.
    a. Fever
    b. Vasodilation
    c. Leukocytosis
    d. Decreased capillary permeability

122. A system response to acute inflammation is:
    a. fever.
    b. vasodilation.
    c. the development of exudates.
    d. increased capillary permeability.

123. The type of immunity that you acquire by getting a disease and developing immunity afterward is _____ immunity.
    a. natural
    b. acquired
    c. nonspecific
    d. cell-mediated

124. The system that plays a vital role in attracting white blood cells to the site of the infection is called:
    a. bradykinin.
    b. immunocascade.
    c. complement.
    d. macrophage.

125. The role of _____ during inflammation is to engulf foreign matter and bacteria.
    a. phagocytes
    b. monocytes
    c. macrophages
    d. eosinophils

Exam #8 Answer Form

	A	B	C	D		A	B	C	D
1.	❑	❑	❑	❑	34.	❑	❑	❑	❑
2.	❑	❑	❑	❑	35.	❑	❑	❑	❑
3.	❑	❑	❑	❑	36.	❑	❑	❑	❑
4.	❑	❑	❑	❑	37.	❑	❑	❑	❑
5.	❑	❑	❑	❑	38.	❑	❑	❑	❑
6.	❑	❑	❑	❑	39.	❑	❑	❑	❑
7.	❑	❑	❑	❑	40.	❑	❑	❑	❑
8.	❑	❑	❑	❑	41.	❑	❑	❑	❑
9.	❑	❑	❑	❑	42.	❑	❑	❑	❑
10.	❑	❑	❑	❑	43.	❑	❑	❑	❑
11.	❑	❑	❑	❑	44.	❑	❑	❑	❑
12.	❑	❑	❑	❑	45.	❑	❑	❑	❑
13.	❑	❑	❑	❑	46.	❑	❑	❑	❑
14.	❑	❑	❑	❑	47.	❑	❑	❑	❑
15.	❑	❑	❑	❑	48.	❑	❑	❑	❑
16.	❑	❑	❑	❑	49.	❑	❑	❑	❑
17.	❑	❑	❑	❑	50.	❑	❑	❑	❑
18.	❑	❑	❑	❑	51.	❑	❑	❑	❑
19.	❑	❑	❑	❑	52.	❑	❑	❑	❑
20.	❑	❑	❑	❑	53.	❑	❑	❑	❑
21.	❑	❑	❑	❑	54.	❑	❑	❑	❑
22.	❑	❑	❑	❑	55.	❑	❑	❑	❑
23.	❑	❑	❑	❑	56.	❑	❑	❑	❑
24.	❑	❑	❑	❑	57.	❑	❑	❑	❑
25.	❑	❑	❑	❑	58.	❑	❑	❑	❑
26.	❑	❑	❑	❑	59.	❑	❑	❑	❑
27.	❑	❑	❑	❑	60.	❑	❑	❑	❑
28.	❑	❑	❑	❑	61.	❑	❑	❑	❑
29.	❑	❑	❑	❑	62.	❑	❑	❑	❑
30.	❑	❑	❑	❑	63.	❑	❑	❑	❑
31.	❑	❑	❑	❑	64.	❑	❑	❑	❑
32.	❑	❑	❑	❑	65.	❑	❑	❑	❑
33.	❑	❑	❑	❑	66.	❑	❑	❑	❑

Exam #8 Answer Form

	A	B	C	D			A	B	C	D
67.	❏	❏	❏	❏		97.	❏	❏	❏	❏
68.	❏	❏	❏	❏		98.	❏	❏	❏	❏
69.	❏	❏	❏	❏		99.	❏	❏	❏	❏
70.	❏	❏	❏	❏		100.	❏	❏	❏	❏
71.	❏	❏	❏	❏		101.	❏	❏	❏	❏
72.	❏	❏	❏	❏		102.	❏	❏	❏	❏
73.	❏	❏	❏	❏		103.	❏	❏	❏	❏
74.	❏	❏	❏	❏		104.	❏	❏	❏	❏
75.	❏	❏	❏	❏		105.	❏	❏	❏	❏
76.	❏	❏	❏	❏		106.	❏	❏	❏	❏
77.	❏	❏	❏	❏		107.	❏	❏	❏	❏
78.	❏	❏	❏	❏		108.	❏	❏	❏	❏
79.	❏	❏	❏	❏		109.	❏	❏	❏	❏
80.	❏	❏	❏	❏		110.	❏	❏	❏	❏
81.	❏	❏	❏	❏		111.	❏	❏	❏	❏
82.	❏	❏	❏	❏		112.	❏	❏	❏	❏
83.	❏	❏	❏	❏		113.	❏	❏	❏	❏
84.	❏	❏	❏	❏		114.	❏	❏	❏	❏
85.	❏	❏	❏	❏		115.	❏	❏	❏	❏
86.	❏	❏	❏	❏		116.	❏	❏	❏	❏
87.	❏	❏	❏	❏		117.	❏	❏	❏	❏
88.	❏	❏	❏	❏		118.	❏	❏	❏	❏
89.	❏	❏	❏	❏		119.	❏	❏	❏	❏
90.	❏	❏	❏	❏		120.	❏	❏	❏	❏
91.	❏	❏	❏	❏		121.	❏	❏	❏	❏
92.	❏	❏	❏	❏		122.	❏	❏	❏	❏
93.	❏	❏	❏	❏		123.	❏	❏	❏	❏
94.	❏	❏	❏	❏		124.	❏	❏	❏	❏
95.	❏	❏	❏	❏		125.	❏	❏	❏	❏
96.	❏	❏	❏	❏						

Life Span Development

1. The average weight of a newborn at birth is:
   a. 2.5–3.0 kg.
   b. 3.0–3.5 kg.
   c. 4.0–4.5 kg.
   d. 4.5–5.0 kg.

2. During the first week of life, a baby will lose _____ % of its body weight due to excretion of extracellular fluid present at birth.
   a. 2–5
   b. 5–10
   c. 10–15
   d. 15–20

3. The average weight of an infant is double its birth weight by what age?
   a. 1 year
   b. 3 months
   c. 4–6 months
   d. 9–12 months

4. When a newborn's cardiovascular system has made the shift from fetal circulation to normal infant circulation, which of the following has occurred?
   a. The foramen ovale has opened.
   b. The ductus venosus has opened.
   c. The ductus arteriosus has opened.
   d. The ductus arteriosus has closed.

5. Infants are primarily obligate nose breathers until what age?
   a. 4 weeks
   b. 3 months
   c. 6 weeks
   d. 6 months

6. Of the following statements about the infant's pulmonary system, which is true?
   a. Diaphragmatic breathing causes the airways to be more easily obstructed.
   b. Accessory muscles of respiration are prone to barotraumas.
   c. The alveoli are numerous with increased collateral ventilation.
   d. The ribs are positioned horizontally, causing diaphragmatic breathing.

7. At what age do the posterior fontanelles close on an infant?
   a. 3 months
   b. 6 months
   c. 12 months
   d. 18 months

8. At what age do the anterior fontanelles usually close on an infant?
   a. 3–6 months
   b. 6–9 months
   c. 9–18 months
   d. 2 years

9. Which of the following factors can lead to abnormally fast bone growth in an infant?
   a. poor general health
   b. abnormal sleep cycle
   c. abnormal thyroid hormone levels
   d. formula supplemented with calcium and iron

10. What is the average annual weight gain, in kilograms, for a toddler?
    a. 1
    b. 2
    c. 3
    d. 4

11. A 4-year-old boy puts on his father's golf shoes and attempts to take a few practice swings with one of his father's golf clubs. In psychological terms, what type of behavior is the child displaying?
    a. magical thinking
    b. modeling
    c. separation anxiety
    d. sibling rivalry

12. In which age group do children primarily develop self-esteem?
    a. toddler
    b. preschool
    c. school age
    d. adolescence

13. When a young teenage male experiences a change in voice quality, this is an example of a typical stage of:
    a. primary sexual development.
    b. secondary sexual development.
    c. a growth spurt.
    d. menarche.

14. Which of the following statements is true about endocrine system changes that take place during adolescence?
    a. Gonadotropins released by the pituitary gland promote the production of testosterone.
    b. Interstitial cell-stimulating hormone causes acne.
    c. Muscle mass increases from the release of lutenizing hormone.
    d. Body fat decreases from the release of follicle-stimulating hormone.

15. Changes that occur during late adulthood within the respiratory system that lead to decreased respiratory function include a(n):
    a. decrease in elasticity of the diaphragm.
    b. increase in chest wall compliance.
    c. decrease in alveolar pressures.
    d. increase in pulmonic vascular strength.

16. The elderly often have an ineffective cough reflex caused by:
    a. exposure to cigarette smoke.
    b. weakening of the chest wall.
    c. lower production of cortisol.
    d. atrophy of the pituitary gland.

17. A major change in the endocrine system function during late adulthood is a(n):
    a. increase in insulin production.
    b. decrease in insulin production.
    c. increase in thyroid hormone production.
    d. decrease in red blood cell (RBC) production.

18. Older adults are often prescribed medications in lower doses than younger adults because of changes in metabolism caused by:
    a. increased acid reflux.
    b. increased GI obstruction.
    c. vitamin deficiencies.
    d. changes in renal function.

19. You are transferring an elderly nursing home resident to the hospital for an injury from a fall. The patient is lying in bed, conscious, and complaining of pain in her right wrist. The wrist is swollen and bruised. As you transfer the patient to the stretcher, you see that she is wearing an adult diaper. One of the primary reasons elderly adults lose control of their bowels is that:
    a. they are prone to fluid retention.
    b. they are prone to urinary tract infections.
    c. their muscular sphincters become less effective with age.
    d. they are unable to digest food as effectively as younger patients.

20. Which of the following statements about adolescent growth spurts is most accurate?
    a. More boys than girls experience growth spurts.
    b. Growth spurts begin with enlargement of the chest and trunk.
    c. Growth spurts begin with enlargement of the feet and hands.
    d. Most boys are finished growing before most girls.

21. In which age group are the kidneys unable to concentrate urine?
    a. infancy
    b. toddler
    c. adolescence
    d. late adulthood

22. Many aging adults are at risk of developing problems with their joints due to a condition called:
    a. hemophilia.
    b. osteoarthritis.
    c. osteomyelitis.
    d. Addison's disease.

23. At birth, the infant immune system is relatively undeveloped. Antibodies transferred from the mother help the child maintain passive immunity through what age?
    a. 6 months
    b. 1 year
    c. 18 months
    d. 2 years

24. A heart rate of less than _____ bpm in a newborn is abnormal.
    a. 140
    b. 120
    c. 110
    d. 100

25. You have just assisted in the delivery of a newborn, and the respiratory rate after 1 minute is 20. This is considered a(n) _____ finding.
    a. normal
    b. abnormal
    c. critical
    d. insignificant

26. You are assessing an infant that is 11 months old. You do not know the child's exact weight, but you can estimate that the child's weight is _____ its birth weight.
    a. double
    b. triple
    c. quadruple
    d. five times

27. Baby teeth begin to erupt at _____ months.
    a. 1–3
    b. 5–7
    c. 12–18
    d. 18–24

28. The amount of time remaining in a person's life before he is expected to die is referred to as the life:
    a. span.
    b. profile.
    c. expansion.
    d. expectancy.

29. What is the leading cause of death among early adults?
    a. cancer
    b. accidents
    c. ACS
    d. suicide

30. In what age group does cardiovascular disease become a major concern?
    a. adolescent
    b. early adulthood
    c. middle adulthood
    d. late adulthood

31. Aging adults tend to experience memory problems as a result of:
    a. inadequate compensatory mechanisms.
    b. increased peripheral vascular resistance.
    c. an increase in falls leading to brain injuries.
    d. a decrease in the number of neurons in the brain.

32. _____ is the total duration of one life, from birth to death.
    a. Life expectancy
    b. Life profile
    c. Development
    d. Life span

33. With the effects of aging, the baroreceptors within blood vessels lose their sensitivity. As a result, late adults are more sensitive to _____ changes.
    a. climate
    b. orthostatic
    c. elevation
    d. nutritional

34. It is not uncommon for a blood pressure reading to be falsely high in late adults because of the effects of:
    a. arteriosclerosis.
    b. postural hypotension.
    c. orthostatic changes.
    d. gravity.

35. As the heart ages, the myocardium is less able to respond to exercise because the muscle is:
    a. dehydrated.
    b. hypertrophied.
    c. less elastic.
    d. more elastic.

36. Degeneration of the cardiac conduction system may lead to a combination of brady- and tachydysrhythmias, often called "tachy–brady" syndrome or _____ syndrome.
    a. Wolff–Parkinson–White
    b. sick sinus
    c. Wilson–Mikity
    d. witzelsucht

37. With aging, there is a decreased functional blood volume and a decrease in the levels of RBCs caused by:
    a. polypharmacy.
    b. poor nutrition and malabsorption.
    c. dehydration.
    d. hypothyroidism.

38. _____ is a common problem in the elderly population because of dehydration, lack of exercise, and lower-fiber diets.
   a. Cancer
   b. Diarrhea
   c. Constipation
   d. GI bleeding

39. Which of the following statements is true about the changes in the respiratory system in late adulthood?
   a. There is an increase in generalized lung capacity.
   b. There is a decrease in upper respiratory infections.
   c. There is an increase in normal mucous membrane linings.
   d. There is a loss in normal mucous membrane linings.

40. As a person ages, atherosclerosis increases the narrowing of the lumen of large vessels putting them at risk for:
   a. aneurysms.
   b. significant weight gain.
   c. developing atrial fibrillation.
   d. developing hypothermia.

41. Normal changes in the nervous system during late adulthood result in disturbances of the:
   a. sleep–wake cycle.
   b. myelin sheath.
   c. psychosomatic process.
   d. leukapheresis cycle.

42. You are transporting an elderly female to the hospital for a local infection that is in need of immediate care. The patient is alert and, during the ride, your conversation turns to a discussion about the patient's height. She tells you that she is several inches shorter than she was as a young adult. What is one of the primary reasons for the change in height that comes with aging?
   a. perpetual hypocalcemia
   b. trauma injury to the spine
   c. osteoporosis of the spine
   d. loss of neurons and neurotransmitters

43. In which age group does the body reach peak physical conditioning?
   a. school age
   b. adolescence
   c. early adulthood
   d. middle adulthood

44. Normal behavioral "milestones," such as the development of self-concept, self-esteem, and morals typically occur in which age group?
   a. preschool
   b. school age
   c. adolescence
   d. early adulthood

45. At what age does the hearing sense reach peak (maturity) levels?
   a. 1–2 years
   b. 3–4 years
   c. 5–6 years
   d. 7–8 years

46. Which one of the four parenting styles described by psychologists is characterized by the parent(s) showing tolerance toward the child's impulses and using a minimal amount of punishment, while making few demands on the child to act maturely?
   a. authoritarian
   b. authoritative
   c. permissive–indulgent
   d. permissive–indifferent

47. Which of the following is true of young adolescent development?
   a. Growth spurts usually will occur in boys first.
   b. Growth in the torso typically occurs first.
   c. Growth in the limbs typically occurs first.
   d. In girls, menstruation typically precedes the onset of the growth spurt.

48. _____ is a term for normal hearing loss caused by aging.
   a. Tympanitis
   b. Osteomyelitis
   c. Kinesthesia
   d. Presbycusis

49. The late adult is less equipped to handle bodily stresses such as severe infection because of:
   a. an increase in thyroid hormone production.
   b. an increase in insulin production.
   c. a decrease in cortisol production.
   d. a decrease in financial status.

50. Changes in myocardium in a late adult include:
   a. loss of normal cardiac pacemaker cells.
   b. enhanced automaticity.
   c. increased syncytium.
   d. decreased syncytium.

Exam #9 Answer Form

	A	B	C	D			A	B	C	D
1.	❏	❏	❏	❏		26.	❏	❏	❏	❏
2.	❏	❏	❏	❏		27.	❏	❏	❏	❏
3.	❏	❏	❏	❏		28.	❏	❏	❏	❏
4.	❏	❏	❏	❏		29.	❏	❏	❏	❏
5.	❏	❏	❏	❏		30.	❏	❏	❏	❏
6.	❏	❏	❏	❏		31.	❏	❏	❏	❏
7.	❏	❏	❏	❏		32.	❏	❏	❏	❏
8.	❏	❏	❏	❏		33.	❏	❏	❏	❏
9.	❏	❏	❏	❏		34.	❏	❏	❏	❏
10.	❏	❏	❏	❏		35.	❏	❏	❏	❏
11.	❏	❏	❏	❏		36.	❏	❏	❏	❏
12.	❏	❏	❏	❏		37.	❏	❏	❏	❏
13.	❏	❏	❏	❏		38.	❏	❏	❏	❏
14.	❏	❏	❏	❏		39.	❏	❏	❏	❏
15.	❏	❏	❏	❏		40.	❏	❏	❏	❏
16.	❏	❏	❏	❏		41.	❏	❏	❏	❏
17.	❏	❏	❏	❏		42.	❏	❏	❏	❏
18.	❏	❏	❏	❏		43.	❏	❏	❏	❏
19.	❏	❏	❏	❏		44.	❏	❏	❏	❏
20.	❏	❏	❏	❏		45.	❏	❏	❏	❏
21.	❏	❏	❏	❏		46.	❏	❏	❏	❏
22.	❏	❏	❏	❏		47.	❏	❏	❏	❏
23.	❏	❏	❏	❏		48.	❏	❏	❏	❏
24.	❏	❏	❏	❏		49.	❏	❏	❏	❏
25.	❏	❏	❏	❏		50.	❏	❏	❏	❏

CHAPTER

10

Principles of Pharmacology and Medication Administration

1. Any chemical substance that, when taken into a living organism, produces a biologic response affecting one or more of that organism's processes or functions is a:
   a. solution.
   b. drug.
   c. antigen.
   d. antibody.

2. The term for the study of how a drug is altered as it travels through the body is:
   a. pharmacokinetics.
   b. pharmacodynamics.
   c. pharmaceutics.
   d. antagonism.

3. The study of how and why a drug works, specifically its biochemical and physiologic effects, is called:
   a. pharmacodynamics.
   b. pharmaceutics.
   c. pharmacokinetics.
   d. pharmacopoeia.

4. The chemical breakdown of a drug while in the body is called:
   a. absorption.
   b. distribution.
   c. elimination.
   d. biotransformation.

5. The general properties of a drug include all of the following, *except*:
   a. therapeutic.
   b. prophylactic.
   c. diagnostic.
   d. research.

6. Drug-induced physiologic changes in a body function or process are known as a(n):
   a. drug action.
   b. side effect.
   c. half-life.
   d. idiosyncrasy.

7. A drug that stimulates a receptor is called a(n):
   a. agonist.
   b. antagonist.
   c. sympatholytic.
   d. sympathomimetic.

8. The major mechanism by which a drug affects the body is by joining with receptors located on the:
   a. red blood cells.
   b. target organs or tissues.
   c. white blood cells.
   d. mast cells.

9. A drug that mimics the functions of the sympathetic nervous system is called a(n):
   a. agonist.
   b. antagonist.
   c. sympatholytic.
   d. sympathomimetic.

10. An example of an emergency-use drug that is also a sympathetic nervous system neurotransmitter is:
    a. dopamine.
    b. amiodarone.
    c. dobutamine.
    d. procainamide.

11. ACLS drugs, such as epinephrine, dopamine, and dobutamine, belong to a group of drugs called:
    a. fibrins.
    b. ionospheres.
    c. sympatholytics.
    d. sympathomimetics.

12. Antiadrenergic drugs that block the function of the sympathetic nervous system are called:
    a. fibrins.
    b. ionospheres.
    c. sympatholytics.
    d. sympathomimetics.

13. Cholinergic receptors respond to the neurotransmitter:
    a. acetylcholine.
    b. epinephrine.
    c. norepinephrine.
    d. nortriptyline.

14. Drugs that block cholinergic receptors and parasympathetic response are called parasympatholytics. In the prehospital setting, the most commonly used parasympatholytic is:
    a. metoprolol.
    b. atenolol.
    c. dobutamine.
    d. atropine.

15. For a drug to get inside a cell or body part, the two primary means of transportation are active and passive transport. The difference between the two is that active transport requires:
    a. energy produced through a chemical reaction.
    b. a change in homeostasis.
    c. the formation of genetic repressors.
    d. energy to produce and displace phosphatide.

16. When repeated doses of a drug lead to toxicity in a patient, this condition is known as a:
    a. side effect.
    b. habituation.
    c. hypersensitivity.
    d. cumulative effect.

17. When a patient takes a medication and has an unexpected response that most patients would *not* have, this is called a(n):
    a. idiosyncrasy.
    b. side effect.
    c. toxicity.
    d. cumulative effect.

18. A physiologic blockade that protects the brain from exposure to various drugs is called:
    a. cerebral spinal fluid.
    b. blood-brain barrier.
    c. meninges.
    d. collateral barrier.

19. The name of a drug that is assigned by the U.S. Adopted Name Council is the _____ name.
    a. official
    b. generic
    c. trade
    d. brand

20. Angiotensin-converting enzyme (ACE) inhibitors work primarily by inhibiting:
    a. renin from releasing sodium.
    b. angiotensin I from converting angiotensin II.
    c. sodium and water retention.
    d. acetylcholine.

21. Chemical assay is a test that determines a drug's:
    a. ingredients.
    b. reliability.
    c. half-life.
    d. mechanism of injury.

22. The Pure Food and Drug Act of 1906 required drug manufacturers to:
    a. test a drug for effectiveness.
    b. test a drug for safety.
    c. label all ingredients.
    d. label all dangerous ingredients in drug products.

23. The Federal Drug Administration (FDA) is responsible for all of the following, *except*:
    a. testing of drugs.
    b. marketing of drugs.
    c. availability of drugs.
    d. drug enforcement.

24. Most pediatric medication doses are administered according to body weight because:
    a. children metabolize drugs faster than adults.
    b. the total body weight affects the distribution of the drug.
    c. children require more medication than adults because of immature liver function.
    d. children require more medication than adults because of immature kidney function.

25. A drug's ability to join with a receptor is known as:
    a. affinity.
    b. ability.
    c. selective response.
    d. agonist.

26. A drug that joins partially with a receptor and prevents a reaction is called a(n):
    a. partial antagonist.
    b. partial agonist.
    c. agonist.
    d. antagonist.

27. The two types of sympathetic receptors in the body are:
    a. dopaminergic and adrenergic.
    b. adrenergic and cholinergic.
    c. iatrogenic and dopaminergic.
    d. cholinergic and inhibitory.

28. Diffusion, filtration, and osmosis are all means of:
    a. drug actions.
    b. precipitation.
    c. active transport.
    d. passive transport.

29. The pressure that develops when two solutions of different concentrations are separated by a semipermeable membrane is called _____ pressure.
    a. osmotic
    b. hydrostatic
    c. hypertonic
    d. hypotonic

30. The term for the combined effect of drugs taken at the same time altering the expected therapeutic effect of each is known as:
    a. systemic action.
    b. therapeutic antagonism.
    c. drug interaction.
    d. mechanism of action.

31. When two drugs are used together to produce a desired effect that is much better than what only one drug alone could produce, this is referred to as what type of synergism?
    a. additive effect
    b. potentiation
    c. competitive effect
    d. physiologic effect

32. You are interviewing a patient and find that the patient has been taking barbiturates regularly. Today he has also been drinking alcohol. What type of synergistic effect would you expect to find in this patient?
    a. additive
    b. potentiation
    c. competitive
    d. therapeutic

33. A patient who has ingested poison was given activated charcoal. The charcoal will bind and absorb toxins present in the GI tract to inactivate and then excrete them. This chemical process is known as:
    a. loading dose.
    b. tolerance.
    c. hypersensitivity.
    d. antagonism.

34. A paramedic is about to administer adenosine to a patient experiencing SVT. The paramedic chooses a large venous access and will administer this medication in a *rapid* IV push, followed by a rapid flush, to achieve the correct therapeutic effect. Which of the following terms best refers to the specific reason for this therapeutic effect?
    a. idiosyncrasy
    b. adverse reaction
    c. half-life
    d. side effect

35. The Harrison Narcotic Act of 1914 was the first act passed by a nation that:
    a. controlled the sale of narcotics and drugs that cause dependence.
    b. required drug manufacturers to label certain dangerous ingredients on the packages.
    c. empowered the government to enforce safety standards on the production of narcotics.
    d. required proof of both safety and efficacy before a new narcotic could be approved for use.

36. Controlled substances are divided into five schedules depending on their potential for abuse. Which of the following schedules would a cough preparation containing an opioid be listed in?
    a. I
    b. II
    c. IV
    d. V

37. Before a new drug is approved by the FDA for use, the drug has to complete _____ phases to ensure its safety and efficacy.
    a. three
    b. four
    c. six
    d. eight

38. Defects in drug products can result in lawsuits. For drug product liability to exist, which of the following criteria must be met?
   a. The defect occurred after it left the manufacturer.
   b. The defect occurred before it left the manufacturer.
   c. The product was not used for its intended purpose.
   d. The defect was reported by a health-care professional.

39. Drugs are classified by their chemical class, mechanism of action, or:
   a. potency.
   b. therapeutic effect.
   c. solid or liquid form.
   d. potential for abuse.

40. Drugs that are administered in higher doses often have:
   a. the tendency to delay hepatic metabolism.
   b. a slower absorption rate than lower doses.
   c. a quicker absorption rate than lower doses.
   d. the same absorption rate as lower doses.

41. What is the difference between a loading dose and a maintenance dose of a drug?
   a. A loading dose is typically a single dose of a drug.
   b. A loading dose is typically administered by IV drip.
   c. A maintenance dose will never lose its half-life.
   d. A maintenance dose is only administered by IV drip.

42. You are assessing a patient with an altered mental status (AMS), and you find that the patient takes Lasix, potassium, and Colace. The potassium bottle is old and empty. Based only on the medications of the patient, what might be the cause of the patient's AMS?
   a. dehydration
   b. hypertension
   c. diabetes
   d. thyroid

43. A 66-year-old female patient is experiencing severe side effects (slow heart rate and low blood pressure) from a new medication. Her past medical history (PMH) includes stroke, COPD, kidney failure, and diverticulitis. Based on her PMH, which of the following is the probable cause of the side effects?
   a. decreased pulmonary function
   b. decreased renal function
   c. neurologic dysfunction
   d. decreased GI motility

44. A drug reference, and the only official book of drug standards in the United States that only lists drugs that have met high standards of quality, purity, and strength, is the:
   a. Physician's Desk Reference (PDR).
   b. U.S. Pharmacopoeia.
   c. Hospital Formulary (HF).
   d. FDA's Drug Reference.

45. Because the stomach has a pH of approximately 1.4 and the small intestine a pH of 5.3, a drug's chemical acidity will determine where it is absorbed. Which drugs will be better absorbed in the stomach than in the intestine?
   a. All drugs are absorbed in the intestine.
   b. Drugs that are neutral.
   c. Drugs with a weak base.
   d. Drugs with weak acidity.

46. IM drug administration should be avoided in the patient suspected of having an ACS because:
   a. the pain of injection may worsen the MI.
   b. it may elevate diagnostic enzyme levels.
   c. the drug will not be absorbed fast enough to be of benefit.
   d. total drug volumes are too large for cardiac patients.

47. You are administering an aerosolized medication to a patient for an asthma attack. How can you avoid inhaling the medication yourself?
   a. Have the patient take deep breaths and hold them.
   b. Wear a face mask.
   c. Ask the patient to exhale in a direction away from you.
   d. Plug the end of the nebulizer oxygen tubing.

48. Drugs are metabolized in the body by various organs and tissues. Which of the following is not involved in this process?
   a. liver
   b. lungs
   c. heart muscle
   d. intestinal mucosa

49. The adverse mental or physical condition affecting a patient through the outcome of treatment by a practitioner is called:
   a. iatrogenic.
   b. assay.
   c. disregard.
   d. identity crises.

50. The method for making sure a drug dosage and reliability are accurate is called:
    a. standardization.
    b. classification.
    c. cataloging.
    d. bioassay.

51. You are working the v-fib algorithm on a patient in cardiac arrest; you have intubated, started an IV, given shocks, and administered 1-mg epinephrine, and now you call medical control for further direction. Up to this point, all the skills you have performed have been done as:
    a. direct orders of medical control.
    b. indirect orders of medical control.
    c. quality management.
    d. quality improvement.

52. The "six rights of medication administration" are used by health-care providers in an effort to:
    a. avoid making medication administration errors.
    b. gain patient consent for emergency treatment.
    c. assure that the patient is informed of his rights.
    d. remember when to document a PCR.

53. A chemical product designed for topical application to kill bacteria is a(n):
    a. antimicrobial.
    b. antibiotic.
    c. antiseptic.
    d. disinfectant.

54. A chemical or physical agent approved by the Environmental Protection Agency (EPA) to prevent infection by killing bacteria is a(n):
    a. antimicrobial.
    b. antibiotic.
    c. antiseptic.
    d. disinfectant.

55. Which of the following is an example of a sharp?
    a. an open vial
    b. an open ampule
    c. a used angiocatheter
    d. a three-way stop cock

56. Which of the following is the most common complication associated with drawing blood samples?
    a. local infection
    b. systemic infection
    c. nerve or muscle damage
    d. miscannulation of an artery instead of a vein

57. You are looking at a patient's prescription medication bottle and the dose reads 40 mg b.i.d. How often should the medication be taken?
    a. once a day
    b. four times a day
    c. twice a day
    d. twice a night

58. Which of the following routes of drug administration injects the medication under the dermis into connective tissue or fat?
    a. enteral
    b. epidural
    c. subcutaneous
    d. intramuscular

59. The three systems of measure used for drug administration include the metric system, the apothecary system, and the _____ method.
    a. household
    b. English
    c. Mayan
    d. Egyptian

60. In the metric system of measure, the basic unit of mass (weight) is the:
    a. kilo.
    b. ounce.
    c. gram.
    d. pound.

61. You are adjusting your drip rate to run approximately one drop every 2 seconds. This is the standard rate used when an IV is kept in place for purposes other than replacing fluids and is often referred to as:
    a. KVO.
    b. TKO.
    c. either KVO or TKO.
    d. neither KVO or TKO.

62. One of the primary advantages of giving drugs by parenteral route in emergencies is that:
    a. it is most convenient.
    b. it is the most economical.
    c. IV access is always available.
    d. absorption effects are more predictable.

63. When a drug is administered to be dissolved between the cheek and gum, what type of route is this?
    a. buccal
    b. ingestion
    c. sublingual
    d. intra-atricular

64. When diazepam is administered per rectum, by what route of administration has this drug been given?
    a. enteral
    b. parenteral
    c. transdermal
    d. subcutaneous

65. The injection of a drug into the spinal canal on or outside the dura mater that surrounds the spinal column is called a(n):
    a. subdural.
    b. epidural.
    c. intrapleural.
    d. intravenous.

66. Convert 3,500 mg to grams.
    a. 0.35 grams
    b. 3.5 grams
    c. 35 grams
    d. 350 grams

67. Convert 1,200 mcg to grams.
    a. 0.0012 grams
    b. 0.012 grams
    c. 0.12 grams
    d. 1.2 grams

68. Convert 2.5 liters to milliliters.
    a. 2.5 ml
    b. 25 ml
    c. 250 ml
    d. 2,500 ml

69. Convert a patient's weight of 198 pounds to kilograms.
    a. 86 kg
    b. 92 kg
    c. 90 kg
    d. 99 kg

70. Convert 66 kilograms to pounds.
    a. 140 lb
    b. 142 lb
    c. 145 lb
    d. 146 lb

71. You need to administer 1.5 mg/kg of lidocaine to your patient who weighs 176 pounds. The drug comes packaged as 100 mg in 10 ml. How much lidocaine do you need to administer?
    a. 265 mg
    b. 120 mg
    c. 100 mg
    d. 80 mg

72. In reference to question 71, how many milliliters of the lidocaine will you need to administer to deliver 1.5 mg/kg?
    a. 20.65
    b. 12
    c. 10
    d. 4

73. Medical control gives you an order to administer a 300-ml bolus over 30 minutes using a 10-gtt drip set. How many drops per minute will it take to infuse the bolus?
    a. 10 gtt/min
    b. 100 gtt/min
    c. 30 gtt/min
    d. 300 gtt/min

74. You are to administer D-50 to an unresponsive diabetic patient. The D-50 comes in a 50-ml (preload) syringe, and you will administer all of it. How many grams of dextrose will you administer?
    a. 5
    b. 25
    c. 50
    d. 500

75. Medical control advises you to administer D-25 to a diabetic pediatric patient. The only dextrose you have on hand is D-50. What do you need to do to administer the proper concentration?
    a. Hang a drip of D-50.
    b. Infuse half the dose of D-50 without diluting.
    c. Dilute the D-50 by one-half, then administer.
    d. Tell medical control you cannot help the patient.

76. Following a bolus of lidocaine, you now need to set up an IV drip of 3 mg per minute. You have 200 mg of lidocaine, a 50-ml bag of normal saline, and a 60-gtt drip set. How many drops (gtts) per minute will you need to run to administer a 3 mg/min drip?
    a. 15 gtts
    b. 30 gtts
    c. 45 gtts
    d. 60 gtts

77. You are given an order to administer 5 mg of morphine sulfate to a patient. You have on hand two vials, each containing 4 mg in 2 ml. How many ml of the drug will you have remaining after administering the correct dose?
    a. 0.5 ml
    b. 1 ml
    c. 1.5 ml
    d. 2 ml

78. Convert a temperature of 98.6° Fahrenheit to Celsius and select the correct answer.
   a. 37°
   b. 39.5°
   c. 40.2°
   d. 41.6°

79. A drug package that is a small glass container with a rubber stopper by which the drug is withdrawn by a needle and syringe is a(n):
   a. ampule.
   b. vial.
   c. preloaded cartridge.
   d. small volume nebulizer.

80. Which of the following medications is administered enterally in the prehospital setting?
   a. epinephrine
   b. nitro paste
   c. nitro spray
   d. aspirin

81. Which of the following is least accurate about medication administration by (PO) oral route?
   a. The absorption rate is fast.
   b. The absorption rate is slow.
   c. NPO in the field is common due to nausea and vomiting.
   d. PO medications are easy to take.

82. Which of the following is true about medication administration by (PR) rectal route?
   a. PR is the preferred route for pediatric medications.
   b. PR is the preferred route for seizure patients.
   c. PR allows for rapid absorption.
   d. The absorption rate is unpredictable.

83. When reviewing your paperwork, you realize you made an error while charting a medication administration dose. The proper way to correct this error is to:
   a. erase the error and rewrite the correct dose.
   b. use a single line to mark out the error, make the change, and initial it.
   c. write over the error to fix it.
   d. never change or correct medications errors.

84. When using a blood pressure cuff as a tourniquet to start an IV, the cuff is inflated to occlude venous blood flow, but not arterial flow. What is the appropriate range of inflation for this procedure?
   a. 140–160 mmHg
   b. 120–130 mmHg
   c. 90–110 mmHg
   d. 70–80 mmHg

85. You have administered 25 mg of Benadryl® IVP to a patient experiencing an allergic reaction to a bee sting. Suddenly the patient becomes hypotensive. The hypotension is probably a result of:
   a. an incorrect dose of Benadryl®.
   b. a reaction from the bee sting.
   c. the incorrect route of medication administration.
   d. a potentiation effect of the medication.

86. Which of the following metric units is the largest prefix?
   a. kilo
   b. micro
   c. centi
   d. milli

87. Medical control has given you an order to administer an amiodarone drip. The order is for 150 mg of amiodarone into a 50-ml bag, to be run in over 10 minutes with a macro 10-gtt drip set. How many drops per minute will you need to run?
   a. 15 gtt/min
   b. 45 gtt/min
   c. 50 gtt/min
   d. 150 gtt/min

88. You have a patient in severe bronchospasm, and medical control has given you an order for a magnesium sulfate drip. The order is 2 grams into 50 ml over 20 minutes with a macro 10-gtt drip set. How many drops per minute will you need?
   a. 4 gtt/min
   b. 25 gtt/min
   c. 40 gtt/min
   d. 250 gtt/min

89. You have a 500-ml bag of IV D5W. How many grams of dextrose (sugar) are in this bag?
   a. 5
   b. 20
   c. 25
   d. 50

90. Medical control gives you an order to run a dopamine drip at 5 mcg/kg/min. The patient weighs 100 kg and you have a concentration of 1,600 mcg/ml mixed in a 250-ml bag with a micro drip set. How many drips per minute do you run?
   a. 19
   b. 30
   c. 45
   d. 63

91. Medical control gives you the order to administer 0.02 mg/kg of atropine to a child who weighs 12 pounds. The minimum loading dose of atropine is 0.1 mg. What is the correct dose for this child?
   a. 0.1 mg
   b. 0.15 mg
   c. 1.0 mg
   d. 1.5 mg

92. You are running a micro drip at one drop every 2 seconds. How many minutes will it take for a 50-ml bag of normal saline to run out completely?
   a. 25
   b. 30
   c. 50
   d. 100

93. You are running a 1-liter bag of normal saline through a 10-gtt administration set at 60 gtt/min. During a 20-minute transport time to the hospital, how much fluid will be infused?
   a. 10 ml
   b. 20 ml
   c. 60 ml
   d. 120 ml

94. You are going to administer 0.25 mg/kg of diltiazem over 2 minutes to a patient with an uncontrolled atrial fibrillation. The patient weighs 200 pounds, and the package of medication has 25 mg in 5 ml. How many milligrams will you administer?
   a. 4 mg
   b. 8 mg
   c. 16 mg
   d. 23 mg

95. In reference to question 44, what is the smallest size of syringe you can use to administer the entire dose in one injection?
   a. 1 cc
   b. 5 cc
   c. 20 cc
   d. 30 cc

96. You are going to administer 150 mg of lidocaine over 10 minutes. How many mg per minute will you infuse?
   a. 10
   b. 15
   c. 1.0
   d. 1.5

97. A male patient is bleeding from a traumatic injury and has lost 3.5 pints of blood. If his total blood volume is 6 quarts, what percent of his blood volume has he lost?
   a. 10
   b. 20
   c. 25
   d. 30

98. You have started an IV with a macro drip set at 10 gtt/ml. Medical control tells you to give 1-liter bag at a rate of 250 ml/hr. How many drops per minute will you need to infuse?
   a. 4 gtt/min
   b. 10 gtt/min
   c. 33 gtt/min
   d. 42 gtt/min

99. You are administering oxygen via a non-rebreather mask to a patient at 12 lpm. The tank contained 350 liters of oxygen when you began. How many minutes can you continue at the current rate before running completely out of oxygen?
   a. 25
   b. 29
   c. 33
   d. 39

100. You are going to give a subcutaneous injection to a patient. Which of the following needles would be the most appropriate for this administration?
   a. 19-ga and 1.5-inch needle
   b. 23-ga and 0.5-inch needle
   c. 18-ga angio
   d. 20-ga biopsy needle

Exam #10 Answer Form

	A	B	C	D			A	B	C	D
1.	❏	❏	❏	❏		31.	❏	❏	❏	❏
2.	❏	❏	❏	❏		32.	❏	❏	❏	❏
3.	❏	❏	❏	❏		33.	❏	❏	❏	❏
4.	❏	❏	❏	❏		34.	❏	❏	❏	❏
5.	❏	❏	❏	❏		35.	❏	❏	❏	❏
6.	❏	❏	❏	❏		36.	❏	❏	❏	❏
7.	❏	❏	❏	❏		37.	❏	❏	❏	❏
8.	❏	❏	❏	❏		38.	❏	❏	❏	❏
9.	❏	❏	❏	❏		39.	❏	❏	❏	❏
10.	❏	❏	❏	❏		40.	❏	❏	❏	❏
11.	❏	❏	❏	❏		41.	❏	❏	❏	❏
12.	❏	❏	❏	❏		42.	❏	❏	❏	❏
13.	❏	❏	❏	❏		43.	❏	❏	❏	❏
14.	❏	❏	❏	❏		44.	❏	❏	❏	❏
15.	❏	❏	❏	❏		45.	❏	❏	❏	❏
16.	❏	❏	❏	❏		46.	❏	❏	❏	❏
17.	❏	❏	❏	❏		47.	❏	❏	❏	❏
18.	❏	❏	❏	❏		48.	❏	❏	❏	❏
19.	❏	❏	❏	❏		49.	❏	❏	❏	❏
20.	❏	❏	❏	❏		50.	❏	❏	❏	❏
21.	❏	❏	❏	❏		51.	❏	❏	❏	❏
22.	❏	❏	❏	❏		52.	❏	❏	❏	❏
23.	❏	❏	❏	❏		53.	❏	❏	❏	❏
24.	❏	❏	❏	❏		54.	❏	❏	❏	❏
25.	❏	❏	❏	❏		55.	❏	❏	❏	❏
26.	❏	❏	❏	❏		56.	❏	❏	❏	❏
27.	❏	❏	❏	❏		57.	❏	❏	❏	❏
28.	❏	❏	❏	❏		58.	❏	❏	❏	❏
29.	❏	❏	❏	❏		59.	❏	❏	❏	❏
30.	❏	❏	❏	❏		60.	❏	❏	❏	❏

Exam #10 Answer Form

	A	B	C	D		A	B	C	D
61.	❏	❏	❏	❏	81.	❏	❏	❏	❏
62.	❏	❏	❏	❏	82.	❏	❏	❏	❏
63.	❏	❏	❏	❏	83.	❏	❏	❏	❏
64.	❏	❏	❏	❏	84.	❏	❏	❏	❏
65.	❏	❏	❏	❏	85.	❏	❏	❏	❏
66.	❏	❏	❏	❏	86.	❏	❏	❏	❏
67.	❏	❏	❏	❏	87.	❏	❏	❏	❏
68.	❏	❏	❏	❏	88.	❏	❏	❏	❏
69.	❏	❏	❏	❏	89.	❏	❏	❏	❏
70.	❏	❏	❏	❏	90.	❏	❏	❏	❏
71.	❏	❏	❏	❏	91.	❏	❏	❏	❏
72.	❏	❏	❏	❏	92.	❏	❏	❏	❏
73.	❏	❏	❏	❏	93.	❏	❏	❏	❏
74.	❏	❏	❏	❏	94.	❏	❏	❏	❏
75.	❏	❏	❏	❏	95.	❏	❏	❏	❏
76.	❏	❏	❏	❏	96.	❏	❏	❏	❏
77.	❏	❏	❏	❏	97.	❏	❏	❏	❏
78.	❏	❏	❏	❏	98.	❏	❏	❏	❏
79.	❏	❏	❏	❏	99.	❏	❏	❏	❏
80.	❏	❏	❏	❏	100.	❏	❏	❏	❏

CHAPTER

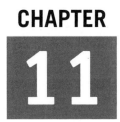

11

Emergency Medications

1. You are assessing a conscious and alert 22-year-old male who has ingested a large quantity of a noncorrosive but toxic liquid. He is approximately 220 lbs. Which of the following medications will you consider in your treatment plan?
   a. Zofran, 25 mg
   b. Haldol, 5 mg
   c. Activated Charcoal, 200 grams
   d. Phenergan, 50 mg

2. You are treating a 70-year-old male patient who has PSVT with heart palpitations and dizziness. Which medication would be most appropriate to administer this patient in an IV bolus?
   a. Lidocaine, 100 mg
   b. Adenosine, 6 mg
   c. Diphenhydramine, 25 mg
   d. Lopressor, 5 mg

3. You are treating a 33-year-old female who is complaining of breathing difficulty and would benefit from a drug that is a smooth-muscle relaxer in the bronchial tree as well as the peripheral vasculature. What medicine would be best to administer?
   a. Amiodarone, 300 mg
   b. Atropine Sulfate, 0.5 mg
   c. Albuterol, 2.5 mg
   d. Furosemide, 0.5–1 mg/kg

4. You are treating a 59-year-old male who was found in cardiac arrest. High-quality CPR has been provided and his ECG was initially ventricular fibrillation. After two shocks, separated by 2 minutes of CPR, the patient is again pulseless in VF. Aside from chest compressions and preparing to shock, which antidysrhythmic medication would be appropriate for this patient?
   a. Lidocaine, 200 mg
   b. Magnesium Sulfate, 2 grams
   c. Vasopressin, 40 units
   d. Amiodarone, 300 mg

5. Your 55-year-old male patient is complaining of substernal chest pain for the past 20 minutes since an argument he had with his spouse. He states he has a cardiac history and has experienced this pain before. He denies any allergies and has not taken any medication as yet. Aside from oxygen, what medication from the list below should you consider administering right away?
   a. Atenolol, 5 mg
   b. Aspirin, 160 to 325 mg (chewed)
   c. Diazepam, 5 mg
   d. Nitropaste, 1 inch

6. Of the following medications, which would be inappropriate to administer to the 65-year-old female patient with a stable tachydysrhythmia?
   a. Oxygen, 12 L per minute
   b. Diazepam, 5 mg
   c. Diphenhydramine, 25 mg
   d. Atropine Sulfate, 0.5 mg

7. What side effect does each of the drugs Dexamethasone, Aspirin, and Clopidogrel have in common?
   a. They all cause hypotension.
   b. They can cause GI bleeding.
   c. The all cause fluid retension.
   d. They will each speed up the heart.

8. You are treating a 26-year-old male patient who just had his third seizure without regaining consciousness. Of the following medications, which would be the most appropriate to treat him with?
   a. Diltiazem, 0.25 mg/kg
   b. Diphenhydramine, 50 mg
   c. Diazepam, 5 to 10 mg
   d. Etomidate, 0.2 to 0.6 mg/kg

9. A calcium channel blocker that is often administered to patients to control rapid ventricular rate due to atrial dysrhythmias (i.e., atrial fibrillation, atrial flutter, re-entry SVT) is:
   a. Fentanyl Citrate, 50 to 100 ug.
   b. Epinephrine, 1 mg.
   c. Diltiazem, 0.25 mg/kg.
   d. Haloperidol Lactate, 2 to 5 mg.

10. Your patient states she is having a reaction to a new medication she started taking last night. She has hives across the top of her chest and arms and is complaining of nausea, the sniffles, and watery eyes. Which medicine would be your first choice, provided her vital signs are stable?
    a. Epinephrine, 1 mg
    b. Diphenhydramine, 25 to 50 mg
    c. Dobutamine Hydrochloride, 2 to 20 ug/kg/min drip
    d. Metaproterenol Sulfate, 2 to 3 inhalations

11. You are treating a patient who has a low cardiac output after experiencing his third MI. To help improve his blood pressure it would be appropriate to consider administering which medication?
    a. Epinephrine, 1 mg
    b. Diltiazem, 0.25 mg/kg
    c. Dopamine Hydrochloride, 2 to 20 ug/kg/min drip
    d. Dolasetron, 12.5 mg IV

12. Of the following drugs, which is not a sympathomimetic class of drug?
    a. Dobutamine Hydrochloride
    b. Dopamine Hydrochloride
    c. Etomidate
    d. Epinephrine

13. You are treating a 22-year-old male patient who is experiencing a severe reaction to bee sting he obtained when he moved his lawn mower into a bee hive. He complains of tightening of the throat, difficulty breathing, nausea, and dizziness. Which drug will be needed to treat this patient?
    a. Fentanyl, 1 ug/kg
    b. Epinephrine, 1 mg
    c. Naloxone Hydrochloride, 0.4 to 2 mg
    d. Ondansetron Hydrochloride, 4 mg

14. You are treating a 22-year-old male who fell out of a tree and broke both arms. He is in severe pain and his vital signs are stable at this point. He is approximately 85 kg. To help relieve his pain, it would be appropriate to administer:
    a. Etomidate, 40 mg IV
    b. Flumazenil, 2 mg
    c. Fentanyl Citrate, 85 ug IV
    d. Morphine Sulfate, 45 mg

15. A loop diuretic that has been used to increase urine output in CHF patients with pulmonary edema and pedal edema would be:
    a. Heparin Sodium, 60 U/kg.
    b. Furosemide, 0.5 to 1 mg/kg.
    c. Labetalol, 10 mg.
    d. Levalbuterol, 1.25 to 2.5 mg.

16. You are treating a 35-year-old female who has a history of Type I diabetes. Today she has an altered mental status and is argumentative and combative with a blood sugar of 60 g/dL. If you cannot immediately find an IV site, what would be an appropriate medication to administer?
    a. Fosphenytoin, 10 to 20 mg
    b. Haloperidol Lactate, 2 to 5 mg IM
    c. Lorazepam, 2 to 4 mg IM
    d. Glucagon, 0.5 to 1 mg IM

17. You are treating a patient who is extremely anxious and extremely combative. With some assistance from the police, you manage to physically restrain him and could choose to chemically restrain him with the drug:
    a. Haloperidol Lactate, 2 to 5 mg IM.
    b. Morphine Sulfate, 5 mg IM.
    c. Midazolam Hydrochloride, 5 mg IM.
    d. Glucagon, 0.5 to 1 mg IM.

18. You are at a fire and you are treating a patient who you suspect was exposed to cyanide. One medication that has been used to treat this type of poisoning is called:
    a. Naloxone, 1 mg.
    b. Promethazine Hydrochloride, 1 to 3 mg.
    c. Hydroxocobalamin, 5 grams.
    d. Vecuronium Bromide, 0.1 to 0.2 mg/kg.

19. Of the following medications, the one most commonly used for patients presenting with persistent bronchospasms would be:
    a. Ketorolac Tromethamine, 30 mg.
    b. Ipratropium, 250 to 500 ug via nebulizer.
    c. Magnesium Sulfate, 1 to 4 grams.
    d. Meperidine Hydrochloride, 50 to 100 mg IM.

20. Which of the following drugs is not used to assist the patient having severe pain?
    a. Levalbuterol
    b. Meperidine Hydrochloride
    c. Morphine Sulfate
    d. Fentanyl Citrate

Exam #11 Answer Form

	A	B	C	D
1.	❏	❏	❏	❏
2.	❏	❏	❏	❏
3.	❏	❏	❏	❏
4.	❏	❏	❏	❏
5.	❏	❏	❏	❏
6.	❏	❏	❏	❏
7.	❏	❏	❏	❏
8.	❏	❏	❏	❏
9.	❏	❏	❏	❏
10.	❏	❏	❏	❏

	A	B	C	D
11.	❏	❏	❏	❏
12.	❏	❏	❏	❏
13.	❏	❏	❏	❏
14.	❏	❏	❏	❏
15.	❏	❏	❏	❏
16.	❏	❏	❏	❏
17.	❏	❏	❏	❏
18.	❏	❏	❏	❏
19.	❏	❏	❏	❏
20.	❏	❏	❏	❏

CHAPTER 12

Airway Management, Respiration, and Artificial Ventilation

1. Which of the following structures is(are) considered to be part of the lower airways?

    a. alveoli

    b. vocal cords

    c. cricoid ring

    d. thyroid cartilage

2. In the pediatric patient, the smallest diameter of the airway is located at the:

    a. epiglottis.

    b. pyriform fossae.

    c. ring in the trachea.

    d. cricothyroid membrane.

3. Which of the following is most correct about the differences between adult and pediatric airways?

    a. Infants and children have a more flexible trachea than adults.

    b. The epiglottis of infants and children is more rigid than an adult's.

    c. The mouth and nose of an adult are more easily obstructed than an infant's or child's.

    d. The epiglottis of an adult is proportionately larger and floppier than a pediatric epiglottis.

4. Which of the following is most correct about the tongues of infants and children?

    a. The tongue is difficult to manipulate during intubation.

    b. The tongue is easy to manipulate during intubation.

    c. They are proportionately smaller and take up less space in the mouth.

    d. They are proportionately larger and take up more space in the mouth.

5. Which of the following structures is considered part of the upper airway?

    a. carina

    b. trachea

    c. cricoid ring

    d. ethmoid bone

6. The function of the upper airway is to:

    a. warm, filter, and humidify the air we breathe.

    b. facilitate oxygenation at the cellular level.

    c. support pulmonary circulation through ventilation.

    d. exchange oxygen and carbon dioxide in the nares.

7. The function of the lower airway is to:

    a. warm, filter, and humidify the air we breathe.

    b. facilitate conversion of oxygen to energy.

    c. exchange oxygen and carbon dioxide at the cellular level.

    d. equalize pulmonary pressures.

8. _____ is the movement of carbon dioxide out of the lungs, and _____ is the movement of oxygen into the lungs.

    a. Ventilation; oxygenation

    b. Ventilation; perfusion

    c. Perfusion; ventilation

    d. Oxygenation; ventilation

9. The combined pressure of all atmospheric gases is the total pressure. At sea level the pressure, measured in torr, should add up to _____ torr, and the percentage should equal _____ %.

    a. 100; 90

    b. 100; 75

    c. 760; 100

    d. 760; 96

10. An alternative to intubation in airway management, the King Airway (LT-D) is designed to:
    a. fit into any size patient.
    b. be used in any unconscious patient.
    c. be inserted into the trachea and seal it off.
    d. be inserted into the esophagus and seal it off.

11. Cheyne–Stokes respirations gradually increase in rate and tidal volume, which increase to a maximum point and then gradually decrease and repeat in pattern. This pattern occurs when:
    a. there is a COPD exacerbation.
    b. the brain stem has been injured.
    c. the patient has increased intracranial pressure.
    d. the patient is experiencing diabetic ketoacidosis.

12. The major controlling factors over the respiratory rate are the central nervous system (CNS) and the:
    a. patient's mental status.
    b. patient's metabolic status.
    c. age of the patient.
    d. patient's heart rate.

13. Which area in the CNS is the primary involuntary respiratory center?
    a. medulla
    b. vagus nerve
    c. chemoreceptor
    d. baroreceptor

14. The pons has the secondary control center of respirations called the _____ center.
    a. secondary
    b. backup
    c. chemoreceptor
    d. apneustic

15. Chemoreceptors control respiration by measuring the pH of the blood and:
    a. surfactant.
    b. pulmonary pressure.
    c. cerebral spinal fluid.
    d. blood pressure.

16. Chemoreceptors are most plentiful in the carotid sinus and:
    a. aortic arch.
    b. medulla.
    c. pons.
    d. pneumotaxic center.

17. Normally the primary stimulus to breathe is a _____ in the blood.
    a. low concentration of carbon dioxide
    b. high concentration of carbon dioxide
    c. low concentration of oxygen
    d. high concentration of oxygen

18. In chronic COPD patients, the normal stimulus to breathe may fail because of:
    a. the use of steroids.
    b. excessive mucus production.
    c. trapped or retained CO_2.
    d. excessive surfactant production.

19. You are assessing a 56-year-old female with a complaint of sudden onset of difficulty breathing. She has a history of COPD and is on oxygen 24/7 by cannula at 2 lpm. She is alert and denies chest pain but gets dizzy when standing. The physical exam shows skin that is cyanotic, warm, and dry; lung sounds are clear; and the distal pulse is tachy/regular. She has retractions of the sternocleidomastoid muscles but no peripheral edema or jugular vein distention. Select the statement that is most accurate about this patient.
    a. There is a great possibility that this patient will need to be intubated.
    b. Long-term use of high-flow oxygen will not be harmful to this patient.
    c. The risk of under-oxygenating this patient is less than the risk of suppressing the stimulus to breathe.
    d. This patient would most likely do well with CPAP.

20. Your patient is a 59-year-old male with shortness of breath. He states that he has been sick for several days, and each day he feels worse. It is obvious that he is a smoker, but he denies having a COPD history. After your physical exam, you begin treatment and transport to rule out pneumonia. How can cigarette smoking be a direct contributing factor to developing pneumonia for this patient?
    a. Smoking causes bronchospasm and bronchoconstriction.
    b. Smoking inhibits the normal movement of mucus out of the lung.
    c. Smoking causes inflammation of the lung tissue, blocking the small airways.
    d. Smoking causes overgrowth of mucus glands and excess secretion of mucus that blocks the airway.

21. The condition that is characterized by a lack of oxygen in the tissues of the body is called:
    a. anaerobic metabolism.
    b. anoxia.
    c. hypoxemia.
    d. hypoxia.

22. _____ is a lack of oxygen in the blood.
    a. Anaerobic metabolism
    b. Anoxia
    c. Hypoxemia
    d. Hypoxia

23. The paramedic should consider any patient with a neurologic emergency to be _____ until proven otherwise.
    a. hyperventilating and alkalotic
    b. hypoventilating and hypoxemic
    c. obstructed
    d. acidotic

24. The paramedic is attempting to intubate a patient who is unconscious with no obvious cause and was unsuccessful in the first attempt. He did see the patient's vocal cords in the first attempt; however, in the second attempt, the vocal cords appear to have closed. What is the paramedic seeing?
    a. epiglotitis
    b. fractured larynx
    c. laryngeal spasm
    d. foreign body airway obstruction

25. In response to a call for difficulty breathing, you are assessing a patient whom you suspect has pneumonia. What should be your first consideration when dealing with this patient?
    a. The patient is contagious.
    b. The patient may deteriorate to respiratory arrest.
    c. Pneumonia can precipitate congestive heart failure.
    d. The patient requires high-flow oxygen immediately.

26. Your ambulance has been dispatched to a restaurant for a choking. When you arrive, there is a person administering abdominal thrusts to an unconscious elderly adult. A witness reports the patient started choking on his dinner, a trained bystander gave abdominal thrusts until the victim became unconscious, and she has continued without successfully removing the obstruction. What is your first action?
    a. Begin CPR.
    b. Check for a pulse.
    c. Take over abdominal thrusts.
    d. Open the airway, assess for breathing.

27. The bulb syringe, V-Vac®, or foot pump unit are all examples of _____ devices.
    a. battery-powered airway
    b. oxygen-powered suction
    c. manual suction
    d. AC- or DC-powered suction

28. Oxygen-powered suction units work well, but the biggest disadvantage is that they:
    a. are difficult to clean.
    b. are expensive.
    c. are heavy and difficult to carry.
    d. deplete your oxygen source rapidly.

29. Sterile suction technique is necessary when:
    a. performing any type of patient suctioning.
    b. suctioning the nose only.
    c. suctioning the tracheobronchial region.
    d. the patient has an OPA in place.

30. Suctioning can cause vagal stimulation by:
    a. changing the intrathoracic pressure.
    b. tickling the back of the throat.
    c. creating a hypoxic state.
    d. irritating the carotid sinuses.

31. Oral airways are hard plastic tubes designed to:
    a. prevent the tongue from obstructing the glottis.
    b. facilitate oral suctioning.
    c. facilitate oral tracheal intubation.
    d. guarantee that the airway will remain open.

32. One major disadvantage of using the nasopharyngeal airway (NPA) is that:
    a. you cannot suction through them.
    b. they do not provide a secured airway.
    c. they cannot be used on a conscious patient.
    d. they can only be used on an unconscious patient.

33. Which of the following is correct about the bevel on the end of a nasal airway?
    a. The bevel helps to facilitate suctioning.
    b. The bevel is designed to face the nasal septum.
    c. The bevel is a measuring device.
    d. The bevel follows the natural curvature of the nasopharynx.

34. Only water-soluble jelly is used when lubricating airway tubes, because other products are not biodegradable and can:
    a. cause laryngeal edema.
    b. cause excessive slipping of the airway adjuncts.
    c. collect in the lung tissue, causing chemical aspiration pneumonia.
    d. interfere with surfactant production.

35. Pulsus paradoxus is present when the _____ BP drops more than 10 mmHg with _____
    a. systolic; inspiration.
    b. systolic; expiration.
    c. diastolic; inspiration.
    d. diastolic; expiration.

36. Pulsus paradoxus is seen in COPD patients and patients with pericardial tamponade, and may occur:

    a. in an allergic reaction.

    b. during an asthma attack.

    c. with pneumonia.

    d. with a URI.

37. A cough, sneeze, and hiccup are all examples of:

    a. abnormal breathing patterns.

    b. temporary impairment of the respiratory muscles.

    c. protective reflexes used by patients to modify their respirations.

    d. inadequate ventilation associated with impairment of the nervous system.

38. ___ is an involuntary deep breath that increases opening of alveoli, preventing atelectasis. This occurs, on average, once every hour.

    a. Coughing

    b. Sighing

    c. Hiccuping

    d. A gag reflex

39. Your unit has been called for an ALS transport of a patient with kidney failure. As you listen to the verbal report from the nurse, you observe that the patient is unconscious and has deep, gasping respirations. What respiratory pattern is most likely occurring with this patient?

    a. Biot's

    b. agonal

    c. Kussmaul's

    d. Cheyne–Stokes

40. It is 4:00 P.M. when you respond to a call for a patient in severe respiratory distress. The patient is a 66-year-old female who is sitting on the edge of her chair in a sniffing position, working hard to breathe. She has a nasal cannula on and is cyanotic with sternal retractions. You hear audible wet gurgling and wheezing. She is in this position because it:

    a. helps to make it easier to breathe.

    b. increases the opening of the alveoli.

    c. gradually increases the tidal volume.

    d. aids in the clearing of the bronchi and bronchioles.

41. Gastric distention results when a rescuer is giving too much ventilatory volume or when the:

    a. patient has an inspiratory effort.

    b. airway is not properly opened.

    c. patient aspirates.

    d. patient is not intubated.

42. Gastric distention increases the risk of regurgitation and potential for aspiration as well as:

    a. creating resistance to bag mask ventilation.

    b. making an intubation more difficult.

    c. increasing the potential for laryngospasm.

    d. increasing the potential for bronchospasm.

43. The noninvasive method for managing gastric distention includes being prepared for the patient to vomit and:

    a. slowly applying pressure to the epigastric region.

    b. rapidly suctioning the hypopharynx until the patient is relieved.

    c. stimulating the gag reflex with the rigid suction tip.

    d. performing cricoid pressure and pressing on the stomach.

44. Which of the following statements regarding the use of a gastric tube is most accurate?

    a. It interferes with intubation.

    b. It is tolerated by conscious patients.

    c. It is only used on unconscious patients.

    d. It causes severe esophageal irritation and bleeding.

45. Naso- or orogastric intubation causes vagus nerve stimulation and may lead to:

    a. atrial flutter.

    b. heart block.

    c. atrial fibrillation.

    d. supraventricular tachycardia.

46. While inserting a nasogastric tube in a patient with severe gastric distention, you observe that the patient's heart rate is decreasing significantly. Which of the following would be appropriate to correct the problem?

    a. Terminate the procedure.

    b. Continue the procedure and then hyperventilate the patient.

    c. Ask the patient to stop talking.

    d. Administer Zofran for nausea.

47. If your efforts to correct the bradycardia in the patient described in question 46 have not worked and the heart rate remains low, your next step would involve:

    a. administering atropine.

    b. terminating the procedure.

    c. administering Zofran for nausea.

    d. asking the patient to cough.

48. Managing the airway of a patient can be hazardous because of the:
    a. potential for a spinal injury.
    b. potential for breaking teeth.
    c. potential lawsuit by the patient when harm is done.
    d. exposure to body fluids.

49. Oxygen tanks are pressurized vessels that can be very dangerous if dropped. The weakest point is the _____, which could break and send the pressurized vessel flying like a missile.
    a. bottom of the tank
    b. valve stem
    c. hydrostat plate
    d. spine of the tank

50. Oxygen cylinders need to be hydrostatically tested every 5 years. However, if the tank has a star after the test date, it is good for a(n) ___-year period.
    a. 8
    b. 10
    c. 12
    d. 15

51. When handling oxygen cylinders, the use of adhesive tape to mark or label tanks is not recommended because the materials in these products may:
    a. react with the oxygen, causing a fire.
    b. react with the oxygen and cause an explosion.
    c. cause the pressurized vessel to fly like a missile.
    d. make the tank sticky and difficult to handle.

52. Select the statement that is most accurate about oxygen tanks, pressure, and regulators.
    a. High-pressure regulators are used to transfer oxygen directly to patients.
    b. The pressure of the tank is usually around 3,500 psi when the tank is full.
    c. A therapy regulator is designed to be attached to the cylinder stem or wall of the ambulance.
    d. A therapy regulator is generally set at 100 PSI, and the actual delivery to the patient is adjustable to liters per minute.

53. The maximum pressure recommended for positive pressure ventilation should not exceed _____ cm of water pressure.
    a. 15
    b. 30
    c. 50
    d. 100

54. On which of the following patients would a demand-valve device be most appropriate?
    a. trauma arrest patient
    b. respiratory arrest patient
    c. medical cardiac arrest patient
    d. exacerbated congestive heart failure patient

55. On a call for a patient with respiratory distress, you are caring for a patient with a laryngectomy. Select the most accurate statement about the airway management for this patient.
    a. When ventilating a partial laryngectomy patient, you need to cover the mouth.
    b. When ventilating a *complete* laryngectomy patient, you do not need to cover the mouth.
    c. When performing rescue breathing on a laryngectomy patient, you give ventilations into the mouth.
    d. The end of the stoma should never be removed, nor should any airway adjuncts be attached.

56. What is the potential hazard of using a bag mask device with a pop-off valve?
    a. Pop-off valves are difficult to close and open.
    b. Pop-off valves are difficult to size to patients.
    c. Ventilations can exit through the pop-off valve without getting air into the patient.
    d. It is more difficult to get a mask seal.

57. After a cervical collar is applied to a patient, it can be removed for intubation or to correct a problem in the airway only when:
    a. two hands provide manual in-line immobilization.
    b. a second paramedic is available to assist.
    c. the head is taped to a long backboard.
    d. the front of a collar is removed.

58. Which of the following is an indication for the use of intermittent positive pressure breathing (IPPB)?
    a. when a patient is noncompliant or combative
    b. when a patient has poor tidal volume
    c. when a patient needs a high volume of high-concentration oxygen
    d. when the patient is a small child

59. One of the advantages of using IPPB is that:
    a. it allows for an easy mask seal.
    b. it reduces the risk of overinflation.
    c. there is no chance for barotrauma.
    d. there is no chance for gastric distention.

60. You are treating a 72-year-old resident in a nursing home for difficulty breathing. The staff tells you that she was fine in the morning and suddenly had deterioration in mental status and respiratory effort. The patient is alert to voice and is pale, warm, and dry. Lung sounds are diminished in the bases, and wheezing is present in the apices. Distal pulse is tachy/irregular, and her blood pressure is 18/100 mmHg. You put her on a non-rebreather mask while your partner sets up a nebulizer treatment. You start an IV, and after a few minutes of treatment, her SpO_2 has increased from the low 80s to the low 90s. The patient denies chest pain and tells you with difficulty that she doesn't feel much better. What noninvasive airway management/ventilation device or technique would be most comfortable and most likely effective for this patient?

a. biphasic positive airway pressure

b. nasal cannula with a partial-rebreather mask

c. assisted ventilations with a bag mask device

d. small volume nebulizer attached to a bag mask device

61. _____ improve(s) ventilation in both intubated and non-intubated patients as compared with other devices.

a. Mouth-to-mask

b. Bag mask devices

c. Manually triggered devices

d. Automatic transport ventilators (ATV)

62. Which of the following is an indication for the use of an ATV?

a. conscious patients who are combative

b. patient with an obstructed airway

c. patient with a pneumothorax

d. unconscious patients who are sedated

63. _____ refers to positive pressure ventilation as a treatment on a patient using either a tight-fitting nasal or face mask, but without endotracheal intubation.

a. Continuous inflation flow

b. Esophageal obturator

c. Noninvasive ventilation

d. Noninvasive transthoracic perfusion

64. The major advantage to the use of CPAP and BiPAP devices is that:

a. intubation may be avoided where it may have previously been required.

b. there is no wasting of oxygen.

c. it is available to all prehospital providers.

d. it does not require continuing education.

65. Collapse of the smaller airways and alveoli caused by hypoventilation or obstruction is called:

a. pneumotaxis.

b. atelectasis.

c. hemostaxis.

d. pneumothorax.

66. Which of the following patient conditions is a common cause of the condition described in question 65?

a. epistaxis

b. fractured ribs

c. allergic reaction

d. a pediatric on a ventilator

67. When inserted too far, why is the ET tube more likely to slide into the right main stem bronchus than the left?

a. The left main stem is harder to see.

b. The left main stem is often occluded with mucus.

c. The right main stem bronchus is straighter.

d. The right main stem is more rigid than the left.

68. The 68-year-old male in severe respiratory distress went into respiratory arrest and was successfully intubated. During the transport to the hospital, he is improving and now is attempting to pull on the endotracheal tube. What action is most appropriate at this point?

a. Sedate the patient.

b. Physically restrain the patient.

c. Prepare to extubate the patient.

d. Note the patient's $EtCO_2$ and SpO_2 readings.

69. _____ is the volume of air inspired or expired during each normal, quiet breath and in an adult male is normally _____ ml.

a. Tidal volume; 500

b. Alveolar volume; 350

c. Dead Space Volume; 150

d. Total lung capacity; 6,000

70. During a lengthy extrication process of an unconscious patient who was trapped in a vehicle, you intubated and started an IV. En route to the nearest trauma center 10 minutes away, the patient begins to awaken and attempts to pull out the endotracheal tube. What is the most significant risk for the patient who attempts to extubate herself?

a. hemothorax

b. pneumothorax

c. aspiration of vomitus

d. tension pneumothorax

71. What is the complication associated with performing the Sellick maneuver?
    a. When pressure is applied improperly, airway obstruction results.
    b. When performed improperly, atelectasis may develop.
    c. The early release of pressure can result in obstruction.
    d. The late release of pressure can result in aspiration.

72. When performing the Sellick maneuver, pressure is applied on the _____ of the cartilages and maintained until after the ET tube is inserted and _____.
    a. lateral edge; the tube is measured
    b. top edge; the cuff is inflated
    c. bottom edge; the tube is measured
    d. lateral edge; the cuff is inflated

73. The use of the laryngeal mask airway (LMA) should be avoided when the patient:
    a. is elderly.
    b. has chest trauma.
    c. has been sedated.
    d. is an infant or small child.

74. Which of the following airway devices is considered a direct, rather than an indirect, method of advanced airway device?
    a. EOA
    b. PTL
    c. LMA
    d. ETT

75. Digital or tactile intubation is a technique that may be helpful when:
    a. there is a suspected cervical spine injury.
    b. the tongue is extra large.
    c. secretions are copious.
    d. bleeding into the airway is uncontrolled.

76. Retrograde intubation is a technique that should only be performed by properly trained providers and:
    a. involves an invasive procedure beyond intubation.
    b. requires the use of an uncuffed endotracheal tube.
    c. can only be performed with the use of rapid sequence induction.
    d. should only be considered for patients with suspected cervical spine injury.

77. Pulse oximetry is a noninvasive technique that uses a(n) _____ light beam to measure the oxygen saturation of the blood.
    a. effervescent
    b. luminescent
    c. infrared
    d. ultraviolet

78. Pulse oximetry is known to provide false readings under certain conditions. Which of the following is the correct explanation for the false readings?
    a. Any condition that impairs venous blood flow will cause false readings.
    b. When the skin is too thick to absorb the luminescent light, a false reading will occur.
    c. Any condition that causes an altered hemoglobin molecule can cause a false reading.
    d. The principle of pulse oximetry assumes blood temperature is normothermic, so abnormally high temperatures cause false readings.

79. You are treating a patient who called EMS because she has been vomiting blood (bright red blood clots). She is pale and diaphoretic and tells you that she has been sick for a week. Her vital signs are respiratory rate of 24/nonlabored, pulse rate of 130/irregular, BP of 88/50 mmHg, and SpO_2 of 99 percent. Why is the pulse oximetry reading likely to be unreliable?
    a. The hemoglobin concentration is low due to shock.
    b. Pale and diaphoretic skin can impede the light beam reading.
    c. Low blood pressure enhances the light beam through the fingertip.
    d. Low blood pressure diminishes the light beam through the fingertip.

80. Which of the following devices is used for detection of exhaled CO_2 via the paper filter method?
    a. pulse oximetry
    b. colorimetric device
    c. capnography
    d. capnometer

81. For the cardiac arrest patient who has been intubated, prior to obtaining an accurate end-tidal CO_2 reading, it is recommended that the patient be ventilated five to six times to:
    a. wash out any residual $EtCO_2$ that may be present in the esophagus.
    b. rule out the presence of a pulmonary embolism.
    c. give the meter a chance to warm up.
    d. make sure the patient is hyperoxygenated.

82. COPD patients have raised CO_2 levels and depend on a deficiency of oxygen to stimulate respiration. This mechanism is called:

    a. apnea.

    b. hypoxic drive.

    c. ventilation–perfusion mismatch.

    d. central neurogenic hyperventilation.

83. A(n) _____ is a syringe-like device that may be helpful in verifying tracheal versus esophageal intubation.

    a. esophageal gastric tube airway

    b. esophageal intubation detector

    c. Beck airway flow monitor

    d. esophageal obturator airway

84. During transport to the hospital with a cardiac arrest patient, you observe that the patient has become difficult to ventilate. Which of the following should you check first?

    a. Verify lung sounds.

    b. Check the pulse oximeter reading.

    c. Check the capnograph reading.

    d. Check the pulse.

85. The fire department is working on a vehicle extrication with an unconscious young male driver who is trapped. Your primary assessment reveals that the patient has a large contusion on the forehead, his teeth are clenched, he is breathing abnormally, and he has a weak and rapid distal pulse. You begin ventilations with a bag mask device as your partner prepares your equipment to nasally intubate the patient. The major advantage of using nasotracheal intubation for this patient is that:

    a. the technique does not require the use of a laryngoscope.

    b. correct tube placement is more effectively verified than an orally placed tube.

    c. the patient cannot pull the tube or accidentally dislodge it once it is secured.

    d. the tube is more easily placed in a patient with a suspected spinal injury than an orally placed tube.

86. The major disadvantage of nasotracheal intubation is that it:

    a. is a blind technique.

    b. is more difficult to verify tube placement.

    c. does not work with spinal cord injured patients.

    d. often has a false-positive capnography reading.

87. Devices such as the Beck Airway Airflow Monitor (BAAM) and the Endotrol® tube are effective in the facilitation of:

    a. orotracheal intubation.

    b. nasotracheal intubation.

    c. sterile suctioning.

    d. CO_2 monitoring.

88. _____ is a last resort airway technique when a patient has a complete airway obstruction or in whom endotracheal intubation is otherwise impossible.

    a. Laryngeal mask airway (LMA)

    b. Needle decompression

    c. Needle cricothyrotomy

    d. Rapid sequence intubation

89. Translaryngeal cannula ventilation (TLCV) is a means of providing ventilation through a large-bore needle that is directly inserted:

    a. through the cricothyroid membrane.

    b. in the second intercostal space on the midclavicular chest.

    c. in the fifth intercostal space on the midaxillary chest.

    d. in the laryngectomy patient's stoma.

90. The neuromuscular blocking agent succinylcholine (SUX) is contraindicated in patients with massive tissue injury because of the:

    a. side effects associated with hypovolemia.

    b. effects of prolonged muscular tremors.

    c. risk of hypokalemia.

    d. risk of hyperkalemia.

91. Your patient is a 2-year-old infant in respiratory arrest. Your partner is ventilating with a bag mask device while you prepare to intubate the child. You choose an uncuffed tube for this intubation because:

    a. cuffed tubes make visualization of the vocal cords more difficult.

    b. uncuffed tubes are easier to place than cuffed tubes.

    c. the cricoid cartilage narrows in the trachea and serves as a functional cuff.

    d. it is easier to verify tube placement with an uncuffed tube.

92. The patient you are evaluating for a syncopal event has started to seize, and his teeth are clenched. Which of the following airway devices is appropriate for this patient?

    a. LMA

    b. nasotracheal intubation

    c. nasal airway

    d. nasogastric tube

93. Which of the following situations would most likely invite a paramedic to the courtroom?

    a. use of the wrong size LMA that resulted in laryngitis

    b. use of a pediatric pop-off device that prevented adequate oxygenation of a patient

    c. recognition of a misplaced endotracheal tube, which was subsequently extubated in the field by the paramedic in charge

    d. documentation of a normal pulse oximetry reading by the paramedic on a patient who was really sick

94. An elderly female fell down a flight of stairs in her home and sustained a serious head injury. She has an altered mental status, has clenched teeth, and is at risk of vomiting and possible aspirating. Which of the following airway management techniques is the safest for both the patient and the paramedic?

    a. NPA with CPAP

    b. nasotracheal intubation

    c. rapid sequence intubation

    d. NPA with an automatic transport ventilation

95. Further evaluation of the patient described in question 94 reveals that he is unresponsive to painful stimuli and has slow, shallow, and stridorous respiration at a rate of 10 bpm. His distal pulse is rapid and weak, and his skin is ashen and cool. What action should you take next?

    a. Suction the airway and insert a nasal airway.

    b. Place a cervical collar and perform a rapid extrication.

    c. Insert an oral airway and start an IV prior to extrication.

    d. Have your partner contact medical control to obtain an order for a possible emergency needle cricothyrotomy.

96. Your EMS service is conducting an update on advanced airway devices. One of the devices that is being discussed is the LMA. A significant benefit of the use of the LMA as an advanced airway device is that:

    a. it has no face mask seal to maintain.

    b. it can be used on conscious patients.

    c. it increases anatomical dead air space.

    d. once properly inserted, it completely protects against aspiration.

97. Your patient is a 24-year-old female asthmatic in severe respiratory distress. She called EMS when she could not get relief from her metered dose inhalers (Combivent and albuterol). The patient appears exhausted and cyanotic, and auscultation of her lungs reveals no air movement on inspiration or expiration. What should you do next?

    a. Obtain a pulse oximetry reading.

    b. Administer a nebulizer treatment through a non-rebreather mask.

    c. Insert an oral airway and provide rapid ventilations with a bag mask device.

    d. Assist ventilations with a bag mask device slowly and gently over 2 seconds.

98. Rapid sequence induction (RSI) can be a safe way of providing airway access and is an ideal airway management procedure for which type of patient?

    a. traumatic cardiac arrest patient

    b. conscious, uncooperative patient in respiratory failure

    c. unconscious, hypothermic patient with slow and shallow respirations

    d. unresponsive patient in respiratory arrest preceded by an asthma attack

99. The RSI can produce muscular tremors called fasciculations, which are produced by:

    a. narcotic sedatives.

    b. temporary hypoxia.

    c. benzodiazepine sedatives.

    d. neuromuscular blocking agents.

100. Which of the following airway devices is not an appropriate device for a patient with high airway pressures?

    a. LMA

    b. Combitube

    c. orotracheal tube

    d. nasotracheal tube

Exam #12 Answer Form

	A	B	C	D		A	B	C	D
1.	❏	❏	❏	❏	31.	❏	❏	❏	❏
2.	❏	❏	❏	❏	32.	❏	❏	❏	❏
3.	❏	❏	❏	❏	33.	❏	❏	❏	❏
4.	❏	❏	❏	❏	34.	❏	❏	❏	❏
5.	❏	❏	❏	❏	35.	❏	❏	❏	❏
6.	❏	❏	❏	❏	36.	❏	❏	❏	❏
7.	❏	❏	❏	❏	37.	❏	❏	❏	❏
8.	❏	❏	❏	❏	38.	❏	❏	❏	❏
9.	❏	❏	❏	❏	39.	❏	❏	❏	❏
10.	❏	❏	❏	❏	40.	❏	❏	❏	❏
11.	❏	❏	❏	❏	41.	❏	❏	❏	❏
12.	❏	❏	❏	❏	42.	❏	❏	❏	❏
13.	❏	❏	❏	❏	43.	❏	❏	❏	❏
14.	❏	❏	❏	❏	44.	❏	❏	❏	❏
15.	❏	❏	❏	❏	45.	❏	❏	❏	❏
16.	❏	❏	❏	❏	46.	❏	❏	❏	❏
17.	❏	❏	❏	❏	47.	❏	❏	❏	❏
18.	❏	❏	❏	❏	48.	❏	❏	❏	❏
19.	❏	❏	❏	❏	49.	❏	❏	❏	❏
20.	❏	❏	❏	❏	50.	❏	❏	❏	❏
21.	❏	❏	❏	❏	51.	❏	❏	❏	❏
22.	❏	❏	❏	❏	52.	❏	❏	❏	❏
23.	❏	❏	❏	❏	53.	❏	❏	❏	❏
24.	❏	❏	❏	❏	54.	❏	❏	❏	❏
25.	❏	❏	❏	❏	55.	❏	❏	❏	❏
26.	❏	❏	❏	❏	56.	❏	❏	❏	❏
27.	❏	❏	❏	❏	57.	❏	❏	❏	❏
28.	❏	❏	❏	❏	58.	❏	❏	❏	❏
29.	❏	❏	❏	❏	59.	❏	❏	❏	❏
30.	❏	❏	❏	❏	60.	❏	❏	❏	❏

Exam #12 Answer Form

	A	B	C	D		A	B	C	D
61.	❏	❏	❏	❏	81.	❏	❏	❏	❏
62.	❏	❏	❏	❏	82.	❏	❏	❏	❏
63.	❏	❏	❏	❏	83.	❏	❏	❏	❏
64.	❏	❏	❏	❏	84.	❏	❏	❏	❏
65.	❏	❏	❏	❏	85.	❏	❏	❏	❏
66.	❏	❏	❏	❏	86.	❏	❏	❏	❏
67.	❏	❏	❏	❏	87.	❏	❏	❏	❏
68.	❏	❏	❏	❏	88.	❏	❏	❏	❏
69.	❏	❏	❏	❏	89.	❏	❏	❏	❏
70.	❏	❏	❏	❏	90.	❏	❏	❏	❏
71.	❏	❏	❏	❏	91.	❏	❏	❏	❏
72.	❏	❏	❏	❏	92.	❏	❏	❏	❏
73.	❏	❏	❏	❏	93.	❏	❏	❏	❏
74.	❏	❏	❏	❏	94.	❏	❏	❏	❏
75.	❏	❏	❏	❏	95.	❏	❏	❏	❏
76.	❏	❏	❏	❏	96.	❏	❏	❏	❏
77.	❏	❏	❏	❏	97.	❏	❏	❏	❏
78.	❏	❏	❏	❏	98.	❏	❏	❏	❏
79.	❏	❏	❏	❏	99.	❏	❏	❏	❏
80.	❏	❏	❏	❏	100.	❏	❏	❏	❏

CHAPTER

13

Scene Size-Up and Primary Assessment

1. Of the components listed, the second component of an assessment in the field is:
   a. scene size-up.
   b. primary assessment.
   c. opening the airway.
   d. providing high-flow oxygen.

2. One step the paramedic can take at the scene of a residential call in order to make it safe is to:
   a. make use of doorstops.
   b. quickly suction the patient's airway.
   c. notify dispatch of estimated scene time.
   d. take and maintain C-spine stabilization.

3. Which of the following MOIs is nonsignificant for most adult and pediatric patients?
   a. near drowning
   b. gunshot wound (GSW)
   c. fall from a height of 30 feet
   d. trip and fall from a standing position

4. The injury pattern commonly seen in children who have been hit by a motor vehicle, which includes injury to the legs, chest, and head, is known as:
   a. Waddell's triad.
   b. Cushing's blow.
   c. Warren's impact.
   d. Ryan's compression.

5. Getting a general impression of a patient is sometimes referred to as:
   a. the look test.
   b. the patient interview.
   c. prioritizing.
   d. the nature of illness.

6. The acronym AVPU is used in the primary assessment to determine the:
   a. patient's mental status.
   b. patient's chief complaint.
   c. need for an additional ambulance.
   d. mechanism of injury (MOI).

7. The first and foremost priority for the paramedic on call is:
   a. dispatching information accuracy.
   b. the patient's chief complaint.
   c. recognizing hazards and your safety.
   d. the patient's mechanism of injury (MOI).

8. You are on the scene of a call and you are beginning to suspect there may be hazardous materials involved in this scene. Which of the following clues indicates there may be hazardous materials involved in the incident?
   a. The family's pet dog is barking at the front door.
   b. Three out of four family members are complaining of a headache.
   c. Power lines are down on the scene of a motor vehicle collision.
   d. There is advance notice of infestation at the scene of a call.

9. What does the term "secure" scene mean?
   a. The area is closed off to the public.
   b. The media is barred from entering the scene.
   c. The area is a crime scene.
   d. A potentially violent scene is safe for EMS.

10. Which of the following examples is a potential threat to a paramedic in a typical residential area?

    a. a 3:00 a.m. response to a house that has no lights on

    b. a response to a house with no one to let you in, but a woman is calling out "I can't get up"

    c. a standby at a fire scene of a fully involved structure fire

    d. a response to a suicide attempt with police on scene

11. You and your crew are working with the fire department to extricate the driver of a midsized vehicle who is trapped under the steering wheel after striking a tree with great force. The patient is in respiratory distress with a rapidly decreasing mental status. The decision has been made to rapidly extricate the patient; during the move, a handgun falls from the patient's clothing. What immediate action should be taken to keep the scene safe?

    a. Back away from the patient and let the police officer remove the gun.

    b. Continue to remove the patient and do not let anyone touch the gun.

    c. Assign a firefighter to remove the gun from the vehicle and continue to move the patient.

    d. Immediately remove the patient's clothing to assure no other weapons are present prior to moving him any further.

12. Before a scene is secure, where should EMS respond?

    a. to the staging area around the corner

    b. to the standby in quarters

    c. to the restocking station nearest to the call

    d. to the nearest police department

13. Which of the following is an example of a potentially infectious process at the scene that may involve a hazard to the paramedic?

    a. a crying baby

    b. a patient with a productive cough

    c. the odor of vomitus at the scene

    d. the presence of insulin syringes at the scene

14. Which of the following is an example of an unstable scene that the paramedic can easily stabilize, if recognized?

    a. Put out a small engine fire with a fire extinguisher.

    b. Engage the emergency brake on a car that has been left in neutral.

    c. Disarm a perpetrator at a crime scene.

    d. Stand between a wife and her abusive husband.

15. Of the hazards to the paramedic listed below, which presents the greatest hazard?

    a. needle stick injuries

    b. exposure to TB

    c. exposure to hazardous materials

    d. working in traffic at the scene of a collision

16. A common MOI associated with sports such as basketball, skiing, soccer, and racquetball is:

    a. ejection.

    b. penetration.

    c. twisting of the knee.

    d. a rapid acceleration force.

17. Which of the following examples depicts a mechanism of injury (MOI) rather than a common nature of illness (NOI) that a paramedic would recognize during the scene size-up and primary assessment of a 44-year-old male?

    a. seizure

    b. poisoning

    c. attempted hanging

    d. altered mental status

18. When the paramedic understands the _____, he can make some predictions or be more attuned to specific injury patterns.

    a. past medical history (PMH)

    b. chief complaint (CC)

    c. mechanism of injury (MOI)

    d. nature of illness (NOI)

19. The _____ is your first impression of the patient as you approach her and has been referred to as the "assessment from the doorway."

    a. scene size-up

    b. general impression

    c. primary assessment

    d. MOI

20. While working in an incident command situation, which of the following actions is inappropriate for the paramedic to take?

    a. Report to the incident commander upon arrival.

    b. Obtain a quick report and assignment for your crew.

    c. Complete the assignment and search for the next patient.

    d. Complete the assignment and report back to command.

21. You are assessing the level of consciousness of a patient who is wearing a helmet and appears to have been involved in a serious motorcycle collision. The patient's eyes are closed, and he has abnormal breathing. When you speak to him, he does not answer, but when you touch him, he moans and tries to move his arms. The patient's initial level of consciousness should be recorded as:
    a. alert.
    b. verbal.
    c. painful.
    d. unresponsive.

22. While assessing a patient for a painful response, which of the following is an appropriate response?
    a. withdrawing from pain
    b. no response
    c. flexing the arm
    d. extending the arm

23. The level of consciousness or mental status of an infant is best assessed by:
    a. calling medical control to consult for advice.
    b. using the Broselow tape for pediatrics.
    c. how loud the infant cries.
    d. asking the parent or caregiver to determine if the response is normal.

24. _____ is the degree of alertness, wakefulness, or arousibility of the patient.
    a. Mental response
    b. Level of consciousness
    c. Emotion
    d. Reaction

25. Decerebrate neurologic posturing is illustrative of _____ brain functioning.
    a. absence of
    b. low-level
    c. mid-level
    d. high-level

26. Neurologic posturing is most commonly caused by herniation and compression of the brainstem or by:
    a. the effects of advanced Alzheimer's.
    b. metabolic causes.
    c. hyperventilation by the patient.
    d. injury to the lumbar spine.

27. Even if a patient is responsive and alert, he may still have serious airway compromise, such as a(n):
    a. broken jaw.
    b. abscessed tooth.
    c. cervical spine injury.
    d. postnasal drip.

28. Anytime a patient has received a high-energy impact from the clavicles or superior to the clavicles, the paramedic must consider the possibility of:
    a. low blood sugar.
    b. hypoxia.
    c. neck injury.
    d. hypovolemia.

29. You are assessing your patient during the primary survey. The _____ is the appropriateness of the patient's thinking and is described with AVPU.
    a. mental status
    b. level of response
    c. emotion
    d. reaction

30. The volume of gas inspired or expired by your patient each minute is called the:
    a. adequate volume.
    b. dead space volume.
    c. tidal volume.
    d. minute volume.

31. The neck of an infant should not be hyperextended when opening the airway, as this can:
    a. cause the infant to swallow the tongue.
    b. close the airway.
    c. interfere with nose breathing.
    d. cause cervical spinal injury.

32. During the primary assessment of an unconscious child, the pulse is taken at the _____ for the "quick check" to determine if the patient has a pulse.
    a. radial artery
    b. brachial artery
    c. carotid artery
    d. carotid vein

33. Assessing the _____ pulse is more useful in the primary assessment of a patient because it gives information about the effectiveness of the _____ circulation.
    a. radial; distal
    b. brachial; central
    c. carotid; central
    d. femoral; core

34. What is assessed about the patient's skin during the primary assessment?
    a. color and pigmentation
    b. color, temperature, and condition
    c. pulse oximetry
    d. the presence of urticaria

35. You are assessing a 55-year-old male patient who has no immediate threats to life. Which of the following skin colors is considered an abnormal finding associated with hepatic or renal failure?

   a. red

   b. pale

   c. jaundice

   d. cyanosis

36. When assessing the skin of patients with varying degrees of skin pigmentation, the paramedic should look at the _____, as the normal skin color is similar in most persons.

   a. ears

   b. axilla

   c. tongue

   d. palms or soles

37. In recent years, the use of capillary refill has been limited to certain groups of patients. In which of the following is capillary refill still considered a reliable sign?

   a. a 55-year-old male with COPD

   b. a 25-year-old female with anemia

   c. a 14-year-old male with hypothermia

   d. a 3-year-old asthmatic

38. The main reason the paramedic should prioritize the patient for treatment and transportation at the completion of the primary assessment is:

   a. to identify and manage immediate life-threatening conditions.

   b. that this task has the highest priority in the first few minutes of a call.

   c. to determine the need for rapid transport and definitive care at the hospital.

   d. to determine when a critical patient should be stabilized on scene or transported rapidly.

39. You are on the scene of a 22-year-old male patient who sustained a high-speed motorcycle crash. Where should severe trauma, such as this patient sustained, be stabilized?

   a. on the scene prior to transport

   b. in the ambulance en route to the local hospital

   c. in the emergency department

   d. in the operating room by a surgeon

40. You are treating a critical patient who was thrown from his car during a high-speed collision. Which of the following steps may be skipped or expedited during the care of a critical trauma patient?

   a. use of a short board immobilization device

   b. use of a long board immobilization device

   c. bleeding control for life-threatening external bleeding

   d. airway control

41. The _____ is a name for what is done in the ambulance en route to the hospital and includes serial vital signs and checking interventions you have already administered.

   a. detailed assessment

   b. focused assessment

   c. reassessment

   d. vectored exam

42. A _____ exam is an examination that attempts to look at a specific patient problem and not examine every body part, which could take a long time and not be in the patient's best interest.

   a. detailed

   b. focused

   c. reassessment

   d. primary

43. The primary assessment is repeated in the reassessment in cases where the patient's:

   a. condition may be changing rapidly.

   b. condition shows an improved mental status from the baseline.

   c. condition includes a nonsignificant MOI.

   d. blood glucose returns to normal.

44. _____ is establishing a pattern of assessment findings, which will help the paramedic determine if the patient's condition is getting worse or better.

   a. Diagnosing

   b. Trending

   c. Documenting

   d. Prioritizing

45. Medical patients are classified into two groups within the medical category of assessment-based management. These two groups are:

   a. significant and nonsignificant.

   b. responsive and unresponsive.

   c. critical and noncritical.

   d. adult and child.

46. Trauma patients are classified into two groups within the trauma category of assessment-based management. These two groups are _____ MOI.

   a. significant and nonsignificant

   b. conscious and unconscious

   c. adult and child

   d. alpha and delta

47. Your patient is a 37-year-old male who you have decided has both a medical problem and an injury. When a patient has both a medical and a trauma problem, which is treated first?

    a. medical

    b. trauma

    c. any immediate threat to life

    d. medical control decides

48. What is the best treatment the paramedic can provide for the patient with internal bleeding?

    a. Start two large-bore IVs.

    b. Apply MAST/PASG pants and inflate.

    c. Administer analgesia for pain.

    d. Provide rapid transport to an OR.

49. You are assessing a 43-year-old female patient and have decided to prioritize her as critical. Which of the following injuries or conditions is she most likely to have?

    a. low-grade fever

    b. sickle cell crisis

    c. productive cough

    d. possible cervical neck injury

50. You have prioritized your patient as stable. Of the following injuries or conditions, which is most likely the condition of your patient?

    a. patella dislocation

    b. respiratory distress

    c. compensated shock

    d. rising intracranial pressure

Exam #13 Answer Form

	A	B	C	D		A	B	C	D
1.	❏	❏	❏	❏	26.	❏	❏	❏	❏
2.	❏	❏	❏	❏	27.	❏	❏	❏	❏
3.	❏	❏	❏	❏	28.	❏	❏	❏	❏
4.	❏	❏	❏	❏	29.	❏	❏	❏	❏
5.	❏	❏	❏	❏	30.	❏	❏	❏	❏
6.	❏	❏	❏	❏	31.	❏	❏	❏	❏
7.	❏	❏	❏	❏	32.	❏	❏	❏	❏
8.	❏	❏	❏	❏	33.	❏	❏	❏	❏
9.	❏	❏	❏	❏	34.	❏	❏	❏	❏
10.	❏	❏	❏	❏	35.	❏	❏	❏	❏
11.	❏	❏	❏	❏	36.	❏	❏	❏	❏
12.	❏	❏	❏	❏	37.	❏	❏	❏	❏
13.	❏	❏	❏	❏	38.	❏	❏	❏	❏
14.	❏	❏	❏	❏	39.	❏	❏	❏	❏
15.	❏	❏	❏	❏	40.	❏	❏	❏	❏
16.	❏	❏	❏	❏	41.	❏	❏	❏	❏
17.	❏	❏	❏	❏	42.	❏	❏	❏	❏
18.	❏	❏	❏	❏	43.	❏	❏	❏	❏
19.	❏	❏	❏	❏	44.	❏	❏	❏	❏
20.	❏	❏	❏	❏	45.	❏	❏	❏	❏
21.	❏	❏	❏	❏	46.	❏	❏	❏	❏
22.	❏	❏	❏	❏	47.	❏	❏	❏	❏
23.	❏	❏	❏	❏	48.	❏	❏	❏	❏
24.	❏	❏	❏	❏	49.	❏	❏	❏	❏
25.	❏	❏	❏	❏	50.	❏	❏	❏	❏

CHAPTER

14

History Taking

1. When the paramedic is caring for a patient who does not communicate in the same language as he/she, the paramedic should:
   a. wait for an interpreter.
   b. rely exclusively on body language.
   c. allow twice as much interview time.
   d. assess and care for the patient without communicating.

2. The best way to assess the mental status of your patient, to see if he is conversing normally, is to:
   a. speak with him.
   b. obtain a glucose reading.
   c. obtain a pulse oximetry reading.
   d. ask a family member if the patient is acting normal.

3. _____ is an effective technique for improving cross-cultural communication.
   a. Active listening
   b. Very slow talking
   c. Lengthy conversations
   d. Joking and keeping things light

4. A _____ history is all the medical events and conditions that have ever occurred to the patient.
   a. complete health
   b. focused
   c. past medical
   d. SAMPLE

5. A focused history is the chronologic history of the patient's:
   a. surgeries.
   b. present illness.
   c. medication use.
   d. family history.

6. During the patient interview, the paramedic should attempt to obtain the following information about a patient's current event.
   a. What is the patient's marital status?
   b. What is the patient's general outlook?
   c. Is this event similar to any previous events?
   d. Will a similar event occur in the near future?

7. The acronym OPQRST is used to remember the set of questions used to obtain information about the patient's:
   a. past medical history.
   b. complete health history.
   c. use of OTC medications.
   d. present illness or injury.

8. _____ is one technique used to create a rapport between two people across cultures and it focuses on the vocal pitch and body language.
   a. Mirror and matching
   b. Using motivating words
   c. Using the patient's name
   d. Cross-over matching

9. Which of the following pieces of patient information is irrelevant to the paramedic in the field?
   a. recent surgery
   b. recent illness
   c. change in daily living activities
   d. tonsillectomy in childhood

10. For the paramedic, the goal of obtaining the patient's medical history is to:
    a. develop a treatment plan.
    b. make a medical diagnosis.
    c. establish a paramedic–patient relationship.
    d. get the patient to talk endlessly in a rambling manner.

11. Why is it important for the paramedic to be empathetic when obtaining a health history?
    a. Showing empathy helps to obtain more cooperation from the patient.
    b. Empathy helps the family to trust you with the patient.
    c. It is a way of showing respect to the patient.
    d. It helps the patient to communicate with the next health care provider.

12. Which of the following is a disrespectful use of terms for the patient?
    a. using the patient's proper name
    b. calling the patient "honey"
    c. using the patient's nickname with permission
    d. using the patient's first name with permission

13. Although paramedics are taught to ask direct questions of the patient, which of the following is an example of a good open-ended question to ask a patient?
    a. What hospital have you been to?
    b. Why did you call us here today?
    c. How does that make you feel?
    d. Why do you feel that your doctor is unable to help you?

14. When you are not getting the answer to questions that appear obvious, consider that the patient may be:
    a. pregnant.
    b. falsely reassured.
    c. not ill or injured.
    d. embarrassed.

15. During an interview with a patient having chest pain, you ask the patient, "How is the pain different today?" This is an example of a(n) _____ question.
    a. direct
    b. closed
    c. leading
    d. open-ended

16. When is it better to ask direct questions of the patient?
    a. when a behavioral problem is suspected
    b. when specific information is required
    c. when the patient's family is present
    d. when the patient has no specific complaint

17. Which of the following cultures may consider direct eye contact during an interview to be impolite or aggressive?
    a. Italian
    b. German
    c. Native American
    d. New Yorker

18. Why should the paramedic avoid providing false reassurance to a patient in distress?
    a. The patient will sue if she finds out the truth.
    b. The patient will suffer harm.
    c. The paramedic could lose her certification.
    d. The paramedic could lose the patient's trust.

19. Which of the following is an example of a leading question?
    a. Are you pregnant?
    b. Do you have sharp chest pain?
    c. Do you have a history of diabetes?
    d. When did you last take your medication?

20. Which of the following is an example of a condescending question to be avoided during an interview?
    a. How much did you have to drink tonight?
    b. You don't smoke, do you?
    c. Do you take your medications every day?
    d. When was your last menstrual period?

21. In an effort to keep a patient from becoming more anxious during a patient interview, the paramedic should:
    a. shun nonverbal communication.
    b. avoid facilitation whenever possible.
    c. stay away from silence as an interview technique.
    d. avoid the use of complicated medical terminology.

22. An example of a negative communication technique that the paramedic should avoid with patients and their families is:
    a. reflection.
    b. inattentiveness.
    c. asking for clarification when a patient's response is ambiguous.
    d. being conscious of the amount of physical space between you and the patient.

23. _____ is the way you speak, and how your posture and your actions are used to encourage the patient to say more.
    a. Empathy
    b. Confrontation
    c. Facilitation
    d. Reflection

24. To repeat or echo the patient's own words as a way of encouraging the flow of conversation without interrupting the patient's concentration is referred to as:
    a. interpretation.
    b. clarification.
    c. facilitation.
    d. reflection.

25. _____ is reasoning based not on what you observed from the patient, but on what you have concluded from the information you have compiled.
    a. Interpretation
    b. Clarification
    c. Empathy
    d. Silence

26. Which of the following conditions is least likely to be an obstacle during a patient interview?
    a. a patient who is blind
    b. a patient who is overly talkative
    c. a patient who is symptomatic
    d. a patient who is developmentally disabled

27. A rolled piece of paper (scroll style) in a plastic container, which contains medical information about a patient is a(n):
    a. MedicAlert® tag.
    b. prescription bottle.
    c. Vial of Life®.
    d. Emergency Lifeline®.

28. When treating a patient who only speaks a foreign language that you do not, and no interpreter is immediately available, which of the following can you do to best facilitate care?
    a. Use positive body language while you begin care.
    b. Wait for a translator before initiating care.
    c. Ask police for assistance.
    d. Call the paramedic supervisor.

29. While caring for a blind patient, it is appropriate to announce yourself, to explain as much as possible, and to:
    a. secure the seeing eye dog for your protection.
    b. speak while facing the patient.
    c. interact with the patient the same way as with a seeing patient.
    d. ask permission to touch the patient before actually touching him.

30. You are caring for a patient who is very angry and is taking his anger out on you. Which of the following should you avoid doing?
    a. getting angry in return
    b. doing a quick pat down for weapons
    c. keeping the situation calm
    d. requesting police

31. Sleep disorders, appetite disturbances, the inability to concentrate, and lack of energy are all signs of:
    a. fear.
    b. confusion.
    c. depression.
    d. abuse.

32. When interviewing a patient who is extremely talkative, but is not providing you with the information you need, which of the following techniques might be useful in obtaining what you need?
    a. Ignore the patient.
    b. Ask the patient to stop talking and listen.
    c. Try using diversion tactics.
    d. Try using direct "yes" or "no" questions.

33. _____ and history taking are a significant portion of the patient interview.
    a. Dispatch information
    b. A rapid response time
    c. Establishing a rapport with the patient
    d. Professional appearance

34. During an interview with a patient in severe respiratory distress, you ask the patient to "nod yes or shake no" to answer your questions. This is an example of asking questions that are:
    a. direct.
    b. leading.
    c. patronizing.
    d. open-ended.

35. Which of the following is not considered part of a health history?
    a. religious beliefs
    b. career status
    c. daily living activities
    d. current vital signs

36. Information obtained from the patient or bystanders about the current event, including what led up to it, is called:
    a. chief complaint.
    b. focused history.
    c. signs and symptoms.
    d. positive feedback.

37. _____ is part of the communication process rather than a communication technique.
    a. Silence
    b. Encoding
    c. Listening
    d. Explanation

38. _____ may be found on necklaces, bracelets, and anklets and provide vital medical information such as a medical condition or reaction.
    a. Dog tags®
    b. Lucky charms®
    c. MedicAlert tags®
    d. Coils

39. Once you have arrived at the ED with a hearing-impaired patient, the _____ requires that the hospital provide a sign interpreter within 30 minutes of the patient's arrival.

    a. American's with Disabilities Act (ADA)
    b. Veteran's Administration (VA)
    c. Centers for Disease Control (CDC)
    d. American Sign Language (ASL) bill

40. When caring for a hearing-impaired patient, be sure to face the patient when you are speaking and to:

    a. speak very slowly.
    b. use a family member to communicate.
    c. exaggerate your speech.
    d. look to see if his hearing aid is on.

Exam #14 Answer Form

	A	B	C	D			A	B	C	D
1.	❏	❏	❏	❏		21.	❏	❏	❏	❏
2.	❏	❏	❏	❏		22.	❏	❏	❏	❏
3.	❏	❏	❏	❏		23.	❏	❏	❏	❏
4.	❏	❏	❏	❏		24.	❏	❏	❏	❏
5.	❏	❏	❏	❏		25.	❏	❏	❏	❏
6.	❏	❏	❏	❏		26.	❏	❏	❏	❏
7.	❏	❏	❏	❏		27.	❏	❏	❏	❏
8.	❏	❏	❏	❏		28.	❏	❏	❏	❏
9.	❏	❏	❏	❏		29.	❏	❏	❏	❏
10.	❏	❏	❏	❏		30.	❏	❏	❏	❏
11.	❏	❏	❏	❏		31.	❏	❏	❏	❏
12.	❏	❏	❏	❏		32.	❏	❏	❏	❏
13.	❏	❏	❏	❏		33.	❏	❏	❏	❏
14.	❏	❏	❏	❏		34.	❏	❏	❏	❏
15.	❏	❏	❏	❏		35.	❏	❏	❏	❏
16.	❏	❏	❏	❏		36.	❏	❏	❏	❏
17.	❏	❏	❏	❏		37.	❏	❏	❏	❏
18.	❏	❏	❏	❏		38.	❏	❏	❏	❏
19.	❏	❏	❏	❏		39.	❏	❏	❏	❏
20.	❏	❏	❏	❏		40.	❏	❏	❏	❏

Secondary Assessment: Medical Patient

1. The secondary assessment of the conscious medical patient is performed:
   a. immediately after the scene size-up has been performed.
   b. after the primary assessment has been completed.
   c. before the ABCs are managed.
   d. before the chief complaint has been attained.

2. The objective of the focused physical examination is to direct the assessment to:
   a. the patient's ABCs.
   b. gather a SAMPLE history.
   c. the patient's chief complaint.
   d. establish consent to treat the patient.

3. Your patient fell and possibly experienced a loss of consciousness while in the bathroom. She is alert and oriented when you perform your primary assessment, but she tells you that when she was on the floor she could not move or cry out for help. You suspect that the patient may have experienced a(n):
   a. TIA.
   b. ACS.
   c. hypertensive event.
   d. hypoglycemic event.

4. You have responded to a call for an unconscious female in the shopping mall. Security leads you to a department store restroom, where a conscious 45-year-old female is lying on the floor complaining of abdominal pain and nausea. How should you proceed?
   a. Begin a secondary assessment.
   b. Obtain a SAMPLE and focused history.
   c. Begin a focused physical exam of the abdomen.
   d. Determine if there is trauma associated with this event.

5. Obtaining the SAMPLE history of a medical patient will provide the paramedic with information about:
   a. a presumptive diagnosis.
   b. the need for a rapid physical exam.
   c. the events that preceded this episode.
   d. pertinent positive and negative findings.

6. While obtaining the focused history from a patient, the paramedic should gather a SAMPLE history, a history of the present illness (HPI), and:
   a. a list of the patient's possessions that she will be taking to the hospital.
   b. positive findings and pertinent negatives.
   c. a history of childhood vaccinations.
   d. the date of the patient's last tetanus shot.

7. A paramedic interviewing a patient has asked about chest pain associated with breathing, orthopnea, prolonged bed rest, and activity at onset. Based on these questions, what is most likely the patient's chief complaint?
   a. dizziness
   b. nausea and vomiting
   c. chest tightness
   d. difficulty breathing

8. For a patient with a chief complaint of difficulty breathing, the paramedic should assess lung sounds, perform pulse oximetry, and:
   a. orthostatic assessment.
   b. assess breath odors.
   c. look for peripheral edema.
   d. obtain a blood glucose reading.

9. The acronym AEIOU-TIPS is helpful to the paramedic when considering the causes of:
   a. chest pain.
   b. altered mental status.
   c. abdominal pain.
   d. shortness of breath.

10. While interviewing and performing the secondary assessment on an elderly patient, it is typical to discover:
    a. traumatic injury.
    b. shingles.
    c. concurrent medical problems.
    d. poisoning.

11. When a medical patient is discovered to be unconscious, the paramedic performs the primary assessment followed by the:
    a. rapid physical examination.
    b. focused history.
    c. reassesssment.
    d. SAMPLE history.

12. A 54-year-old male has shortness of breath and chest pain with deep inspiration. His skin color, temperature, and condition are pale, warm, and moist. Auscultation of the lungs reveals clear and dry sounds in all fields. Vitals are pulse of 100 bpm and slightly irregular, blood pressure of 130/68 mm Hg, and respiratory rate of 30 and labored. The paramedic begins treatment for this patient by providing high-flow oxygen and a(n):
    a. diuretic.
    b. nitrate.
    c. bronchodilator.
    d. analgesic.

13. A patient with respiratory distress has denied having chest pain, loss of consciousness, or a productive cough. These are all examples of:
    a. past medical history.
    b. pertinent positive findings.
    c. pertinent negative findings.
    d. events leading up to this episode.

14. The frequency of performing reassessments is usually based on:
    a. medical versus trauma patient.
    b. good clinical judgment and experience.
    c. age of patient.
    d. past medical history.

15. During the patient interview, a patient admitted to having a fever and productive cough for 2 days in addition to a chief complaint of chest pain. This information, aside from the chief complaint, is referred to as:
    a. the SAMPLE history.
    b. provocation.
    c. associated signs and symptoms.
    d. stimulus.

16. A 24-year-old male has a chief complaint of dizziness, but only when he moves his head. He also has nausea, and his vital signs are stable. The only other significant history is that of a recent head cold that lasted several days. On which of the following areas should the paramedic focus the exam?
    a. cardiac
    b. respiratory
    c. neurologic
    d. behavioral

17. During the typical time a paramedic has patient contact, she must attempt to quickly establish a positive rapport with the patient in order to:
    a. make a patient transport decision.
    b. demonstrate professionalism to the patient.
    c. gain trust and cooperation from the patient.
    d. identify immediate life-threatening conditions.

18. The secondary assessment of a patient having an allergic reaction includes assessing the face and airway for swelling, listening to lung sounds, and:
    a. examining the body for urticaria.
    b. smelling the breath for unusual odor.
    c. asking about excessive thirst or hunger.
    d. asking about blood in the urine or stool.

19. A 78-year-old female is complaining of weakness, dizziness, and nausea. She denies having chest pain or shortness of breath and is not diabetic. Which of the following body systems should the paramedic focus on first?
    a. gastrointestinal
    b. genitourinary
    c. cardiac
    d. neurologic

20. The paramedic should focus the physical examination on:
    a. the scene size-up and baseline vital signs.
    b. priority dispatch, scene size-up, and the presence of a DNAR.
    c. findings in the primary assessment and absence of a DNAR.
    d. chief complaint and findings in the primary assessment.

21. In many cases, making a precise diagnosis in the field is difficult; therefore, the paramedic should strive to recognize emergent signs and symptoms and then:
    a. begin transport and initiate treatment en route.
    b. stabilize and transport.
    c. transport to the nearest facility.
    d. contact medical control and transport.

22. During the primary assessment of an adult patient complaining of chest tightness, weakness, and light-headedness, you find that he is pale and hypotensive. When you apply oxygen and lay him down, you feel that his skin is warm and dry. As your partner obtains vital signs, you begin to focus your physical exam in which direction?

    a. neurologic

    b. pulmonary

    c. abdominal

    d. cardiothoracic

23. In reference to question 22, as part of the focused physical exam the paramedic would:

    a. assess speech and facial symmetry.

    b. assess lung sounds and color of sputum.

    c. auscultate and palpate the abdomen.

    d. obtain an ECG and pulse quality.

24. When obtaining information about a presenting condition that is causing pain or discomfort for a patient, which of the following acronyms is commonly used by EMS providers?

    a. OPQRST

    b. SAMPLE

    c. DCAP-BTLS

    d. AEIOU-TIPS

25. A paramedic is assessing a patient who has had a loss of bowel control, decreased sensation in the legs bilaterally, and impaired coordination. Based on these problems, for what type of medical problem might this patient be further evaluated?

    a. cardiac

    b. neurologic

    c. behavioral disorder

    d. respiratory

26. A paramedic is assessing a patient who has a chief complaint of headache, nausea, and dizziness. The focused history revealed that the patient has had these symptoms for several days, and that the spouse and children have had similar complaints (but less severe). From the information obtained in the focused history, the paramedic should consider these to be associated symptoms of:

    a. food poisoning.

    b. possible CO poisoning.

    c. infestation in the home.

    d. family history of mental disorders.

27. When assessing a patient, the mnemonic DCAP-BTLS is used to help the paramedic remember to look for specific information about the patient's:

    a. skin.

    b. mental status.

    c. respiratory effort.

    d. trauma status.

28. In which of the following cases would the paramedic most likely perform a rapid physical examination?

    a. an unresponsive 40-year-old male

    b. a 55-year-old female with crushing chest pain

    c. an 18-month-old who is postictal after a seizure and crying

    d. a 16-year-old experiencing an acute asthma attack

29. The secondary assessment of an unconscious patient with no signs of traumatic injury begins with:

    a. looking for medical ID tags or devices.

    b. obtaining a history from any bystanders.

    c. a rapid assessment of the entire body.

    d. vitals signs and blood glucose reading.

30. When a paramedic assesses a patient for weakness or the ability of the patient to move a body part, which focused assessment is she making?

    a. behavioral

    b. neurologic

    c. head-to-toe

    d. rapid physical exam

31. Your patient has a chief compliant of severe nausea and vomiting. As you proceed to ask the patient more questions regarding his chief complaint, which of the following statements should you consider?

    a. Vomiting is always preceded by nausea.

    b. The vomiting reflex is located in the cerebral cortex.

    c. Intracranial pressure can stimulate the vomiting reflex.

    d. Nausea and vomiting are associated with very few disorders.

32. The difference between true vertigo and dizziness is that:

    a. vertigo is a vestibular disorder.

    b. there is no difference.

    c. only adults experience vertigo.

    d. vertigo is not associated with nausea.

33. The patient is complaining of lower-back pain and dysuria. Which of the following body systems should the paramedic focus on first?
    a. gastrointestinal
    b. genitourinary
    c. cardiac
    d. neurologic

34. During your secondary assessment of a cardiac patient, you review his medication list and note that he takes a stool softener. The patient denies having any stomach problems. So, why would he have this medication?
    a. to reduce vagal stimulation
    b. he has an enlarged prostate
    c. to prevent diverticulosis
    d. to prevent diverticulitis

35. When conducting a secondary assessment on a young adult and you find orthostatic changes with no obvious reason, the most likely cause is:
    a. internal bleeding.
    b. prolonged bed rest.
    c. the patient is a diabetic.
    d. the patient is taking a blood thinner.

36. In the unconscious medical patient, vitals signs should be obtained:
    a. after the rapid physical exam.
    b. prior to the primary assessment.
    c. before the rapid physical exam.
    d. after gathering a PMHx from family or bystanders.

37. You respond to a residence for a 29-year-old male who fell in the bathroom. He has a laceration on the back of his head with active bleeding. His wife tells you that he was shaving when she heard him fall, and that he was unconscious for about 90 seconds. The first treatment step is to:
    a. take C-spine precautions.
    b. stop the bleeding.
    c. administer oxygen.
    d. obtaining a blood glucose reading.

38. In reference to question 37, the patient denies having chest pain or shortness of breath, but states that he felt dizzy just before passing out. The most likely cause of the fall may be from what type of syncope?
    a. pharmacologic
    b. neurologic
    c. vasovagal
    d. respiratory

39. When considering the reason why your patient "passed out," you recall that _____ is a cause of noncardiac syncope.
    a. angina
    b. aortic stenosis
    c. vasovagal stimulation
    d. Stokes–Adams syndrome

40. When considering all the medications that could cause a patient to "pass out," remember that _____ is the most common drug classification that causes syncope.
    a. beta-blocker
    b. cold medication
    c. antacid
    d. antibiotic

41. An alert patient is complaining of a severe headache after experiencing a seizure for the first time. No apparent trauma is visible from the seizure, pulse is 80 and regular, and respirations are 20 and nonlabored. The patient stated that he checked his sugar 30 minutes ago, and the blood sugar was 110 mg/dl. In continuing with the focused history and physical examination, what should the paramedic consider obtaining next?
    a. repeat blood glucose
    b. ECG
    c. breath sounds
    d. blood pressure

42. Vomiting, in itself, is not a medical diagnosis; however, prolonged or frequent vomiting can lead to serious complications such as:
    a. GI bleeding.
    b. limbic system disorders.
    c. cardiac stress.
    d. endogenous infections.

43. The secondary assessment of the patient with a neurological problem includes examining for facial drop, unilateral weakness, evidence of a seizure or loss of consciousness, and:
    a. sacral edema.
    b. peripheral edema.
    c. speech problems.
    d. jugular vein distention.

44. One of the most common rooms in the home in which a patient becomes ill or injured is the:
    a. bathroom.
    b. garage.
    c. basement.
    d. attic.

45. During the secondary assessment of a patient complaining of "almost passing out," the paramedic identifies a life-threatening condition. Which of the following did the paramedic most likely identify?

    a. nystagmus
    b. blood sugar of 80 mg/dl
    c. heart block
    d. orthostatic changes

46. When performing a rapid physical exam on an unconscious medical patient, the paramedic should:

    a. assess the pupils first.
    b. assess the chest first and back last.
    c. assess the patient from head to toe.
    d. obtain an ECG, pulse oximetry, and blood glucose reading.

47. When assessing a patient who had experienced a syncope, the paramedic should consider the most common causes of syncope are vasovagal faint, positional orthostatic hypotension, and:

    a. cardiac dysrhythmias.
    b. micturition.
    c. neurologic induced.
    d. dehydration.

48. During the secondary assessment of a patient complaining of generalized weakness, you learn that the patient has been urinating excessively without pain or blood in the urine and has been drinking water in excess but is always thirsty. Which exam should the paramedic now focus on?

    a. GI/GU
    b. endocrine
    c. neurologic
    d. cardiothoracic

49. Orthostatic vital signs are not always significant or reliable, because most people will normally have subtle vital sign changes when going from a supine or sitting position to a standing position. A more significant finding is:

    a. an abnormal pulse oximetry reading.
    b. positional symptoms.
    c. the age of the patient.
    d. the presence of edema.

50. After interviewing a patient with a chief complaint of chest pain that increases with movement and palpation of the chest, the paramedic obtained a history that included smoking, lack of exercise, and a family history of hypertension. What should the paramedic focus on during the physical exam?

    a. vital signs
    b. recent chest trauma
    c. cardiothoracic
    d. position of the patient

Exam #15 Answer Form

	A	B	C	D			A	B	C	D
1.	❏	❏	❏	❏		26.	❏	❏	❏	❏
2.	❏	❏	❏	❏		27.	❏	❏	❏	❏
3.	❏	❏	❏	❏		28.	❏	❏	❏	❏
4.	❏	❏	❏	❏		29.	❏	❏	❏	❏
5.	❏	❏	❏	❏		30.	❏	❏	❏	❏
6.	❏	❏	❏	❏		31.	❏	❏	❏	❏
7.	❏	❏	❏	❏		32.	❏	❏	❏	❏
8.	❏	❏	❏	❏		33.	❏	❏	❏	❏
9.	❏	❏	❏	❏		34.	❏	❏	❏	❏
10.	❏	❏	❏	❏		35.	❏	❏	❏	❏
11.	❏	❏	❏	❏		36.	❏	❏	❏	❏
12.	❏	❏	❏	❏		37.	❏	❏	❏	❏
13.	❏	❏	❏	❏		38.	❏	❏	❏	❏
14.	❏	❏	❏	❏		39.	❏	❏	❏	❏
15.	❏	❏	❏	❏		40.	❏	❏	❏	❏
16.	❏	❏	❏	❏		41.	❏	❏	❏	❏
17.	❏	❏	❏	❏		42.	❏	❏	❏	❏
18.	❏	❏	❏	❏		43.	❏	❏	❏	❏
19.	❏	❏	❏	❏		44.	❏	❏	❏	❏
20.	❏	❏	❏	❏		45.	❏	❏	❏	❏
21.	❏	❏	❏	❏		46.	❏	❏	❏	❏
22.	❏	❏	❏	❏		47.	❏	❏	❏	❏
23.	❏	❏	❏	❏		48.	❏	❏	❏	❏
24.	❏	❏	❏	❏		49.	❏	❏	❏	❏
25.	❏	❏	❏	❏		50.	❏	❏	❏	❏

CHAPTER 16

Secondary Assessment: Trauma Patient

1. An example of a life-threatening situation that requires immediate intervention is:
   a. any auto–pedestrian collision.
   b. any burn injury.
   c. an injury that affects the ABCs.
   d. all motorcycle collisions.

2. Critical trauma patients have the best chance for survival if they can be stabilized in a surgical suite within _____ of the onset of injury.
   a. 1 hour
   b. 90 minutes
   c. 2 hours
   d. 4 hours

3. The maximum time the paramedic should spend on scene with a critical trauma patient, barring any lengthy extrication, is _____ minutes.
   a. 10
   b. 15
   c. 20
   d. 30

4. For the noncritical trauma patient, the concerns are similar to the critical trauma patient; however, _____ may not be required.
   a. determining the mechanism of injury (MOI)
   b. the primary assessment
   c. assessment of the ABCs
   d. rapid transport

5. A thorough evaluation of the _____ by the paramedic can help predict injuries that may or may not be obvious at the first impression.
   a. patient's ABCs
   b. MOI
   c. patient's mental status
   d. vital signs

6. _____ is the abbreviation used to remember what is assessed about the patient's soft tissues.
   a. BTLS
   b. DCAP-BTLS
   c. GCS
   d. MOI

7. On which of the following patients would it be most appropriate for the paramedic to perform the secondary assessment en route to the hospital rather than on the scene?
   a. a 28-year-old female complaining of neck pain due a low-speed rear-end motor vehicle collision
   b. a 36-year-old male who required decontamination after falling into chlorine containers and breaking his ankle
   c. a 32-year-old female at 34 weeks' gestation complaining of abdominal cramping after falling in her home
   d. a 43-year-old male inmate at a correctional facility with facial injuries and neck pain

8. When should transport of the critical trauma patient be delayed to wait for ALS to arrive?
   a. when the patient is conscious
   b. only when the patient is fully immobilized
   c. when the patient needs to be intubated using medications
   d. transportation should not be delayed to wait for ALS to arrive

9. The transportation decision is usually made after the scene assessment for MOI and the _____ have been completed.
   a. cervical collar application
   b. primary assessment
   c. radio report
   d. immobilization

10. You are assessing a trauma patient for a possible cervical injury; which of the following criteria would you give the most consideration when deciding to apply a cervical immobilization collar?
    a. the MOI
    b. the age of the patient
    c. the patient denies neck pain
    d. the patient had a loss of consciousness

11. How often should the reassessment of the noncritical trauma patient be repeated?
    a. every 5 minutes
    b. every 15 minutes
    c. only when a change in mental status is noted
    d. only when the patient becomes critical

12. A level _____ trauma center may be a clinic rather than a hospital where the goal is to provide initial stabilization of the patient and then transfer to a higher-level trauma center.
    a. I
    b. II
    c. III
    d. IV

13. A level _____ trauma center is a regional center that serves as a leader in trauma care for a specific geographic area.
    a. I
    b. II
    c. III
    d. IV

14. Which one of the following patients should be transported to the nearest hospital even if it is not a level I trauma center?
    a. severe burns
    b. pediatric trauma
    c. pregnant trauma patient
    d. traumatic cardiac arrest

15. You are at the scene with a trauma patient who was involved in an MVC with a lengthy extrication. The patient is a conscious but confused 20-year-old male who was unconscious when you first arrived. The airway is open and he is breathing adequately, and he has a distal pulse that is 100/regular. His skin is pale, warm, and dry, and his BP is 150/100 mmHg. Both lower legs are fractured, and the left is an open fracture. Transport to the trauma center takes 45 minutes. Which of the following criteria would you use to request aeromedical transport for this patient?
    a. the fractures
    b. the transport time
    c. the age of the patient
    d. the loss of consciousness

16. The _____ is a numeric grading system that combines the GCS and measurements of cardiopulmonary function as a gauge of the severity of injury and a predictor of survival after blunt injury to the head.
    a. Cincinnati score
    b. trauma score
    c. CUPS
    d. traumatic brain injury scale

17. If a patient fell from a height of 20 feet and landed feet first, which of the following injuries could you predict the patient might have?
    a. fractures of the heels, ankles, and hips
    b. fractures of the heels, ankles, and clavicles
    c. lower-extremity fractures and head injury
    d. lower- and upper-extremity fractures

18. Which of the following steps cannot be skipped or omitted during the care of a critical trauma patient?
    a. full spinal immobilization
    b. short board spinal immobilization
    c. bleeding control for venous bleeding
    d. hand fracture immobilization

19. Trauma is the number one killer of _____ in the United States.
    a. men
    b. women
    c. children
    d. geriatrics

20. Special consideration for assessment of the elderly trauma patient includes an understanding that decreased:
    a. brain mass lessens the risk for brain injury.
    b. body fat minimizes the body's protection (padding) against traumatic injury.
    c. stroke volume in the elderly helps to slow bleeding associated with traumatic injury.
    d. calcification of cartilage can increase pain tolerance, and it may take longer for the patient to develop pain when injury is present.

21. _____ is the most common cause of death in children.
    a. Spinal cord injury
    b. Head injury
    c. Abdominal trauma
    d. Chest trauma

22. The most common MOI in children is:
    a. falls.
    b. bicycle accidents.
    c. MVC.
    d. auto–pedestrian collisions.

23. Special consideration for assessment of the pediatric trauma patient includes an understanding that:

 a. the presence of rib fractures is a critical finding.

 b. the airway is less prone to obstruction than adults.

 c. growth plate injuries are rare and, when present, increase the risk of mortality.

 d. the abdomen is large and well padded, decreasing the risk of internal injuries.

24. When caring for the pregnant trauma patient, the paramedic must consider that pregnancy slows peristalsis, which increases the risk of:

 a. abdominal trauma.

 b. vomiting.

 c. hypotension.

 d. abruptio placenta.

25. In the third trimester pregnant trauma patient, a blood loss of _____ can occur before any signs of shock begin to develop.

 a. 10 percent

 b. 20 percent

 c. 30 percent

 d. 40 percent

26. When the MOI is a rapid, head-first impact, the paramedic must consider the possibility of primary injuries to the cranium, cervical spine, and:

 a. aorta.

 b. trachea.

 c. ribs.

 d. sternum.

27. You are assessing an unrestrained driver of a vehicle whose front end struck a tree. There is a foot of intrusion into the engine compartment, and the patient was found down and under the steering column. What predictable injury pattern is associated with this type of collision?

 a. chest and abdomen

 b. face, neck, and chest

 c. spine, knee, and lower legs

 d. head, humerus, ribs, and pelvis

28. As you assess a patient involved in an MVC, which of the following items that you observed as part of the scene size-up leads you to suspect underlying injuries to the patient?

 a. flat tires

 b. no air bag deployment

 c. broken steering wheel

 d. intrusion into the engine compartment

29. Striking one side of the head often causes blunt trauma to the brain in the area that was struck as well as the opposite area of the brain. What type of injury is this called?

 a. contra coup

 b. coup-contracoup

 c. traumatic brain ischemia

 d. contra coup constriction

30. _____ is an injury pattern in children, when struck by a vehicle, involving the legs, chest, and head.

 a. Waddell's triad

 b. SCIWORA

 c. Crushing

 d. Whipple's triad

31. The momentary acceleration of tissue laterally away from the projectile tract of a bullet in the body, which explains why exit wounds are usually larger than entrance wounds, is called:

 a. tumble.

 b. fragmentation.

 c. profile.

 d. cavitation.

32. It is estimated that the chance of a spinal injury increases up to _____ times by being ejected from a vehicle while not wearing a seat belt.

 a. 30

 b. 300

 c. 1,300

 d. 3,000

33. Striking the "temples" of the cranium with a blunt object can cause the middle meningeal artery to bleed and a(n) _____ to develop.

 a. neoplasm

 b. leak of CSF in the ears

 c. subdural hematoma

 d. epidural hematoma

34. Secondary injuries from an MVC, where the driver went up and over the steering column/dash, include:

 a. face and head.

 b. head and neck.

 c. chest and abdomen.

 d. cervical spine.

35. You are caring for a critical trauma patient. Which of the following can be used to move the patient safely and quickly to minimize scene time?

 a. long backboard

 b. Kendrick extrication device (KED)

 c. short backboard

 d. blanket

36. You have responded to a motorcycle crash where police are on scene and report that the driver denied any injury after crashing but is acting strange. When you approach the patient he is uncooperative and quarrelsome. There are no signs that he has been drinking. What do you suspect is causing the patient to act the way he is?

    a. The patient has something to hide.

    b. The patient has an altered mental status.

    c. The patient is angry because his bike is damaged.

    d. The patient is uninjured and it is his normal disposition.

37. Criteria for the designated transportation destination of trauma patients for a specific EMS agency can usually be found in:

    a. regional protocols.

    b. EMT and paramedic texts.

    c. hospital rules.

    d. state law.

38. Which of the following unique physiologic responses do children have to shock trauma?

    a. Children in shock decompensate slower than adults.

    b. Children in shock appear worse than they actually are.

    c. Children compensate for shock better than adults in late shock.

    d. Children compensate for shock better than adults in early shock.

39. Your patient is a 5-year-old female who was struck by a car backing out of a driveway while she was riding her bike. The child is wearing a helmet, which is cracked. She is unconscious and breathing abnormally. What action(s) must be completed first?

    a. Suction the airway.

    b. Remove the helmet.

    c. Perform a rapid trauma exam.

    d. Immobilize the C-spine and open the airway.

40. You are assessing an alert 84-year-old female who fell backwards and struck her head on the way to the bathroom in the middle of the night. Staff called EMS when they heard her call for help. She states she lost her balance and denies losing consciousness. She complains of pain on the back of her head and neck pain. Her vital signs are skin warm and dry, respiratory rate 18/nonlabored, pulse rate 58 regular, and BP 140/80 mmHg. What information must be obtained to help you determine the priority for this patient?

    a. the medication list

    b. has the patient fallen before and, if so, when

    c. ECG, pulse oximetry, and blood glucose readings

    d. is the patient nauseous

41. You are assessing a belted passenger involved in a moderate-speed MVC. Initially, the patient had no complaint of injury or pain. Twenty minutes after the collision, the patient states that he feels dizzy, and he looks pale and diaphoretic. What condition do you suspect the patient has?

    a. potential spinal injury

    b. head injury

    c. intra-abdominal hemorrhage

    d. neurogenic shock

42. While responding to a call for a self-inflicted GSW, dispatch advises that the injury was to the head and face as reported by police. What do you anticipate will be the priority of care for this patient?

    a. blood loss

    b. rapid transport

    c. complicated airway

    d. spinal immobilization

43. A patient who was burned in a house fire sustained multiple injuries. Which of the following is the primary concern for the paramedic?

    a. third-degree burns on both hands

    b. first- and second-degree burns on the face and neck

    c. clothing charred into the chest and back

    d. wheezing present with a hoarse voice

44. After responding to the scene of a diving accident in a backyard pool, you are treating a male patient who is unable to move any part of his body below the neck. You have him fully immobilized and are ready for transport. Where should you take him?

    a. the nearest hospital

    b. level I trauma center

    c. level II trauma center

    d. level III trauma center

45. While en route to the hospital with the patient from question 44, you determine that he has sensation to the shoulders but none below. Where do you suspect the spinal injury is?

    a. C1 and C2

    b. C3 and C4

    c. C6 and C7

    d. T1 and T2

Exam #16 Answer Form

	A	B	C	D		A	B	C	D
1.	❏	❏	❏	❏	24.	❏	❏	❏	❏
2.	❏	❏	❏	❏	25.	❏	❏	❏	❏
3.	❏	❏	❏	❏	26.	❏	❏	❏	❏
4.	❏	❏	❏	❏	27.	❏	❏	❏	❏
5.	❏	❏	❏	❏	28.	❏	❏	❏	❏
6.	❏	❏	❏	❏	29.	❏	❏	❏	❏
7.	❏	❏	❏	❏	30.	❏	❏	❏	❏
8.	❏	❏	❏	❏	31.	❏	❏	❏	❏
9.	❏	❏	❏	❏	32.	❏	❏	❏	❏
10.	❏	❏	❏	❏	33.	❏	❏	❏	❏
11.	❏	❏	❏	❏	34.	❏	❏	❏	❏
12.	❏	❏	❏	❏	35.	❏	❏	❏	❏
13.	❏	❏	❏	❏	36.	❏	❏	❏	❏
14.	❏	❏	❏	❏	37.	❏	❏	❏	❏
15.	❏	❏	❏	❏	38.	❏	❏	❏	❏
16.	❏	❏	❏	❏	39.	❏	❏	❏	❏
17.	❏	❏	❏	❏	40.	❏	❏	❏	❏
18.	❏	❏	❏	❏	41.	❏	❏	❏	❏
19.	❏	❏	❏	❏	42.	❏	❏	❏	❏
20.	❏	❏	❏	❏	43.	❏	❏	❏	❏
21.	❏	❏	❏	❏	44.	❏	❏	❏	❏
22.	❏	❏	❏	❏	45.	❏	❏	❏	❏
23.	❏	❏	❏	❏					

Monitoring Devices and Vital Signs

1. You are assessing a 25-year-old male adult with a chief complaint of chest pain for the past 20 minutes. Which of the following would not be a routine vital sign to take on this patient with this complaint?
   a. pulse rate
   b. respiration rate
   c. blood sugar level
   d. blood pressure

2. Of the following pulse rates, which would be the most appropriate for a 50-year-old female patient?
   a. 50 to 60 bpm
   b. 65 to 75 bpm
   c. 95 to 105 bpm
   d. 110 to 120 bpm

3. Of the following respiration rates, which would be most appropriate for a 65-year-old male patient found sitting on the couch, alert, and in little distress?
   a. 12 per minute
   b. 18 per minute
   c. 26 per minute
   d. 34 per minute

4. If you have not memorized all the vital sign rates for each age group, a useful resource to use with small children would be to:
   a. carry the textbook in your ambulance.
   b. ask the family what the normal vital signs should be.
   c. utilize a length-based tape to determine.
   d. double the normal adult rates for a child.

5. What is the expected body temperature of an adult male patient complaining of chills?
   a. 85°F
   b. 99°F
   c. 102°F
   d. 106°F

6. When a patient has a pulse rate over 100 bpm, this is called:
   a. bradycardia.
   b. a normal pulse.
   c. hypertension.
   d. tachycardia.

7. When a patient has a systolic BP of 146 mmHg, this is referred to as:
   a. hypotension.
   b. tachycardia.
   c. hypertension.
   d. systolic murmur.

8. An alert 35-year-old male patient who is in respiratory distress is likely to have a breathing rate of:
   a. 12 times a minute.
   b. 16 times a minute.
   c. 18 times a minute.
   d. 28 times a minute.

9. An $EtCO_2$ monitoring device measures the amount of _____ during each breath at the end of _____.
   a. carbon dioxide; inspiration
   b. carbon monoxide; inspiration
   c. carbon dioxide; exhalation
   d. carbon monoxide; exhalation

10. In which of the following patients would the pulse oximetry reading be most useful to the paramedic?
    a. SpO_2 98% in a 35-year-old male complaining of weakness and who has a history of anemia
    b. SpO_2 88% in a 4-year-old having an asthma attack
    c. SpO_2 96% in a 62-year-old female complaining of exertional dyspnea and who has a history of COPD
    d. SpO_2 100% in a 22-year-old male who just attempted suicide by CO exposure

11. The method of obtaining a blood pressure by palpation is often used by the paramedic because:
    a. ambient noise is too loud to hear pulse sounds.
    b. the paramedic often does not carry a stethoscope.
    c. taking the BP by auscultation takes too long.
    d. a trained provider is not available to take it.

12. While taking a blood pressure, the sounds heard with a stethoscope that indicate the systolic and diastolic readings are called:
    a. pulse pressures.
    b. pulsus paradoxus.
    c. apical pulse.
    d. Korotkoff sounds.

13. When checking for the pulse on an unconscious patient, the paramedic should assess the _____ pulse.
    a. radial
    b. brachial
    c. carotid
    d. femoral

14. When checking for the pulse on an alert patient, the paramedic should assess the _____ pulse.
    a. radial
    b. brachial
    c. carotid
    d. femoral

15. When a patient has rapid respirations, this is referred to as:
    a. apnea.
    b. hypernea.
    c. tackypnea.
    d. eupnea.

16. For a child who is of preschool age (3 to 6 years), a normal heart rate range would include:
    a. 70 bpm.
    b. 90 bpm.
    c. 150 bpm.
    d. 160 bpm.

17. For a child who is of toddler age (1 to 3 years), a normal heart rate range would include:
    a. 80 bpm.
    b. 100 bpm.
    c. 155 bpm.
    d. 165 bpm.

18. For child of school age (6 to 12 years), a normal systolic BP range would include:
    a. 60 mm Hg.
    b. 70 mm Hg.
    c. 110 mm Hg.
    d. 120 mm Hg.

19. When assessing the skin of a patient, you locate patchy skin discoloration due to vasoconstriction or vasodilation. This is called:
    a. cyanosis.
    b. pallor.
    c. ashen.
    d. mottling.

20. Which monitoring device should be used for all patients presenting with cardiac-related signs and symptoms?
    a. noninvasive BP
    b. blood glucose monitoring
    c. continuous ECG monitoring
    d. waveform capnography

21. Of the following reasons, which is a key reason for 12-lead ECG acquisition by the paramedic in the field?
    a. It can shorten the door-to-treatment interval for cardiac patients.
    b. It can rule out life-threatening angina.
    c. It can help determine if the patient will survive the transport to the hospital.
    d. It can help to increase the field time of the patient being managed.

22. When applying the 12-lead ECG in the field, where should V3 be placed on the patient's chest?
    a. fourth intercostal space at the right sternal border
    b. midaxillary line on the same horizontal plane as V4
    c. equidistant between V2 and V4
    d. anterior axillary line on the same horizontal plane as V4

23. When applying the 12-lead ECG in the field, where should V4 be placed on the patient's chest?
    a. fourth intercostal space at the left sternal border
    b. fifth intercostal space in left midclavicular line
    c. midaxillary line on the same horizontal plane as V5
    d. equidistant between V3 and V6

24. Which device is the standard for prehospital confirmation and monitoring of endotracheal tube placement?
    a. colorimetric CO_2 detector
    b. EZ-IV device
    c. waveform capnography device
    d. the tube-check® device

25. When the decision is made to assess the blood of a patient who has an altered mental status with a glucometer, which reading would indicate the need for dextrose administration in the field?
    a. 90 g/dl
    b. 70 g/dl
    c. 60 mg/L
    d. 180 units/kg

26. Each of the following are examples of monitoring devices used in the field, *except*:
    a. CO monitor.
    b. pulse oximeter.
    c. capnography.
    d. ECG calipers.

27. If you are assessing and managing a patient with a suspected stroke, which two monitoring devices should be used in addition to monitoring the BP?
    a. pulse oximeter and cardiac enzymes
    b. 12-lead ECG and glucometer
    c. pH and enzymes
    d. ICP and MAP

28. When assessing a patient who has been outdoors in the cold rain without the appropriate clothing, you find he is severely shivering. If you took his body temperature, what would be the most likely temperature?
    a. 102.6°F
    b. 98.6°F
    c. 95°F
    d. 88°F

29. On an ECG, a normal QRS complex should be:
    a. 0.12 to 0.20 seconds.
    b. less than or equal to 0.12 seconds.
    c. less than or equal to 0.04 seconds.
    d. 0.36 to 0.44 seconds.

30. On an ECG, a normal PR interval should be:
    a. 0.12 to 0.20 seconds.
    b. less than or equal to 0.12 seconds.
    c. less than or equal to 0.04 seconds.
    d. 0.36 to 0.44 seconds.

Exam #17 Answer Form

	A	B	C	D		A	B	C	D
1.	❏	❏	❏	❏	16.	❏	❏	❏	❏
2.	❏	❏	❏	❏	17.	❏	❏	❏	❏
3.	❏	❏	❏	❏	18.	❏	❏	❏	❏
4.	❏	❏	❏	❏	19.	❏	❏	❏	❏
5.	❏	❏	❏	❏	20.	❏	❏	❏	❏
6.	❏	❏	❏	❏	21.	❏	❏	❏	❏
7.	❏	❏	❏	❏	22.	❏	❏	❏	❏
8.	❏	❏	❏	❏	23.	❏	❏	❏	❏
9.	❏	❏	❏	❏	24.	❏	❏	❏	❏
10.	❏	❏	❏	❏	25.	❏	❏	❏	❏
11.	❏	❏	❏	❏	26.	❏	❏	❏	❏
12.	❏	❏	❏	❏	27.	❏	❏	❏	❏
13.	❏	❏	❏	❏	28.	❏	❏	❏	❏
14.	❏	❏	❏	❏	29.	❏	❏	❏	❏
15.	❏	❏	❏	❏	30.	❏	❏	❏	❏

CHAPTER

18

Reassessment and Clinical Decision Making

1. Which statement is most accurate about reassessing the patient prior to arriving at the hospital?
   a. Sometimes there is not enough time to reassess the patient.
   b. Reassessing the patient will correct any life-threatening conditions.
   c. Trending will help the paramedic identify changes in the patient's condition.
   d. The patient care report cannot be completed without the information of the reassessment.

2. The hormonal "fight or flight" response to stress can affect the paramedic in which of the following ways?
   a. increased concentration
   b. improved muscular strength
   c. decreased visual senses
   d. improved critical thinking

3. Lights and sirens, pagers, phones, and traffic are all examples of:
   a. stimulants that improve critical thinking.
   b. stimulants of the "fight or flight" response for paramedics.
   c. distractions in the standard approach to patient care.
   d. distractions for patients, which provide structure for the paramedic.

4. Which of the following factors is most likely to alter the reassessment in an unstable patient?
   a. short transport time
   b. the patient's gender
   c. an obvious injury pattern
   d. the patient's chief complaint

5. Which of the following statements about repeating the reassessment is most correct?
   a. Reassessment should only be repeated by a paramedic for critical patients.
   b. Reassessment should be repeated every 10 minutes for the critical trauma patient.
   c. Reassessment should be repeated every 10 minutes for the noncritical trauma patient.
   d. The time interval for reassessing the critical trauma patient is the same for the critical medical patient.

6. _____ is the process of obtaining a baseline assessment and then repeating the assessment for comparison.
   a. Trending
   b. Palpation
   c. Pairing off
   d. Serial processing

7. During the management of the patient en route to the hospital, the early indicators of deterioration of a patient are often:
   a. subtle changes in the patient's blood pressure.
   b. subtle changes in the patient's mental status.
   c. changes in skin color.
   d. changes in the lung sounds.

8. Which of the following statements about measurements or observations obtained during management of the patient is most accurate?
   a. Isolated measurements are generally less helpful than changes over time.
   b. Isolated observations are significantly more helpful than acute changes over time.
   c. Treatment protocols are specifically designed for patients with acute changes.
   d. Treatment protocols help the paramedic to identify deterioration of a patient's mental status.

9. The cornerstone of being an effective paramedic is having the ability to:

a. reassess the patient on a bumpy street.

b. avoid conflict with family members.

c. drive all types of emergency vehicles.

d. think and work under pressure.

10. One of the essential concepts of clinical decision making is:

a. being a mentor to an EMT student.

b. evaluating and processing information.

c. scrutinizing the actions of the emergency medical responders.

d. gathering the patient's belongings for the transport.

11. You are treating a 64-year-old female with an acute onset of severe dyspnea. She is developing chest pressure while you are assessing her. You have given her oxygen, aspirin, and started an IV. Her respiratory rate is 28, shallow, and labored; pulse rate is 130, with sinus tachycardia and depressed T wave in aVL and V2; BP is 98/58 mmHg. After 5 minutes, her symptoms have not improved and her BP is now 72/44 mmHg, so you lay her down and raise her legs. What action(s) would you apply before reassessing her again?

a. get her insurance information

b. interpret the response to the initial treatment

c. collect more history and process the information

d. start a dopamine drip and reassess the blood pressure

12. Which of the following is a major difference between patient care in the out-of-hospital setting and inhospital setting?

a. Patients open up more to the ED staff than they do to paramedics.

b. The hospital is a relatively controlled environment.

c. Paramedics can perform skills that nurses cannot.

d. Reassessment is a different skill in the hospital.

13. You are treating a patient in cardiogenic shock and have hung a dopamine (Intropin) drip. After running the drip for a few minutes, what do you want to reassess?

a. lung sounds

b. repeat the 12 lead ECG

c. the patient's blood pressure

d. level of discomfort

14. You are treating a 52-year-old male patient with a complaint of chest pain of severity 8/10 that radiates down the left arm. Vital signs are respiratory rate of 22/nonlabored, pulse rate of 68/irregular, BP of 124/70 mmHg, SpO_2 of 100%, and skin CTC is pale and moist. You have provided oxygen, administered aspirin and nitroglycerin, established an IV, and obtained a 12 lead ECG. You are now ready to transport. Which of the following aspects is most valuable to you when you reassess the patient?

a. repeating the ECG

b. the patient's blood pressure

c. the patient's level of discomfort

d. the patient's oxygen saturation

15. One of the fundamental elements of critical thinking for the paramedic working in the out-of-hospital setting is:

a. improving reflexes and muscular strength.

b. avoiding distractions that impair critical thinking.

c. following written protocols and never utilizing online medical control.

d. achieving and maintaining an adequate body of medical knowledge.

16. You are assessing a patient having moderate to severe difficulty breathing. She is a smoker with a productive cough, has a history of COPD and CHF, and recently finished a script of antibiotics for a respiratory infection. She has decreased breath sounds in the bases and wheezing in the apices. Her skin is very warm and dry, respiratory rate is 28/labored, pulse is 112/irregular, BP 170/100 mmHg, and SpO_2 92%. You give her a treatment of nebulized bronchodilator. What action(s) should be completed next?

a. Assess for JVD, peripheral edema, and start an IV.

b. Determine whether there is a DNR and/or healthcare proxy.

c. Obtain a medication history and set up your CPAP equipment.

d. Prepare to intubate as the patient is likely to deteriorate to respiratory arrest.

17. During a call for an allergic reaction, you realize that you have forgotten the new standing order dose for Benadryl®. Which of the following is the most appropriate action?

a. Use the old standing order dose.

b. Guess the dose, because it is too embarrassing to ask medical control.

c. Look up the correct dose in your protocols.

d. Just give the epinephrine and say that you are out of Benadryl®.

18. _____ is one of the fundamental elements of critical thinking for the paramedic.
    a. Learning a second language
    b. Focusing on one task at a time
    c. Improving visual and auditory acuity
    d. Identifying and managing medical ambiguity

19. One of the benefits of protocols, standing orders, and patient care algorithms is that they:
    a. clearly define performance parameters.
    b. cover all aspects of the critically ill patient.
    c. cover all aspects of the critically injured patient.
    d. provide a solid, legal, defensible back for the paramedic.

20. Which of the following is an advantage of protocols and standing orders?
    a. They do not usually cover multisystem failures or nonspecific complaints.
    b. They do not usually cover concurrent disease processes.
    c. They can speed the application of critical interventions.
    d. They usually cover the "textbook" patient injury or illness.

21. Working a patient in cardiac arrest requires many hands working together to complete treatments steps in the correct order. The paramedic must coordinate the team to make sure each task is managed well. To gain proficiency with this type of care, the paramedic must:
    a. identify the causes of cardiac arrest.
    b. reassess vital signs after each intervention.
    c. practice the same scenario frequently.
    d. call medical control for consultation.

22. You are assessing a male in his 20s who is lying on a couch and appears to be having a focal seizure. His eyes are open and he is staring to one side. He does not respond to you as you place an oxygen mask on his face. Which sequence of critical-thinking components should you follow with this patient?
    a. Collect information and formulate concepts, interpret and process information, apply treatment, reevaluate, and reflect.
    b. Apply treatment, reevaluate, reflect, collect information and formulate concepts, and interpret and process information.
    c. Interpret and process information, reflect, apply treatment, reevaluate, and collect information and formulate concepts.
    d. Reflect, reevaluate, apply treatment, collect information and formulate concepts, and interpret and process information.

23. When multiple stimuli on the scene of a call start to cloud critical thinking, the paramedic can use which of the following mental tricks to avoid panicking?
    a. Stop and think before acting.
    b. Obtain insurance information.
    c. Reflect on what has occurred so far.
    d. Be optimistic and hope for the best outcome.

24. Behaviors that can aid the paramedic to make good decisions while working under pressure include using a systematic assessment process and:
    a. planning for the worst scenario.
    b. planning for the best possible outcome.
    c. reviewing the performance after the call.
    d. asking the patient to provide his past medical history.

25. Which of the following is an example of a potential teaching moment for the paramedic?
    a. an unrestrained victim of an MVC sustaining facial lacerations on the windshield
    b. a 3-year-old child experiencing an anaphylactic reaction to a bee sting
    c. a 55-year-old having an acute myocardial infarction
    d. an asthmatic having a severe asthma attack after 3 months without an attack

26. Which of the following acronyms is used to help paramedics determine treatment and transportation priority decisions?
    a. CUPS
    b. ALS
    c. PHTLS
    d. PALS

27. As the paramedic gains more experience over time, it is expected that she will be better able to:
    a. manage similar experiences.
    b. transport the patient to the nearest facility.
    c. work with less manpower on difficult calls.
    d. limit the amount of turnaround time at the hospital.

28. Key aspects of reassessment include:
    a. observing the MOI.
    b. trending mental status and vital signs.
    c. starting an IV.
    d. obtaining a baseline ECG.

29. When a paramedic becomes overwhelmed and critical thinking becomes clouded, which of the following is advised?

    a. Take a deep breath and revert back to assessing the ABCs.

    b. Call for a backup crew to transport the patient.

    c. Utilize the paramedic supervisor as a mentor.

    d. Call the paramedic supervisor and request to go home for the day.

30. You are interviewing a 23-year-old male with a chief complaint of 8/10 chest pain. The pain increases with movement, coughing, and palpation. He also feels dizzy, short of breath, and is nauseous. His ECG shows ischemia in the lateral leads V5 and V6. Skin is warm and dry with good color, respiratory rate is 20 with clear lung sounds, pulse rate is 72/regular, and SpO_2 is 100%. You are not sure to treat this patient for a cardiac problem, muscular problem, or pleuritic problem so you:

    a. consult medical control.

    b. administer oxygen, aspirin, and transport.

    c. administer oxygen, start an IV, and transport.

    d. reassess vital signs in 5 minutes and formulate a treatment plan.

Exam #18 Answer Form

	A	B	C	D			A	B	C	D
1.	❏	❏	❏	❏		16.	❏	❏	❏	❏
2.	❏	❏	❏	❏		17.	❏	❏	❏	❏
3.	❏	❏	❏	❏		18.	❏	❏	❏	❏
4.	❏	❏	❏	❏		19.	❏	❏	❏	❏
5.	❏	❏	❏	❏		20.	❏	❏	❏	❏
6.	❏	❏	❏	❏		21.	❏	❏	❏	❏
7.	❏	❏	❏	❏		22.	❏	❏	❏	❏
8.	❏	❏	❏	❏		23.	❏	❏	❏	❏
9.	❏	❏	❏	❏		24.	❏	❏	❏	❏
10.	❏	❏	❏	❏		25.	❏	❏	❏	❏
11.	❏	❏	❏	❏		26.	❏	❏	❏	❏
12.	❏	❏	❏	❏		27.	❏	❏	❏	❏
13.	❏	❏	❏	❏		28.	❏	❏	❏	❏
14.	❏	❏	❏	❏		29.	❏	❏	❏	❏
15.	❏	❏	❏	❏		30.	❏	❏	❏	❏

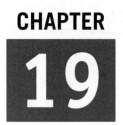

CHAPTER

19

Critical Thinking and Assessment-Based Management

1. _____ is the cornerstone of patient care.
   a. Past medical history
   b. Assessment
   c. Field impression
   d. Scene size-up

2. It is estimated that 80 percent of a medical diagnosis is based on the:
   a. physical examination.
   b. medications.
   c. history.
   d. chief complaint.

3. You and your crew have been dispatched to a supermarket for a patient with an unknown problem. Upon your arrival, the store manager tells you that the patient has been wandering around the store acting confused and slurring his words. He brings you to an aisle where a male in his late 50s is sitting on a wheeled cart. He is conscious but confused, and he does have slurred speech. He cannot answer your questions. His skin is warm and dry with good color, and he has a strong distal pulse. Which of the following factors could impede a proper field assessment of this patient?
   a. gender
   b. environment
   c. advanced directives
   d. past medical history

4. (Continuing with the patient in question 3) You assist him onto your stretcher and your crew obtains vital signs: respiratory rate is 20/nonlabored; pulse rate is 66, strong/regular; and BP is 144/100 mmHg. There is no obvious injury, but the patient smells of body odor and dried urine. Where should you focus your assessment next?
   a. possible head injury
   b. rule out hypothermia
   c. rule out hypoglycemia
   d. behavioral emergency

5. Which of the following is an example of "labeling" a patient?
   a. frequent flyer
   b. unstable head injury
   c. gut instinct
   d. diabetic neuropathy

6. When obtaining a history from a patient, the paramedic should focus on the:
   a. organ systems associated with the complaint.
   b. family preference for treatment and hospital destination.
   c. length of time the patient has waited for treatment.
   d. medical conditions the patient's family members may have.

7. Which of the following statements about injury pattern recognition for the trauma patient is most correct?
   a. The paramedic's knowledge base of injury patterns needs to be similar to that of a trauma surgeon's.
   b. Recognition of various injury patterns can help the paramedic be better prepared to provide the proper emergency care.
   c. To become proficient in pattern recognition, a paramedic's knowledge base needs to be similar to an emergency physician's.
   d. It is the responsibility of the EMS agency's medical director to provide expanded and continuous training in injury pattern recognition.

8. What is the essential equipment that should initially be brought to the side of every patient?
   a. clipboard, pen, and stethoscope
   b. PPE, stethoscope, blood pressure cuff, and penlight
   c. equipment to conduct the primary assessment of the patient's ABCs
   d. cardiac monitor/AED, stretcher, blood pressure cuff, and oxygen administration equipment

9. It is important for the paramedic to understand that protocols are intended as:

    a. the gold standard and should never be deviated from.

    b. guidelines for care.

    c. the basis of an action plan for all patients.

    d. a cookbook list of what the paramedic must do.

10. Which of the following is a factor that could impede decision making or proper field assessment by the paramedic?

    a. having a bias against people who do not have a background similar to hers

    b. having insufficient access to the patient's medical insurance records

    c. taking the time to listen to the patient's associated complaints

    d. treating distracting injuries after correcting life threats

11. When the paramedic has _____, he may miss vital pieces of information, which may short-circuit the information-gathering process.

    a. insufficient manpower

    b. a partner with less training or experience

    c. a biased or prejudicial "attitude"

    d. concerned family at the scene

12. The team leader is usually the paramedic who will:

    a. talk to the family and bystanders.

    b. act as the triage group leader in an MCI.

    c. drive the crew to the hospital.

    d. accompany the patient through definitive care.

13. Roles of the patient care provider member of the team usually include any of the following, *except*:

    a. obtaining vital signs.

    b. performing skills as designated by the team leader.

    c. acting as the initial EMS command in an MCI.

    d. gathering patient information.

14. A sign or symptom that suggests the patient may have a serious injury or medical condition is often referred to as a:

    a. presenting problem.

    b. red flag.

    c. historical indicator.

    d. comorbidity factor.

15. If a paramedic gives a poor oral presentation when giving a report on a patient, the paramedic suggests to the receiving health-care provider that:

    a. a poor assessment and care were made.

    b. there is really nothing wrong with the patient.

    c. the paramedic has other tasks of more importance.

    d. the paramedic failed to establish trust and credibility with the patient.

Exam #19 Answer Form

	A	B	C	D			A	B	C	D
1.	❏	❏	❏	❏		9.	❏	❏	❏	❏
2.	❏	❏	❏	❏		10.	❏	❏	❏	❏
3.	❏	❏	❏	❏		11.	❏	❏	❏	❏
4.	❏	❏	❏	❏		12.	❏	❏	❏	❏
5.	❏	❏	❏	❏		13.	❏	❏	❏	❏
6.	❏	❏	❏	❏		14.	❏	❏	❏	❏
7.	❏	❏	❏	❏		15.	❏	❏	❏	❏
8.	❏	❏	❏	❏						

CHAPTER
20

Medical Overview

1. An insulin-dependent diabetic patient is presenting with an altered mental status and a low blood sugar reading. Which of the following pieces of information from the SAMPLE history obtained from a family member is most important to the paramedic immediately?
   a. A—allergies
   b. M—medications
   c. P—past medical history
   d. L—last meal

2. When assessing a patient who has an obvious medical problem and has no one else present, and you are not sure if the problem is new or old, how should you proceed?
   a. Proceed as if the condition is new.
   b. Proceed as if the condition is chronic.
   c. Call dispatch to see if there is a prior history at the residence.
   d. Attempt to locate a neighbor who might be able to provide information.

3. To avoid the appearance of confusion when working with multiple crew members, the paramedic should:
   a. have and practice a preplan.
   b. ignore non-life-threatening, distracting injuries.
   c. carry the least amount of equipment to the patient.
   d. consider the family's concern for the patient's welfare.

4. Staging of the events and actions of a call so that they happen smoothly is called:
   a. choreography.
   b. algorithms.
   c. a protocol.
   d. an advanced directive.

5. Tunnel vision may have obstructed the assessment process in which of the following cases?
   a. Responding to an anaphylactic call where the patient forgot to administer his Epipen®.
   b. Seeing a local drug abuser and immediately blaming his disorientation on the drugs rather than looking for a medical problem.
   c. Assessing a patient's MS-ABCs before attending to an open femur fracture with gross angulation.
   d. Assuming EMS command at the scene of an MCI where the fire department is on scene first.

6. In order to _____ the paramedic must gather information as well as evaluate and synthesize that information.
   a. diagnose a patient's illness,
   b. provide definitive care for the patient,
   c. educate the patient's family on future 9-1-1 calls for assistance,
   d. make the appropriate management decisions,

7. You must proceed through the patient assessment in an organized fashion because:
   a. it is necessary in order to explain each step to the patient.
   b. this approach will help you to follow protocols and standing orders.
   c. this approach will help you to limit the amount of time spent on scene.
   d. an unorganized approach can lead to important information being overlooked.

8. Following an assessment sequence is most efficient because:
   a. the crew will know what they should do next.
   b. the patient will cooperate more easily.
   c. it allows for a complete and smooth assessment.
   d. it is easier to write up on the PCR.

9. Treatment decisions should be based on the data gathered in the focused history, the physical exam, and:
   a. emergency medical dispatch procedures.
   b. existing treatment protocols.
   c. third-party caller information.
   d. the paramedic's ability to make a definitive field diagnosis.

10. The quality of the patient's history is effected by the:
    a. patient's knowledge about the health care system.
    b. paramedic's knowledge of a disease and its assessment findings.
    c. local protocols and patient algorithms of a specific illness.
    d. medical director's level of involvement in QI/QA.

11. The value of a complete physical examination includes:
    a. building trust with the patient.
    b. understanding important information can be missed by performing a cursory exam.
    c. impressing the physician with a complete physical exam.
    d. a complete physical exam that will keep you from being sued.

12. An important aspect of the job is for the paramedic to think her patients are customers and to:
    a. ask them to rate your medical performance.
    b. impress them with the amount of equipment you can carry.
    c. inform the patient about all the training you have completed.
    d. provide excellent customer service through good people skills.

13. Two paramedics are working as a team. With simultaneous information gathering and management, care can be:
    a. more efficient.
    b. less efficient.
    c. confusing to the patient.
    d. a problem for establishing patient rapport.

14. The paramedic can improve scene choreography by:
    a. utilizing distance learning.
    b. taking a course in MCI leadership.
    c. watching training videos.
    d. preplanning and practicing with her crew.

15. The patient care provider is responsible for providing scene "cover" by:
    a. shutting the ambulance and taking the keys out of the ignition.
    b. setting up a cover for the crew working in the rain.
    c. watching everyone's back to make sure no one gets hurt.
    d. establishing a rehab sector for fire standbys.

Exam #20 Answer Form

	A	B	C	D			A	B	C	D
1.	❏	❏	❏	❏		9.	❏	❏	❏	❏
2.	❏	❏	❏	❏		10.	❏	❏	❏	❏
3.	❏	❏	❏	❏		11.	❏	❏	❏	❏
4.	❏	❏	❏	❏		12.	❏	❏	❏	❏
5.	❏	❏	❏	❏		13.	❏	❏	❏	❏
6.	❏	❏	❏	❏		14.	❏	❏	❏	❏
7.	❏	❏	❏	❏		15.	❏	❏	❏	❏
8.	❏	❏	❏	❏						

CHAPTER

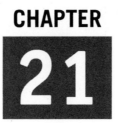

Respiratory

1. The process where oxygenated blood is pumped to the tissues, and waste products returned to the lungs, is called:
   a. respiration.
   b. ventilation.
   c. diffusion.
   d. perfusion.

2. _____ refers specifically to the exchange of carbon dioxide, whereas _____ refers only to the exchange of oxygen.
   a. Ventilation; oxygenation
   b. Oxygenation; ventilation
   c. Diffusion; oxygenation
   d. Perfusion; ventilation

3. A shift in the oxyhemoglobin saturation curve indicates a change in the affinity of hemoglobin for oxygen. A(n) _____ shift decreases it, whereas a _____ shift of the curve increases the binding (affinity) of oxygen to hemoglobin.
   a. upward; rightward
   b. downward; leftward
   c. rightward; leftward
   d. leftward; rightward

4. When a person develops a fever, the cell's metabolic rate increases and so:
   a. a leftward shift of the oxyhemoglobin saturation curve occurs.
   b. does his oxygen need.
   c. does his hemoglobin need.
   d. a downward shift of the oxyhemoglobin saturation curve occurs.

5. Which of the following factors causes a shift in the oxyhemoglobin curve, decreasing the tissue oxygen delivery?
   a. decreased body temperature
   b. increased body temperature
   c. acidosis
   d. increased metabolic rate

6. The pCO_2 measures ventilation (exchange of carbon dioxide). Normal levels of pCO_2 are _____ mm Hg.
   a. 7.35–7.45
   b. 7.40–7.50
   c. 35–40
   d. 40–45

7. pCO_2 is a respiratory:
   a. side effect.
   b. alkali.
   c. basic.
   d. acid.

8. For every 10-mm Hg change of the pCO_2, either up or down, the result is a _____ change in the pH in the opposite direction.
   a. 0.1
   b. 1.0
   c. 1.5
   d. 10.0

9. The pO_2 measures oxygenation at sea level and should normally run greater than _____ mm Hg.
   a. 30
   b. 50
   c. 70
   d. 80

10. Which of the following statements about blood gases is correct?
    a. Changes in pO_2 always occur when there is a change in pCO_2.
    b. The only predictable and reproducible relation in blood gases is between the pH and the pCO_2.
    c. Hypoventilation leads to decreased pO_2 and decreased pCO_2.
    d. Hyperventilation raises the pCO_2 and the pO_2.

11. In respiratory acidosis, CO_2 retention leads to increased levels of:
    a. O_2.
    b. pO_2.
    c. pCO_2.
    d. SpO_2.

12. A patient who is hypoventilating because of a heroin overdose is most likely experiencing which acid–base disorder?
    a. respiratory acidosis
    b. respiratory alkalosis
    c. metabolic acidosis
    d. metabolic alkalosis

13. Which of the following is a possible cause of an upper airway obstruction?
    a. tonsillitis
    b. pleural effusion
    c. pulmonary embolus
    d. bronchoconstriction

14. When the paramedic discovers his patient has _____ he should consider that the patient could have a chronic respiratory or heart or gastrointestinal disease and ask specific questions to that point in the patient interview.
    a. signs of infection,
    b. an ashtray in the residence,
    c. clubbing of the fingers or toes,
    d. past prescriptions for antibiotics,

15. Which of the following is an example of a perfusion-related factor that may impair gas exchange in the lungs?
    a. FBAO
    b. anemia
    c. epiglottitis
    d. smooth muscle spasm

16. A person with multiple sclerosis or muscular dystrophy may, because of her disease, experience respiratory abnormalities that affect ventilation by:
    a. foreign body airway obstruction.
    b. impairment of circulatory blood flow.
    c. impairment of chest wall movement.
    d. developing inadequate hemoglobin levels.

17. A patient who experiences a severe illness or trauma is at risk for developing _____, which affects both lungs and is associated with a high death rate.
    a. embolism
    b. cystic fibrosis
    c. foreign body airway obstruction
    d. acute respiratory distress syndrome

18. The presence of grunting is usually a sign of respiratory distress that occurs primarily in infants and small toddlers when the child breathes:
    a. in against a partially closed epiglottis.
    b. in against an airway obstruction.
    c. out against a partially closed epiglottis.
    d. out against an airway obstruction.

19. The school nurse called EMS to transport a student because the parent could not. The student is a 16-year-old female who has a sore throat, difficulty swallowing, fever, and headache. She denies dyspnea and was recently treated for an ear infection. What do you suspect is her problem today?
    a. pneumonia
    b. epiglotitis
    c. pharyngitis
    d. mononucleosis

20. You are reassessing an adult patient having an asthma attack after administering one nebulized treatment of albuterol and Atrovent. The patient initially was pale and had bilateral wheezing in the apices, and her SpO_2 was in the 90s. She looks no better, and her SpO_2 is now 89, but she is no longer wheezing. Assessment of which of the following can best guide your continued treatment plan with this patient?
    a. pulse rate
    b. mentation
    c. SpO_2 reading
    d. patient's position of comfort

21. When obtaining a focused history from a patient with a pulmonary disease, history of previous intubation is:
    a. a possible clue to a history of severe pulmonary disease.
    b. a nonspecific finding associated with respiratory distress.
    c. an indication that you will need to intubate the patient.
    d. not suggestive that intubation may be required again.

22. Certain medications, such as _____, can affect the ability of the sympathetic nervous system to cause bronchodilation and may cause or worsen obstructive lung disease.
    a. antianginals
    b. beta-blockers
    c. inhaled steroids
    d. oral corticosteroids

23. Typical findings associated with _____ include acute chest pain on the affected side, increased respiratory rate, and coughing.

    a. lung cancer

    b. pulmonary edema

    c. upper-respiratory infection

    d. spontaneous pneumothorax

24. The most common cause of spontaneous pneumothorax in an adult is:

    a. COPD.

    b. menstruation.

    c. a congenital bleb.

    d. lung disease involving the connective tissue of the lung.

25. In the face of a respiratory problem, _____ is an ominous sign of severe hypoxemia and suggests imminent cardiac arrest.

    a. a low SpO_2 reading

    b. tachypnea

    c. tachycardia

    d. bradycardia

26. The respiratory pattern that is characterized by alternating periods of apnea and deep, rapid breathing is called:

    a. eupnea.

    b. central neurogenic hyperventilation.

    c. Kussmaul breathing.

    d. Cheyne–Stokes respiration.

27. The type of breathing characterized by a series of several short inspirations followed by long, irregular periods of apnea, and associated with increased intracranial pressure is called _____ breathing.

    a. ataxic

    b. apneustic

    c. Cheyne–Stokes

    d. central neurogen hyperventilation.

28. The most common types of abnormal respiratory patterns seen in the field include tachypnea, bradypnea, apnea, and:

    a. eupnea.

    b. Biot's.

    c. Kussmaul's.

    d. Cheyne–Stokes'.

29. Many forms of lung disease cause increased resistance to blood flow in the lungs, causing the right heart to work harder. The heart compensates initially, but later is unable to maintain compensatory efforts resulting in:

    a. right heart failure.

    b. left heart failure.

    c. pursed-lip breathing.

    d. decreased pulmonary resistance.

30. You have been dispatched to a nursing home for a patient with severe respiratory distress. The patient is a 78-year-old female with low SpO_2 readings (in the 80s). You perform a physical exam and find that the patient has distended neck veins (JVD), wet crackles in the bases of her lungs, peripheral edema, and ascites. Her vital signs are: respiratory rate, 40; pulse rate, 90/irregular; BP, 176/98 mmHg; and skin CTC is cyanotic, warm, and dry. Based on your findings, what is this patient's primary problem?

    a. pneumonia

    b. lung cancer

    c. right-sided heart failure

    d. obstructive airway disease

31. The _____ deformity seen in some COPD and asthma patients is caused by _____ expiratory resistance to flow and air trapping.

    a. barrel chest; increased

    b. pigeon chest; increased

    c. barrel chest; decreased

    d. pigeon chest; decreased

32. When fluid accumulates in the airway, in the interstitial tissue, or both, the adventitious breath sounds you are likely to hear are:

    a. crackles.

    b. friction rubs.

    c. wheezes.

    d. stridors.

33. _____ spasm is a spasmodic contraction of the hands, wrists, feet, and ankles, which is associated with decreased levels of carbon dioxide.

    a. Hypocarpopedal

    b. Carbonix

    c. Carpopedal

    d. Carbon dorsal

34. Continuous positive airway pressure face masks improve oxygenation in many diseases, including asthma, COPD, and:

    a. sleep apnea.

    b. neoplasm of the lung.

    c. tension pneumothorax.

    d. spontaneous pneumothorax.

35. Capnography measures _____, or how much carbon dioxide is exhaled.

    a. end-tidal CO_2

    b. pO_2

    c. pCO_2

    d. peak flow

36. The most common obstructive airway diseases include asthma and:
    a. URI.
    b. COPD.
    c. cystic fibrosis.
    d. Legionnaires' disease.

37. You have successfully intubated a patient who was in near respiratory arrest as a result of a severe asthma attack. En route to the hospital, the patient is becoming alert and is attempting to pull on the endotracheal tube. Which of the following actions should you take now?
    a. Administer Versed 0.05 mg/kg.
    b. Prepare to extubate the patient.
    c. Administer Solu Medrol 125 mg IV.
    d. Administer magnesium 2 grams IV in 50 ml NS over 10 minutes.

38. During bronchospasm, the tiny muscle layers surrounding the bronchioles go into spasm and narrow the lumen of the airways. The result is:
    a. irritation.
    b. wheezing.
    c. snoring.
    d. coughing.

39. During an acute asthma attack, mucus production is increased because of _____ in the bronchial airways.
    a. irritation
    b. wheezing
    c. snoring
    d. coughing

40. _____ are the most common asthma triggers.
    a. Chewing tobaccos
    b. Car fumes
    c. Respiratory infections
    d. Flower spores

41. Exercise or fast breathing is a trigger for asthma attacks, especially during _____ weather.
    a. hot
    b. cold
    c. humid
    d. rainy

42. Any condition that leads to _____ may cause carpopedal spasm.
    a. respiratory acidosis
    b. respiratory alkalosis
    c. metabolic acidosis
    d. metabolic alkalosis

43. _____ is a highly specific diagnosis consisting of high-permeability pulmonary edema, due to any of several causes, and the inability to adequately oxygenate the blood despite 100% FiO_2.
    a. Status asthmaticus
    b. Ventilation–perfusion mismatch
    c. Adult respiratory distress syndrome
    d. Chronic obstructive pulmonary disease

44. _____ is a severe, prolonged asthma attack that does not respond to standard medications.
    a. Acute bronchial asthma
    b. Status asthmaticus
    c. Allergy-induced asthma
    d. Exercise-induced asthma

45. Death rates from asthma continue to soar despite all of the current knowledge about asthma. Two factors that underlie the fatal trend include decreased airway sensitivity and:
    a. inadequate use of anti-inflammatory medication.
    b. the lack of peak flow meter use.
    c. increased use of antibiotics.
    d. increased exposure to the Lyme-carrying tick.

46. _____ results from overgrowth of the airway mucus glands and excess secretion of mucus that blocks the airway.
    a. Asthma
    b. Chronic bronchitis
    c. Emphysema
    d. Exacerbation

47. _____ results from destruction of the walls of the alveoli, which leads to a decrease in elastic recoil.
    a. Asthma
    b. Chronic bronchitis
    c. Emphysema
    d. Legionnaires' disease

48. Which of the following is the major cause of COPD?
    a. air pollution
    b. cigarette smoking
    c. tuberculosis
    d. asbestos

49. Victims of asthma attacks will have symptoms that _____, as compared with persons with COPD.
    a. are wheezing in nature
    b. are associated with smoking
    c. progressively worsen over several days
    d. come on relatively quickly

50. A young child is presenting with acute respiratory distress and audible wheezing. He has no history of asthma and takes no medications. Which of the following do you attempt to rule out first?
    a. FBAO
    b. COPD
    c. toxic inhalation
    d. asthma

51. Epinephrine, terbutaline, and albuterol all have _____ effects, which are potentially useful in the treatment of obstructive lung disease.
    a. bronchoconstricting
    b. bronchodilating
    c. vasoconstricting
    d. anti-inflammatory

52. Steroids are beneficial in the chronic treatment of nearly all asthma patients and many COPD patients because of the _____ effects.
    a. smooth muscle relaxing
    b. bronchodilating
    c. vasoconstricting
    d. anti-inflammatory

53. The inhaled steroids used in the first line of the treatment of asthma and COPD patients result in _____ side effects than the oral preparations.
    a. more
    b. fewer
    c. the same
    d. different

54. Some EMS systems administer steroids, because these drugs:
    a. take at least 1 or 2 hours to work.
    b. work immediately.
    c. are of no benefit after the first 39 minutes of intervention of respiratory distress.
    d. are of minimal benefit after the first 30 minutes of intervention of respiratory distress.

55. _____ is(are) one of the major inflammation-causing compounds produced in asthma.
    a. Glucocorticoids
    b. Latex
    c. Leukotrienes
    d. Leukocytes

56. Magnesium sulfate has been shown to be of some benefit to some asthmatic patients, primarily because of its _____ effects.
    a. smooth muscle relaxing
    b. bronchodilating
    c. vasoconstricting
    d. anti-inflammatory

57. The accumulation of carbon dioxide in blood is the major stimulus that normally causes:
    a. altered mental status.
    b. hormonal secretions.
    c. a healthy person to breathe.
    d. fluid retention.

58. Cigarette smoke directly inhibits the normal:
    a. movement of mucus via bronchial cilia out of the lungs.
    b. response to breathing in teenagers.
    c. immune response in the elderly.
    d. hormonal response in postmenopausal women.

59. Chronic alcoholics have an increased risk of respiratory infections because of:
    a. decreased thermoregulatory systems.
    b. weakened immune systems caused by ethanol.
    c. increased exposure to hypothermia.
    d. decreased hepatic functions.

60. _____ is a life-threatening genetic disease that causes mucus to accumulate and clog certain organs in the body, particularly the lungs and pancreas.
    a. Asthma
    b. Emphysema
    c. Cystic fibrosis
    d. Chronic bronchitis

61. Which of the following statements about pneumonia is most correct?
    a. Most pneumonias are caused by viruses.
    b. The clinical approach to viral or bacterial pneumonia is the same.
    c. The clinical approach to viral or bacterial pneumonia is different.
    d. It is possible to tell the difference between viral and bacterial pneumonia in the prehospital setting.

62. A secondary mechanism that stimulates breathing is a lack of oxygen in the blood and is called:
    a. carbon dioxide drive.
    b. hypoxic drive.
    c. bicarboxic force.
    d. bicarbonic influence.

63. Which of the following is an atypical finding associated with pneumonia?
    a. productive cough
    b. pleuritic chest pain
    c. nonproductive cough
    d. decreased breath sounds

64. A 22-year-old female called EMS because she is coughing up blood. She has had cold-like symptoms that have lasted longer than 1 week, but the blood is new and she is frightened. What action should the paramedic complete first?
    a. Get a good history of the present condition.
    b. Take standard precautions for a contagious condition.
    c. Start the patient on nebulized albuterol and atrovent.
    d. Listen to lung sounds and obtain vital signs including temperature.

65. The patient in the previous question states she has had a mild fever, runny nose, and is having difficulty sleeping at night due to coughing fits. Her lung sounds are clear, respiratory rate is 20 non-labored, pulse rate is 78/regular, BP is 128/68 mmHg, and SpO2 is 98%. What do you suspect is causing the patient's symptoms?
    a. pertussis
    b. pneumonia
    c. common cold
    d. pulmonary embolism

66. Out-of-hospital treatment for respiratory distress with drug therapy of _____ may be helpful, especially if the patient has accompanying obstructive lung disease.
    a. Ventolin
    b. antibiotics
    c. aspirin
    d. calcium

67. Influenza is a specific type of _____ infection that may affect both the upper and lower respiratory tracts.
    a. viral
    b. bacterial
    c. fungal
    d. spore

68. It is impossible to differentiate viral upper respiratory infection (URI) from a bacterial URI without:
    a. a good past medical history.
    b. cultures.
    c. the presence of an elevated temperature.
    d. a visit to the emergency department.

69. Most patients with URIs have spontaneous resolution of their symptoms within 7 days:
    a. only when they go to the ED.
    b. only when they see their own MD.
    c. with or without antibiotics.
    d. with or without an underlying disease.

70. Select the statement that is most accurate about URIs.
    a. Some URIs cause bronchoconstriction.
    b. The terms URI and influenza are nearly interchangeable.
    c. URIs are self-limiting and rarely develop into serious complications.
    d. Only people with underlying disease experience two or more URIs a year.

71. A patient who presents with URI and has had his _____ removed is at grave risk for a life-threatening illness.
    a. lung
    b. appendix
    c. spleen
    d. gallbladder

72. The most common cause of primary lung tumors is:
    a. coal miner's lung.
    b. asbestosis.
    c. cigarette smoking.
    d. heredity.

73. Patients with massive pulmonary emboli often suffer a syncopal spell or _____ as the first symptom(s) of the illness.
    a. cardiac arrest
    b. nausea and vomiting
    c. high-pressure pulmonary edema
    d. high-permeability pulmonary edema

74. A patient who just received treatment with chemotherapy for lung cancer would most likely have which of the following complaints?
    a. nausea, vomiting, and weakness
    b. diaphoresis and shortness of breath
    c. chest pain
    d. vision and equilibrium disturbances

75. A patient who, earlier in the day, received treatment with radiotherapy for lung cancer would most likely experience which of the following symptoms?
    a. fever and chills
    b. dizziness and chest pain
    c. dry cough or shortness of breath
    d. nausea, vomiting, and weakness

76. What should be the primary concern for the paramedic when treating a patient who may have pneumonia?
    a. respiratory distress
    b. respiratory failure
    c. exposure to a contagious patient
    d. severe dehydration

77. Persons with acute pulmonary edema caused by _____ have "severe congestive heart failure," but not all patients with "severe congestive heart failure" have pulmonary edema.
   a. ARDS
   b. scorpion bites
   c. pericarditis
   d. cardiac ischemia

78. The primary difference between pulmonary edema and congestive heart failure (CHF) is:
   a. pulmonary edema develops progressively, and CHF does not.
   b. only pulmonary edema is associated with ARDS.
   c. CHF is a spectrum of conditions associated with decreases in cardiac function.
   d. only CHF can be exacerbated by asthma or COPD.

79. Patients with CHF or pulmonary edema may have orthopnea because:
   a. the recumbent position increased venous return to the heart.
   b. the recumbent position decreased venous return to the heart.
   c. these patients have a decreased preload mechanism.
   d. these patients are usually obese, and this increases pulmonary resistance.

80. The role of nitroglycerine in the treatment of patients with acute pulmonary edema is:
   a. to dilate the veins.
   b. to dilate the arteries.
   c. vasodilation of both veins and arteries.
   d. decreasing lymphatic flow from the lungs.

81. A patient with cystic fibrosis called 9-1-1 for transport to the emergency department for exacerbation of a respiratory infection. He is having difficulty breathing, has green productive cough, and is fatigued. His lung sounds are diminished bilaterally and his SpO_2 is 90% with his oxygen by cannula at 2 lpm. What treatment will be most helpful during transport?
   a. CPAP
   b. IV fluid bolus
   c. nebulized Ventolin
   d. oxygen 4 lpm by cannula

82. Besides the analgesic effect, morphine sulfate also has which of the following effects on the patient with acute pulmonary edema?
   a. reduces cardiac preload and afterload
   b. increases cardiac preload and afterload
   c. increases cerebral diuresis
   d. has an amnesic effect

83. ACE inhibitors have been used to treat hypertension and CHF for years. The way they work is by blocking:
   a. the hormone aldosterone on the kidneys.
   b. the conversion of angiotensin I to angiotensin II in the lungs.
   c. the collapse of portions of the lung and improving overall ventilation.
   d. vasoconstriction of cardiac arteries.

84. The role of simple positive pressure in the treatment of patients with respiratory distress is to:
   a. decrease intrathoracic pressure.
   b. increase intrathoracic pressure.
   c. regulate pulmonary pressures independently.
   d. regulate pulmonary pressure.

85. A 33-year-old male suddenly develops sharp chest pain and shortness of breath. His wife tells you that the patient has been sick with a cold for a nearly a week. He has been coughing more frequently since the pain began; he states that the pain is stabbing and points to the left chest. Except for smoking, the patient denies any significant past medical history. Vital signs are respiratory rate, 34/diminished on the right side; pulse rate, 112/regular; BP 140/80 mmHg; and skin CTC is warm, moist, and good color. What do you suspect is the patient's problem?
   a. pulmonary embolism
   b. acute myocardial infarction
   c. spontaneous pneumothorax
   d. new onset of bronchial asthma

86. The use of oral contraceptives increases the risk of a woman developing a pulmonary embolism because they:
   a. produce emboli of fat.
   b. produce emboli of tumor tissue.
   c. affect levels of natural anticoagulants in the blood.
   d. cause the kidneys to retain certain proteins, which produce emboli.

87. The pathology of a pulmonary embolism includes the emboli becoming lodged in:
   a. pulmonary arterial circulation.
   b. pulmonary venous circulation.
   c. deep veins.
   d. the right heart.

88. The occlusion that results from a pulmonary embolism not only results in decreased blood supply to the affected area but also leads to the release of histamines, which causes _____ in the region of the clot.
   a. bronchospasm
   b. ACS
   c. bronchodilation
   d. tissue necrosis

89. Which of the following conditions can mimic a pulmonary embolism?
    a. hypertensive crisis
    b. ACS
    c. labor
    d. hypoglycemia

90. Which of the following has more significance in the differential diagnosis of a pulmonary embolism than the others?
    a. the presence or absence of pleuritic chest pain
    b. history of a recent URI
    c. use of diuretics
    d. smoking history

91. The most common physical finding associated with pulmonary embolism includes tachypnea and:
    a. cyanosis.
    b. wheezing.
    c. peripheral edema.
    d. tachycardia.

92. Which of the following profiles is most often associated with spontaneous pneumothorax?
    a. elderly, obese, male smoker
    b. elderly, thin, female smoker
    c. young, tall, male smoker
    d. young, petite, female smoker

93. The pathology of hyperventilation results in _____ levels of carbon dioxide and _____ the pH.
    a. low; increases
    b. low; decreases
    c. high; increases
    d. high; decreases

94. What is the major risk in caring for a patient presenting with hyperventilation?
    a. recognizing that the patient is hypoxic
    b. understanding that hyperventilation is caused by many illnesses
    c. assuming that the patient is experiencing a simple anxiety attack
    d. providing high-flow oxygen to a patient in a state of hypocapnea

95. You are treating a patient who is experiencing acute pulmonary edema, but the patient is refusing to wear an oxygen mask. Which of the following is most appropriate for the patient?
    a. Insist that the patient needs the oxygen, and apply the mask anyway.
    b. Offer the patient a nasal cannula.
    c. Consider the need for a ventilator.
    d. Ask medical control for authorization to perform RSI.

96. Your patient is a 36-year-old male who has a c/c of acute non-exertional dyspnea that is getting progressively worse. Wheezing is heard on auscultation, but there is no PMHx of any obstructive respiratory or cardiac diseases. The only medication he takes is O-T-C Motrin® for pain in the leg from a fracture 2 months ago. Which of the following conditions do you suspect is causing the dyspnea?
    a. pulmonary embolism
    b. spontaneous pneumothorax
    c. hyperventilation syndrome
    d. early CHF

97. When considering the pathology for the cause of the dyspnea described in question 96, which of the following is the most likely cause?
    a. fat embolus from bone marrow
    b. ruptured congenital bleb
    c. anxiety
    d. ACS

98. A slender 24-year-old male is complaining of an acute onset of non-exertional sharp chest pain on the right side and shortness of breath. He is a smoker with a history of a nonproductive cough for 2 days. Breath sounds are decreased on the right side and vital signs are R/R 36, H/R 116, and B/P 100/80 mmHg. Which of the following conditions do you suspect?
    a. pneumonia
    b. pulmonary embolus
    c. spontaneous pneumothorax
    d. AMI

99. You are dispatched to an office building for a 28-year-old female complaining of dizziness and numbness in her hands and legs. Coworkers tell you that the patient has been under a lot of stress, and today she has been especially anxious. The patient denies S.O.B., chest pain, or any recent illnesses, and her vital signs are stable. Based on the initial findings, what do you suspect is the cause of the patient's extremity numbness?
    a. CVA
    b. TIA
    c. psychologic
    d. carpopedal spasm

100. Further information about the patient described in question 99 confirms that the patient was hyperventilating prior to EMS arriving. The patient has a PMHx of asthma but has not had an attack in months. Your initial management of this patient includes:
    a. providing high-flow oxygen and watching for changes in mental status.
    b. withholding oxygen to see if the numbness resolves.
    c. beginning an albuterol treatment.
    d. calling medical control for advice.

Exam #21 Answer Form

	A	B	C	D			A	B	C	D
1.	❏	❏	❏	❏		31.	❏	❏	❏	❏
2.	❏	❏	❏	❏		32.	❏	❏	❏	❏
3.	❏	❏	❏	❏		33.	❏	❏	❏	❏
4.	❏	❏	❏	❏		34.	❏	❏	❏	❏
5.	❏	❏	❏	❏		35.	❏	❏	❏	❏
6.	❏	❏	❏	❏		36.	❏	❏	❏	❏
7.	❏	❏	❏	❏		37.	❏	❏	❏	❏
8.	❏	❏	❏	❏		38.	❏	❏	❏	❏
9.	❏	❏	❏	❏		39.	❏	❏	❏	❏
10.	❏	❏	❏	❏		40.	❏	❏	❏	❏
11.	❏	❏	❏	❏		41.	❏	❏	❏	❏
12.	❏	❏	❏	❏		42.	❏	❏	❏	❏
13.	❏	❏	❏	❏		43.	❏	❏	❏	❏
14.	❏	❏	❏	❏		44.	❏	❏	❏	❏
15.	❏	❏	❏	❏		45.	❏	❏	❏	❏
16.	❏	❏	❏	❏		46.	❏	❏	❏	❏
17.	❏	❏	❏	❏		47.	❏	❏	❏	❏
18.	❏	❏	❏	❏		48.	❏	❏	❏	❏
19.	❏	❏	❏	❏		49.	❏	❏	❏	❏
20.	❏	❏	❏	❏		50.	❏	❏	❏	❏
21.	❏	❏	❏	❏		51.	❏	❏	❏	❏
22.	❏	❏	❏	❏		52.	❏	❏	❏	❏
23.	❏	❏	❏	❏		53.	❏	❏	❏	❏
24.	❏	❏	❏	❏		54.	❏	❏	❏	❏
25.	❏	❏	❏	❏		55.	❏	❏	❏	❏
26.	❏	❏	❏	❏		56.	❏	❏	❏	❏
27.	❏	❏	❏	❏		57.	❏	❏	❏	❏
28.	❏	❏	❏	❏		58.	❏	❏	❏	❏
29.	❏	❏	❏	❏		59.	❏	❏	❏	❏
30.	❏	❏	❏	❏		60.	❏	❏	❏	❏

Exam #21 Answer Form

	A	B	C	D
61.	❑	❑	❑	❑
62.	❑	❑	❑	❑
63.	❑	❑	❑	❑
64.	❑	❑	❑	❑
65.	❑	❑	❑	❑
66.	❑	❑	❑	❑
67.	❑	❑	❑	❑
68.	❑	❑	❑	❑
69.	❑	❑	❑	❑
70.	❑	❑	❑	❑
71.	❑	❑	❑	❑
72.	❑	❑	❑	❑
73.	❑	❑	❑	❑
74.	❑	❑	❑	❑
75.	❑	❑	❑	❑
76.	❑	❑	❑	❑
77.	❑	❑	❑	❑
78.	❑	❑	❑	❑
79.	❑	❑	❑	❑
80.	❑	❑	❑	❑

	A	B	C	D
81.	❑	❑	❑	❑
82.	❑	❑	❑	❑
83.	❑	❑	❑	❑
84.	❑	❑	❑	❑
85.	❑	❑	❑	❑
86.	❑	❑	❑	❑
87.	❑	❑	❑	❑
88.	❑	❑	❑	❑
89.	❑	❑	❑	❑
90.	❑	❑	❑	❑
91.	❑	❑	❑	❑
92.	❑	❑	❑	❑
93.	❑	❑	❑	❑
94.	❑	❑	❑	❑
95.	❑	❑	❑	❑
96.	❑	❑	❑	❑
97.	❑	❑	❑	❑
98.	❑	❑	❑	❑
99.	❑	❑	❑	❑
100.	❑	❑	❑	❑

Cardiovascular

1. The semilunar valves include the _____ valves.
   a. pulmonic and aortic
   b. pulmonic and mitral
   c. mitral and tricuspid
   d. tricuspid and aortic

2. When one or more valves become narrowed because of congenital damage, the valve is said to be:
   a. stenotic.
   b. murmured.
   c. regurgitant.
   d. intrinsic.

3. The coronary sinus, a portion of the coronary circulation, is a large vein that opens into the:
   a. aorta.
   b. right atrium.
   c. vena cava.
   d. left ventricle.

4. While assessing a 65-year-old female with atrial fibrillation, you discover that her radial pulse is less than her apical pulse. This finding is called:
   a. pulsus paradoxus.
   b. pulsus alternans.
   c. pulse deficit.
   d. pulse differential.

5. You are assessing the pulse rate and quality on a 23-year-old male experiencing an asthma attack. You find that the pulse is strong, regular, and tachy; however, the pulse decreases considerably during inspiration. This phenomenon is called:
   a. pulsus paradoxus.
   b. pulsus alternans.
   c. pulse deficit.
   d. pulse differential.

6. The normal heart sound S1 is caused by vibrations that occur with the closure of the _____ valves at the start of ventricular systole.
   a. pulmonic and aortic
   b. pulmonic and mitral
   c. mitral and tricuspid
   d. tricuspid and aortic

7. The abnormal heart sound S3, though sometimes present in healthy young persons, most commonly is associated with moderate to severe:
   a. asthma.
   b. pulmonary embolism.
   c. stroke.
   d. heart failure.

8. The abnormal heart sound that occurs when inflammation is present in the parietal and visceral pericardium is a(n):
   a. murmur.
   b. pericardial friction rub.
   c. S4.
   d. S3.

9. The layer of the heart that lines the chambers of the heart and is continuous with the intima is the:
   a. epicardium.
   b. myocardium.
   c. endocardium.
   d. visceral pericardium.

10. Following a severe steering wheel chest impact, the pericardial space can rapidly accumulate fluid, resulting in pericardial tamponade. In the average-size adult, tamponade can occur with as little as _____ milliliters of fluid.
    a. 25
    b. 50
    c. 75
    d. 100

11. A potentially fatal bacterial infection typically affecting the heart valves is:
    a. epicarditis.
    b. myocarditis.
    c. endocarditis.
    d. scarlet fever.

12. The majority of coronary artery blood flow and myocardial perfusion occurs during which phase of the cardiac cycle?
    a. systole
    b. diastole
    c. asystole
    d. effusion

13. The relationship between increased stroke volume and increased ventricular end-diastolic volume for a given intrinsic contractility is called:
    a. Beck's triad.
    b. Iowa pressure articulation.
    c. autoregulation.
    d. Starling's law of the heart.

14. When a drug's specific action is a negative chronotropic effect, what effect will it have on the heart?
    a. increased heart rate
    b. decreased heart rate
    c. increased force of muscular contractility
    d. decreased force of muscular contractility

15. When a drug has a positive inotropic effect, the drug will affect the heart in which of the following ways?
    a. increased heart rate
    b. decreased heart rate
    c. increased force of muscular contractility
    d. decreased force of muscular contractility

16. A _____ is the formation of a blood clot in the deep vein within the leg or pelvis.
    a. stroke
    b. thrombosis
    c. phlebitis
    d. pulmonary embolism

17. A 25-year-old female is complaining of abdominal pain that she describes as intermittent and cramping. What type of pain is the patient most likely experiencing?
    a. somatic
    b. idiopathic
    c. visceral
    d. neurotic

18. Some diabetic patients experience an altered pain perception from a chronic nerve condition called:
    a. dyspepsia.
    b. neuropathy.
    c. parathesia.
    d. ghost pain.

19. People with the preexisting medical condition _____ are more likely to experience a "silent ACS" than those without it.
    a. hypertension
    b. diabetes
    c. Parkinson's
    d. esophageal reflux

20. When there is inadequate blood flow to an organ, such as the heart, _____ occurs initially.
    a. ischemia
    b. infarction
    c. stroke
    d. embolus

21. Fibrinolytics and blood thinners are used to treat occlusions of coronary arteries due to thrombi after an acute MI in an effort to restore blood flow. They are also used to treat:
    a. Marfan syndrome.
    b. pulmonary embolism.
    c. congestive heart failure.
    d. abdominal aortic aneurysm.

22. Pain that is felt at a site that is different from that of the injured or diseased part of the body is called:
    a. referred pain.
    b. irritation.
    c. inflammation.
    d. musculoskeletal.

23. The three primary components used for diagnosis of an acute MI include cardiac enzyme analysis, abnormal ECG and/or ECG changes, and:
    a. vital signs.
    b. daily use of aspirin.
    c. history.
    d. prehospital treatment.

24. An atypical form of chest pain caused by vasospasm of otherwise normal coronary arteries is called _____ angina.
    a. stable
    b. unstable
    c. Wicket's
    d. Prinzmetal's

25. The most frequent cause of acute myocardial infarction (MI) is:
   a. coronary thrombosis.
   b. hypertension.
   c. trauma.
   d. use of recreational drugs.

26. Which of the following symptoms associated with ischemic chest pain is considered atypical for a 40-year-old male?
   a. dyspnea
   b. weakness
   c. diaphoresis
   d. indigestion

27. The ECG wave form that represents the impulse generated as the ventricles depolarize prior to contraction is the:
   a. PR interval.
   b. QRS complex.
   c. J point.
   d. QT interval.

28. ALS was dispatched for an unconscious 72-year-old male. When you arrive, he is conscious, pale, diaphoretic, and supine on the floor. A bystander tells you that he complained of chest pain after waking up. Now the patient describes the pain as 8/10. While your partner administers oxygen, you determine that he is hypotensive, has a BP of 70/34 mmHg, and has a third-degree heart block with a rate of 38 bpm. Which of the following interventions is most appropriate to apply first?
   a. Administer a fluid bolus and aspirin.
   b. Start an IV and administer a dose of atropine.
   c. Sedate the patient and begin transcutaneous pacing.
   d. Administer aspirin and nitroglycerin for the chest pain.

29. ST elevation is usually a sign of severe myocardial injury. However, other common causes of ST elevation that may be confused with ACS are:
   a. myocarditis and gout.
   b. syncope and pleurisy.
   c. acute pericarditis and Prinzmetal's angina.
   d. CHF and pleural effusion.

30. Patients with right ventricular infarcts often have problems with hypotension and decreased cardiac output and are very sensitive to drugs that reduce preload, such as:
   a. nitroglycerin.
   b. aspirin.
   c. dopamine.
   d. fentanyl.

31. A 12 lead ECG analysis can help to identify the size and location of the infarct that occurs during an ACS, thus helping to guide treatment. A patient experiencing an inferior wall MI of the left ventricle may have abnormalities in which leads?
   a. V_1 and V_2
   b. V_3 and V_4
   c. II, III, and aVF
   d. I, aVL, V_5, and V_6

32. A patient experiencing an acute anterior wall MI of the left ventricle may have abnormalities in which leads?
   a. V_1 and V_2
   b. V_3 and V_4
   c. II, III, and aVF
   d. I, aVL, V_5, and V_6

33. A patient experiencing a septal wall MI may have abnormalities in which leads?
   a. V_1 and V_2
   b. V_3 and V_4
   c. II, III, and aVF
   d. I, aVL, V_5, and V_6

34. Claudication is a painful, cramping feeling in the legs that usually occurs after walking and resolves with rest and is caused by:
   a. ulcers.
   b. deep vein thrombosis.
   c. peripheral artery disease.
   d. chronic hypertension.

35. You are interviewing a 74-year-old woman who had a syncopal event while at the market with her daughter. Both the patient and daughter confirm that the patient has a history of periodic loss of consciousness caused by a heart block. They cannot remember what this condition is called, but you suspect which of the following conditions?
   a. unstable syncope
   b. unstable angina
   c. Wolff–Parkinson–White syndrome
   d. Adams–Stokes syndrome

36. Synchronized cardioversion is a timed shock delivered to the heart to convert abnormal rhythms to a normal rhythm. Synchronization is preferred over defibrillation in patients with a pulse because synchronization reduces the energy required to convert and:
   a. reduces the chance of post-shock dysrhythmias.
   b. increases the period of an extra-conduction pathway.
   c. reduces the possibility of pre-excitation syndrome.
   d. increases the stimulation of the relative refractory phase.

37. When injury to the myocardium affects the automaticity and the heart is no longer able to produce the normal pace or rhythm, the treatment of choice in the prehospital setting is:
    a. atropine.
    b. isoproterenol.
    c. external pacing.
    d. defibrillation.

38. When an ECG displays a short PR interval and a wide QRS complex, which characteristically shows early QRS widening referred to as a "delta wave," this is a clue that the patient has:
    a. a hypoxic heart.
    b. myocardial ischemia.
    c. Adams–Stokes syndrome.
    d. Wolff–Parkinson–White syndrome.

39. You are performing a focused history and physical examination for possible ACS on a 55-year-old patient complaining of substernal chest pain and exertional dyspnea. Which of the following pieces of information from the patient's past medical history will rule out this patient as a candidate for reperfusion therapy?
    a. stable angina
    b. kidney disease
    c. mild hypertension
    d. appendectomy 18 months ago

40. Cardiac muscle tissue has the ability to contract without neural stimulation. This property is called:
    a. self-excitation.
    b. automaticity.
    c. syncytium.
    d. depolarization.

41. Cardiac muscle tissue has the ability to conduct impulses much quicker than regular muscle cells, a property called:
    a. self-excitation.
    b. automaticity.
    c. syncytium.
    d. repolarization.

42. Many patients who take diuretics such as Lasix also take potassium to prevent _____, which is an excessive loss of potassium that occurs with diuresis.
    a. hypokalemia
    b. hyperkalemia
    c. hyponatremia
    d. hypercalcemia

43. When cardiac muscle tissue gets an altered amount of potassium, the effect on the heart is a(n):
    a. increased force of contraction.
    b. decreased force of contraction.
    c. slow heart rate.
    d. fast heart rate.

44. Cardiac muscle tissue uses three primary cations to effect depolarization and repolarization of the heart. These three include potassium, sodium, and:
    a. phosphate.
    b. gluconate.
    c. citrate.
    d. calcium.

45. While working as part of a medic team standing by at a marathon, you are treating a runner who is exhausted. The patient's vital signs are R/R 16, BP 102/50 mm Hg, and H/R 42. After obtaining a focused history from the patient, which of the following is the most likely cause of the slow heart rate?
    a. use of supplemental salt tablets
    b. dehydration from overexertion
    c. heat stroke
    d. hypoglycemia

46. The pacemaker cells in the _____ of the heart normally initiate the electrical impulses that start the sequence of excitation and conduction through the heart.
    a. SA node
    b. AV node
    c. bundle branches
    d. Purkinje fibers

47. If the primary pacemaker of the heart failed, the next backup pacemaker should take over changing the normal look of the complexes in the ECG to reflect:
    a. ST elevation.
    b. ST depression.
    c. a widened QRS.
    d. absent or abnormal P waves.

48. Acetylcholine, a neurotransmitter released by parasympathetic motor neurons, has which of the following effects on the heart?
    a. regulates normal contractions
    b. lowers stroke volume
    c. increases heart rate
    d. enhances automaticity

49. Three neurotransmitters that stimulate the sympathetic response and are also cardiac medications are epinephrine, norepinephrine, and:
   a. cardizem.
   b. dopamine.
   c. dobutamine.
   d. amiodarone.

50. Sympathetic nerves are located throughout the heart. The parasympathetic nerves are located primarily in the:
   a. bundle of His.
   b. Purkinje fibers.
   c. bundle branches.
   d. SA and AV nodes.

51. An irregular connection between the atria and the ventricles that bypasses the AV node is called a(n):
   a. reentry.
   b. aberration.
   c. accessory pathway.
   d. PVC.

52. When conduction of electrical impulses in the heart experiences an alteration of the repolarization wave from its normal direction, which is blocked, to another direction that is not blocked, this is known as:
   a. reentry.
   b. an aberration.
   c. accessory pathway.
   d. PVC.

53. When the heart muscle is injured and the ventricles can no longer pump effectively, the arterial pressures begin to change and:
   a. only the preload is affected.
   b. only the afterload is affected.
   c. the preload and afterload are directly affected.
   d. the preload and afterload are indirectly affected.

54. Hypertension is a devastating disease that places an increased workload on the heart. Specifically, the extra workload causes the left ventricle to:
   a. dystrophy.
   b. myotrophy.
   c. atrophy.
   d. hypertrophy.

55. The primary types of damage that occur with chronic hypertension are aneurysm, stroke, and:
   a. nausea.
   b. deep vein thrombosis.
   c. headache.
   d. renal failure.

56. The treatment plan for hypertensive crisis is to reduce the patient's blood pressure within 1 or 2 hours to avoid:
   a. an ACS.
   b. permanent organ damage.
   c. sudden death.
   d. atherosclerosis.

57. A normal defense mechanism designed to maintain cerebral perfusion after an insult such as a stroke or head injury is called:
   a. cerebral autoregulation.
   b. Beck's triad.
   c. hypotension.
   d. hypertension.

58. A normal property of the brain that maintains cerebral perfusion within a fairly wide range of mean arterial blood pressures is known as:
   a. cerebral autoregulation.
   b. Beck's triad.
   c. Frank–Starling law.
   d. homeostasis.

59. An inflammation of a vein causing pain in the affected part of the body, which is accompanied by stiffness and edema is called:
   a. phlebitis.
   b. ascites.
   c. thrombosis.
   d. angioedema.

60. A patient affected with Marfan syndrome may experience sudden death at an early age, usually from which of the following mechanisms?
   a. congestive heart failure
   b. spontaneous papillary rupture
   c. spontaneous pneumothorax
   d. spontaneous rupture of the aorta

61. You are called to transport a 65-year-old male for evaluation of severe pain in the left calf. The patient tells you the pain began suddenly while he was taking his daily walk, but now that he is sitting, the pain is subsiding. Which of the following conditions do you suspect?
   a. edema
   b. ascites
   c. claudication
   d. muscle cramp

62. In a cardiac contraction, the degree of stretch of the contraction muscle is called the:
    a. atrial pressure point.
    b. ventricular pressure point.
    c. preload.
    d. afterload.

63. The major problems that occur with heart failure are that cardiac output decreases and _____ develop(s).
    a. venous congestion
    b. vasospasms
    c. bradycardia
    d. autoregulation

64. In the early stages of heart failure, the body senses the decrease in cardiac output and attempts to compensate through stimulation of the:
    a. vagus nerve.
    b. sympathetic nervous system.
    c. renal buffer system.
    d. pulmonic system.

65. Left heart failure is more common than right heart failure because the left ventricle is more often affected by:
    a. smoking.
    b. diabetes.
    c. obesity.
    d. chronic hypertension.

66. Prehospital management of cardiogenic shock begins with treating the patient for:
    a. respiratory arrest.
    b. shock.
    c. sepsis infection.
    d. severe dehydration.

67. Chronic right heart failure may present with signs and symptoms of tachycardia, peripheral edema, and:
    a. ascites.
    b. syncope.
    c. back pain.
    d. leg pain.

68. When the heart suddenly becomes so weak that it cannot effectively pump enough blood throughout the body, the condition is called:
    a. endocarditis.
    b. pericardial tamponade.
    c. cardiogenic shock.
    d. acute myocardial infarction.

69. You were dispatched to a patient found unresponsive in the park. It is early morning and 25°F. The patient appears to be in his late sixties, smells of urine and alcohol, and is apneic and pulseless. You and your crew administer 2 minutes of high-quality CPR, determine the rhythm is V-fib, and continue CPR following the V-fib algorithm. After 15 minutes the rhythm remains V-fib. Which of the following factors is most likely the reason the patient's rhythm is resistant to defibrillation?
    a. age
    b. alcohol use
    c. hypothermia
    d. prolonged downtime

70. The goal in the treatment of CHF is to improve oxygenation and ventilation by:
    a. increasing afterload.
    b. decreasing preload.
    c. administering IV fluid therapy.
    d. stopping the possible infarction.

71. When a patient with a history of chronic heart failure rapidly progresses to a state of severe pulmonary edema, more aggressive treatment such as _____ is needed to manage the patient.
    a. external pacing
    b. fluid replacement
    c. ventilatory support
    d. obtaining a 12 lead ECG

72. The most severe form of heart failure, resulting in inadequate cardiac output caused by left ventricular malfunction, is called:
    a. cardiogenic shock.
    b. ischemic shock.
    c. sudden death.
    d. cardiomyopathy.

73. To help differentiate between congestive heart failure (CHF) and acute pulmonary edema (APE), the paramedic should assess for:
    a. shortness of breath.
    b. wet lung sounds.
    c. ECG changes.
    d. past medical history of heart disease.

74. Which of the following is a life-threatening condition with a pathology of an accumulation of fluids in the pericardial sac?
    a. pericarditis
    b. cardiac tamponade
    c. pneumopericardium
    d. myocarditis

75. You are assessing a 59-year-old female with a chief complaint of dyspnea. Your primary assessment findings reveal an R/R of 34 and labored crackles in the bases of the lungs, SpO_2 of 90%, P/R of 112/irregular, and BP of 140/100 mmHg, and she is afebrile. PMHx includes HTN and COPD. Your first differential diagnosis is:

    a. CHF versus APE.

    b. pneumonia versus URI.

    c. CHF versus pneumonia.

    d. APE versus URI.

76. The initial signs and symptoms of cardiogenic shock are the same as seen with:

    a. neurogenic shock.

    b. ACS.

    c. APE.

    d. CVA.

77. Peripheral edema is more likely to be present with _____ because it takes several hours to days to develop.

    a. chronic CHF

    b. pneumonia

    c. acute myocardial infarction

    d. bronchitis

78. When treating a patient with CHF, which of the following is paramount to improve oxygenation and ventilation?

    a. positioning the patient supine

    b. positioning the patient upright

    c. starting an IV

    d. intubating the patient

79. You have been called to manage a 72-year-old female who awoke suddenly from sleep with shortness of breath and diaphoresis. She tells you that she has a history of heart failure. You suspect that she is presenting with:

    a. anxiety.

    b. exacerbation of COPD.

    c. bronchitis.

    d. paroxysmal nocturnal dyspnea.

80. You are dispatched to the residence of a 45-year-old male who had a seizure. The patient is conscious but confused, and he complains of severe headache and nausea. His family tells you that he had one seizure and was vomiting earlier. You administer oxygen while your partner obtains vital signs: skin is warm, dry, and flushed in the face; respirations 16/nonlabored; pulse 90/irregular; BP 240/140 mmHg; and SpO_2. Which additional diagnostic information will be most helpful before providing additional treatment?

    a. 12 lead ECG

    b. $EtCO_2$

    c. temperature

    d. blood glucose

81. (Continuing with question 80) You now have the following diagnostic information: 12 lead ECG is sinus rhythm with PACs; $EtCO_2$ is 42 mm Hg; temperature is 98.4°F (37.3°C); and blood glucose is 150 mg/dL. This patient is most likely experiencing:

    a. meningitis.

    b. a dysrhythmia.

    c. a diabetic problem.

    d. hypertensive emergency.

82. Chronic hypertension weakens arterial blood vessels due to excessive pressures and the three primary types of damage that occur are stroke, aneurysm, and:

    a. blindness.

    b. renal failure.

    c. neuropathy.

    d. liver failure.

83. When a blood clot forms in the deep vein of the leg and then moves to another part of the body it is called:

    a. an embolism.

    b. deep vein thrombosis.

    c. pericardial tamponade.

    d. peripheral artery disease.

84. Aneurysms often go unrecognized until the bulging of the sac grows so large that the pressure it exerts on other structures causes symptoms such as:

    a. pain.

    b. hypotension.

    c. hypertension.

    d. syncope.

85. If an abdominal aortic aneurysm goes unrecognized or untreated it may grow and burst, usually resulting in:
    a. ACS.
    b. CVA.
    c. paralysis.
    d. sudden death.

86. Prehospital management of aortic abdominal aneurysm (AAA) is limited to suspicion or recognition of the condition, supportive care, and:
    a. rapid transport.
    b. stabilization prior to transport.
    c. definitive treatment.
    d. localized treatment.

87. Clinical signs and symptoms associated with hypertensive crisis include:
    a. headache, backache, and dizziness.
    b. headache, vision disturbance, and confusion.
    c. vision disturbance, nausea, and shortness of breath.
    d. chest pain, confusion, and vomiting.

88. Marfan's syndrome is a connective tissue disease in which the features are found primarily in the:
    a. brain.
    b. bones and joints.
    c. heart and blood vessels.
    d. lungs, brain, and heart.

89. You are taking care of an elderly female whom you have discovered has accidentally taken an overdose of her potassium medication. Knowing that potassium has important effects on cardiac function, what clinical finding would you expect to be present in this patient?
    a. bradycardia
    b. tachycardia
    c. PVCs
    d. PACs

90. You are evaluating an 82-year-old woman who has had an episode of syncope. She is short of breath, complaining of numbness in both legs, and has back pain. Her husband tells you that, before passing out, she had complained of lower-back pain. She has a history of diabetes and hypertension. Her vital signs are skin pale, cool, and dry; respirations 22/shallow; pulse 114/irregular; BP 78/40 mmHg; and 12 lead ECG is NRS with inverted T waves in leads II and III. This patient is most likely experiencing:
    a. silent MI.
    b. urinary tract infection.
    c. gastrointestinal bleeding.
    d. dissecting abdominal aortic aneurysm.

91. Aspirin is given to patients with acute chest pain to thin the blood in an effort to:
    a. relieve chest pain.
    b. restore perfusion.
    c. increase myocardial workload.
    d. differentiate angina from ACS.

92. _____ sign is a paradoxical filling of the neck veins during inspiration and suggests a right ventricular infarction, massive pulmonary embolism, or pericarditis.
    a. Beck's
    b. Kussmaul's
    c. Cushing's
    d. Levine's

93. Several types of pacemakers are available for patients with irreversible heart damage. The type of pacemaker a patient receives depends on the:
    a. size of the heart.
    b. sex of the patient.
    c. age of the patient.
    d. location of the damage.

94. While interviewing a patient, she tells you that she has an implanted pacemaker. During your physical examination of the patient, where would you expect to see a scar for the site of the implantation?
    a. left-upper back
    b. right-lower abdomen
    c. left chest area
    d. right thigh

95. When the heart muscle becomes hypoxic, the myocardium becomes irritable and may cause:
    a. systemic ischemia.
    b. blood loss.
    c. ACS.
    d. dysrhythmias.

96. When a person experiences a heart attack that damages the muscle affecting the heart's electrical system, which of the following conditions is most likely to occur?
    a. heart block
    b. myocarditis
    c. pericarditis
    d. atrial fibrillation

97. The definitive treatment of cardiac tamponade is to:
    a. place a chest tube.
    b. relieve cardiac compression.
    c. decompress the chest.
    d. administer IV antibiotic therapy.

98. You are treating a 74-year-old female complaining of 10/10 chest pain after awakening from a syncopal episode. Her vital signs are respirations 24/labored, pulse 38/irregular, and BP is 78/40 mmHg. Which treatment must be applied first?

    a. IV and amiodarone
    b. external pacemaker
    c. IV fluids and atropine
    d. aspirin and nitroglycerin

99. You are dispatched to a call for severe respiratory distress. Upon arrival, you are brought to a hospice patient with leukemia. A friend called EMS because the patient is too weak to be driven to the hospital. The patient tells you that he becomes short of breath when ambulating, and he denies chest pain. His vital signs are skin pale, warm, and dry; respirations 22/nonlabored; pulse 56/irregular; and BP 130/76 mmHg. Your partner administers oxygen while you obtain the ECG. The rhythm is a very narrow complex with a P wave after each QRS complex, and the rate fluctuates between 40 and 60. What is the rhythm?

    a. sinus bradycardia
    b. junctional escape
    c. accelerated junctional
    d. controlled atrial fibrillation

100. (Continuing with the patient from question 99) Four minutes after you begin transport to the hospital, the patient tells you that he now has nausea and chest pain 8/10 that radiates into his neck and back. He states that the pain feels like his angina. His vital signs and ECG are unchanged from the baseline set. What action should you take next?

    a. Obtain a 12 lead ECG.
    b. Administer nitroglycerine and aspirin.
    c. Observe only, because he is a hospice patient.
    d. Administer an antiemetic and call medical control.

Exam #22 Answer Form

	A	B	C	D			A	B	C	D
1.	❏	❏	❏	❏		31.	❏	❏	❏	❏
2.	❏	❏	❏	❏		32.	❏	❏	❏	❏
3.	❏	❏	❏	❏		33.	❏	❏	❏	❏
4.	❏	❏	❏	❏		34.	❏	❏	❏	❏
5.	❏	❏	❏	❏		35.	❏	❏	❏	❏
6.	❏	❏	❏	❏		36.	❏	❏	❏	❏
7.	❏	❏	❏	❏		37.	❏	❏	❏	❏
8.	❏	❏	❏	❏		38.	❏	❏	❏	❏
9.	❏	❏	❏	❏		39.	❏	❏	❏	❏
10.	❏	❏	❏	❏		40.	❏	❏	❏	❏
11.	❏	❏	❏	❏		41.	❏	❏	❏	❏
12.	❏	❏	❏	❏		42.	❏	❏	❏	❏
13.	❏	❏	❏	❏		43.	❏	❏	❏	❏
14.	❏	❏	❏	❏		44.	❏	❏	❏	❏
15.	❏	❏	❏	❏		45.	❏	❏	❏	❏
16.	❏	❏	❏	❏		46.	❏	❏	❏	❏
17.	❏	❏	❏	❏		47.	❏	❏	❏	❏
18.	❏	❏	❏	❏		48.	❏	❏	❏	❏
19.	❏	❏	❏	❏		49.	❏	❏	❏	❏
20.	❏	❏	❏	❏		50.	❏	❏	❏	❏
21.	❏	❏	❏	❏		51.	❏	❏	❏	❏
22.	❏	❏	❏	❏		52.	❏	❏	❏	❏
23.	❏	❏	❏	❏		53.	❏	❏	❏	❏
24.	❏	❏	❏	❏		54.	❏	❏	❏	❏
25.	❏	❏	❏	❏		55.	❏	❏	❏	❏
26.	❏	❏	❏	❏		56.	❏	❏	❏	❏
27.	❏	❏	❏	❏		57.	❏	❏	❏	❏
28.	❏	❏	❏	❏		58.	❏	❏	❏	❏
29.	❏	❏	❏	❏		59.	❏	❏	❏	❏
30.	❏	❏	❏	❏		60.	❏	❏	❏	❏

Exam #22 Answer Form

	A	B	C	D		A	B	C	D
61.	❏	❏	❏	❏	81.	❏	❏	❏	❏
62.	❏	❏	❏	❏	82.	❏	❏	❏	❏
63.	❏	❏	❏	❏	83.	❏	❏	❏	❏
64.	❏	❏	❏	❏	84.	❏	❏	❏	❏
65.	❏	❏	❏	❏	85.	❏	❏	❏	❏
66.	❏	❏	❏	❏	86.	❏	❏	❏	❏
67.	❏	❏	❏	❏	87.	❏	❏	❏	❏
68.	❏	❏	❏	❏	88.	❏	❏	❏	❏
69.	❏	❏	❏	❏	89.	❏	❏	❏	❏
70.	❏	❏	❏	❏	90.	❏	❏	❏	❏
71.	❏	❏	❏	❏	91.	❏	❏	❏	❏
72.	❏	❏	❏	❏	92.	❏	❏	❏	❏
73.	❏	❏	❏	❏	93.	❏	❏	❏	❏
74.	❏	❏	❏	❏	94.	❏	❏	❏	❏
75.	❏	❏	❏	❏	95.	❏	❏	❏	❏
76.	❏	❏	❏	❏	96.	❏	❏	❏	❏
77.	❏	❏	❏	❏	97.	❏	❏	❏	❏
78.	❏	❏	❏	❏	98.	❏	❏	❏	❏
79.	❏	❏	❏	❏	99.	❏	❏	❏	❏
80.	❏	❏	❏	❏	100.	❏	❏	❏	❏

CHAPTER

23

Neurology

1. The major function of the nervous system is to:
   a. monitor internal changes of the body.
   b. circulate nutrients to all body cells.
   c. regulate the neurons.
   d. provide support for the body structures.

2. The largest part of the brain is divided into right and left hemispheres and is called the:
   a. cerebellum.
   b. cerebrum.
   c. diencephalon.
   d. brain stem.

3. The _____ is the location in the brain of higher cognitive functions such as learning and language.
   a. corpus callosum
   b. telencephalon
   c. diencephalon
   d. thalamus

4. Blood enters the brain from the two internal carotid arteries and the:
   a. jugular artery.
   b. iliac artery.
   c. basilar artery.
   d. subclavian artery.

5. The structure that forms a circle around the stalk of the pituitary gland and works as a backup mechanism for complications with cerebral blood flow is called the:
   a. foramen magnum.
   b. arch of atlas.
   c. circle of Willis.
   d. cerebral spinal canal.

6. The structures within the brain stem, from top (superior) to bottom (inferior), are the:
   a. pituitary, midbrain, and pons.
   b. midbrain, pons, and medulla oblongata.
   c. pons, midbrain, and medulla oblongata.
   d. medulla oblongata, pituitary, midbrain, and pons.

7. The _____ regulates the biologic clock of the body.
   a. pineal body
   b. medulla
   c. thalamus
   d. optic chiasma

8. The section of the brain responsible for maintaining posture, balance, and voluntary coordination of skilled movements is the:
   a. midbrain.
   b. diencephalon.
   c. cerebellum.
   d. brain stem.

9. Cerebrospinal fluid (CSF) is present in the spinal cord, cavities, and canals of the brain as well as the:
   a. temporal gap.
   b. parietal shelf.
   c. epidural space.
   d. subarachnoid space.

10. CSF has several functions, one of which is to:
    a. help with coordination and balance.
    b. help regulate the biological clock of the body.
    c. oxygenate tissues in the brain and spinal cord.
    d. help the brain to recognize changes in CO_2 levels.

11. _____ is an increase in the amount of CSF, from either a blockage or decrease in normal reabsorption.
    a. Cerebrosis
    b. Hydrocephalus
    c. Cerebroma
    d. Cephalophora

12. Which of the meninges is the highly vascular covering of the brain and spinal cord?
    a. dura mater
    b. pia mater
    c. arachnoid membrane
    d. falx cerebelli

13. Meningitis is a potentially life-threatening infection of both the _____ and meninges.
    a. spinal cord
    b. white matter
    c. CSF
    d. gray matter

14. The major difference between gray matter and white matter is that gray matter is:
    a. not covered with myelinated fibers.
    b. covered with myelinated fibers.
    c. ashen colored because of anaerobic metabolism.
    d. there really is no major difference.

15. The fundamental component of the nervous system is the:
    a. myelin.
    b. neuron.
    c. spinal cord.
    d. nerve impulse.

16. The _____ is the part of the nerve cell that is responsible for the supply of energy in the form of ATP (adenosine triphosphate).
    a. axon
    b. nucleus
    c. dendrite
    d. mitochondrium

17. Nervous tissue requires a tremendous amount of metabolic energy. For this to occur, it is essential that there is a constant supply of oxygen and:
    a. potassium.
    b. sodium.
    c. glucose.
    d. carbon dioxide.

18. A disease process that destroys the myelin sheath and infects the nerve fibers, impairing nerve function, is called:
    a. multiple sclerosis.
    b. Parkinson's disease.
    c. epilepsy.
    d. Lou Gehrig's disease.

19. Nerve cells communicate with each other primarily through the:
    a. peripheral system.
    b. flow of acetylcholine.
    c. limbic system.
    d. synapses.

20. High in the brain stem is the _____, which is responsible for maintaining consciousness.
    a. reticular activating system
    b. limbic system
    c. autonomic nervous system (ANS)
    d. central nervous system (CNS)

21. The twelve pairs of cranial nerves are a component of which part of the nervous system?
    a. autonomic
    b. peripheral
    c. structural
    d. functional

22. _____ is a disorder of the CNS, named after the famous baseball player Lou Gehrig. It has a rapidly progressive deterioration leading to atrophy of all body muscles and death.
    a. Bell's palsy
    b. Amyotrophic lateral sclerosis (ALS)
    c. Cerebral palsy
    d. Parkinson's disease

23. The term for a chronic, progressive disease of the CNS characterized by exacerbation and remission of assorted multiple neurologic symptoms is:
    a. epilepsy.
    b. Bell's palsy.
    c. multiple sclerosis.
    d. Parkinson's disease.

24. Which of the following is an abnormal condition related to a structural problem within the brain, rather than an infectious disease of the nervous system?
    a. tetanus
    b. encephalitis
    c. poliomyelitis
    d. hydrocephalus

25. You are assessing a 28-year-old male complaining of a severe headache. Just before losing consciousness in front of you, he tells you that it came on very suddenly after he experienced a loud sound like a bang in his head. Which of the following conditions do you suspect was the cause of this event?
    a. CVA
    b. TIA
    c. ruptured aneurysm
    d. meningitis

26. You are looking at the chart of an elderly nursing home resident with a diagnosis of dementia. Also included in the history are possible causes of the dementia. Which of the following is most likely the cause of this patient's dementia?

    a. concussion

    b. atherosclerosis

    c. retrograde amnesia

    d. anterograde amnesia

27. Ischemia, ICP, cerebral edema, and brain herniation are all _____ injuries from traumatic brain injury.

    a. primary

    b. secondary

    c. tertiary

    d. irreversible

28. A mild closed head injury that results in a transient loss of brain function with or without a loss of consciousness is called:

    a. amnesia.

    b. contusion.

    c. concussion.

    d. contra-coup.

29. With the help of the fire department, your patient has been extricated from a vehicle with significant damage following a collision. The patient has been unconscious the entire time, and you strongly suspect that he has a traumatic brain injury. Which of the following can you do to significantly reduce the patient's morbidity?

    a. Administer steroids.

    b. Hyperventilate the patient.

    c. Rapidly transport the patient to a trauma center.

    d. Assess for CSF leakage from the nose and ears.

30. You are assessing a conscious patient with a known condition that causes low levels of dopamine in the parts of the brain that control voluntary movement. Today he has weakness and muscle rigidity in addition to his normal irregular gait and fine resting tremor. What is your impression of this patient?

    a. This is a common neurological emergency.

    b. This is an uncommon neurological emergency.

    c. This is a chronic disorder that does not require emergency care.

    d. This is a chronic disorder that requires prompt emergency care.

31. The major difference between a stroke and a TIA is that:

    a. a TIA always precedes a stroke.

    b. a stroke always precedes a TIA.

    c. the TIA has no lasting effect.

    d. the stroke is considered a warning sign.

32. An undiagnosed TIA is a very high risk factor for:

    a. hypertension.

    b. a major stroke.

    c. new-onset diabetes.

    d. heart disease.

33. A sudden, temporary change in behavior, sensory, or motor activity caused by an excessive or chaotic electrical discharge of one or more groups of neurons in the brain is known as a:

    a. TIA.

    b. CVA.

    c. seizure.

    d. palsy.

34. _____ headaches occur in men more than women and are severe with pain on one side of the head and often produce a nasal congestion, watery eyes, and runny nose on the same side as the pain.

    a. Sinus

    b. Cluster

    c. Tension

    d. Migraine

35. A seizure characterized by impairment of consciousness, including an aura, is a(n) _____ seizure.

    a. simple partial

    b. complex partial

    c. absence

    d. complete motor

36. Prolonged or repeated seizures are true emergencies because:

    a. brain damage can occur.

    b. the patient can swallow the tongue.

    c. the patient forgets to breathe.

    d. the acid in the blood decreases.

37. Noncardiac syncope often occurs in patients with no underlying disease, usually from a stressor such as pain, emotion, or:

    a. heat.

    b. cold.

    c. medication.

    d. strobe lights.

38. How is a patient's mental status best assessed?

    a. by speaking with the patient

    b. by assessing the cranial nerves

    c. by checking for symmetry of motor response

    d. by checking for deficits in coordination and reflexes

39. What is the most significant aspect of a neurologic assessment?

    a. performing serial assessments

    b. a positive Babinski sign

    c. absence of seizure activity

    d. medication compliance

40. First developed in 1974, the _____ is an objective measure of the patient's level of consciousness.

    a. Glasgow coma scale (GCS)

    b. AVPU

    c. Babinski sign

    d. CT scan

41. A respiratory pattern in which an extended inspiratory effort or gasping with a brief expiration, caused by pressure, damage, or surgical removal of the pons in the area of CN IV, is called:

    a. ataxic.

    b. Biot's respiration.

    c. cluster breathing.

    d. apneusis.

42. While assessing an unconscious, head-injured victim of an MVC, you observe the patient's respiratory effort as a pattern of cycles of apnea and hyperventilation. You recognize this pattern as:

    a. autisms.

    b. Kussmaul's breathing.

    c. Cheyne–Stokes respirations.

    d. apneusis.

43. Involuntary neurologic activities such as yawning, hiccupping, coughing, and vomiting are called:

    a. ataxics.

    b. autisms.

    c. clusters.

    d. central neurologic initiations.

44. _____ breathing often precedes agonal breathing (gasping) and apnea and has no pattern or rhythm with depth or rate.

    a. Biot's

    b. Kussmaul's

    c. Ataxic

    d. Cluster

45. The term for normal visual function of the eyes that depends on the ability of both eyes to fix on the same subject is:

    a. diplopia.

    b. binocular vision.

    c. medial gaze.

    d. vergence reflex.

46. The term _____ refers to the adjustment of the eyes to variations in distance.

    a. accommodation

    b. acuity

    c. conjugate gaze

    d. divergence

47. An involuntary movement of the eyes that can be in any direction, but more often is either vertical or horizontal, is:

    a. doll's eyes.

    b. dysconjugate gaze.

    c. nystagmus.

    d. diplopia.

48. An abnormal constriction of the pupils, caused by certain types of infection and some types of drug overdose, is called:

    a. anisocoria.

    b. glaucoma.

    c. dystonia.

    d. meiosis.

49. Nearly 10 percent of the population has a congenital inequality of their pupil sizes. The term for this condition is:

    a. anisocoria.

    b. glaucoma.

    c. akinesia.

    d. meiosis.

50. A brief involuntary movement of distal extremities and facial muscles, which often occurs in Huntington's disease, Parkinson's disease, and thyrotoxicosis, is:

    a. chorea.

    b. ballism.

    c. myclonus.

    d. tics.

51. The condition of slow and irregular involuntary winding movements of the extremities, as seen in cerebral palsy, encephalitis, and some drug side effects is:

    a. akinesia.

    b. athetosis.

    c. dystonia.

    d. dyskinesia.

52. A disorder with characteristics of lack of muscle coordination, involuntary muscle movement, tics, incoherent grunts, barks, and cursing is called:

    a. tremors.

    b. Creutzfeldt–Jakob's disease.

    c. Tourette's syndrome.

    d. Wernicke syndrome.

53. Assessing extraocular movements (EOMs) is the best single method for measuring brain stem integrity. Which of the following is a test for checking EOMs?

    a. Assess for palmar drift.

    b. Assess the patient's gait.

    c. Assess the six cardinal positions of gaze.

    d. Assess discriminative touch, dull versus sharp.

54. While assessing a patient presenting with new stroke symptoms such as dysphasia, difficulty swallowing, and chewing, which cranial nerve do you suspect is being affected?

    a. X

    b. VIII

    c. VI

    d. V

55. _____ is an abnormal gait characterized by unsteady, uncoordinated, wide at the base steps, as seen with drunkenness, heavily medicated persons, or certain medical conditions.

    a. Steppage

    b. Ataxia

    c. Festination

    d. Spastic hemiparesis

56. The loss of sensory and motor function below certain levels of the spine defines a(n):

    a. spinal cord injury.

    b. frontal lobe lesion.

    c. injury to Broca's area.

    d. precursor to ICP.

57. Patients experiencing cerebral vascular accidents including stroke, intracerebral, or subarachnoid hemorrhage can present with typical signs of _____, which can make diagnosis of the underlying problem difficult.

    a. hypothermia

    b. heat stroke

    c. hyperglycemia

    d. memory loss

58. The most common signs of brain dysfunction are AMS and:

    a. hyperglycemia.

    b. loss of motor control.

    c. speech deficits.

    d. behavioral changes.

59. You have been called to care for an unconscious patient with a known brain tumor. The patient presents with the jaws clenched and arms and legs extended. You suspect the lesion is located in the diencephalon, midbrain, or:

    a. pons.

    b. medulla.

    c. thalamus.

    d. insula.

60. _____ posturing, also referred to as flexion, is associated with a lesion at or above the upper brain stem.

    a. Broca's

    b. Wernicke's

    c. Decorticate

    d. Decerebrate

61. Cushing's triad is a(n) _____ sign of rising ICP.

    a. early

    b. late

    c. unreliable

    d. insufficient

62. Babinski's reflex is a test to assess for spinal cord dysfunction, specifically in the _____ portion of the motor control system.

    a. pyramidal

    b. extrapyramidal

    c. ipsilateral

    d. lateral

63. Both sides of the brain communicate via _____ to carry out many complex functions.

    a. the corpus callosum

    b. Broca's area

    c. Wernicke's area

    d. the island of Reil

64. The _____ lobe of the brain receives and translates somatic sensations of pain, touch, pressure, heat and cold, and body position.

    a. frontal

    b. parietal

    c. occipital

    d. temporal

65. The _____ links the nervous and endocrine systems as well as the mind (psyche) and body.

    a. thalamus

    b. insula

    c. pineal body

    d. hypothalamus

66. CSF is produced in the _____ and is completely replaced several times each day.
    a. spine
    b. epidural space
    c. ventricles of the brain
    d. arachnoid space

67. Wernicke's encephalopathy is caused by a lack of vitamin B_1 and causes brain damage in the:
    a. cerebrum.
    b. cerebellum.
    c. medulla oblongata.
    d. thalamus and hypothalamus.

68. What type of bleeding occurs in a subdural hematoma?
    a. venous
    b. arterial
    c. systemic
    d. metabolic

69. A 26-year-old female called 9-1-1 because 30 minutes ago she started drooling and felt numbness in her face. She walked out to the ambulance as you drove up and stated that she thinks she is having a stroke. Her speech is clear and appropriate and she is walking with no problem. In the ambulance you see that the left side of her face appears stiff and paralyzed, rather than drooping. She denies having a headache and her BP is 112/60 mmHg. What do you suspect is her problem?
    a. stroke
    b. Bell's palsy
    c. encephalitis
    d. meningitis

70. _____ are extensions of the nerve cell body with branches that conduct impulses to the cell body, relaying information to the neuron.
    a. Axons
    b. Dendrites
    c. DNA
    d. RNA

71. The layer or coating around the axon that protects the axon process and increases the conduction of nerve impulses is the:
    a. myelin.
    b. stratum.
    c. swathe.
    d. jacket.

72. The two most common hematomas that may develop within the brain are:
    a. temporal and parietal.
    b. epidural and subdural.
    c. cerebral and epidural.
    d. subdural and cerebral.

73. The most common developmental defect of the CNS occurring while in utero is:
    a. hydrocephalus.
    b. shingles.
    c. spina bifida.
    d. polio.

74. _____ is a viral infection causing inflammation of the gray matter of the spinal cord that may temporarily or permanently affect neurologic functions.
    a. Poliomyelitis
    b. Abscess
    c. Spina bifida
    d. Meningitis

75. Which of the following conditions may be seen with a head CT scan?
    a. concussion
    b. contusion
    c. amnesia
    d. aphasia

76. _____ is the type of amnesia that affects the ability to recall memories from the past.
    a. Aphasic
    b. Non-phasic
    c. Anterograde
    d. Retrograde

77. A 45-year-old male is complaining, "I am having the worst headache of my life." He is lying on his couch in the dark. The headache came on suddenly without trauma. His vital signs are skin warm and dry, respirations 22 nonlabored, pulse rate 98/regular, and BP is 144/92 mmHg. What do you suspect is causing the headache?
    a. meningitis
    b. migraine
    c. hypertension
    d. subarachnoid hemorrhage

78. (Continuing with the previous question) What information should the paramedic obtain that will be most valuable prior to arriving at the hospital?
    a. blood glucose reading
    b. results of a stroke exam
    c. 12 ECG and SpO$_2$ reading
    d. history of recent trauma

79. You are using a thrombolytic checklist on a patient presenting with stroke symptoms. Which of the following is an exclusion criterion for the use of fibrinolytics?
    a. alert mental status
    b. able to give consent
    c. uncontrolled hypertension
    d. onset of symptoms < 3 hours

80. When the paramedic finds a patient with dilated pupils, she must look at the medications the patient is taking and consider if a medication is causing the dilation. Which classifications of drugs will produce dilated pupils?
    a. anticholinergics
    b. antihypertensives
    c. anticoagulants
    d. antidiabletics

81. The _____ test is used in comatose patients to assess for brain stem or oculomotor injury, after neck injury has been ruled out.
    a. accommodation
    b. doll's-eye maneuver
    c. drop-foot
    d. pronator drift

82. The difference of _____ millimeter(s) or more in the size of the pupils is an abnormal finding.
    a. 1
    b. 2
    c. 3
    d. 4

83. _____ is the loss of ability to speak because of a defect in or loss of language function.
    a. Ataxia
    b. Aphasia
    c. Dysarthria
    d. Dysphonia

84. The primary problem with rising intracranial pressure is that this condition can damage the brain or spinal cord by:
    a. causing seizures.
    b. causing infection.
    c. restricting blood flow into the brain.
    d. inhibiting reuptake of dopamine.

85. When describing the patient's mental status, avoid terms such as *stupor*, *lethargic*, and *obtunded* because they:
    a. all mean the same thing.
    b. mean different things to different people.
    c. are difficult to spell.
    d. are not real medical terms.

86. An unconscious 36-year-old patient was seen seizing by his family. They tell you that the seizure lasted approximately 2 minutes, and that he has no history of seizures. You open the airway, administer high-concentration oxygen, complete a primary assessment, and quickly obtain vital signs and a blood glucose reading. Which of the following findings suggests a neurologic deficit?
    a. blood around the mouth
    b. irregular breathing pattern
    c. withdrawing from painful stimulus
    d. blood glucose reading of 180 mg/dl

87. Loss of lateral eye movement is an early sign of:
    a. vision loss.
    b. rising ICP.
    c. decreasing ICP.
    d. an orbital fracture.

88. You are assessing the driver of an automobile that was rear-ended at a moderate speed. The patient was complaining of severe pain in the left leg immediately after the collision, but there is no apparent trauma to the leg. Which of the following do you suspect?
    a. herniated disc
    b. spinal fracture
    c. muscle cramp
    d. faking

89. A functional disorder of the CNS, characterized by unilateral facial paralysis caused by compression of cranial nerve VII (facial nerve) is called:
    a. a brain abscess.
    b. a neoplasm.
    c. Bell's palsy.
    d. ALS.

90. During what part of the day do thrombotic strokes typically occur?

a. late morning

b. early afternoon

c. early evening

d. during sleep

91. The parents of a 6-month-old infant called EMS when the baby had a seizure for the first time. They were extremely upset as they described the baby rolling his eyes back into his head and how it appeared as if he had stopped breathing for a few seconds. Which of the following is the least likely cause of the patient's seizure?

a. epilepsy

b. infection

c. congenital defect

d. electrolyte abnormality

92. The phase of a seizure characterized by a loss of consciousness with muscle contraction is called:

a. preictal.

b. aura.

c. tonic.

d. clonic.

93. A _____ event is a transient loss of consciousness caused by a decreased blood supply to the brain.

a. TIA

b. CVA

c. syncopal

d. seizure

94. The term _____ means new growth and is used synonymously with tumor.

a. abscess

b. migraine

c. neoplasm

d. foci

95. Which of the following is a possible sign associated with a neurologic disorder, rather than the neurologic disorder itself?

a. seizures

b. shingles

c. hypertension

d. Alzheimer's

96. Tic douloureux is pain in one or more of the three branches of the _____ cranial nerve that runs along the face.

a. III

b. V

c. VIII

d. XII

97. Glaucoma can occur as a congenital defect or as a result of another eye disorder and is associated with:

a. heredity.

b. trauma.

c. hyperthyroidism.

d. female gender.

98. You are assessing a 62-year-old male who called EMS because he has severe eye pain. The pain came on suddenly while the patient was watching TV. The eye is red, the pupil is dilated, and he tells you his vision is blurred. He also feels nauseated. The patient has no significant medical history and no vision disorders. What could be the cause of his sudden ailment?

a. stroke

b. glaucoma

c. Bell's palsy

d. trigeminal neuralgia

99. Your patient is a 32-year-old male who suddenly lost function in his legs while at home. He has history of chronic back pain, but no recent trauma, illness, or surgery. His vital signs are stable. What do you suspect is causing his problem?

a. back spasm

b. meningitis

c. blood clot from a deep vein

d. compression on the spinal cord

100. (Continuing with the patient in the previous question) What is the most appropriate treatment?

a. splinting the legs

b. pain management

c. spinal immobilization

d. position of comfort

Exam #23 Answer Form

	A	B	C	D			A	B	C	D
1.	❏	❏	❏	❏		31.	❏	❏	❏	❏
2.	❏	❏	❏	❏		32.	❏	❏	❏	❏
3.	❏	❏	❏	❏		33.	❏	❏	❏	❏
4.	❏	❏	❏	❏		34.	❏	❏	❏	❏
5.	❏	❏	❏	❏		35.	❏	❏	❏	❏
6.	❏	❏	❏	❏		36.	❏	❏	❏	❏
7.	❏	❏	❏	❏		37.	❏	❏	❏	❏
8.	❏	❏	❏	❏		38.	❏	❏	❏	❏
9.	❏	❏	❏	❏		39.	❏	❏	❏	❏
10.	❏	❏	❏	❏		40.	❏	❏	❏	❏
11.	❏	❏	❏	❏		41.	❏	❏	❏	❏
12.	❏	❏	❏	❏		42.	❏	❏	❏	❏
13.	❏	❏	❏	❏		43.	❏	❏	❏	❏
14.	❏	❏	❏	❏		44.	❏	❏	❏	❏
15.	❏	❏	❏	❏		45.	❏	❏	❏	❏
16.	❏	❏	❏	❏		46.	❏	❏	❏	❏
17.	❏	❏	❏	❏		47.	❏	❏	❏	❏
18.	❏	❏	❏	❏		48.	❏	❏	❏	❏
19.	❏	❏	❏	❏		49.	❏	❏	❏	❏
20.	❏	❏	❏	❏		50.	❏	❏	❏	❏
21.	❏	❏	❏	❏		51.	❏	❏	❏	❏
22.	❏	❏	❏	❏		52.	❏	❏	❏	❏
23.	❏	❏	❏	❏		53.	❏	❏	❏	❏
24.	❏	❏	❏	❏		54.	❏	❏	❏	❏
25.	❏	❏	❏	❏		55.	❏	❏	❏	❏
26.	❏	❏	❏	❏		56.	❏	❏	❏	❏
27.	❏	❏	❏	❏		57.	❏	❏	❏	❏
28.	❏	❏	❏	❏		58.	❏	❏	❏	❏
29.	❏	❏	❏	❏		59.	❏	❏	❏	❏
30.	❏	❏	❏	❏		60.	❏	❏	❏	❏

Exam #23 Answer Form

	A	B	C	D		A	B	C	D
61.	❏	❏	❏	❏	81.	❏	❏	❏	❏
62.	❏	❏	❏	❏	82.	❏	❏	❏	❏
63.	❏	❏	❏	❏	83.	❏	❏	❏	❏
64.	❏	❏	❏	❏	84.	❏	❏	❏	❏
65.	❏	❏	❏	❏	85.	❏	❏	❏	❏
66.	❏	❏	❏	❏	86.	❏	❏	❏	❏
67.	❏	❏	❏	❏	87.	❏	❏	❏	❏
68.	❏	❏	❏	❏	88.	❏	❏	❏	❏
69.	❏	❏	❏	❏	89.	❏	❏	❏	❏
70.	❏	❏	❏	❏	90.	❏	❏	❏	❏
71.	❏	❏	❏	❏	91.	❏	❏	❏	❏
72.	❏	❏	❏	❏	92.	❏	❏	❏	❏
73.	❏	❏	❏	❏	93.	❏	❏	❏	❏
74.	❏	❏	❏	❏	94.	❏	❏	❏	❏
75.	❏	❏	❏	❏	95.	❏	❏	❏	❏
76.	❏	❏	❏	❏	96.	❏	❏	❏	❏
77.	❏	❏	❏	❏	97.	❏	❏	❏	❏
78.	❏	❏	❏	❏	98.	❏	❏	❏	❏
79.	❏	❏	❏	❏	99.	❏	❏	❏	❏
80.	❏	❏	❏	❏	100.	❏	❏	❏	❏

CHAPTER

24

Endocrine Diseases

1. The most common of the endocrine emergencies is
   _____, which occur(s) more frequently than all the
   rest combined.
   a. fluid imbalance
   b. altered mental status
   c. diabetic problems
   d. respiratory problems

2. Which of the following is not a risk factor predisposing to endocrine disease?
   a. hyperlipidemia
   b. heredity
   c. hypothyroidism
   d. hypopituitarism

3. _____ is the leading cause of adult blindness,
   end-stage kidney failure, and nontraumatic lower
   extremity amputations.
   a. Diabetes
   b. Hypopituitarism
   c. Hypothyroidism
   d. Hyperthyroidism

4. The endocrine system is an integrated _____ and
   coordination system enabling reproduction, growth
   and development, and regulation of energy.
   a. chemical
   b. fluid
   c. muscle
   d. nerve

5. The endocrine system, together with the _____
   system, maintains internal homeostasis of the body
   and coordinates responses to environmental changes
   and stress.
   a. GI
   b. integumentary
   c. biofeedback
   d. nervous

6. _____ regulate many body functions, such as
   growth, reproduction, temperature, metabolism, and
   blood pressure.
   a. Stem cells
   b. Hormones
   c. Receptors
   d. Emotions

7. Endocrines are called "ductless glands" because they
   secrete their chemical hormones directly into the:
   a. brain.
   b. heart.
   c. lungs.
   d. blood.

8. The only known cure for type I diabetes is:
   a. an adrenal transplant.
   b. a pancreas transplant.
   c. suppression of the adrenals with medication.
   d. suppression of the thyroid gland with medication.

9. The _____ gland, sometimes known as the "master
   gland," is located at the base of the brain in the cranial
   cavity.
   a. parathyroid
   b. adrenal
   c. pituitary
   d. gonad

10. Which of the following endocrine glands is
    responsible for maintaining normal levels of calcium
    in the blood?
    a. parathyroid
    b. adrenal
    c. pituitary
    d. ovaries

11. The _____ is considered an organ of both the digestive and the endocrine systems.
    a. thyroid
    b. parathyroid
    c. pancreas
    d. testes

12. The _____ gland(s) is(are) responsible for secretion of the hormones vital to maintaining the body's water and salt balance.
    a. pancreas
    b. insulin
    c. pituitary
    d. adrenal

13. _____ is one of the major reasons a patient develops an endocrine emergency.
    a. Hyperthermia
    b. Excessive hormone production
    c. Excessive sympathetic stimulation
    d. Disproportionate parasympathetic stimulation

14. In the body's normal regulation of the blood sugar level, insulin is released from the pancreas together with:
    a. epinephrine and glucagon.
    b. glucagon.
    c. amino acids.
    d. fatty acids.

15. Insulin moves sugar molecules from the blood into the cell, where they are:
    a. stored.
    b. bathed.
    c. reconstituted.
    d. broken down.

16. _____ occurs as a result of a viral infection of the pancreas, leading to the formation of antibodies to pancreatic beta-cells that produce insulin.
    a. Type I diabetes
    b. Type II diabetes
    c. Obesity
    d. Insulin receptor resistance

17. Diabetic patients do not always have the classic symptoms of myocardial ischemia, such as crushing substernal chest pain, because:
    a. glucose is the sole source of oxidative metabolism for the CNS.
    b. insulin numbs the pain.
    c. many diabetics have some form of neuropathy.
    d. elevated blood lipid levels alter sensation.

18. Hypoglycemia of more than 20 to 30 minutes' duration results in the production of toxic compounds in the brain that cause:
    a. cardiac arrest.
    b. excessive levels of heat production.
    c. a decrease in the thyroid function.
    d. permanent neuronal damage.

19. Many patients with hyperglycemia are significantly _____; therefore, _____ is(are) part of the primary treatment.
    a. hyperthermic; cooling
    b. hypothermic; heat
    c. dehydrated; fluids
    d. altered in mental status; insulin

20. Diabetic patients lack the normal effects of insulin; therefore, sugar and other substances such as _____ fail to enter the cells properly.
    a. amino acids
    b. glycogen
    c. proteins
    d. triglycerides

21. Diabetic ketoacidosis (DKA) is a metabolic condition consisting of hyperglycemia, dehydration, and the accumulation of _____ in the body.
    a. uric acid
    b. free fatty acids
    c. amino acids
    d. ketones and ketoacids

22. The effects of osmotic diuresis in diabetic patients cause frequent urination. At times, this can lead to dehydration. Depending on the severity of her condition, the patient may also be deficient in:
    a. ketones and ketoacids.
    b. neurons.
    c. calcium.
    d. total body potassium.

23. The most common reason a diabetic patient develops DKA is because of:
    a. excess glucagon.
    b. infection.
    c. too much insulin.
    d. too little insulin.

24. Which of the following statements about DKA is most accurate?
    a. All patients with hyperglycemia have DKA.
    b. Not every patient with hyperglycemia will have DKA.
    c. Hypoglycemic patients who lapse into a coma will also be in shock.
    d. Distinguishing between hyperglycemia and DKA in the field is relatively easy.

25. During periods of insulin deficiency, _____ is(are) broken down to provide energy.
    a. ketones
    b. glucagon
    c. stored fats
    d. epinephrine

26. Ketoacidosis develops when the level of ketones in the _____ is too _____.
    a. blood; high
    b. pancreas; high
    c. blood; low
    d. pancreas; low

27. The diabetic emergency that occurs from a relative insulin deficiency that leads to marked hyperglycemia, but with the absence of ketones and acidosis is called:
    a. hypoosmolar hyperglycemic nonketotic coma.
    b. hyperosmolar hyperglycemic nonketotic coma.
    c. nonketotic mellitus.
    d. nonketotic osmolitis.

28. Many long-standing diabetic patients remain asymptomatic until their sugar level drops low enough to result in loss of consciousness. This occurs because:
    a. early warning signs from the counter-regulatory hormones fail.
    b. they have acquired dysfunction of the peripheral nervous system.
    c. they develop a tolerance to symptoms.
    d. early warning signs from the beta-cells are inactivated.

29. Which of the following substances can increase a person's sensitivity to hypoglycemia, which may result in a person feeling hypoglycemic symptoms at blood sugar levels not usually associated with causing problems?
    a. poppy seeds
    b. chocolate
    c. peanuts
    d. caffeine

30. The production of glucagon and epinephrine stimulates enzymes that break down glycogen to glucose. This process is called:
    a. homeostasis.
    b. Harada's syndrome.
    c. gluconeogenesis.
    d. glycogenolysis.

31. Hyperglycemia is common in _____ due to insulin resistance and increased glycogenolysis.
    a. massive head trauma
    b. Cushing's syndrome
    c. thyrotoxicosis
    d. myxedema coma

32. Signs and symptoms of new-onset thyrotoxicosis in a 55-year-old female include:
    a. atrial fibrillation and fever.
    b. hypothermia and hypoglycemia.
    c. muscle weakness and hirsuitism.
    d. weight loss and brown pigmentation of the skin.

33. Before the diagnosis of _____ is established, patients often have fatigue, lethargy, and gradual weight gain for years.
    a. hyperthyroidism
    b. hypothyroidism
    c. myxedema coma
    d. Cushing's syndrome

34. An elderly female patient with a recent history of infection and a past medical history of thyroid disease is found with an altered mental status. She is breathing slow and shallow and feels cold to the touch in a warm environment. Which endocrine disorder is this patient exhibiting?
    a. hyperthyroidism
    b. myxedema coma
    c. Cushing's syndrome
    d. hypoglycemia

35. You are doing an ALS transfer from one medical facility to another for a patient in full myxedema coma. What dysrhythmia is most common for a patient in this condition?
    a. tachycardia
    b. atrial fibrillation
    c. sinus bradycardia
    d. sick sinus syndrome

36. _____ is a metabolic syndrome resulting from hypersecretion of the glucocorticoid hormone, cortisol, which affects carbohydrate, protein, and lipid metabolism.
    a. Cushing's syndrome
    b. Adrenal insufficiency
    c. Addison's disease
    d. Graves' disease

37. _____ is an endocrine disorder associated with excess growth of body hair, abnormal pattern of fat distribution, adult-onset acne, and purple or dark stretch marks.
    a. Thyrotoxicosis
    b. Exophthalmus
    c. Hypothyroidism
    d. Cushing's syndrome

38. In many cases, the chronic overproduction of hormones from the adrenal glands is a result of:
    a. heredity.
    b. antihypertensives.
    c. electrolyte imbalance.
    d. tumors in the adrenal glands.

39. Autoimmune destruction of the adrenal glands is the most common cause of adrenal insufficiency and is called:
    a. Cushing's syndrome.
    b. thyroid storm.
    c. Addison's disease.
    d. Graves' disease.

40. Adrenal insufficiency is inadequate production of adrenal hormones, primarily _____, for any of a number of reasons.
    a. adrenocortical
    b. cortisol and aldosterone
    c. follicle-stimulating hormone (FSH)
    d. parathyroid hormone (PTH)

41. The pathophysiology of adrenal insufficiency is that the normal feedback loop between the hypothalamus, pituitary gland, and adrenal gland is suppressed because of:
    a. the use of oral or inhaled steroids.
    b. daily injections of insulin.
    c. the use of oral hypoglycemic agents.
    d. daily estrogen use.

42. Signs and symptoms of chronic adrenal insufficiency include:
    a. weight loss, fatigue, and joint pain.
    b. weight gain, overeating, and weakness.
    c. cold intolerance, constipation, and hypertension.
    d. increased thirst, frequent urination, and increased libido.

43. Acute adrenal insufficiency, sometimes called an Addisonian crisis, presents as hypotension, hypoglycemia, and severe:
    a. hypovolemia.
    b. hypercarbia.
    c. weight loss.
    d. muscle and joint pain.

44. Protrusion of the eyeballs (exophthalmus) is a common physical finding in patients with:
    a. hyperthyroidism.
    b. hypothyroidism.
    c. myxedema coma.
    d. Cushing's syndrome.

45. Oral diabetic agents work by:
    a. decreasing caloric intake.
    b. increasing the amount of glucose in the blood.
    c. stimulating the pancreas to secrete more insulin.
    d. inhibiting the pancreas from releasing too much insulin.

46. The onset of action is faster and duration is shorter with _____ insulin preparations.
    a. beef
    b. pork
    c. human
    d. chicken

47. Insulin is a protein secreted from the pancreas in healthy individuals. When the pancreas can no longer release insulin, the effect is:
    a. hypoglycemia.
    b. fluid retention.
    c. a state of cell starvation.
    d. an uptake of free fatty acids.

48. Your patient has a nontraumatic altered mental status. His vital signs are H/R 110, BP 74/44 mmHg, R/R 20, and his skin is warm and moist. His spouse tells you that he is not diabetic, but he does have asthma and uses steroid inhalers daily. You check his glucose level, and it is 40 mg/dl. After assuring that his airway and breathing are adequate, what would be the next appropriate step in care?
    a. Administer glucagon.
    b. Give fluid boluses.
    c. Administer IV dextrose.
    d. Administer thiamine.

49. As hypoglycemia alone does not typically result in hypotension, which of the following conditions is the patient discussed in question 48 most likely experiencing?
    a. acute adrenal insufficiency
    b. Cushing's syndrome
    c. myxedema
    d. thyrotoxicosis

50. Cushing's syndrome is caused by the hypersecretion of glucocorticoids by the _____ gland(s).
    a. adrenal
    b. thymus
    c. reproductive
    d. pancreas

51. You are assessing a 22-year-old male with insulin-dependent diabetes mellitus (IDDM) who is having a diabetic event. His girlfriend called because she could not get him up this morning, and says he has been sick with a bad cold for several days. The patient's eyes are open, but he cannot verbalize a response. His breathing is deep and rapid, his skin is warm and dry, and he looks dehydrated. Vital signs are R/R 40, BP 84/50 mmHg, and P/R 118. While you are checking his glucose level, which diabetic emergency do you suspect?

a. hypoglycemia

b. hyperglycemia

c. HHNC

d. acute adrenal insufficiency

52. What is the significance of the respirations of the patient described in question 51?

a. He is hyperventilating because of dehydration.

b. This is the body's response to hypoosmolarity and high pH.

c. Deep respirations are a response to increased acid levels from ketones.

d. The deep and rapid breathing is caused by the congestion from his cold.

53. Insulin release is stimulated by glucose, amino acids, and:

a. hunger.

b. ketones.

c. glucagon and thiamine.

d. glucagon, epinephrine, and growth hormone.

54. The spouse of an unresponsive diabetic male called EMS when she found her husband lying on the kitchen floor in the morning. His initial blood sugar reading is 26 mg/dL, and his vital signs are skin CTC cool, dry, and pale; respirations 20/puffing and snoring; pulse 70/regular; and BP 110/68 mmHg. After administering oxygen, starting an IV, and giving 25 grams of dextrose, the patient is still unresponsive and his blood sugar reading is 44 mg/dL. What would be the most appropriate treatment at this point?

a. Intubate.

b. Begin rapid transport.

c. Administer glucagon IM.

d. Administer another 25 grams of dextrose.

55. You have responded to a suburban residence for a 60-year-old male with an altered mental status. A neighbor called EMS because the patient is having stroke symptoms and is unable to get out of bed today. The patient is conscious but very confused. His responses are slow, and he feels week. He denies any pain or history of diabetes, his vital signs are R/R 20, BP 100/50 mmHg, P/R 62, and his skin is warm and dry. Which of the following conditions do you suspect first?

a. CVA

b. diabetic emergency

c. ACS

d. all of the above

56. Further evaluation of the patient described in question 55 reveals that his medications include beta-blocker and antihypertensive meds. His SpO2 is 99% with oxygen. Before you begin transport, which of the following would be of most value to make a differential diagnosis?

a. 12 lead ECG

b. glucose reading

c. neurologic examination

d. medication changes

57. What is the significance of the medications for the patient described in question 55?

a. Beta-blockers will conceal compensatory signs of shock.

b. Antihypertensives may precipitate hypoglycemia.

c. Antihypertensives may conceal hyperglycemia.

d. Beta-blockers may precipitate a stroke.

58. How fast an injection of glucagon works on a hypoglycemic patient primarily depends on:

a. the age, gender, and weight of the patient.

b. the amount of glycogen reserves in the liver.

c. whether the patient is type I or type II diabetic.

d. the other types of medications the patient is taking.

59. Which of the following hormones produced in the pancreas stimulates an increase in blood sugar?

a. insulin

b. glucagon

c. beta-cell

d. cortisone

60. Chronic high blood sugar < 140 mg/dl can produce:
    a. atrial fibrillation.
    b. temporary hair loss.
    c. permanent hair loss.
    d. permanent nerve damage.

61. You respond to a call for a patient who fell and cannot get up. You find a 47-year-old female who fell while getting out of bed. She has no specific pain, but is complaining of increased weakness over the last week. You immediately recognize that she has one of the classic physical findings associated with Cushing's syndrome, _____.
    a. moon face
    b. bulging eyes
    c. extreme peripheral edema
    d. fruity breath odor

62. You assist the patient described in question 61 to a chair, and she allows you to assess her and take her vital signs. You find that her arms and legs appear to be wasting, compared to the rest of her body. She also has unusual stretch marks on her skin. You attribute these findings to be _____ with Cushing's disease.
    a. typical findings associated
    b. noncompliance of medications associated
    c. side effects of medications associated
    d. none of the findings associated

63. Which of the following conditions is characterized by the body breaking down fat rather than glucose as its energy source?
    a. hypoglycemia
    b. DKA
    c. pancreatitis
    d. insulin shock

64. Which of the following gland(s) is(are) the only one(s) with both endocrine and exocrine functions?
    a. thyroid
    b. parathyroids
    c. pancreas
    d. adrenals

65. Which of the following gland(s) is(are) responsible for the secretion of antidiuretic hormone?
    a. ovaries
    b. testes
    c. thymus
    d. pituitary

Exam #24 Answer Form

	A	B	C	D		A	B	C	D
1.	❏	❏	❏	❏	34.	❏	❏	❏	❏
2.	❏	❏	❏	❏	35.	❏	❏	❏	❏
3.	❏	❏	❏	❏	36.	❏	❏	❏	❏
4.	❏	❏	❏	❏	37.	❏	❏	❏	❏
5.	❏	❏	❏	❏	38.	❏	❏	❏	❏
6.	❏	❏	❏	❏	39.	❏	❏	❏	❏
7.	❏	❏	❏	❏	40.	❏	❏	❏	❏
8.	❏	❏	❏	❏	41.	❏	❏	❏	❏
9.	❏	❏	❏	❏	42.	❏	❏	❏	❏
10.	❏	❏	❏	❏	43.	❏	❏	❏	❏
11.	❏	❏	❏	❏	44.	❏	❏	❏	❏
12.	❏	❏	❏	❏	45.	❏	❏	❏	❏
13.	❏	❏	❏	❏	46.	❏	❏	❏	❏
14.	❏	❏	❏	❏	47.	❏	❏	❏	❏
15.	❏	❏	❏	❏	48.	❏	❏	❏	❏
16.	❏	❏	❏	❏	49.	❏	❏	❏	❏
17.	❏	❏	❏	❏	50.	❏	❏	❏	❏
18.	❏	❏	❏	❏	51.	❏	❏	❏	❏
19.	❏	❏	❏	❏	52.	❏	❏	❏	❏
20.	❏	❏	❏	❏	53.	❏	❏	❏	❏
21.	❏	❏	❏	❏	54.	❏	❏	❏	❏
22.	❏	❏	❏	❏	55.	❏	❏	❏	❏
23.	❏	❏	❏	❏	56.	❏	❏	❏	❏
24.	❏	❏	❏	❏	57.	❏	❏	❏	❏
25.	❏	❏	❏	❏	58.	❏	❏	❏	❏
26.	❏	❏	❏	❏	59.	❏	❏	❏	❏
27.	❏	❏	❏	❏	60.	❏	❏	❏	❏
28.	❏	❏	❏	❏	61.	❏	❏	❏	❏
29.	❏	❏	❏	❏	62.	❏	❏	❏	❏
30.	❏	❏	❏	❏	63.	❏	❏	❏	❏
31.	❏	❏	❏	❏	64.	❏	❏	❏	❏
32.	❏	❏	❏	❏	65.	❏	❏	❏	❏
33.	❏	❏	❏	❏					

CHAPTER

25

Allergies and Immunology

1. When protective cells are able to recognize infections as they enter the body and destroy them prior to causing harm, this is called an:
   a. antigen.
   b. antibody.
   c. immune response.
   d. immunity.

2. An _____ is an overreaction by the body's immune response to normally harmless foreign substances, which causes damage to body tissues.
   a. immune response
   b. antibody
   c. allergic reaction
   d. allergy

3. When an antigen and the IgE antibody react, the combination leads to the release of mediators from:
   a. basophils and mast cells.
   b. histamines.
   c. leukotrienes.
   d. antibodies.

4. Swelling of the skin caused by leakage of fluid from the blood vessels into the interstitial and subcutaneous tissues is called:
   a. urticaria.
   b. angioneurotic edema.
   c. angiocerebral edema.
   d. perisacral edema.

5. The most common causes of anaphylaxis include drugs, insect stings, food, and:
   a. pollen.
   b. animal hair.
   c. animal dander.
   d. blood products.

6. An atypical finding in a patient suspected of a severe allergic reaction is:
   a. dyspnea.
   b. tachycardia.
   c. bradycardia.
   d. hypotension.

7. When a patient is experiencing an allergic reaction that develops into severe signs and symptoms, the paramedic will see changes affecting the:
   a. skin.
   b. GI tract.
   c. endocrine system.
   d. renal system.

8. The epinephrine auto-injector contains _____ mg for adults and _____ mg for children.
   a. 0.5; 0:25
   b. 0.5; 0:05
   c. 0.3; 0.33
   d. 0.3; 0.15

9. Besides epinephrine, what other medication classification does the paramedic administer to a patient in anaphylaxis?
   a. beta-blocker
   b. antihistamine
   c. antidiuretic
   d. ACE inhibitor

10. A person who has a latex allergy is likely to have sensitivity to foods such as potatoes, tomatoes, bananas, or apricots because:
    a. latex is used in the pesticides to grow these foods.
    b. farmers and food handlers wear latex during harvesting.
    c. latex sap is chemically related to these fruits and vegetables.
    d. supermarkets wash these foods with equipment that contains latex.

11. When is epinephrine appropriate for IV use over SQ injection for the patient in anaphylaxis?

    a. when the patient's auto-injector is empty

    b. when the patient has an AMS

    c. when the patient has taken PO Benadryl® prior to EMS arriving

    d. when peripheral circulation is so poor that SQ injections will be ineffective

12. Which of the following would be the most helpful for the paramedic to determine what type of snake or spider bite a patient has sustained?

    a. the size of the bite

    b. the shape of the bite

    c. the markings of the animal

    d. the time of the bite

13. A 34-year-old female was stung by a bee. She has a known sensitivity to bee stings and has started wheezing even after using her epinephrine auto injector and taking Benedryl®. Her vital signs are: skin warm and dry without hives, respiratory rate 26 and labored, pulse 118 and regular, BP 132/88 mmHg, and SpO$_2$ 98%. What treatment option is most appropriate at this point?

    a. Administer IV epinephrine.

    b. Administer IV solumedrol.

    c. Administer nebulized albuterol.

    d. Administer epinephrine, 3-mg IM injection.

14. Patients in anaphylaxis may be given corticosteroids because they:

    a. slow histamine release.

    b. have a fast-acting effect.

    c. help to produce immunity.

    d. stimulate the antigen effect.

15. The natural hormone _____ regulates inflammation of the immune response. This is why corticosteroids are given to patients with severe allergic reactions.

    a. adenosine

    b. adrenaline

    c. cortisol

    d. progestine

16. A newborn's immunity is acquired primarily from its mother's antibodies and secondarily:

    a. transferred from breast milk.

    b. through initial immune responses.

    c. through cell-mediated immunity.

    d. from immunoglobulins after fetal circulation stops.

17. Diphenhydramine is given to patients for allergic reactions because it:

    a. increases heart rate and strength of contractions.

    b. will mediate IgE.

    c. competes with histamine at the receptor sites, blocking the effects of histamine.

    d. stimulates the antigen effect.

18. The difference between allergic reaction and anaphylaxis is:

    a. anaphylaxis always produces hives.

    b. allergic reaction is preventable, anaphylaxis is not.

    c. allergic reaction is a mild, whole body reaction.

    d. anaphylaxis is a severe, whole body allergic reaction.

19. Beta agonists help to reverse some of the _____ associated with anaphylaxis.

    a. edema

    b. bronchospasm

    c. nausea

    d. vasodilation

20. When the body releases histamine in response to exposure to an antigen, the body is trying to:

    a. vasoconstrict bronchial muscles.

    b. increase dilation of the capillaries.

    c. decrease permeability of the arterioles.

    d. minimize exposure to the antigen.

21. Your patient is a 6-year-old male who is having an allergic reaction to a known substance (nuts). The exposure occurred 30 minutes ago, and he now has wheezing and hives on his torso. His parents gave him 25 mg of Benadryl® PO just before calling EMS. Your primary concern for this patient is:

    a. the airway.

    b. histamine release.

    c. vasodilation.

    d. IV access.

22. Your management of the patient described in question 21 includes a calm approach with oxygen administration and:

    a. IV epinephrine 0.1 mg/kg (1:10,000).

    b. IM epinephrine 1.0 mg/kg (1:1,000).

    c. SC epinephrine 0.01 mg/kg (1:1,000).

    d. SC epinephrine 0.1 mg/kg (1:1,000).

23. Which of the following emergency pharmacologic agents is the primary bronchodilator used to treat a patient experiencing an anaphylactic reaction?
    a. albuterol
    b. Solu Medrol®
    c. epinephrine
    d. diphenhydramine

24. The speed of an anaphylactic reaction depends on the route of exposure and the:
    a. degree of sensitivity.
    b. level of consciousness.
    c. patient's age.
    d. preexisting medical conditions.

25. You are halfway through an interfacility transport with a patient on a ventilator and an IV pump when you observe that the patient has developed urticaria around the neck and face. The IV pump has two medications running at a preset rate. When you were given a report prior to transport, you were told that the patient has just started a new IV antibiotic, and the chart indicates the same. You suspect that the patient is having a reaction to the new medication. What action do you take next?
    a. Administer 0.5 mg epinephrine SQ.
    b. Adjust the pump to stop the flow of antibiotic.
    c. Call the origination facility to obtain new orders.
    d. Call ahead to the destination facility to advise them of the problem.

26. The patient you are treating for an anaphylactic reaction is wheezing, hypotensive, and tachycardic 5 minutes after you have administered epinephrine. Which of the following should the patient receive next?
    a. albuterol
    b. repeat epinephrine and give fluid boluses
    c. Benadryl®
    d. dopamine

27. The patient described in question 26 continues to be hypotensive and tachycardic despite the efforts of your previous treatment. How would you manage the patient en route to the hospital?
    a. Initiate a rapid transport.
    b. Administer a vasopressor drip.
    c. Prepare for a difficult intubation.
    d. Repeat epinephrine and fluid boluses.

28. Urticaria, or hives, occur as a result of the fluid shift that happens when:
    a. blood vessels dilate and become permeable.
    b. the interstitial spaces overflow into the capillaries.
    c. the intracellular spaces constrict.
    d. antihistamines are no longer effective.

29. What is the mechanism by which Benadryl® helps to clear up hives?
    a. Antihistamines stimulate histamines to withdraw into mast cells.
    b. Antihistamines block H_2 receptors in the skin.
    c. Histamines are destroyed when antihistamines block H_1 receptor sites.
    d. Antihistamines block H_1 receptors in blood vessels.

30. Which of the following effects from the medication dopamine is not desired in anaphylaxis?
    a. increased cardiac contractibility
    b. increased peripheral vasoconstriction
    c. renal and mesentery artery vasodilation
    d. maintenance of systolic pressure

Exam #25 Answer Form

	A	B	C	D		A	B	C	D
1.	❏	❏	❏	❏	16.	❏	❏	❏	❏
2.	❏	❏	❏	❏	17.	❏	❏	❏	❏
3.	❏	❏	❏	❏	18.	❏	❏	❏	❏
4.	❏	❏	❏	❏	19.	❏	❏	❏	❏
5.	❏	❏	❏	❏	20.	❏	❏	❏	❏
6.	❏	❏	❏	❏	21.	❏	❏	❏	❏
7.	❏	❏	❏	❏	22.	❏	❏	❏	❏
8.	❏	❏	❏	❏	23.	❏	❏	❏	❏
9.	❏	❏	❏	❏	24.	❏	❏	❏	❏
10.	❏	❏	❏	❏	25.	❏	❏	❏	❏
11.	❏	❏	❏	❏	26.	❏	❏	❏	❏
12.	❏	❏	❏	❏	27.	❏	❏	❏	❏
13.	❏	❏	❏	❏	28.	❏	❏	❏	❏
14.	❏	❏	❏	❏	29.	❏	❏	❏	❏
15.	❏	❏	❏	❏	30.	❏	❏	❏	❏

Abdominal, Gastrointestinal, Genitourinary, and Renal

1. The three major types of acute abdominal pain are visceral, somatic, and:
   a. involuntary.
   b. voluntary.
   c. referred.
   d. diffuse.

2. _____ pain is caused by stimulation of nerve fibers in the parietal peritoneum by chemical or bacterial inflammation.
   a. Visceral
   b. Somatic
   c. Biliary
   d. Radiating

3. _____ pain is caused by sudden stretching or distention of a hollow organ.
   a. Visceral
   b. Somatic
   c. Biliary
   d. Radiating

4. You are assessing a 28-year-old male complaining of acute abdominal pain radiating around the right side to the back and angle of the scapula. Which of the following is most likely the cause of the pain?
   a. pancreas
   b. gallbladder
   c. kidney stone
   d. duodenal ulcer

5. Possible conditions associated with left-lower quadrant pain of the abdomen include:
   a. pelvic inflammatory disease (PID), diverticulitis, and ovarian cyst.
   b. acute coronary syndrome (ACS), appendicitis, and pancreatitis.
   c. cholecystitis, duodenal ulcer, and bowel obstruction.
   d. gallbladder, lesion, and pyelonephritis.

6. A 65-year-old male with cardiac disease is complaining of a sudden onset of pain in his upper thighs and lumbosacral area. You suspect the cause of the pain to be a(n):
   a. ACS.
   b. pulled muscle.
   c. ruptured aneurysm.
   d. appendicitis.

7. Which of the following conditions can mimic a serious GI bleed?
   a. bowel obstruction
   b. ectopic pregnancy
   c. Mallory-Weiss tear
   d. swallowed blood from epistaxis

8. Which of the following conditions is a common cause of upper GI bleeding?
   a. tumors
   b. polyps
   c. fissures
   d. esophageal varices

9. Which of the following conditions is a common cause of lower GI bleeding?
   a. esophagitis
   b. diverticulosis
   c. acute gastritis
   d. peptic ulcer disease

10. You are assessing a 30-year-old male who is in tears and complaining of acute non-traumatic abdominal pain that radiates into the groin and external genitalia. You suspect the cause of the pain to be:
    a. sexually transmitted disease (STD).
    b. renal colic.
    c. appendicitis.
    d. bowel obstruction.

11. While preparing to transport a nursing home resident to the ED for evaluation, the staff reports that the patient has had a melena bowel movement today. What was unusual about the stool?
    a. It appeared tarry and black.
    b. It smelled of vomitus.
    c. Bright red blood was present.
    d. It was yellowish in color.

12. Initial treatment of any patient with GI bleeding, regardless of the location, begins with the administration of high-flow oxygen and:
    a. rapid transport to the ED.
    b. treatment for shock.
    c. treatment for pain control.
    d. nasogastric tube placement.

13. _____ is an acute inflammation of the gallbladder, usually caused by gallstones.
    a. Colitis
    b. Cholecystitis
    c. Crohn's disease
    d. Diverticulitis

14. Your partner is assessing a 35-year-old male with symptoms of malaise, nausea, vomiting, and tenderness on palpation of the upper-right quadrant of the abdomen. After moving the patient to the ambulance, you notice the patient's sclera look yellow. What do you suspect is the patient's problem?
    a. reflux esophagitis
    b. diverticulitis
    c. gastroenteritis
    d. acute hepatitis

15. Benign prostatic hyperplasia (BPH) is a condition in males of an enlarged prostrate that:
    a. is cancerous.
    b. is not cancerous.
    c. is a life-threatening condition.
    d. only occurs in men over 50 years old.

16. Which of the following causes of abdominal pain is not an immediate life threat?
    a. ACS
    b. ruptured ectopic pregnancy
    c. ruptured viscus
    d. reflux esophagitis

17. The _____ is the most important part of the diagnosis in acute abdominal pain.
    a. blood pressure
    b. history
    c. patient's age
    d. type of pain

18. A slow onset of abdominal pain is more commonly associated with which of the following conditions?
    a. appendicitis
    b. ectopic pregnancy
    c. renal infarction
    d. splenic infarction

19. During the interview with a 38-year-old female complaining of GI distress, she tells you the pain began shortly after eating lunch. The lunch consisted of fatty food from a fast-food take-out place. Which of the following conditions do you suspect is the cause of the abdominal pain?
    a. cholecystitis
    b. pancreatitis
    c. gastroenteritis
    d. obstruction

20. A 40-year-old male with severe abdominal pain, which began the day before and has progressively worsened, is lying completely still. The patient is very distressed when any attempt is made to move him. What do you suspect is the nature of his distress?
    a. muscle spasms
    b. colic
    c. peritoneal inflammation
    d. obstruction

21. Which of the following characteristics of bowel sounds is the most significant in the field?
    a. decreased sounds
    b. increased sounds
    c. absence of sounds
    d. abnormal sounds

22. The presence of rebound tenderness in the abdomen during the physical examination indicates:
    a. colic.
    b. obstruction.
    c. shock.
    d. peritoneal irritation.

23. A 12-year-old male is complaining of pain in the groin on the left side. There is swelling in the groin and an abnormal bulge in the scrotum. What condition is most likely present in this patient?
    a. prostatitis
    b. epididymitis
    c. inguinal hernia
    d. enlarged prostate

24. Probably the most common GI abnormality, which includes symptoms of bloating, pain, and often violent diarrhea, is:
    a. acute gastroenteritis.
    b. acute cholecystitis.
    c. lactose intolerance.
    d. bowel obstruction.

25. A condition that is most frequently found in young adults and is characterized by recurrent abdominal pain, usually crampy in nature, and diarrhea, alternating with periods of constipation, is known as:
    a. acute gastroenteritis.
    b. lactose intolerance.
    c. renal colic.
    d. irritable bowel syndrome.

26. The fluid wave test is performed on the abdomen to assess for the presence of:
    a. tenderness.
    b. ascites.
    c. masses.
    d. edema.

27. Patients that are being treated for acute GI emergencies get nothing by mouth (NPO) because they may need an empty stomach for emergency surgery and:
    a. a full stomach impedes diagnostic testing.
    b. the release of digestive enzymes often worsens the condition.
    c. pain management is contraindicated on a full stomach.
    d. their medication only works on an empty stomach.

28. _____ is a general term for a method, involving a semipermeable membrane, used to separate smaller particles from larger ones in a liquid mixture.
    a. Sifting
    b. DPL
    c. Osmosis
    d. Dialysis

29. A petite 20-year-old female has abdominal pain with nausea and vomiting. The pain began the day before as cramping in the periumbilical area and has persisted. Today she feels worse, has not eaten, and has been vomiting. The patient has no significant medical history and is currently menstruating. Her vital signs are: skin CTC pale, warm, and dry; respirations 22/nonlabored; pulse 100/regular; and BP 108/60 mmHg. What initial treatment steps should you begin?
    a. oxygen by cannula, IV fluids, and morphine
    b. oxygen by mask, position of comfort, and IM Zofran
    c. oxygen as tolerated, IV fluids, IV Zofran, and morphine
    d. left lateral recumbent with legs flexed, IM morphine, and Zofran

30. (Continuing with question 29) Your physical exam of the patient's abdomen reveals that the pain has radiated to the right-lower quadrant. She has generalized rigidity and tenderness in that area, but no masses or distention. What do you suspect is the source of her problem?
    a. appendicitis
    b. bowel obstruction
    c. ectopic pregnancy
    d. new onset of Crohn's disease

31. Special considerations for care of the dialysis patient with an acute problem include:
    a. avoiding taking a BP in any extremity with a fistula.
    b. only taking a BP in the extremity with a graft.
    c. accessing medical control for orders to start an IV.
    d. never asking advice from the dialysis technician.

32. You are transporting a nursing home resident to the hospital for evaluation of dysuria, frequency, urgency, and suprapubic pain. The patient has had the symptoms for 2 days. What do you suspect is the problem?
    a. kidney stone
    b. urinary tract infection (UTI)
    c. bowel obstruction
    d. bladder obstruction

33. A 20-year-old female is complaining of abdominal pain and acute urinary retention. Which of the following conditions must be ruled out first?
    a. UTI
    b. ectopic pregnancy
    c. kidney stone
    d. pyelonephritis

34. You are called to a local high school for a male complaining of acute abdominal pain. Upon arrival and primary assessment, you have found that the patient was playing basketball when suddenly he felt severe pain in his left testicle. He denies having abdominal pain but feels nausea. You suspect which of the following?
    a. torsion of the testicle
    b. kidney stone
    c. renal infection
    d. UTI

35. When the liver becomes scarred from disease to the point where it cannot function normally, this condition is called:
    a. cirrhosis.
    b. hepatitis B.
    c. hepatitis C.
    d. alcoholism.

36. One of the functions of the urinary system is:
    a. to maintain proper balance between water and salts in the blood.
    b. to produce aldosterone.
    c. to excrete potassium to solidify waste products.
    d. to help the body eliminate sugar.

37. You are treating a 56-year-old male patient with a complaint of exertional chest pain. Your thorough history taking has revealed that the patient took Viagra® last night. Which of the following treatments would be most appropriate for the relief of this patient's chest pain?
    a. oxygen only
    b. oxygen and nitroglycerin
    c. oxygen and morphine
    d. morphine only

38. The most common STDs in both genders are gonorrhea, syphilis, and:
    a. hepatitis B.
    b. chlamydia.
    c. HIV.
    d. herpes.

39. During your assessment of a 30-year-old male complaining of acute severe abdominal pain that radiates into the right flank area, you discover that the patient has a history of kidney stones. The patient tells you this pain is just like when he had a kidney stone before. After attention to the ABCs, your management plan for this patient includes:
    a. rapid transport.
    b. pain management.
    c. supportive care only.
    d. treating for shock.

40. _____ is a condition of swelling of the tube that connects the testicle with the vas deferens.
    a. Prostatitis
    b. Epididymitis
    c. Enlarged prostate
    d. Rectal abscess

41. Which of the following statements about the presence of bright red discoloration in the stool is most correct?
    a. This condition may indicate obstructive jaundice.
    b. This condition only occurs with lower GI bleeding.
    c. This condition may be caused by a malabsorption syndrome.
    d. Bright red blood can occur with bleeding in the lower or upper GI tract.

42. _____ pain is pain from one area that is being sensed in another as a result of embryologic nerve distribution patterns.
    a. Referred
    b. Acute
    c. Guarded
    d. Reflex

43. A(n) _____ GI bleed is bleeding proximal to the duodenojejunal junction.
    a. upper
    b. lower
    c. acute
    d. non-traumatic

44. Which of the following is a definition for the term *hematochezia*?
    a. vomiting bright red blood
    b. bright red blood in the stool
    c. tarry, sticky black stool
    d. vomiting "coffee grounds" digested blood

45. A 23-year-old male is complaining of abdominal pain in the upper-left quadrant. He has had the pain for a week. He says the pain gets worse after he eats and he ate 20 minutes ago. The pain is 10/10 and radiates to the shoulder blade and this is different. What condition do you suspect is causing the pain?
    a. appendicitis
    b. pancreatitis
    c. ischemic bowel
    d. kidney stone

46. Appendicitis is inflammation of the appendix caused by occlusion of the lumen by a:
    a. small tumor.
    b. small piece of stool.
    c. blood clot.
    d. large lesion.

47. Cholecystitis is an acute inflammation of the gallbladder that blocks the lumen, interfering with:
    a. blood flow.
    b. bile flow.
    c. insulin production.
    d. urine production.

48. _____ is a general term indicating inflammation of the colon for any of a number of reasons.
    a. Diverticulitis
    b. Diverticulosis
    c. Colitis
    d. Gastritis

49. Dilations of the veins of the esophagus secondary to increased portal vein pressures result in:
    a. cirrhosis.
    b. peptic ulcer.
    c. gastric ulcer.
    d. varices.

50. Dilations of the veins in the lower portion of the colon result in:
    a. tumors.
    b. hemorrhoids.
    c. colitis.
    d. varices.

Exam #26 Answer Form

	A	B	C	D			A	B	C	D
1.	❏	❏	❏	❏		26.	❏	❏	❏	❏
2.	❏	❏	❏	❏		27.	❏	❏	❏	❏
3.	❏	❏	❏	❏		28.	❏	❏	❏	❏
4.	❏	❏	❏	❏		29.	❏	❏	❏	❏
5.	❏	❏	❏	❏		30.	❏	❏	❏	❏
6.	❏	❏	❏	❏		31.	❏	❏	❏	❏
7.	❏	❏	❏	❏		32.	❏	❏	❏	❏
8.	❏	❏	❏	❏		33.	❏	❏	❏	❏
9.	❏	❏	❏	❏		34.	❏	❏	❏	❏
10.	❏	❏	❏	❏		35.	❏	❏	❏	❏
11.	❏	❏	❏	❏		36.	❏	❏	❏	❏
12.	❏	❏	❏	❏		37.	❏	❏	❏	❏
13.	❏	❏	❏	❏		38.	❏	❏	❏	❏
14.	❏	❏	❏	❏		39.	❏	❏	❏	❏
15.	❏	❏	❏	❏		40.	❏	❏	❏	❏
16.	❏	❏	❏	❏		41.	❏	❏	❏	❏
17.	❏	❏	❏	❏		42.	❏	❏	❏	❏
18.	❏	❏	❏	❏		43.	❏	❏	❏	❏
19.	❏	❏	❏	❏		44.	❏	❏	❏	❏
20.	❏	❏	❏	❏		45.	❏	❏	❏	❏
21.	❏	❏	❏	❏		46.	❏	❏	❏	❏
22.	❏	❏	❏	❏		47.	❏	❏	❏	❏
23.	❏	❏	❏	❏		48.	❏	❏	❏	❏
24.	❏	❏	❏	❏		49.	❏	❏	❏	❏
25.	❏	❏	❏	❏		50.	❏	❏	❏	❏

CHAPTER

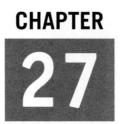

Toxicology

1. The majority of the reported poisoning exposures occur in(on):
   a. the patient's home.
   b. a workplace.
   c. recreational facilities.
   d. the highway.

2. The largest number of poisoning deaths occurs in which age group?
   a. 1–8
   b. 9–19
   c. 35–54
   d. 50–70

3. Which of the following risk factors most predisposes an individual to a toxic emergency?
   a. gender
   b. unattended children
   c. working at an industrial site
   d. having a known allergic reaction

4. An example of a toxic effect on the respiratory system includes:
   a. the inability of the cells to manufacture ATP.
   b. overstimulation of nerve impulses.
   c. the development of pulmonary edema.
   d. increased salivation.

5. Which of the following is an example of a poison exposure by injection?
   a. insect stinger
   b. poison ivy contact
   c. mushroom digestion
   d. physically handling pesticides

6. When a substance enters the body by passing through the skin, this route of exposure is called:
   a. critical.
   b. absorption.
   c. intermittent.
   d. unpredictable.

7. Once a substance enters the body, the effects it has on the body primarily depend on:
   a. the type of poison.
   b. the patient's past medical history.
   c. the patient's tolerance to the substance.
   d. how many times the patient has been previously exposed.

8. Which of the following sea creatures can inject painful venom into a human's skin?
   a. gar
   b. shark
   c. stingray
   d. sea urchin

9. If a person is exposed to a nerve agent, which of the following signs and symptoms would you expect to find?
   a. salivation and nausea
   b. hallucinations and fever
   c. tachycardia and miosis
   d. euphoria and hyperactivity

10. _____ or syndromes are groupings of drugs that present with similar patterns of toxicity.
    a. Toxidromes
    b. Poisonings
    c. Intoxications
    d. Envenomations

11. The poisoned patient who took a large quantity of _____ may become hyperthermic in normal ambient temperatures.
    a. alcohol
    b. a narcotic
    c. a sedative
    d. aspirin

12. A patient who develops digitalis toxicity is very likely to develop:
    a. tachycardia.
    b. bradycardia.
    c. hypertension.
    d. hyperthermia.

13. _____ cause a person's pupils to become large (mydriasis).
    a. Pesticides
    b. Cholinergics
    c. Anticholinergics
    d. Phenothiazines

14. An overdose of narcotics will cause the pupils to be:
    a. fixed.
    b. dilated.
    c. unequal.
    d. constricted.

15. _____ is a rare and potentially deadly form of food poisoning that produces serious CNS symptoms.
    a. *E. coli*
    b. Botulism
    c. *Staphylococci*
    d. Viral food poisoning

16. Common agents that fall into the toxidrome referred to as anticholinergics include:
    a. pesticides and nerve agents.
    b. LSD, PCP, and mescaline.
    c. tricyclic antidepressants and mushrooms.
    d. diet pills, caffeine, and cocaine.

17. Euphoria, hypotension, and respiratory depression are most commonly found with which toxidrome?
    a. sympathomimetic
    b. narcotics
    c. anticholinergics
    d. hallucinogens

18. Tachycardia, diaphoresis, chest pain, and stroke are most commonly caused by which toxidrome?
    a. sympathomimetics
    b. anticholinergics
    c. cholinergics
    d. narcotics

19. What is the most common route of poisoning?
    a. absorption
    b. inhalation
    c. ingestion
    d. injection

20. The first cardinal principle of management for all EMS providers when dealing with a toxicologic emergency is to:
    a. consider specific antidotes.
    b. consider decontamination of the patient.
    c. ensure your own safety first.
    d. maintain an open airway and breathing.

21. The difference between a poisoning and an overdose is:
    a. poisoning involves exposure to a substance that is generally harmful and has no beneficial effects.
    b. overdose suggests an excessive exposure to a substance that is not normally used to treat humans.
    c. there is no difference between the two terms and they are used interchangeably.
    d. the age of the patient.

22. Inducing vomiting may be part of the appropriate treatment in a patient who has ingested:
    a. lye.
    b. acid.
    c. aspirin.
    d. silver nitrate.

23. Vomiting should not be induced if the patient:
    a. has taken pills.
    b. is over 50 years old.
    c. has a decreased mental status.
    d. is a known drug abuser.

24. Induced vomiting in a patient who has ingested _____ should be avoided.
    a. strychnine
    b. an overdose of aspirin
    c. an overdose of MAO inhibitors
    d. an overdose of acetaminophen

25. Gastric dialysis is a mechanism of poison removal aided by the administration of:
    a. activated charcoal.
    b. ipecac syrup.
    c. tincture of benzene.
    d. milk or mild soap.

26. When treating a 27-year-old male patient who has a history of depression, you determine that the patient may have taken 10 to 20 tricyclic antidepressants. His vitals are within normal range, and he is alert at this time. What treatment should be considered?
    a. Administer 2-mg Narcan.
    b. Transport to the poison control center.
    c. Consider administering activated charcoal.
    d. Quickly restrain the patient.

27. Exposure to systemic toxins, such as carbon monoxide, often results in:
    a. hypoxia.
    b. vertigo.
    c. diaphoresis.
    d. edema.

28. For any patient removed from a fire scene, the paramedic should suspect _____ even when the patient has no burns.
    a. cardiovascular collapse
    b. drug overdose
    c. carbon dioxide exposure
    d. carbon monoxide exposure

29. You have been dispatched to transfer a 45-year-old patient from an on-call medical facility to the ED. The patient has accumulated excessive levels of theophylline. Which of the following effects should you be prepared to manage during the transport?
    a. seizures
    b. metabolic acidosis
    c. malignant hypothermia
    d. acute pulmonary edema

30. The herbal supplements ginkgo biloba, garlic, ginger, and vitamin E have the property of:
    a. blood thinners.
    b. chemotherapy.
    c. causing weight loss.
    d. sexual stimulants.

31. The patient taking digitalis for his heart is at increased risk for developing toxicity when he also takes:
    a. narcotics.
    b. steroids.
    c. diuretics.
    d. blood thinners.

32. Used frequently in the late adult population as sleep aids, _____ carry risks for withdrawal, dependency, and rebound insomnia.
    a. antimigraine drugs
    b. thiazides
    c. sulfonamides
    d. sedative hypnotics

33. Your patient is a 22-year-old female who is 7 months pregnant. Apparently she took an overdose of over-the-counter medication designed to relieve abdominal cramping. She is alert and oriented, and her vital signs are within normal range. What is your best course of treatment?
    a. Induce vomiting with syrup of ipecac.
    b. Restrain her, as she may become violent.
    c. Monitor her ABCs and administer oxygen.
    d. Administer activated charcoal and rush her to the ED.

34. What does the pathophysiology of poisoning by inhalation involve?
    a. The substance is absorbed into the bloodstream in the intestines.
    b. The substance is absorbed at the alveolar level, leading to systemic toxicity.
    c. The material is absorbed through the skin into the muscles.
    d. The material moves across the blood-brain barrier into the venous system.

35. What desired effect is most helpful to the patient when the paramedic administers Narcan?
    a. immediate withdrawal symptoms from the overdose
    b. reversal of the hypertension
    c. reversal of the respiratory depression
    d. a heightened sensitivity to the surrounding environment

36. Which clinical use would a patient taking benzodiazepines have?
    a. seizure control
    b. pain management
    c. nausea control
    d. attention deficit

37. If your patient was exposed to a herbicide, which antidote may prove useful if authorized by medical control to administer?
    a. Narcan
    b. atropine
    c. Solu Medrol
    d. nitrous oxide

38. Your patient is a 52-year-old male who was working in the fields of his farm all day. His wife called the ambulance because he has been acting crazy and very shaky, and has been drooling upon returning home. What could be wrong with him?

    a. He has taken an accidental overdose of beta-blocker.
    b. He had an exposure to lithium.
    c. He had an excessive exposure to insecticide.
    d. He is having a stroke.

39. An acquired resistance to the therapeutic effects of typical doses of a drug is referred to as:

    a. addiction.
    b. tolerance.
    c. dependence.
    d. drug abuse.

40. A psychologic craving for, or reliance on, a chemical agent is referred to as a(n):

    a. addiction.
    b. tolerance.
    c. dependence.
    d. drug abuse.

41. What is the source of most illegal drugs in the United States?

    a. smuggling from Colombia
    b. stolen shipments to hospital pharmacies
    c. artificially manufactured in college labs
    d. they are grown and produced in rural areas

42. Prolonged use of nonsteriodal anti-inflammatory drugs (NSAIDs) causes:

    a. seizures.
    b. stomach cancer.
    c. liver and kidney failure.
    d. psychosis and hallucinations.

43. Medications that are often abused, yet are medically prescribed for bed-wetting, seizures, and Tourette's syndrome, include:

    a. narcotics.
    b. tricyclic antidepressants.
    c. cyanide.
    d. sedative-hypnotics.

44. A drug that is frequently abused, which decreases inhibitory synapses in the brain, then excitatory synapses, causing euphoria followed by depression, is called a(n):

    a. opiate.
    b. alcohol.
    c. barbiturate.
    d. mushroom.

45. Which of the following substances has a delayed reaction so that the patient appears fine initially, only to deteriorate later?

    a. cyanide
    b. cocaine
    c. sympathomimetics
    d. tricyclic antidepressants

46. _____ is the use of hydrocarbons and produces CNS alterations, cardiac dysfunction, and liver dysfunction.

    a. Huffing
    b. Freebasing
    c. Snorting
    d. Flat lining

47. A woman has called EMS because her 3-year-old grandson is sick and has been vomiting. She believes he ingested pills from a bottle left out on the table. The child appears ill and is shivering. He is tachycardic and hypotensive. Which of the following substances did the child most likely ingest?

    a. iron
    b. MAOI
    c. antacid
    d. warfarin

48. When a patient is thought to have sustained carbon monoxide poisoning, his management should include high-concentration oxygen and consideration for:

    a. activated charcoal.
    b. syrup of ipecac.
    c. a hyperbaric chamber.
    d. a large dose of atropine.

49. When a patient with a history of hypertension suddenly stops taking his anti-hypertensive, which of the following emergencies is likely to develop?

    a. acute MI
    b. anxiety and tremors
    c. rebound hypertension
    d. profound hypotension

50. You have been called to a housing project where three preschoolers routinely play in the hallways and basement. The building is old, decaying, and sorely in need of repair. The parent of one child states that her son is complaining of a diffuse crampy abdominal pain and has diarrhea. He has been acting uncoordinated and irritable, and he has memory lapses. What could be the cause of this sickness?

    a. carbon monoxide poisoning.
    b. lead poisoning.
    c. hydrocarbon poisoning.
    d. an overdose of cocaine.

Exam #27 Answer Form

	A	B	C	D		A	B	C	D
1.	❏	❏	❏	❏	26.	❏	❏	❏	❏
2.	❏	❏	❏	❏	27.	❏	❏	❏	❏
3.	❏	❏	❏	❏	28.	❏	❏	❏	❏
4.	❏	❏	❏	❏	29.	❏	❏	❏	❏
5.	❏	❏	❏	❏	30.	❏	❏	❏	❏
6.	❏	❏	❏	❏	31.	❏	❏	❏	❏
7.	❏	❏	❏	❏	32.	❏	❏	❏	❏
8.	❏	❏	❏	❏	33.	❏	❏	❏	❏
9.	❏	❏	❏	❏	34.	❏	❏	❏	❏
10.	❏	❏	❏	❏	35.	❏	❏	❏	❏
11.	❏	❏	❏	❏	36.	❏	❏	❏	❏
12.	❏	❏	❏	❏	37.	❏	❏	❏	❏
13.	❏	❏	❏	❏	38.	❏	❏	❏	❏
14.	❏	❏	❏	❏	39.	❏	❏	❏	❏
15.	❏	❏	❏	❏	40.	❏	❏	❏	❏
16.	❏	❏	❏	❏	41.	❏	❏	❏	❏
17.	❏	❏	❏	❏	42.	❏	❏	❏	❏
18.	❏	❏	❏	❏	43.	❏	❏	❏	❏
19.	❏	❏	❏	❏	44.	❏	❏	❏	❏
20.	❏	❏	❏	❏	45.	❏	❏	❏	❏
21.	❏	❏	❏	❏	46.	❏	❏	❏	❏
22.	❏	❏	❏	❏	47.	❏	❏	❏	❏
23.	❏	❏	❏	❏	48.	❏	❏	❏	❏
24.	❏	❏	❏	❏	49.	❏	❏	❏	❏
25.	❏	❏	❏	❏	50.	❏	❏	❏	❏

CHAPTER 28

Infectious Diseases

1. A microorganism capable of causing disease is a(n):
   a. host.
   b. pathogen.
   c. parasite.
   d. infectious agent.

2. Nonpathogenic bacteria that live on the human skin, in the GI tract, and in mucous membranes are called:
   a. normal flora.
   b. protozoa.
   c. fungi.
   d. virus.

3. A single-cell microscopic parasitic organism that causes infection is a:
   a. normal flora.
   b. protozoa.
   c. fungus.
   d. virus.

4. A parasitic organism that can only live within a cell of a living animal or plant is a:
   a. helminth.
   b. host.
   c. fungi.
   d. virus.

5. A significant exposure occurs when blood or body fluids come into contact with broken skin, the eyes, parenteral contact, or:
   a. ingestion.
   b. cutaneous contact.
   c. mucous membranes.
   d. transdermal absorption.

6. When a person is infected with antimicrobial-resistant organisms they:
   a. cannot spread the bacteria.
   b. are less likely to die of the infection.
   c. are more likely to die of the infection.
   d. have no chance of surviving the infection.

7. Which of the following is an example of an external barrier found on the human body?
   a. hair
   b. teeth
   c. skin
   d. earwax

8. The period after an exposure has occurred to a host, when the infection cannot be transmitted to someone else, is the _____ period.
   a. refractory
   b. latency
   c. communicable
   d. disease

9. The duration of time between exposure to a host and the development of signs and symptoms of the disease is the _____ period.
   a. communicable
   b. incubation
   c. immune
   d. inflammatory

10. The duration of time from onset of symptoms to resolution of symptoms or death is called the _____ period.
    a. refractory
    b. resolution
    c. distribution
    d. disease

11. The _____ is responsible for reporting to the county health department communicable diseases seen by prehospital health-care providers.
    a. paramedic
    b. hospital
    c. patient's personal physician
    d. nursing home

12. The Ryan White Act of 1990 requires that exposure notification to emergency responders must be made within _____ hours.
    a. 12
    b. 24
    c. 48
    d. 72

13. OSHA is an example of a _____-level agency involved in disease outbreak.
    a. federal
    b. state
    c. local
    d. private sector

14. The primary mode of transmission of the antibiotic resistant staph infection MRSA is:
    a. blood borne.
    b. droplets in the air.
    c. direct skin to skin contact.
    d. contact with fecal matter.

15. Which of the following infections can be caused by needle stick?
    a. HBV, HCV, and HIV
    b. HBV, HIV, and pneumonia
    c. HIV, UTI, and URI
    d. HIV, TB, and pneumonia

16. The single most important task a health-care provider can do to reduce the transmission of communicable disease is:
    a. to not recap needles.
    b. to dispose of all needles into sharps containers.
    c. to place biohazards in red bags.
    d. hand washing.

17. Which of the following statements is most accurate about receiving a positive titer for HBV?
    a. Another titer is necessary following an exposure.
    b. Follow-up titers are recommended every five years.
    c. No further titers are necessary, even after an exposure.
    d. Additional boosters are recommended every five years.

18. Hantaviruses are spread by contact with:
    a. rodents.
    b. deer ticks.
    c. mosquitoes.
    d. dead birds.

19. What is the most common serious infectious disease in the United States?
    a. HIV
    b. AIDS
    c. hepatitis
    d. TB

20. How many types of hepatitis are there?
    a. five
    b. six
    c. seven
    d. eight

21. A person began the series of three hepatitis B vaccinations but failed to receive the last shot. Now, two years later, he wants to complete the vaccination. How should he complete the series?
    a. Restart the entire series.
    b. Repeat only the second dose.
    c. Complete only the third dose.
    d. Completion is no longer recommended.

22. Primary contraction of HCV is through direct contact with blood, such as a needle stick and:
    a. sexual contact.
    b. airborne droplet.
    c. indirect contact with urine.
    d. indirect contact with feces.

23. Which of the following infectious diseases does not have a known vaccine?
    a. HBV
    b. HCV
    c. chicken pox
    d. pneumococcal disease

24. What is the primary mode of transmission for HAV?
    a. needle stick
    b. oral—fecal
    c. airborne droplet
    d. direct contact with blood

25. What is the most common symptom of active TB?
    a. productive cough
    b. shortness of breath
    c. fever
    d. weakness

26. The transmission of _____ occurs from the saliva transferred through animal bites, most commonly by dogs, cats, bats, raccoons, and skunks.
    a. Lyme disease
    b. rabies
    c. arbovirus
    d. West Nile virus

27. Which of the following is the cause of most stomach ulcers?
    a. stress
    b. spicy foods
    c. stomach acid
    d. bacteria

28. An acute viral infectious disease of the CNS that causes painful muscle spasms in the throat and interferes with swallowing, leading to dehydration and death, is:
    a. salmonella.
    b. rabies.
    c. AIDS.
    d. arbovirus.

29. _____ is usually transmitted to humans by eating foods contaminated with animal feces.
    a. Salmonella
    b. Rabies
    c. Lyme disease
    d. Arbovirus

30. A person infected with _____ can pass on the disease by touching food after using the toilet and not washing her hands.
    a. salmonella
    b. varicella
    c. Lyme disease
    d. arbovirus

31. The two life-threatening conditions that can result from hantavirus infection are:
    a. sepsis and pneumonia.
    b. respiratory and renal failure.
    c. liver failure and meningitis.
    d. blood clots and respiratory failure.

32. Signs and symptoms of _____ include flu-like symptoms, muscle ache, and joint pain, with or without a rash.
    a. chicken pox
    b. rabies
    c. Lyme disease
    d. pneumonia

33. EMS was called by the husband of a 32-year-old female. He states that his wife has been ill with a cold (sore throat and fever) for 3 days. Today she complained of a severe headache, has been vomiting, and is now extremely sleepy; he is unable to get her up. She appears dehydrated; her skin is very warm and flushed, with no sign of rash. Vital signs are: respiratory 16/nonlabored; pulse 100/regular; and BP 100/50 mmHg. Blood sugar is 112 mg/dL, and SpO_2 is 96%. What do you suspect is the cause of her present condition?
    a. influenza
    b. meningitis
    c. Lyme disease
    d. herpes zoster

34. An example of a human internal barrier that protects against infectious diseases is:
    a. normal flora.
    b. an inflammatory response.
    c. Cushing's response.
    d. endorphins.

35. The liaison that is responsible for notification between the hospital and an exposed emergency responder is the EMS agency's:
    a. Medical Director.
    b. designated officer.
    c. chief supervisor.
    d. dispatcher.

36. Lyme disease affects:
    a. only Caucasians.
    b. the skin and joints.
    c. only immunosuppressed people.
    d. the skin, joints, nervous system, and heart.

37. _____ is included in the top ten recommended vaccinations for children.
    a. HAV
    b. Varicella
    c. Influenza
    d. HPV

38. _____ is an approach to infection control, which is based on the assumption that all blood and body fluids are potentially infectious.
    a. Standard precautions
    b. PPE
    c. Hand washing
    d. Biohazard labeling

39. The most commonly spread illnesses passed on by touching droplets from sneezing and coughing are influenza, the common cold, and:

   a. TB.

   b. HPV.

   c. pneumonia.

   d. staph.

40. Biohazardous wastes are placed in _____ bags that are labeled accordingly for disposal.

   a. clear

   b. yellow

   c. red

   d. green

41. All needles and sharps must be discarded in _____ that are properly labeled.

   a. red bags

   b. puncture-proof containers

   c. red containers

   d. unbreakable glass containers

42. A 40-year-old male is complaining of pain and a rash on his left thoracic area. He states that the pain began 2 days ago and has persisted. Today the pain is severe and constant. He denies dyspnea, diaphoresis, nausea, or other GI symptoms. When you examine his chest, you see a unilateral rash on the left thoracic area that spreads around to the back. What do you suspect is the cause of his present condition?

   a. ringworm

   b. shingles

   c. trichinosis

   d. tuberculosis

43. A _____ is a test using a sample of blood to measure the amount of antibody against a particular antigen in that blood.

   a. glucometer

   b. titer

   c. Gram stain

   d. Hemoccult

44. After a paramedic is exposed to HBV while on the job, the _____ must assure and pay for proper medical follow-up.

   a. patient

   b. paramedic

   c. employer

   d. hospital

45. In the United States, _____ is most prevalent in nursing facilities, homeless shelters, prisons, and migrant farm camps.

   a. HBV

   b. HCV

   c. meningitis

   d. tuberculosis

46. _____ is often called the stomach flu. It is incorrectly used to describe many types of infections and irritations of the digestive tract.

   a. Ulcer

   b. Esophageal reflux

   c. Gastroenteritis

   d. Helicobacteria pylori

47. Diseases caused by _____ include the West Nile virus, encephalitis, yellow fever, and dengue.

   a. the Lyme tick

   b. arbovirus

   c. meningitis

   d. the plague

48. Advanced clinical features of _____ include AMS, paralysis, paresthesia, stiff neck, sensitivity to light, dysrhythmia, and chest pain.

   a. varicella

   b. salmonella

   c. Lyme disease

   d. HBV

49. The principal forms of plague are bubonic, septicemic, and:

   a. pneumonic.

   b. pulmonic.

   c. cardiogenic.

   d. enteric.

50. In recent times, the most cases of plague in the United States have been reported in New Mexico, Arizona, California, and:

   a. Alaska.

   b. Colorado.

   c. New York.

   d. Florida.

Exam #28 Answer Form

	A	B	C	D		A	B	C	D
1.	❏	❏	❏	❏	26.	❏	❏	❏	❏
2.	❏	❏	❏	❏	27.	❏	❏	❏	❏
3.	❏	❏	❏	❏	28.	❏	❏	❏	❏
4.	❏	❏	❏	❏	29.	❏	❏	❏	❏
5.	❏	❏	❏	❏	30.	❏	❏	❏	❏
6.	❏	❏	❏	❏	31.	❏	❏	❏	❏
7.	❏	❏	❏	❏	32.	❏	❏	❏	❏
8.	❏	❏	❏	❏	33.	❏	❏	❏	❏
9.	❏	❏	❏	❏	34.	❏	❏	❏	❏
10.	❏	❏	❏	❏	35.	❏	❏	❏	❏
11.	❏	❏	❏	❏	36.	❏	❏	❏	❏
12.	❏	❏	❏	❏	37.	❏	❏	❏	❏
13.	❏	❏	❏	❏	38.	❏	❏	❏	❏
14.	❏	❏	❏	❏	39.	❏	❏	❏	❏
15.	❏	❏	❏	❏	40.	❏	❏	❏	❏
16.	❏	❏	❏	❏	41.	❏	❏	❏	❏
17.	❏	❏	❏	❏	42.	❏	❏	❏	❏
18.	❏	❏	❏	❏	43.	❏	❏	❏	❏
19.	❏	❏	❏	❏	44.	❏	❏	❏	❏
20.	❏	❏	❏	❏	45.	❏	❏	❏	❏
21.	❏	❏	❏	❏	46.	❏	❏	❏	❏
22.	❏	❏	❏	❏	47.	❏	❏	❏	❏
23.	❏	❏	❏	❏	48.	❏	❏	❏	❏
24.	❏	❏	❏	❏	49.	❏	❏	❏	❏
25.	❏	❏	❏	❏	50.	❏	❏	❏	❏

CHAPTER

29

Psychiatric

1. A(n) _____ is a strong feeling, often accompanied by physical signs such as tachycardia and diaphoresis.
   a. disorder
   b. emotion
   c. nightmare
   d. daydream

2. Any disturbance of emotional balance, manifested by maladaptive behavior and impaired function, is called:
   a. insanity.
   b. mental disorder.
   c. normalcy.
   d. malfunction.

3. Which of the following statements about mental illness is true?
   a. In the United States, behavioral and psychiatric disorders incapacitate more people than all other health problems combined.
   b. Mental disorders are most often incurable.
   c. Studies have shown that most mentally disabled patients are unstable and dangerous.
   d. Abnormal behavior is always bizarre.

4. Which of the following statements about mental illness is false?
   a. In many cases, psychiatric illness has an organic basis.
   b. Many patients with mental illness are calm and never present a danger.
   c. Having a mental disorder is cause for embarrassment and shame.
   d. Modern medical and psychotherapeutic techniques can provide stabilized treatment for most mental disorders.

5. Intermittent explosive disorder is an impulse-control disorder in which a person has an impulse to:
   a. pull his own hair out.
   b. defecate in unusual places.
   c. set fires with the use of pyrotechnics.
   d. lose control and become aggressive.

6. Delirium and dementia are examples of _____ disorders.
   a. cognitive
   b. psychotic
   c. mood
   d. somatoform

7. _____ is a type of disorder that involves gross distortions of reality.
   a. Anxiety
   b. Schizophrenia
   c. Substance abuse
   d. Somatoform

8. A mood disorder consisting of alternating periods of depression and mania is called:
   a. dementia.
   b. psychosis.
   c. hallucinations.
   d. bipolar.

9. Panic disorders, phobias, and post-traumatic syndromes are all examples of _____ disorders.
   a. insanity
   b. mood
   c. anxiety
   d. paranoia

10. Dependence is a _____ craving for a chemical agent, resulting from abuse or addiction.
    a. psychologic
    b. physical
    c. neural
    d. spiritual

11. _____ disorders are a group of neurotic disorders with symptoms suggesting physical disease, but with no demonstrable organic causes.
    a. Dissociative
    b. Somatoform
    c. Eating
    d. Factitious

12. A type of neurosis in which emotions are so repressed that a split occurs in the personality is what type of disorder?
    a. dissociative
    b. somatoform
    c. insanity
    d. factitious

13. _____ disorders are a large category of mental disorders characterized by inflexible and maladaptive behavior that impairs a person's ability to function in society.
    a. Dissociative
    b. Impulsive
    c. Personality
    d. Schizophrenic

14. You are the paramedic assigned to assess and manage a 22-year-old male experiencing a behavioral emergency. You should consider:
    a. that the patient is most likely overreacting.
    b. that the patient will raise his voice and become violent.
    c. spending less time with the patient than other types of calls.
    d. spending more time with the patient than other types of calls.

15. With respect to medical legal concerns, the paramedic should be aware of local facilities and procedures for:
    a. alcohol ingestion.
    b. registration of sexual predators.
    c. crisis intervention.
    d. definitive care.

16. The paramedic is responsible for knowing both local protocols and _____ regarding treatment of persons with mental illnesses.
    a. family wishes
    b. state laws
    c. advanced directives
    d. federal briefs

17. Many mental illnesses have been shown to occur from a chemical alteration in the brain. These chemicals are called:
    a. neurons.
    b. antidepressants.
    c. neurotransmitters.
    d. neuters.

18. Just because a person is on a "psych" drug does not mean that he has an emotional illness, as several of these agents are useful in other conditions such as:
    a. diabetes.
    b. toothaches.
    c. acne.
    d. migraine headaches.

19. When a paramedic is assessing a patient displaying abnormal motor activity, she should always consider the possibility of hypoxia, drug intoxification, blood sugar abnormality, and:
    a. pain.
    b. abnormal thought content.
    c. stimulated intellectual function.
    d. mood disorders.

20. During the assessment of a patient, the paramedic should be alert for examples of overt behaviors associated with behavioral and psychiatric disorders such as:
    a. poor hygiene.
    b. hypoglycemia.
    c. a lack of family support.
    d. multiple pets.

21. _____ are irrational, intense, and obsessive fears of a specific thing, such as an object or a physical situation.
    a. Hysterias
    b. Impulses
    c. Anxieties
    d. Phobias

22. Which of the following is an example of when the paramedic may need to transport a patient against his will?
    a. when the patient has no available transportation
    b. when the patient exhibits a danger to others
    c. when emergency dental care is needed
    d. after the patient falls and needs assistance getting up

23. Which of the following conditions can produce symptoms that resemble a psychiatric emergency?
    a. hypoxia
    b. heart attack
    c. pulmonary embolism
    d. allergic reaction

24. The state of incoherent excitement, confused speech, restlessness, and sometimes hallucinations often caused by acute illness or drug intoxication is referred to as:
    a. depression.
    b. delirium.
    c. dementia.
    d. paranoia.

25. The police have just turned a patient over to you after an apparent attempt to harm herself. She is 16 years old, with a history of depression. Today she used a razor blade to make numerous superficial cuts on her arms and thighs. Which of the following approaches should be avoided with this patient?
    a. Ask the patient if she intended to kill herself today.
    b. Ask the patient is she has any specific plans to kill herself.
    c. Ask the patient is there is anyone else she would like to harm.
    d. Assume the patient's actions were not an actual suicide attempt.

26. A _____ is something done by a person intending to ask for help rather than die.
    a. homicide attempt
    b. homicide gesture
    c. suicide attempt
    d. suicide gesture

27. Whenever possible, paramedics of the same sex as the patient experiencing a psychiatric emergency should be utilized:
    a. because it is safer.
    b. so that the patient will be more cooperative.
    c. so as to avoid accusations of sexual misconduct.
    d. because this method helps to keep the patient calm.

28. _____ is when a patient has no conception whatsoever of reality.
    a. Psychosis
    b. Neurosis
    c. Anxiety
    d. Phobia

29. The best way to deal with a patient experiencing hallucinations is:
    a. to use a chemical restraint.
    b. the "talk-down" technique.
    c. to use physical restraint.
    d. to shout at the patient.

30. The paramedic should assist in the physical restraint of a violent or severely agitated patient only when:
    a. the patient has harmed himself.
    b. the patient is threatening to harm himself.
    c. the patient has attempted to harm another.
    d. there are enough personnel to do the job.

31. The most common organic cause of apparent emotional and psychiatric illness in the elderly population is:
    a. inactivity.
    b. alcoholism.
    c. medication.
    d. seasonal weather changes.

32. Mania, or excessive hyperactivity, is an example of a(n) _____ disorder.
    a. impulsive control
    b. eating
    c. personality
    d. mood

33. _____ is a condition characterized by an overwhelming desire to continue taking a drug on which one has become "hooked" through repeated consumption.
    a. Dependence
    b. Intoxication
    c. Addiction
    d. Abuse

34. _____ relates to acute effects of taking a substance and may or may not be related to dependence.
    a. Alcoholism
    b. Intoxication
    c. Addiction
    d. Abuse

35. True _____ is both a psychologic and physical event, whereby the patient has both a physical and psychologic craving for the drug as well as for the effect.
    a. dependence
    b. intoxication
    c. addiction
    d. neurosis

36. As a rule, if a person has a psychiatric disorder and then develops a drug addition or alcoholism, the underlying psychiatric condition:
    a. improves.
    b. worsens.
    c. is cured.
    d. shows no change.

37. With respect to emotional illness, the term for assuming a certain body-language position suggestive of a particular emotion is:
    a. affect.
    b. fear.
    c. mental status.
    d. posture.

38. The term _____ refers to a state of mind in which one is uncertain of the present time, place, or self-identity.
    a. anger
    b. delirium
    c. confusion
    d. bipolar

39. The term _____ refers to the emotional tone behind an expressed emotion or behavior.
    a. fear
    b. anxiety
    c. affect
    d. mental status

40. While interviewing an emotionally disturbed patient, which of the following is a positive therapeutic interview technique the paramedic might use?
    a. Look directly into the patient's eyes.
    b. Promptly interrupt the patient when she becomes too talkative.
    c. Avoid asking questions about the immediate problem.
    d. Engage in active listening.

41. Management of behavioral emergencies begins with maintaining scene and personal safety, and then the paramedic should:
    a. begin the physical exam.
    b. attempt to build a good rapport with the patient.
    c. wait until the crisis team arrives before beginning care.
    d. have the police stand over the patient.

42. If a situation escalates and you become trapped by the patient, what should you do until help arrives?
    a. Scream for help.
    b. Do not say anything.
    c. Keep talking to the patient.
    d. Threaten the patient with bodily harm.

43. The police are attempting to restrain a 25-year-old male who is ranting irrationally and refusing to cooperate with transport. The male was found wandering in the road and appears uninjured. The patient becomes violent and difficult to handcuff. You call medical control and get an order to sedate the patient using:
    a. propofol.
    b. etomidate.
    c. haldol and versed.
    d. valium and morphine.

44. Studies report that the risk of suicide in men is double that of women after experiencing a divorce or marital separation primarily because:
    a. men are mentally weaker than women.
    b. women have better support systems.
    c. men lack certain female hormones.
    d. women tend to remarry more quickly than men.

45. The term _____ refers specifically to physical problems brought about by underlying emotional problems.
    a. somatogenesis
    b. pseudopsychosis
    c. psychosomatic illness
    d. psychogenic disease

46. You are on the scene with police for an "emotionally disturbed person." A 20-year-old female is pacing back and forth in her backyard, bragging about how tough she is, despite just being assaulted by her boyfriend. This patient is exhibiting clues that she:
    a. is bipolar.
    b. may attempt suicide.
    c. may develop violent behavior.
    d. has ingested excessive alcohol.

47. Which of the following statements about neurotic fear is true?
    a. A person with neurosis is probably insane.
    b. People with neurosis are not crazy.
    c. Most people with neurosis cannot cope with their fears.
    d. Neurosis is a normal anxiety reaction to a perceived fear.

48. Elderly persons commonly appear to have organic illnesses such as cardiac conditions when, in reality, they are:
    a. severely depressed.
    b. lonely.
    c. overmedicated.
    d. undermedicated.

49. Which of the following statements best describes how phobias can be unhealthy?
    a. Phobias can cause AMS.
    b. People with phobias are prone to ACS.
    c. Phobias are not unhealthy.
    d. Phobias can interfere with daily living activities.

50. Which of the following statements about the use of "open-ended" questions with behavioral patients is most accurate?
    a. They are used to encourage better patient responses.
    b. They do not tend to lead the patient to a specific answer.
    c. They are more likely to provoke an untoward emotional response.
    d. They do not give the patient the opportunity to express his anger verbally.

Exam #29 Answer Form

	A	B	C	D		A	B	C	D
1.	❏	❏	❏	❏	26.	❏	❏	❏	❏
2.	❏	❏	❏	❏	27.	❏	❏	❏	❏
3.	❏	❏	❏	❏	28.	❏	❏	❏	❏
4.	❏	❏	❏	❏	29.	❏	❏	❏	❏
5.	❏	❏	❏	❏	30.	❏	❏	❏	❏
6.	❏	❏	❏	❏	31.	❏	❏	❏	❏
7.	❏	❏	❏	❏	32.	❏	❏	❏	❏
8.	❏	❏	❏	❏	33.	❏	❏	❏	❏
9.	❏	❏	❏	❏	34.	❏	❏	❏	❏
10.	❏	❏	❏	❏	35.	❏	❏	❏	❏
11.	❏	❏	❏	❏	36.	❏	❏	❏	❏
12.	❏	❏	❏	❏	37.	❏	❏	❏	❏
13.	❏	❏	❏	❏	38.	❏	❏	❏	❏
14.	❏	❏	❏	❏	39.	❏	❏	❏	❏
15.	❏	❏	❏	❏	40.	❏	❏	❏	❏
16.	❏	❏	❏	❏	41.	❏	❏	❏	❏
17.	❏	❏	❏	❏	42.	❏	❏	❏	❏
18.	❏	❏	❏	❏	43.	❏	❏	❏	❏
19.	❏	❏	❏	❏	44.	❏	❏	❏	❏
20.	❏	❏	❏	❏	45.	❏	❏	❏	❏
21.	❏	❏	❏	❏	46.	❏	❏	❏	❏
22.	❏	❏	❏	❏	47.	❏	❏	❏	❏
23.	❏	❏	❏	❏	48.	❏	❏	❏	❏
24.	❏	❏	❏	❏	49.	❏	❏	❏	❏
25.	❏	❏	❏	❏	50.	❏	❏	❏	❏

Hematology

1. What is the name of the body system that produces blood cells?
   a. hepatic
   b. hemophilic
   c. hematopoietic
   d. uremic

2. The key components of the body system described in question 1 include the liver, spleen, and:
   a. kidneys.
   b. bone marrow.
   c. gray matter.
   d. CFS.

3. The majority of the blood cells are formed in the:
   a. spleen.
   b. liver.
   c. lungs.
   d. bone marrow.

4. The average pH of blood is:
   a. 7.30.
   b. 7.35.
   c. 7.40.
   d. 7.45.

5. Men have approximately _____ cc of blood per kg of body weight.
   a. 60
   b. 70
   c. 80
   d. 90

6. During fetal development, red blood cells are produced in the:
   a. lungs.
   b. kidneys.
   c. umbilical cord.
   d. spleen.

7. All the elements in the red cells, white cells, and platelets are derived from the:
   a. leukocytes.
   b. stem cell.
   c. monocytes.
   d. erythrocytes.

8. How many days do mature red blood cells normally circulate in the blood?
   a. 30
   b. 60
   c. 120
   d. 240

9. Hemoglobin by-products are excreted by the body in the form of:
   a. bilirubin.
   b. hemotoxins.
   c. urine.
   d. cytokines.

10. The measure of the number of red blood cells per unit of blood volume is called the:
    a. pulse oximetry.
    b. end tidal CO_2.
    c. hematocrit.
    d. hematacrit.

11. When a patient has a low number of red blood cells, this chronic condition is called:
    a. hematuria.
    b. polycythemia.
    c. hypocythemia.
    d. anemia.

12. The normal range of hematocrit for women is:
    a. 36–46.
    b. 44–49.
    c. 50–54.
    d. 55–60.

13. The normal range of hematocrit for men is:
    a. 36–42.
    b. 40–45.
    c. 41–53.
    d. 50–55.

14. Neutrophils, eosinophils, and basophils are different types of:
    a. platelets.
    b. granulocytes.
    c. leukocytes.
    d. hemoglobins.

15. Cells without intracellular granules are called:
    a. neutrophils.
    b. monocytes.
    c. exudates.
    d. hemocells.

16. The main function of a leukocyte is to:
    a. carry oxygen to body cells.
    b. provide the color for the blood.
    c. maintain host defenses against infection.
    d. keep the blood clean of by-products.

17. When the body's volume feedback systems sense a low number of circulating red and white blood cells and platelets, the _____ stimulate(s) the _____ to manufacture additional cells.
    a. kidneys and spleen; SCF
    b. spleen and liver; kidneys
    c. kidneys and liver; bone marrow
    d. spleen; kidneys and bone marrow

18. Antibody-mediated immunity is also called:
    a. humoral immunity.
    b. anemia.
    c. cellular immunity.
    d. leukemia.

19. When a patient has a low number of white blood cells (WBCs), this is called:
    a. leukopenia.
    b. leukocytosis.
    c. leukemia.
    d. anemia.

20. Platelets circulate in the blood for an average of _____ days before being removed by the spleen.
    a. 2–5
    b. 7–10
    c. 20–28
    d. 30–45

21. The aggregation of platelets may be decreased by:
    a. high cholesterol in foods.
    b. polycythemia.
    c. anti-inflammatory drugs.
    d. chronic anemia.

22. Immediately following a vascular injury, which of the following inflammatory responses occurs first?
    a. Tissues swell and become edematous.
    b. Protein-rich fluid leaks out from the vessels.
    c. Blood vessels dilate and develop increased permeability.
    d. WBCs line up along the inside of the blood vessels' walls.

23. The substance that is the final "glue" that completes the blood clot is:
    a. hemoglobin.
    b. epithelium.
    c. fibrin.
    d. elastin.

24. Human blood groups are determined by the presence or absence of two antigens, A and B, on the surface of _____ cells.
    a. platelet
    b. red blood
    c. white blood
    d. stem

25. During an interfacility transport with a patient receiving a blood transfusion, the patient complains of flank pain and nausea. During the first 15 minutes of transport, the heart rate has increased from 86 to 124 bpm and the blood pressure has dropped from 112/58 mm Hg to 98/40 mm Hg. What do you suspect is the problem?
    a. kidney stone
    b. acute hemolytic reaction
    c. poor reaction to medication
    d. pulmonary embolism

26. (Continuing with the patient in the previous question) What action should the paramedic take first?
    a. Provide pain management.
    b. Stop the blood transfusion.
    c. Administer Benadryl and epinephrine.
    d. Administer a fluid bolus and dopamine drip.

27. People with type _____ have no antigens and are considered universal donors.
    a. A
    b. B
    c. AB
    d. O

28. Which of the following hematologic conditions is associated with shortness of breath and severe abdominal pain?
    a. anemia
    b. sickle cell crisis
    c. leukemia
    d. myeloma

29. The hematologic condition that rarely affects females but is sex-linked by transmission from a mother to a son, and is characterized by excessive bleeding after minor wounds, is:
    a. anemia.
    b. sickle cell disease.
    c. hemophilia.
    d. leukemia.

30. _____ results from a malignant tumor of blood-forming tissues and is characterized by abnormalities of the bone marrow, spleen, lymph nodes, and liver.
    a. Polycythemia
    b. Sickle cell disease
    c. Hemophilia
    d. Leukemia

31. _____ is the body's natural and normal way of preventing excess blood clot formation.
    a. Fibrinolysis
    b. Electrolysis
    c. Plasminolysis
    d. Neutrolysis

32. Leukemia is a form of cancer that causes which of the following leukocyte disorders?
    a. leukopenia
    b. leukocytosis
    c. abnormal WBC function
    d. abnormal WBC destruction

33. Which of the following granulocytes in the blood are important in fighting allergic reactions?
    a. neutrophils
    b. neutrophils and basophils
    c. eosinophils and basophils
    d. neutrophils and eosinophils

34. When a clinician refers to a patient's H & H, she is referring to the patient's hematocrit and:
    a. hypoxia.
    b. hemoglobin.
    c. hematology.
    d. hematuria.

35. _____ is a disease that causes the bone marrow to produce more platelets than the body needs.
    a. Hemophilia
    b. Thrombocythemia
    c. Hemochromatosis
    d. Sickle cell anemia

Exam #30 Answer Form

		A	B	C	D			A	B	C	D
	1.	❏	❏	❏	❏		19.	❏	❏	❏	❏
	2.	❏	❏	❏	❏		20.	❏	❏	❏	❏
	3.	❏	❏	❏	❏		21.	❏	❏	❏	❏
	4.	❏	❏	❏	❏		22.	❏	❏	❏	❏
	5.	❏	❏	❏	❏		23.	❏	❏	❏	❏
	6.	❏	❏	❏	❏		24.	❏	❏	❏	❏
	7.	❏	❏	❏	❏		25.	❏	❏	❏	❏
	8.	❏	❏	❏	❏		26.	❏	❏	❏	❏
	9.	❏	❏	❏	❏		27.	❏	❏	❏	❏
	10.	❏	❏	❏	❏		28.	❏	❏	❏	❏
	11.	❏	❏	❏	❏		29.	❏	❏	❏	❏
	12.	❏	❏	❏	❏		30.	❏	❏	❏	❏
	13.	❏	❏	❏	❏		31.	❏	❏	❏	❏
	14.	❏	❏	❏	❏		32.	❏	❏	❏	❏
	15.	❏	❏	❏	❏		33.	❏	❏	❏	❏
	16.	❏	❏	❏	❏		34.	❏	❏	❏	❏
	17.	❏	❏	❏	❏		35.	❏	❏	❏	❏
	18.	❏	❏	❏	❏						

31

Gynecology

1. Which of the following structures does not form the female external genitalia?

   a. mons pubis

   b. urethra

   c. perineum

   d. urinary meatus

2. Which of the following structures of the female genitalia is responsible for sexual hormone secretion?

   a. ovaries

   b. fallopian tubes

   c. myometrium

   d. fimbriae

3. Which of the following statements about the fallopian tubes and their functions is most correct?

   a. Ova take 21 days to travel through the fallopian tubes.

   b. The fimbriae at the ends of the tubes are connected to the ovaries.

   c. Fertilization of the ovum usually occurs in one of the fallopian tubes.

   d. The fallopian tubes produce hormones that regulate female reproduction.

4. The base of the uterus is called the:

   a. fundus.

   b. cervix.

   c. uterine cavity.

   d. endometrium.

5. Endometrial cells can sometimes migrate to an area in the body other than the uterus. This condition is called:

   a. cystitis.

   b. endometritis.

   c. endometriosis.

   d. ectopic pregnancy.

6. The normal menstrual cycle is 28 days and can be divided into three phases: menses, the proliferative phase, and:

   a. the secretory phase.

   b. the sloughing phase.

   c. premenstrual syndrome (PMS).

   d. post-capillary washout.

7. _____ is a condition that involves both physical and emotional symptoms that occur regularly in many women during the premenstrual phase of their reproductive cycle.

   a. Meiosis

   b. Amenorrhea

   c. Mittelschmerz

   d. Premenstrual dysphoric disorder

8. Some women experience intense feelings of depression, irritability, anxiety, or withdrawal prior to each menses. These women may also feel fatigued and experience temporary weight gain during the same time frame. The treatment for this condition is:

   a. supplemental iron therapy.

   b. estrogen hormone therapy.

   c. testosterone hormone therapy.

   d. aimed at relieving the symptoms.

9. The hormone _____ is responsible for stimulating bone and muscle growth.

   a. estrogen

   b. progesterone

   c. actin

   d. testosterone

10. The hormone responsible for restoring and preparing the uterus for pregnancy after menses is:

    a. estrogen.

    b. progesterone.

    c. oxytocin.

    d. Pitocin.

11. _____ is(are) the leading cause of female infertility and ectopic pregnancy.
    a. Peritonitis
    b. Genital warts
    c. Vaginal yeast infections
    d. PID

12. What is the most common bacterial STD?
    a. syphilis
    b. gonorrhea
    c. pubic lice
    d. chlamydia

13. Of the following conditions, which one does not produce vaginal bleeding?
    a. labor
    b. sexual abuse
    c. urinary tract infection
    d. pelvic inflammatory disease

14. Cystitis is a(n) _____ infection, which often occurs secondary to a urinary tract infection (UTI).
    a. kidney
    b. bladder
    c. urethra
    d. ovarian

15. Which of the following is a secondary injury from a sexual assault?
    a. lacerations to the external genitalia
    b. sexually transmitted disease (STD)
    c. bruising on the mons pubis
    d. rectal tears

16. You and your partner are caring for the victim of a rape. As your partner assesses her wounds and obtains baseline vital signs, you consider how to preserve evidence and take which of the following actions?
    a. Place any items removed from the patient into separate bags.
    b. Place any items removed from the patient into a plastic bag.
    c. Allow the patient to void and change her clothes prior to transport.
    d. Place all of the items belonging to the patient together in the same bag.

17. After assessing and addressing any life-threatening conditions, the management of the victim of a sexual assault is focused on:
    a. preserving evidence of the crime.
    b. providing emotional support.
    c. cleaning superficial wounds.
    d. reporting the crime to the appropriate person.

18. Sexual assault is a crime of violence and can occur in any age group. It is estimated that _____ females is raped during her lifetime.
    a. one in three
    b. one in five
    c. one in ten
    d. one in twenty

19. _____ is the cessation of ovarian function and menstrual activity.
    a. Menarche
    b. Menopause
    c. Amenorrhea
    d. Mittelschmerz

20. Which of the following is an example of a gynecological emergency?
    a. UTI
    b. gallstones
    c. gestational diabetes
    d. ruptured ovarian cyst

21. _____ is characterized by lower abdominal pain experienced by some women at the time of ovulation.
    a. Menarche
    b. Menopause
    c. Amenorrhea
    d. Mittelschmerz

22. _____ is an acute or chronic inflammation of the endometrium caused by bacterial infection.
    a. Endometriosis
    b. Endometritis
    c. Cystitis
    d. Oophritis

23. Immediate complications of vaginal bleeding include:
    a. infection.
    b. tissue scarring.
    c. shock and death.
    d. infertility.

24. Dysfunctional uterine bleeding is abnormal vaginal bleeding related to the menstrual cycle that is caused by:
    a. sexual trauma.
    b. vaginal foreign body.
    c. eating excess amounts of chocolate.
    d. too little or too much estrogen.

25. Vaginal foreign bodies are commonly seen in children, with _____ being the most common foreign body.
    a. tampons
    b. toilet paper
    c. small toys
    d. fruit or vegetables

Exam #31 Answer Form

	A	B	C	D			A	B	C	D
1.	❏	❏	❏	❏		14.	❏	❏	❏	❏
2.	❏	❏	❏	❏		15.	❏	❏	❏	❏
3.	❏	❏	❏	❏		16.	❏	❏	❏	❏
4.	❏	❏	❏	❏		17.	❏	❏	❏	❏
5.	❏	❏	❏	❏		18.	❏	❏	❏	❏
6.	❏	❏	❏	❏		19.	❏	❏	❏	❏
7.	❏	❏	❏	❏		20.	❏	❏	❏	❏
8.	❏	❏	❏	❏		21.	❏	❏	❏	❏
9.	❏	❏	❏	❏		22.	❏	❏	❏	❏
10.	❏	❏	❏	❏		23.	❏	❏	❏	❏
11.	❏	❏	❏	❏		24.	❏	❏	❏	❏
12.	❏	❏	❏	❏		25.	❏	❏	❏	❏
13.	❏	❏	❏	❏						

CHAPTER

Non-Traumatic Musculoskeletal Disorders

1. The general assessment findings and symptoms of non-traumatic musculoskeletal disorders include each of the following, *except*:
   a. swelling.
   b. loss of movement.
   c. uticaria.
   d. circulatory changes.

2. Your patient has a non-traumatic musculoskeletal disorder, which causes her chronic pain. Of the conditions listed below, which is most likely her condition?
   a. seizure disorder
   b. osteomyelitis
   c. preeclampsia
   d. cerebral palsy

3. An overuse syndrome from constantly typing on a keyboard is called:
   a. rhabdomyolysis.
   b. fasciitis.
   c. carpal tunnel syndrome.
   d. myosis.

4. Each of the following is a non-traumatic musculo-skeletal disorder of the joints, *except*:
   a. cauda equina syndrome.
   b. arthritis.
   c. gout.
   d. rheumatoid.

5. An example of a non-traumatic musculoskeletal disorder affecting soft tissue would be:
   a. tendonitis.
   b. bone tumor.
   c. gangrene.
   d. bursitis.

6. When a patient describes pain in his elbow after playing tennis for many hours, this could be due to:
   a. cauda equina syndrome.
   b. gout.
   c. fasciitis.
   d. bursitis.

7. An example of a non-traumatic musculoskeletal disorder that is related to the body's retention of uric acids in the blood, causing inflammation, is called:
   a. myalgia.
   b. gout.
   c. bursitis.
   d. osteoarthritis.

8. The breakdown of muscle fibers from the disease rhabdomyolysis can cause serious damage to the patient's:
   a. refractory.
   b. heart.
   c. liver.
   d. kidneys.

9. The disorder that can be found in workers, such as paramedics, who lift improperly is:
   a. low-back pain.
   b. osteomyelitis.
   c. gout.
   d. paronychia.

10. The symptom of muscle pain or aching is most common in:
    a. disc disorder.
    b. myalgia.
    c. paronychia.
    d. fasciitis.

11. The non-traumatic musculoskeletal disorder which affects the joints is:

    a. myositis.

    b. rhabdomyolysis.

    c. arthritis.

    d. flexor tenosynovitis.

12. The inflammation that can affect the tendons of the fingers is called:

    a. gangrene.

    b. flexor tenosynovitis.

    c. paronychia.

    d. septic gout.

13. Peripheral nerve syndrome is an example of a(n):

    a. joint abnormality.

    b. spine disorder.

    c. muscle abnormality.

    d. overuse syndrome.

14. A skin infection occurring around the nails and cuticle is called:

    a. gangrene.

    b. staph infection.

    c. paronychia.

    d. myalgia.

15. Which of the following non-traumatic musculoskeletal disorders involves tissue necrosis?

    a. gout

    b. gangrene

    c. bursitis

    d. osteoarthritis

Exam #32 Answer Form

	A	B	C	D
1.	❑	❑	❑	❑
2.	❑	❑	❑	❑
3.	❑	❑	❑	❑
4.	❑	❑	❑	❑
5.	❑	❑	❑	❑
6.	❑	❑	❑	❑
7.	❑	❑	❑	❑
8.	❑	❑	❑	❑

	A	B	C	D
9.	❑	❑	❑	❑
10.	❑	❑	❑	❑
11.	❑	❑	❑	❑
12.	❑	❑	❑	❑
13.	❑	❑	❑	❑
14.	❑	❑	❑	❑
15.	❑	❑	❑	❑

Diseases of the Ears, Eyes, Nose, and Throat

1. The white of the eye is a tough, fibrous coat that helps maintain the shape of the eye. It is called the:
   a. cornea.
   b. sclera.
   c. conjunctiva.
   d. iris.

2. The circular adjustable opening within the iris through which light passes to the lens is called the:
   a. retina.
   b. cornea.
   c. pupil.
   d. conjunctiva.

3. A delicate, 10-layered structure of nervous tissue that extends from the optic nerve is called the:
   a. retina.
   b. iris.
   c. sclera.
   d. pupil.

4. The portion of the globe between the lens and the cornea is called the _____ . It is filled with a clear watery fluid called:
   a. posterior chamber; aqueous humor.
   b. anterior chamber; aqueous humor.
   c. anterior chamber; vitreous humor.
   d. posterior chamber; vitreous humor.

5. The purpose of the lacrimal system is to:
   a. drain nasal congestion.
   b. send images to the lens.
   c. secrete and drain tears from the eyes.
   d. send images from the lens to the brain.

6. The components of the lacrimal apparatus include each of the following, except:
   a. lacrimal ducts.
   b. lacrimal sacs.
   c. lacrimal gland.
   d. conjunctivae.

7. The image on the retina is transmitted by the optic nerve to the:
   a. visual cortex of the brain.
   b. lens of the eye.
   c. motor cortex of the brain.
   d. brain stem.

8. When examining the eyes, check the globe for:
   a. reaction to light.
   b. redness, lacerations, and discoloration.
   c. tenderness or pain on palpation.
   d. dolls eyes.

9. The exam for ocular function usually involves each of the following, except:
   a. peripheral vision.
   b. visual acuity.
   c. DCAP-BTLS.
   d. ocular motility.

10. The leading cause of adult blindness is:
    a. glaucoma.
    b. stroke.
    c. diabetes.
    d. chemical burns.

11. When the pupils are not equal in size, this condition is called:
    a. diplopia.
    b. anisocoria.
    c. coma.
    d. adnexa.

12. A 22-year-old female has sustained a burn to the eye from falling asleep in a tanning booth under UV light without the appropriate glasses on. Her eyes are dry and painful. The prehospital treatment should include:
    a. applying Silvadene® burn ointment to the cornea.
    b. covering eyes with sterile moist pad and eye shield.
    c. constant flushing with water for 20 minutes.
    d. flushing with vinegar.

13. Irrigation of an eye which has been exposed to chemicals is best done with:
    a. saline and baking soda.
    b. a hard lens irrigator.
    c. tetracaine and Morgan® lens.
    d. water and vinegar.

14. When the eye gets inflamed and looks pink, this is called:
    a. conjunctivitis.
    b. anisocoria.
    c. retinopathy.
    d. adnexa.

15. Serious injury to the eye from blunt trauma, due to a sport like boxing, can cause:
    a. retinopathy.
    b. retinal detachment.
    c. periorbital cellulitis.
    d. chalazion.

16. The inner ear consists of the semicircular canals and:
    a. ossicles.
    b. cochlea.
    c. tympanic membrane.
    d. auditory nerve.

17. Sound waves enter the ear through the:
    a. tympanic membrane.
    b. ossicles.
    c. cochlea.
    d. pinna.

18. An inner ear disorder usually affecting middle-aged adults with symptoms of hearing loss, ear pressure, vertigo, and dizziness could be:
    a. otitis.
    b. Meniere's disease.
    c. sinusitis.
    d. labyrinthitis.

19. The pressure in your ears, when going up in an elevator in a high-rise building, is equalized by the:
    a. sinus tracts.
    b. paranasal sinus.
    c. Eustachian tubes.
    d. tympanic membrane.

20. Your patient is complaining of thick nasal discharge, facial pressure, headache, and fever. This is most likely:
    a. rhinitis.
    b. Meniere's.
    c. sinusitis.
    d. labyrinthitis.

21. Of the following, which is not a nerve involved in the nerve supply to the mouth and its structures?
    a. hypoglossal nerve
    b. oculomotor nerve
    c. trigeminal nerve
    d. glossopharyngeal nerve

22. A yeast infection that causes white patches in the mouth or on the tongue is called:
    a. leukoplakia.
    b. gingivitis.
    c. canker sores.
    d. thrush.

23. A smoker's disease that causes excess cell growth in the mouth, cheek, or gums and presents as white patches is called:
    a. leukoplakia.
    b. canker sores.
    c. gingivitis.
    d. cold sore.

24. A collection of infected material in the back of the throat caused by a bacterial infection which can be accompanied by facial swelling and chills is likely:
    a. tonsillitis.
    b. pharyngitis.
    c. croup.
    d. a peritonsillar abscess.

25. Causes of temporomandibular joint (TMJ) disorder include:
    a. sleep apnea.
    b. arthritis damage to the joint.
    c. injury to jaw.
    d. muscle fatigue from grinding teeth.

Exam #33 Answer Form

	A	B	C	D		A	B	C	D
1.	❏	❏	❏	❏	14.	❏	❏	❏	❏
2.	❏	❏	❏	❏	15.	❏	❏	❏	❏
3.	❏	❏	❏	❏	16.	❏	❏	❏	❏
4.	❏	❏	❏	❏	17.	❏	❏	❏	❏
5.	❏	❏	❏	❏	18.	❏	❏	❏	❏
6.	❏	❏	❏	❏	19.	❏	❏	❏	❏
7.	❏	❏	❏	❏	20.	❏	❏	❏	❏
8.	❏	❏	❏	❏	21.	❏	❏	❏	❏
9.	❏	❏	❏	❏	22.	❏	❏	❏	❏
10.	❏	❏	❏	❏	23.	❏	❏	❏	❏
11.	❏	❏	❏	❏	24.	❏	❏	❏	❏
12.	❏	❏	❏	❏	25.	❏	❏	❏	❏
13.	❏	❏	❏	❏					

Shock and Resuscitation

1. A patient was shot in the stomach. Upon arrival, after assuring that the police have secured the scene, the paramedic is able to talk directly to the patient, who is alert and complaining of severe pain. The paramedic is unable to obtain a radial pulse. What grade/stage of hemorrhage would you suspect the patient is in?
    a. 1
    b. 2
    c. 3
    d. 4

2. Based on the scenario in question 4, approximately how much blood has the patient lost up to the point of primary assessment by the paramedic?
    a. up to 15%
    b. 15–25%
    c. 25–35%
    d. > 35%

3. What treatment would be appropriate for this patient?
    a. sedate and intubate on scene
    b. two large bore IVs en route
    c. vasopressors
    d. two large bore IVs on scene

4. When the systolic BP drops from a hemorrhage, it is referred to as _____ shock.
    a. hypervolemic
    b. decompensated
    c. irreversible
    d. compensated

5. In the formula $CO = HR \times SV$, the SV is usually approximately _____ per heartbeat in an adult.
    a. 25 cc
    b. 50 cc
    c. 70 cc
    d. 120 cc

6. The body's compensatory mechanism for blood loss in the short term is to increase the cardiac output by:
    a. peripheral vasodilation.
    b. increasing the heart rate.
    c. increasing the stroke volume.
    d. decreasing vascular resistance.

7. What is the objective measure of vasoconstriction during hemorrhage?
    a. increase in systolic pressure
    b. increase in diastolic pressure
    c. decrease in systolic pressure
    d. decrease in diastolic pressure

8. For the long term, how can you increase your SV?
    a. weight loss through healthy diet
    b. take medication to slow the heart rate
    c. aerobic exercise on a regular basis
    d. lift weights on a regular basis

9. When the body's compensatory system signals the sympathetic nervous system to release epinephrine, the alpha-1 effects will cause:
    a. bronchodilation.
    b. vasoconstriction.
    c. positive inotropic effects.
    d. positive chronotropic effects.

10. When the body's compensatory system signals the sympathetic nervous system to release epinephrine, the beta-1 effects will cause:
    a. bronchodilation.
    b. vasoconstriction.
    c. positive dromotropic effects.
    d. smooth muscle dilation in the GI tract.

11. The chemical that is released during shock, which starts to act as an antidiuretic, is called:
    a. insulin.
    b. aldosterone.
    c. arginine vasopressin.
    d. glucagon.

12. A potent vasoconstrictor that promotes sodium reabsorption and decreases urine output in shock states is:
    a. insulin.
    b. aldosterone.
    c. arginine vasopressin.
    d. angiotensin II.

13. Following injury and volume loss, the patient is often:
    a. hypoglycemic.
    b. hyperglycemic.
    c. flushed and warm.
    d. depleted of urine.

14. When the compensatory mechanisms are overwhelmed, all of the following occur, except:
    a. preload decreases.
    b. cardiac output decreases.
    c. myocardial blood supply increases.
    d. capillary and cellular changes.

15. At the cellular level, during low perfusion states when the post-capillary sphincter relaxes, this is called the _____ phase.
    a. ischemia
    b. washout
    c. stagnation
    d. final

16. During low perfusion states, the pre-capillary sphincters relax in response to lactic acid and:
    a. decreased carbon dioxide.
    b. vasomotor center failure.
    c. hypothermia.
    d. aerobic metabolism.

17. _____ shock is characterized by signs and symptoms of late shock, but is refractory to treatment.
    a. Hypovolemic
    b. Distributive
    c. Irreversible
    d. Obstructive

18. You are assessing a 60-year-old male who is very sick with a low blood pressure. Which one of the following signs or symptoms may differentiate cardiogenic shock from hypovolemic shock?
    a. chief complaint of chest pain
    b. presence of tachycardia
    c. absence of diaphoresis
    d. poor CTC

19. Which of the following signs may differentiate distributed shock from hypovolemic shock?
    a. chief complaint of dyspnea
    b. presence of tachycardia
    c. absence of diaphoresis
    d. flushed skin

20. Which of the following signs may differentiate obstructive shock from hypovolemic shock?
    a. chief complaint of abdominal pain
    b. presence of JVD
    c. presence of tachycardia
    d. poor CTC

21. Intravenous volume expanders that have the same tonicity as plasma are the _____ solutions.
    a. isotonic
    b. hypertonic
    c. hypotonic
    d. synthetic

22. When using intravenous volume expanders, it is important to recall that only about _____ of the fluid infused stays in the intravascular space.
    a. 1/4
    b. 1/3
    c. 1/2
    d. 2/3

23. When a crystalloid IV volume expander such as normal saline is used, the amount that shifts out of the intravascular space moves into the _____ within approximately 1 hour.
    a. interstitial space
    b. lungs
    c. intracellular compartment
    d. kidneys

24. Which of the following statements is most correct about intravenous volume expanders?
    a. They should only be used en route to the ED.
    b. Hypertonic solutions are best in the prehospital setting.
    c. Isotonic solutions are not routinely used in or out of the ED.
    d. They do not carry hemoglobin.

25. You are assessing an 18-year-old male who crashed his dirt bike. He has an obvious closed femur fracture and abdominal pain. His mental status is alert, but initially he had a brief loss of consciousness, and his vital signs are R/R 30 and shallow, P/R 110, and BP 116/56 mm Hg. His skin is warm and moist. Which stage of shock is indicated by the pulse and blood pressure?
    a. compensated
    b. decompensated
    c. distributive
    d. obstructive

26. Based on the scenario in question 25, the most likely cause of the shock is:
    a. head injury.
    b. internal bleeding.
    c. substantial vasodilation.
    d. loss of venous capacitance.

27. Baroreceptors located in the carotid sinuses and _____ are stimulated by decreased blood flow.
    a. intestines
    b. aortic arch
    c. cerebellum
    d. medulla

28. When baroreceptors sense decreased blood flow and activate the vasomotor center, there is:
    a. vasodilation of the peripheral vessels.
    b. vasodilation of the great vessels.
    c. vasoconstriction of the peripheral vessels.
    d. vasoconstriction of the central organs.

29. When the sympathetic nervous system is stimulated in response to shock, epinephrine and norepinephrine are secreted from the:
    a. thalamus.
    b. hypothalamus.
    c. adrenal gland.
    d. pituitary gland.

30. Which of the following is an early sign of hypovolemic shock?
    a. narrowing pulse pressure
    b. increased peripheral vascular resistance
    c. increased stroke volume
    d. loss of vasomotor tone

31. When the body senses hypovolemia, several regulatory systems are put into play to try to compensate. These include sympathetic responses, vasoconstriction, and:
    a. endocrine responses.
    b. CO_2 elimination.
    c. metabolic purging.
    d. osmotic channeling.

32. The maximum amount of intravenous volume expanders prudent for field administration is about _____ liters so as to avoid reducing hematocrit from being effective.
    a. 1–2
    b. 2–3
    c. 4–5
    d. 5–6

33. Many regions have limited the use of PASG/MAST at this point. For those that still use the device, the indication for the use of PASG/MAST in _____ is still relatively unchanged.
    a. chest trauma
    b. abdominal hemorrhage
    c. stabilization of pelvic fractures
    d. pregnancy

34. Despite the controversies in the use of PASG/MAST, the _____ still recommends that the suit be available for immediate use in hospital emergency departments.
    a. National Registry
    b. ACEP
    c. JEMS
    d. NHTSA

35. Decreased perfusion can be caused by an event resulting in blood loss, kinking of the great vessels (i.e., tension pneumothorax.), or:
    a. release of antidiuretic hormone.
    b. an allergic reaction.
    c. a failure in the buffer system.
    d. loss of vasomotor tone.

36. _____ defends the fluid volume and reduces urine output by promoting sodium reabsorption and water retention in the kidney.
    a. ACTH
    b. Angiotensin I
    c. Aldosterone
    d. Glucagon

37. Renin is released by _____ and catalyzes the conversion of angiotensinogen to angiotensin I.
    a. arterioles in the kidney
    b. transfer of fatty acids into mitochondria
    c. cells in the adrenal cortex
    d. circulating epinephrine

38. Of the following conditions, which would not be considered a pre-morbid condition in an unhealthy patient?
    a. electrocution
    b. congestive heart failure
    c. drug toxicity
    d. stroke

39. You are treating a healthy 35-year-old male patient who is in cardiac arrest. Of the following reasons, which is the most likely cause of the arrest?

    a. uncontrolled diabetes

    b. obesity

    c. pulmonary embolus

    d. renal failure

40. In respect to the physiology of blood flow during CPR, what is the heart pump theory?

    a. The blood flow during CPR is diminished due to the clotting within the chambers.

    b. Compression of the sternum raised the pressure in the chest.

    c. The heart is squeezed through direct compression between sternum and spinal column.

    d. Blood moves from areas of more blood to areas of less blood within the body.

41. Of the following steps in a resuscitation, which is the most important and often most effective?

    a. the total dose and concentration of epinephrine that was administered

    b. early endotracheal intubation of the patient to assure adequate ventilations

    c. high-quality chest compressions with a minimum of interruptions

    d. the number of shocks that are administered to the patient

42. Your 35-year-old male patient has been in cardiac arrest for about 10 minutes and CPR was started within the first few minutes of the arrest by a citizen. Which medication should be your first consideration once venous access is acquired?

    a. lidocaine

    b. amiodarone

    c. epinephrine

    d. atropine

43. After the first 2 minutes of high-quality CPR, your concern in managing the patient who is in cardiac arrest should turn to:

    a. defibrillating VF.

    b. starting an IV.

    c. inserting an advanced airway.

    d. administering an antidysrhythmic.

44. You have been running a cardiac arrest on a 45-year-old female for the past 7 minutes when you notice that the $ETCO_2$ is beginning to improve. What could this be an indication of?

    a. The ET tube just came out of the trachea.

    b. There is a return of spontaneous circulation.

    c. The patient will need another dose of epinephrine right away.

    d. There is a malfunction with the monitor.

45. Which of the following would be the least likely special consideration for the patient who was found in cardiac arrest after being struck by an automobile?

    a. His electrolytes are abnormal.

    b. He may be bleeding out internally.

    c. He could have a tension pneumothorax.

    d. He may have head trauma.

Exam #34 Answer Form

	A	B	C	D
1.	❏	❏	❏	❏
2.	❏	❏	❏	❏
3.	❏	❏	❏	❏
4.	❏	❏	❏	❏
5.	❏	❏	❏	❏
6.	❏	❏	❏	❏
7.	❏	❏	❏	❏
8.	❏	❏	❏	❏
9.	❏	❏	❏	❏
10.	❏	❏	❏	❏
11.	❏	❏	❏	❏
12.	❏	❏	❏	❏
13.	❏	❏	❏	❏
14.	❏	❏	❏	❏
15.	❏	❏	❏	❏
16.	❏	❏	❏	❏
17.	❏	❏	❏	❏
18.	❏	❏	❏	❏
19.	❏	❏	❏	❏
20.	❏	❏	❏	❏
21.	❏	❏	❏	❏
22.	❏	❏	❏	❏
23.	❏	❏	❏	❏

	A	B	C	D
24.	❏	❏	❏	❏
25.	❏	❏	❏	❏
26.	❏	❏	❏	❏
27.	❏	❏	❏	❏
28.	❏	❏	❏	❏
29.	❏	❏	❏	❏
30.	❏	❏	❏	❏
31.	❏	❏	❏	❏
32.	❏	❏	❏	❏
33.	❏	❏	❏	❏
34.	❏	❏	❏	❏
35.	❏	❏	❏	❏
36.	❏	❏	❏	❏
37.	❏	❏	❏	❏
38.	❏	❏	❏	❏
39.	❏	❏	❏	❏
40.	❏	❏	❏	❏
41.	❏	❏	❏	❏
42.	❏	❏	❏	❏
43.	❏	❏	❏	❏
44.	❏	❏	❏	❏
45.	❏	❏	❏	❏

CHAPTER

35

Trauma Overview

1. The leading cause of work-related fatal injuries in the United States is:
   a. falls.
   b. fires and explosions.
   c. transportation incidents.
   d. exposure to harmful substances.

2. The top three causes of trauma death in order are:
   a. motor vehicle collisions (MVC), fire arms, and falls.
   b. motor vehicle collisions (MVC), homicides, and suicides.
   c. falls, poisonings, and firearms.
   d. falls, drownings, and suicides.

3. Getting a complete and accurate account of the mechanism of injury (MOI) can help emergency care providers identify nearly 95% of the possible injuries sustained in most cases, because:
   a. the patient will not know the extent of his own injuries.
   b. many MOIs have predictable patterns for specific injuries.
   c. serious and life-threatening injuries can always be identified early.
   d. early recognition of possible injuries by the paramedic can save the patient from needing rehabilitation.

4. _____ is(are) the form of trauma most likely to result in permanent disability or death.
   a. Burns
   b. Shock
   c. Orthopedic
   d. Traumatic brain injury (TBI)

5. The two major factors for the extent of traumatic injury a victim may suffer are the amount of energy exchanges to the body and:
   a. the patient's gender.
   b. anatomic structures that are involved.
   c. past medical history (PMH).
   d. the use of any safety restraints.

6. Trauma scoring systems:
   a. convert the severity of an injury into a number.
   b. help to rapidly identify life-threatening injuries.
   c. help the paramedic to stabilize the patient prior to transport.
   d. appreciate predictable injury patterns into measurable numbers.

7. After personal safety and management of the patient's ABCs, _____ is the most important information to obtain about any trauma victim.
   a. MOI
   b. past medical history (PMH)
   c. organ donor status
   d. DNAR status

8. One significant feature of a trauma scoring systems is that they can:
   a. give an objective measure to multisystem trauma.
   b. predict in-hospital mortality for trauma patients.
   c. predict prehospital mortality for trauma patients.
   d. help the paramedic decide whether to bring the patient to a trauma center.

9. The paramedic can make a significant impact on the life or death of a trauma victim by:
   a. wearing the appropriate PPE.
   b. stabilizing the patient prior to transport.
   c. minimizing scene time when appropriate.
   d. transporting the trauma patient to the nearest facility.

10. The paper entitled "Accidental Death and Disability: The Neglected Disease of Modern Society" is also known as the:
    a. Ryan White Act.
    b. Highway Safety Act of 1966.
    c. Trauma Prevention Act.
    d. white paper.

11. The components of a trauma system include injury prevention programs, prehospital care, definitive care, rehabilitation, and:
    a. research.
    b. burn centers.
    c. data collection.
    d. hyperbaric centers.

12. A trauma _____ is a reporting system designed to collect trauma-related data in an effort to improve the quality and cost-effectiveness of care and to aid in outcomes of research.
    a. registry
    b. chronicle
    c. journal
    d. catalog

13. Which of the following statements about trauma centers is most correct?
    a. Any hospital that cares for acutely injured patients is a trauma center.
    b. One specific criterion for trauma center designation is the use of air-medical transport.
    c. Trauma centers must meet strict criteria to be designated a trauma center.
    d. Only one hospital can be designated a level I trauma center for a city.

14. In which of the following patient scenarios should the paramedic transport the patient to the nearest hospital, even if it is not a trauma center?
    a. critical burns
    b. multiple system trauma
    c. traumatic cardiac arrest
    d. pregnant patient involved in a significant MOI

15. Which of the following patient situations is an indication for the use of air-medical transport?
    a. access to a remote area
    b. extremely combative patient
    c. patient with injuries induced by barotrauma
    d. inclement weather too severe for ground ambulance transport

16. Which of the following patient situations is a contraindication for the use of air-medical transport?
    a. traumatic cardiac arrest
    b. patient requires a surgical airway
    c. patient with spinal cord injury from a diving accident
    d. ground transport poses a threat to the patient's survival

17. _____ means that energy cannot be created or destroyed, only transferred or exchanged.
    a. Kinetic energy
    b. Force
    c. Newton's first law of motion
    d. Conservation of energy

18. The concept "An object in motion tends to stay in motion, and an object at rest tends to stay at rest" describes:
    a. kinetic energy.
    b. force.
    c. Newton's first law of motion.
    d. conservation of energy.

19. _____ means that the more speed that is involved, the more energy there is.
    a. Kinetic energy
    b. Force
    c. Newton's first law of motion
    d. Conservation of energy

20. _____ is the creation of a cavity in an object that can be permanent or temporary.
    a. Energy
    b. Force
    c. Cavitation
    d. Puncture

21. Which of the following components of kinetic energy makes the greatest impact on a trauma victim?
    a. mass
    b. velocity
    c. acceleration
    d. deceleration

22. Which of the following are the actual units for kinetic energy?
    a. foot-pounds
    b. mile-grams
    c. meter-liters
    d. inch-ounces

23. When does the golden hour for the trauma victim begin?
    a. when the first responder arrives at the patient's side
    b. when the paramedic arrives on the scene
    c. immediately after the injury is sustained
    d. immediately upon arriving at the ED

24. What is meant by the third collision in the MOI of a trauma victim?
    a. Third collision is the internal organs striking against the body.
    b. This is a triad of injuries involving the head, neck, and spine.
    c. Third collision refers to multiple injuries.
    d. Third collision pertains to children involved in motor vehicle collisions.

25. Why are some bullets designed to tumble when fired from a gun?
    a. Tumbling bullets are faster.
    b. Tumbling decreases the force of impact.
    c. Penetration is streamlined with tumbling.
    d. Tumbling creates greater tissue damage.

26. You are sizing up the scene at an MVC, and you see that the vehicle with the only patient involved was rear-ended, which resulted in her vehicle being pushed off the road and into a ditch. What type of force(s) has this patient experienced in this MOI?
    a. blunt penetrating
    b. rapid acceleration
    c. rapid deceleration
    d. rapid acceleration and deceleration

27. Which of the following MOIs is not usually associated with predictable injury patterns?
    a. motorcycle collisions
    b. auto–pedestrian collisions
    c. falls
    d. gunshot wounds (GSWs)

28. The three phases associated with the blast effect are the primary phase, the secondary phase, and the _____ phase.
    a. late
    b. triage
    c. tertiary
    d. end-stage

29. During the secondary phase of the blast effect, the potential for injury comes from:
    a. the heat wave.
    b. flying articles.
    c. pressure waves.
    d. the patient striking an object.

30. Which of the following penetrating MOIs has the greatest potential for energy exchange?
    a. high-power rifle
    b. knife
    c. shotgun
    d. hanging

31. Which of the following will generate the greatest amount of kinetic energy?
    a. 90-kg patient traveling at 30 mph
    b. 80-kg patient traveling at 40 mph
    c. 70-kg patient traveling at 50 mph
    d. 60-kg patient traveling at 60 mph

32. You are assessing a patient who was a victim of a significant blast injury. He has the clinical findings of a closed pneumothorax. Which of the following is the most likely cause of his injury?
    a. heat wave
    b. compression
    c. flying article
    d. sound wave

33. During the _____ phase of the blast effect, injuries can result from the patient becoming a flying object and striking other objects.
    a. end-stage
    b. secondary
    c. late
    d. tertiary

34. Your patient is the victim of a motorcycle collision and has bilateral femur fractures. What type of impact did the patient most likely sustain?
    a. frontal
    b. rear-end
    c. side
    d. rotational

35. Cervical spine injuries are most common with what type of collision?
    a. frontal
    b. rear-end
    c. primary
    d. secondary

36. Your patient was assisted out of a house fire by a fireman who found him lying on the bedroom floor unconscious. Which of the following pieces of information about the MOI is the most significant for this patient?
    a. cause of the fire
    b. when the fire was started
    c. smoke condition in the room in which the patient was found
    d. presence of a carbon monoxide detector in the house

37. What is the most likely cause of the unconsciousness in the patient described in question 36?
    a. airway burns
    b. super-heated air
    c. CO_2 inhalation
    d. shock

38. The patient you are assessing fell from a tall ladder while at work. Which of the following aspects of the MOI should the paramedic focus on?
    a. point of impact of the body
    b. the distance of the fall
    c. the type of surface of the impact
    d. the combination of forces involved

39. When a projectile such as a bullet passes through the body, it creates a wave of pressure that can compress organs and tissue, causing:
    a. contusion, fracture, or rupture.
    b. liquidation.
    c. collapse and disintegration.
    d. spontaneous combustion.

40. Which of the following aspects of a GSW should the paramedic focus on?
    a. the gender of the shooter
    b. the wind speed at the time of the shooting
    c. the level of gravity at the time of the shooting
    d. the type of empty shell casings

41. Your patient is the victim of a motorcycle collision where he was T-boned at an intersection by a car. Which of the following injury patterns is most associated with lateral impact motorcycle collisions?
    a. bilateral femur fractures
    b. crush injuries
    c. pelvis dislocation
    d. pneumothorax

42. Which of the following is an injury associated with third collision MOI?
    a. brain contusion
    b. fractured pelvis
    c. dislocated knee
    d. neck injury

43. By performing a rapid assessment and life-saving procedures, minimizing scene time to _____ minutes and transporting the patient to an appropriate facility, the paramedic makes the difference between life or death for a trauma patient.
    a. 10
    b. 15
    c. 30
    d. 60

44. As a general rule, the entrance wound of a bullet is usually smaller than the exit wound because of:
    a. proximity of the shooter.
    b. positioning of the patient.
    c. cavitation.
    d. dissection.

45. During the primary phase of the blast effect, there is a pressure wave that can cause major damage to the:
    a. eyes and skin.
    b. lungs and GI tract.
    c. head and neck.
    d. hearing.

46. The pathologic effects of the pressure wave during the blast effect include:
    a. lacerations and bruising.
    b. rupture of an organ or air embolism.
    c. whiplash and sprains.
    d. shattering.

47. During the third phase of an auto–pedestrian collision, the patient can sustain injuries from:
    a. the impact of the vehicle.
    b. the fall onto the hood of the vehicle.
    c. going into the vehicle.
    d. being run over by the vehicle.

48. The victim of a motorcycle collision who does not wear a helmet has a _____% increased risk of brain injury.
    a. 30
    b. 50
    c. 300
    d. 500

49. Which of the following statements about air bags in motor vehicles is most correct?
    a. Air bags do not work without the use of seat belts.
    b. Air bags may produce minor facial and forearm abrasions.
    c. The smoke associated with the discharge of the air bag is noxious.
    d. There is no risk of injury from the protective cover over the air bag upon discharge.

50. Which of the following statements about shoulder restraints is correct?
    a. They prevent hyperflexion of the upper torso.
    b. They do not prevent forward motion of the upper torso in frontal impact collisions.
    c. Neck injuries can still be prevented, even without the use of a lap restraint.
    d. Shoulder restraints provide more benefit when the seat is very close to the dashboard.

Exam #35 Answer Form

	A	B	C	D		A	B	C	D
1.	❏	❏	❏	❏	26.	❏	❏	❏	❏
2.	❏	❏	❏	❏	27.	❏	❏	❏	❏
3.	❏	❏	❏	❏	28.	❏	❏	❏	❏
4.	❏	❏	❏	❏	29.	❏	❏	❏	❏
5.	❏	❏	❏	❏	30.	❏	❏	❏	❏
6.	❏	❏	❏	❏	31.	❏	❏	❏	❏
7.	❏	❏	❏	❏	32.	❏	❏	❏	❏
8.	❏	❏	❏	❏	33.	❏	❏	❏	❏
9.	❏	❏	❏	❏	34.	❏	❏	❏	❏
10.	❏	❏	❏	❏	35.	❏	❏	❏	❏
11.	❏	❏	❏	❏	36.	❏	❏	❏	❏
12.	❏	❏	❏	❏	37.	❏	❏	❏	❏
13.	❏	❏	❏	❏	38.	❏	❏	❏	❏
14.	❏	❏	❏	❏	39.	❏	❏	❏	❏
15.	❏	❏	❏	❏	40.	❏	❏	❏	❏
16.	❏	❏	❏	❏	41.	❏	❏	❏	❏
17.	❏	❏	❏	❏	42.	❏	❏	❏	❏
18.	❏	❏	❏	❏	43.	❏	❏	❏	❏
19.	❏	❏	❏	❏	44.	❏	❏	❏	❏
20.	❏	❏	❏	❏	45.	❏	❏	❏	❏
21.	❏	❏	❏	❏	46.	❏	❏	❏	❏
22.	❏	❏	❏	❏	47.	❏	❏	❏	❏
23.	❏	❏	❏	❏	48.	❏	❏	❏	❏
24.	❏	❏	❏	❏	49.	❏	❏	❏	❏
25.	❏	❏	❏	❏	50.	❏	❏	❏	❏

CHAPTER

36

Bleeding, Soft Tissue Trauma, and Burns

1. The two general locations of severe hemorrhage are:
   a. head and neck.
   b. extremities and back.
   c. internal and external.
   d. chest and pelvis.

2. When a patient has signs of hypovolemia and there are no external reasons, the paramedic should consider:
   a. esophageal varices.
   b. occult GI bleeding.
   c. dehydration.
   d. head trauma.

3. Bleeding described as spurting bright red is usually from a(n):
   a. vein.
   b. artery.
   c. capillary.
   d. vesicle.

4. An example of a closed soft tissue injury that may produce cardiac dysrhythmia is a(n):
   a. crushing injury.
   b. epidural hematoma.
   c. subdural hematoma.
   d. hematoma from a failed IV access attempt.

5. Two common examples of soft tissue trauma that may be fatal are hematomas and:
   a. secondary infections.
   b. abrasions.
   c. genital warts.
   d. insect bites.

6. Any physical activity that increases the exposure of the skin to the environment and _____ will increase the risk of a soft tissue injury.
   a. sea/saltwater
   b. physical forces
   c. bloodborne pathogens
   d. airborne pathogens

7. Which of the following is not a layer of the skin?
   a. cutaneous
   b. subcutaneous
   c. superficial lesion
   d. deep fascia

8. Which section of skin contains the stratum germinativum or basal layer?
   a. dermis
   b. epidermis
   c. subcutaneous lesion
   d. deep fascia

9. Fibroblasts, macrophages, and MAST cells are located in the:
   a. dermis.
   b. epidermis.
   c. superficial fascia.
   d. deep fascia.

10. The _____ is a thick, dense layer of fibrous tissue that provides support and protection for the underlying structures.
   a. dermis
   b. epidermis
   c. superficial fascia
   d. deep fascia

11. The skin follows the contours of the underlying structures, creating a natural stretch in the skin called:
   a. tension lines.
   b. stretch marks.
   c. relief stretch.
   d. strain outlines.

12. _____ is the phase of normal wound healing where clotting begins.
   a. Hemostasis
   b. Epithelialization
   c. Collagen synthesis
   d. Neurovascularization

13. The phase of normal healing that involves fibroblast-forming scar tissue that holds the wound edges together tightly is called:
    a. epithelialization.
    b. collagen synthesis.
    c. stretch marks.
    d. tension lines.

14. _____ is the phase of wound healing through reestablishment of skin layers in the first 12 hours.
    a. Epithelialization
    b. Collagen synthesis
    c. Inflammation
    d. Fibroblast formation

15. Normal wound healing can be altered by which of the following factors?
    a. skin temperature
    b. ambient temperature
    c. body region
    d. dry skin

16. Which of the following medications is known to interfere with the normal wound-healing process?
    a. nitrates
    b. laxatives
    c. corticosteroids
    d. anticonvulsants

17. Which of the following medical conditions does not typically affect normal wound healing?
    a. severe alcoholism
    b. diabetes
    c. acne
    d. cardiovascular disease

18. What types of wounds are considered high risk for healing problems and infections?
    a. slivers
    b. abrasions
    c. human bites
    d. insect stings or bites

19. Excessive accumulation of scar tissue that extends beyond the original wound borders is called a:
    a. keloid scar.
    b. stretch mark.
    c. suture over-healing.
    d. hypertrophic scar.

20. Plastic surgery is often requested for wound closures for the purpose of:
    a. minimizing the number of stitches used.
    b. cosmetically acceptable healing.
    c. closing gaps that are too large for sutures.
    d. closing gaps that are too small for sutures.

21. Which of the following soft tissue injuries often requires sutures?
    a. degloving
    b. abrasions
    c. ulcers
    d. abscesses

22. The most common and dangerous infectious disease that EMS providers are at risk for exposure to when treating patients with external bleeding is:
    a. AIDS
    b. hepatitis
    c. meningitis
    d. tuberculosis

23. In a(n) _____, the epidermis remains intact when cells are damaged and the blood vessels in the dermis are torn, causing swelling and pain. The pain can be delayed for up to 24–48 hours after the injury.
    a. contusion
    b. laceration
    c. abrasion
    d. ulcer

24. A(n) _____ is a break in the skin of varying depth usually caused by very sharp objects, such as a knife.
    a. abrasion
    b. laceration
    c. incision
    d. avulsion

25. A 19-year-old female has sustained an injury causing a flap of torn, loose tissue that may not be viable for reimplantation. This soft tissue injury is called a(n):
    a. abrasion.
    b. amputation.
    c. impalement.
    d. avulsion.

26. A 22-year-old male patient has sustained a jagged wound caused by forceful impact with a sharp object, which may cause the ends to bleed freely. This is called a(n):
    a. laceration.
    b. amputation.
    c. evisceration.
    d. puncture.

27. Which of the following is not a type of amputation?
    a. degloving injury
    b. ring injury
    c. complete
    d. partial

28. During which phase(s) of a blast injury would open soft tissue trauma most likely occur?

  a. primary and secondary

  b. primary and tertiary

  c. secondary only

  d. primary only

29. A(n) _____ injury is an injury from a compressive force sufficient to interfere with the normal metabolic function of the involved tissue.

  a. puncture

  b. crush

  c. impaled

  d. blast

30. Your patient has been pinned under a cement walkway for the past few hours. Rescue personnel are about to lift the weight off the patient. Field management for the patient with crush syndrome is focused on aggressive fluid therapy and the administration of:

  a. oxygen to restore hypoxic tissue.

  b. epinephrine to dilate the vessels.

  c. glucagon to metabolize stores of needed glucose.

  d. sodium bicarbonate to neutralize the buildup of acids.

31. While on vacation, a 20-year-old male broke his arm skiing and subsequently had a cast applied. The next day, the patient awoke to find his fingers swollen and cyanotic. What type of soft tissue injury is associated with an improperly applied cast and has likely occurred with this patient?

  a. puncture

  b. contusion

  c. hematoma

  d. crush injury

32. In a crush syndrome injury, after the initial damage to soft tissue, the cells in the crushed area become starved for oxygen and _____ occurs.

  a. compartment syndrome

  b. anaerobic metabolism

  c. unconsciousness

  d. respiratory acidosis

33. Your 35-year-old male patient was involved in a work-related accident that required extrication and disentanglement from machinery. He is alert and has a closed femur fracture. He is complaining of pain and paresthesia in the affected leg, and you cannot palpate a distal pulse. You suspect he is developing compartment syndrome in the thigh. Without proper intervention, how long does the patient have before cell death can occur?

  a. 90 minutes

  b. 2–4 hours

  c. 4–6 hours

  d. 6–8 hours

34. In the pathophysiology of compartment syndrome, the tissue pressure rises above the _____ pressure, resulting in ischemia to muscle.

  a. venous

  b. arterial

  c. osmotic

  d. capillary hydrostatic

35. The "Ps" of compartment syndrome include all of the following, except:

  a. palpation.

  b. pain.

  c. paresis.

  d. pulselessness.

36. Blast injuries can occur from any explosion, but they are often more serious when they occur:

  a. in a shopping mall.

  b. at a fire scene.

  c. inside a confined space.

  d. in a railroad yard.

37. Initial treatment priorities for soft tissue injuries caused by blasts include:

  a. observing for signs of compartment syndrome.

  b. flushing the patient of combustible materials.

  c. considering that both internal and external injuries are possible.

  d. copious amounts of fluid administration.

38. _____ is the quickest and most efficient means of bleeding control.

  a. Direct pressure

  b. Elevation

  c. Tourniquet application

  d. Pressure points

39. The purpose of controlling a hemorrhage by direct pressure is to limit additional significant blood loss and to:

  a. limit exposure to communicable disease.

  b. promote localized clotting.

  c. stop the arterial blood flow.

  d. avoid the use of indirect pressure.

40. Which of the following is incorrect about the use of pressure dressings?

  a. They provide a continuous mechanical pressure on the wound site.

  b. A circumferential bandage should not be used on the neck.

  c. The bandage should not occlude or impede venous blood flow.

  d. The bandage should not occlude or impede arterial blood flow.

40. In which of the following situations would the use of a pressure dressing be most appropriate?
    a. open wound on the neck
    b. open head wound over a skull depression
    c. pregnant trauma patient with an abdominal evisceration
    d. a wound in which applying a pressure point has not slowed the bleeding

41. Do not apply a tourniquet directly around a knee or elbow, as _____ in that area, and it will not adequately control the bleeding.
    a. serious nerve damage will result
    b. it may cut the skin or tissue
    c. there is too much bone
    d. there is no artery

42. Once a tourniquet is applied, the decision implies that you will:
    a. take if off once bleeding has been controlled.
    b. lose the limb to save the life.
    c. replace it with an air splint when one is available.
    d. loosen it when the patient experiences paresthesia.

43. The difference between a sterile and non-sterile dressing is that a sterile dressing has gone through:
    a. the process to eliminate bacteria from the dressing material.
    b. hermetically sealed packaging.
    c. special quality control regiments.
    d. a process to apply a residue to the gauze.

44. An occlusive dressing does not allow _____ through the dressing.
    a. passage of air
    b. passage of blood
    c. surfactant
    d. embolism to develop

45. The type of dressing that has been designed not to damage the surface of the wound when it is removed is a(n) _____ dressing.
    a. occlusive
    b. sterile
    c. non-sterile
    d. non-adherent

46. The type of dressing that is designed to stick onto a wound surface by incorporating wound exudates into the dressing mesh is called a(n) _____ dressing.
    a. occlusive
    b. adhesive
    c. improperly applied
    d. sterile wrap

47. A properly applied dressing may result in which of the following?
    a. increased tissue damage
    b. ineffective bleeding control
    c. unnecessary patient discomfort
    d. decreased risk of wound infection

48. You are at the residence of a patient who cut herself with a box cutter. The wound is deep in the palm, but you have controlled the bleeding with direct pressure and a pressure dressing. She is refusing transport because she does not have insurance. What can you say to the patient to help persuade her to receive further medical attention right away?
    a. Tell her that having medical insurance is not important.
    b. Explain that a tetanus shot and sutures are necessary.
    c. Explain that the bleeding may resume and become life threatening.
    d. Tell her that cosmetic surgery will be necessary because of the location of the injury.

49. (Continuing with question 48) Despite all of your efforts to convince the patient to go to the hospital, she still refuses. She says that she will go to her own physician later. What instructions can you give her to help minimize the risk of infection until she receives further medical attention?
    a. Change the dressing frequently.
    b. Take aspirin as needed for the pain.
    c. Do not allow the dressing to get wet.
    d. Clean the wound and apply a topical ointment.

50. How often is the immunization for tetanus recommended?
    a. every year
    b. every 5 years
    c. every 10 years
    d. every 12 years

51. The paramedic can minimize the risk of infection for a patient with an open wound by:
    a. covering the wound with a dry, sterile dressing.
    b. covering the wound with a wet, sterile dressing.
    c. cleansing and debriding the wound as needed.
    d. placing an occlusive dressing.

52. Considerations for the treatment of an amputated part include that the amputated part should:
    a. be wrapped in dry, sterile dressing.
    b. be wrapped in a sterile, moist gauze pad.
    c. be placed in a bag with ice.
    d. always be transported with the patient.

53. Hyperbaric oxygen treatment is sometimes recommended to prevent _____ and improve healing in crush injuries.
    a. respiratory acidosis
    b. pulmonary embolus
    c. gangrene
    d. deep vein thrombosis

54. After the ABCs, the most important treatment in the patient with a crush injury is:
    a. the observation of the presence of ECG changes or dysrhythmias.
    b. to administer 20% solution of mannitol.
    c. transport to a hyperbaric treatment facility.
    d. to administer IV fluid therapy using the Parkland formula.

55. The _____, also called the superficial fascia, contains loose connective tissue and fat that provides both insulation and protection from trauma.
    a. cutaneous layer
    b. subcutaneous layer
    c. basal layer
    d. reticular dermis

56. Approximately 80% of the fire- and burn-related deaths that occur in the United States are a result of a(n) _____ fire.
    a. house
    b. automobile
    c. camp
    d. brush

57. Burns are the leading cause of trauma in the _____ age group.
    a. newborn
    b. toddler and preschool
    c. teenage
    d. elderly

58. The elderly are in a high-risk group for burns primarily because of:
    a. forgetting to change batteries in smoke detectors.
    b. elder abuse.
    c. smoking in bed.
    d. impairment of mobility or sensation.

59. Prevention strategies to decrease the number of scalding injuries in children include all of the following, except:
    a. never drinking hot liquids while holding a child.
    b. cooking on backburners whenever possible.
    c. turning down the thermostat on the hot water heater to 120°.
    d. testing the water temperature of a bath before allowing the child to enter.

60. Which of the following is not a pathophysiologic or system complication of a burn injury?
    a. decreased catecholamine release
    b. fluid and electrolyte loss
    c. renal, liver, and heart failure
    d. hypothermia

61. A burn classified as _____ is one that extends to the fascia.
    a. superficial
    b. deep fascia
    c. full thickness
    d. partial thickness

62. Which of the following is not a classification of a burn injury?
    a. superficial
    b. deep fascia
    c. partial thickness
    d. full thickness

63. A _____-degree burn involves the outermost layer of skin, the epidermis, as well as the dermal layer.
    a. first
    b. second
    c. third
    d. fourth

64. The three classifications of burn severity do not include:
    a. minor.
    b. moderate.
    c. eschar.
    d. severe.

65. The "rule of nines" is a method of determining:
    a. body surface area burned.
    b. severity of burn.
    c. classification of burn.
    d. type and degree of burn.

66. Burns on the hands or feet, inhalation burns, and electrical burns are all examples of burn injuries that:
    a. are associated with shock from blood loss.
    b. require transport to the nearest hospital.
    c. require transport to a burn specialty center.
    d. do not have a good prognosis for full recovery.

67. Which of the following does not have a significant impact on the management and prognosis of the burn injured patient?
    a. the patient's age
    b. the patient's gender
    c. preexisiting medical problems
    d. associated trauma injury

68. Preexisting medical problems of (with) _____ can make it very difficult for the burn patient to handle the tremendous movement of body fluids that occurs with a burn injury.
    a. seizures
    b. allergies
    c. the kidneys
    d. hypertension

69. Using the pediatric "rule of nines," estimate the percentage of BSA for a scald burn involving both lower legs, up to the knees.
    a. 12%
    b. 18%
    c. 20%
    d. 24%

70. The phases of "burn" shock include all of the following, except the _____ phase.
    a. fluid shift
    b. compensation
    c. resolution
    d. hypermetabolic

71. During the body's initial response to a burn, there is a _____ in response to the pain from the burn.
    a. fluid shift
    b. release of catecholamines
    c. burst of energy
    d. decrease in cardiac output

72. During the _____ phase of a burn injury, there is a release of vasoactive substances from the burned tissues causing wound edema, fluid loss, and hypovolemia.
    a. emergent
    b. compensation
    c. fluid shift
    d. resolution

73. The _____ phase of burn shock usually occurs within 24 hours of the burn injury. In this phase, the scar tissue is laid down and healing occurs.
    a. emergent
    b. fluid shift
    c. resolution
    d. hypermetabolic

74. In 60–70% of all thermal burn patients who die, there is an associated inhalation injury when these patients either have cyanide intoxication or:
    a. carbon monoxide poisoning.
    b. asbestosis.
    c. nitrogen narcosis.
    d. thermal inhalation.

75. _____ is the thick and nonelastic scab or immediate scar that forms on the skin following a burn.
    a. Epithelialization
    b. Collagen synthesis
    c. Coagulation synthesis
    d. Eschar

76. When a circumferential scar forms around an extremity, _____ can be the resulting complication.
    a. circulatory compromise
    b. severe fluid loss
    c. rebound acidosis
    d. cosmetic uncertainty

77. When obtaining assessment findings of the patient with a thermal burn, which of the following is least significant?
    a. the specific MOI
    b. fluid replacement amounts
    c. preexisting medical conditions
    d. the classification and severity of the burn

78. After managing the ABCs on the patient with a thermal burn, which of the following is appropriate treatment?
    a. Maintain body heat.
    b. Apply topical analgesia.
    c. Remove the patient to a safe area.
    d. Stop the burning process.

79. The Parkland formula is used by many burn centers to _____ for the burn patient.
    a. measure scar formation
    b. determine fluid replacement
    c. determine the prognosis
    d. measure circulatory compromise

80. Which of the following factors can reduce the risk of inhalation injury for the victim involved in a house fire?
    a. screaming for help
    b. standing in a room with flames
    c. crawling on the floor in a room with flames
    d. being within an enclosed area involving a fire

81. Which of the following signs or conditions may indicate that a patient has an inhalation injury?
    a. hoarseness
    b. peripheral edema
    c. pain or paresthesia
    d. skin sloughing on the anterior chest

82. Regardless of the cause, _____ therapy for carbon monoxide inhalation is beneficial as it helps decrease the time it takes for the hemoglobin to become saturated with oxygen instead of CO.
    a. endotracheal intubation
    b. hyperbaric nitrogen
    c. hyperbaric oxygen
    d. positive pressure ventilation

83. Which of the following products will produce the most severe burn?
    a. cement
    b. hot tar
    c. hot grease
    d. pepper spray

84. When a patient has been burned with a dry powder, special considerations include:
    a. washing it off, then determining what it is.
    b. brushing it off and calling the poison control center for decon procedures.
    c. avoiding exposure to the chemical.
    d. waiting for the fire department to do the decon.

85. Which of the following is appropriate management of a chemical injury to the eye?
    a. Provide continuous irrigation.
    b. Cover the affected eye with a dressing.
    c. Allow the patient to rub his eyes to facilitate drainage.
    d. Never remove contact lenses.

86. The burning sensation of tear gas lasts for about _____ hour(s), where as pepper gas lasts about _____ hours.
    a. 1; 2
    b. 4; 2
    c. 5; 4
    d. 6; 4

87. To minimize the effects of tear gas or pepper spray, the paramedic can:
    a. get the patient to blow her nose and spit out any residue.
    b. instruct the patient to rub her eyes.
    c. use circular strokes to sponge off any residue.
    d. avoid using water to flush the skin.

88. When a patient with contact lenses has an eye injury or burn from a chemical agent, the paramedic should:
    a. use the Morgan lens® on the unaffected eye and allow it to drain into the affected eye.
    b. remove the lenses with a gloved hand or assist the patient in doing so.
    c. place the Morgan lens® over the contact and irrigate with normal saline.
    d. never use a Morgan lens® on an eye injury caused by a chemical burn.

89. Select the statement that is most accurate about the severity of electrical burns.
    a. The entrance wound will always be more critical than the exit wound.
    b. The exit wound will always be more critical than the entrance wound.
    c. An electric burn that causes internal injury may eventually cause cancer.
    d. The path of electricity through the body may cause serious complications.

90. In the United States, about _____ people die from electrical shock each year.
    a. 100
    b. 1,000
    c. 10,000
    d. 100,000

91. The very first action to take when responding to a call for an electrocution is to:
    a. determine if there were any witnesses to the electrocution.
    b. determine if the unresponsive patient is in ventricular fibrillation.
    c. identify the source of the electricity prior to approaching the patient.
    d. wait for the fire department or power company to determine if the scene is safe to enter.

92. Direct current (DC), which has zero frequency but may be intermittent or pulsating, is:
    a. more dangerous than alternating current (AC).
    b. less dangerous than AC.
    c. the cause of circumferential burns more often than AC.
    d. the cause of circumferential burns less often than AC.

93. Alternating current at _____ Hz, which is household current, produces muscle tetany and tends to "freeze" the patient to the current source.
    a. 20
    b. 40
    c. 60
    d. 120

94. _____ is a lifesaving or limb-saving procedure used to allow expansion of the chest or restore circulation to an extremity in which the scar has formed a tight circumferential band.
    a. Circumcision
    b. Escharotomy
    c. Mesopexy
    d. Lyophilization

95. Which of the following skin conditions has the least resistance to electrical voltage?

    a. dry, intact skin
    b. wet, intact skin
    c. a thickly calloused palm or sole
    d. moist mucous membrane (mouth)

96 When assessing the victim of an electrical burn, the paramedic should look for an entry and exit point of the current, because:

    a. anything in the path is "fair game" for injury.
    b. both sites are always easy to find.
    c. the exit wound will indicate how much internal damage is present.
    d. the entry wound will indicate how much internal damage is present.

97. Which of the following signs or symptoms is not commonly found in a person who has sustained an electrical burn?

    a. trauma from falling
    b. hearing impairment or vision loss
    c. malocclusion
    d. muscle contractions or pain

98. Your patient is a 40-year-old male who was taken to the first-aid room by his coworkers after he suffered an accidental exposure to superheated gases. He is alert and shows signs of respiratory distress. He is wheezing, complains of difficulty swallowing, and is cyanotic. You suspect that his upper airway is swelling. What can you do to keep his airway from swelling any further?

    a. There is nothing you can do.
    b. Administer humidified oxygen.
    c. Endotracheally intubate the patient.
    d. Administer high-concentration oxygen.

99. Which of the following electrical burns is least likely to produce both an entry and exit wound?

    a. lightning strike
    b. arc injury
    c. direct contact with an electrical source
    d. indirect contact with an electrical source

100. All of the following statements about the management of the patient with an electrical injury are correct, except:

    a. do not touch the patient until you are sure that the power is turned off.
    b. treatment of an electric injury is the same as for a thermal injury.
    c. the potential for internal injury is less than a thermal injury.
    d. monitor the patient's ECG to identify hyperkalemia and cell death.

101. The most common entry point for an electrical burn is the:

    a. head.
    b. heart.
    c. hands.
    d. feet.

102. Which of the following is not a common physiologic dysfunction associated with electrical burns?

    a. involuntary muscular contractions
    b. singed nasal hairs
    c. seizures
    d. respiratory arrest

103. The _____ is(are) the most common exit point for an electrical burn.

    a. head
    b. eyes
    c. rectum
    d. feet

104. Ionizing radiation produces immediate chemical effects, known as _____, on human tissue.

    a. ionization
    b. particle density
    c. radionization
    d. micronization

105. In which of the following circumstances should the paramedic suspect that a burn injury is a possible result of child abuse?

    a. when the history is inconsistent with the injuries
    b. when the burns are located on the front of the body
    c. when the burns are located on the back of the body
    d. when the body surface area of the burn is more than 30%

Exam #36 Answer Form

	A	B	C	D		A	B	C	D
1.	❏	❏	❏	❏	34.	❏	❏	❏	❏
2.	❏	❏	❏	❏	35.	❏	❏	❏	❏
3.	❏	❏	❏	❏	36.	❏	❏	❏	❏
4.	❏	❏	❏	❏	37.	❏	❏	❏	❏
5.	❏	❏	❏	❏	38.	❏	❏	❏	❏
6.	❏	❏	❏	❏	39.	❏	❏	❏	❏
7.	❏	❏	❏	❏	40.	❏	❏	❏	❏
8.	❏	❏	❏	❏	41.	❏	❏	❏	❏
9.	❏	❏	❏	❏	42.	❏	❏	❏	❏
10.	❏	❏	❏	❏	43.	❏	❏	❏	❏
11.	❏	❏	❏	❏	44.	❏	❏	❏	❏
12.	❏	❏	❏	❏	45.	❏	❏	❏	❏
13.	❏	❏	❏	❏	46.	❏	❏	❏	❏
14.	❏	❏	❏	❏	47.	❏	❏	❏	❏
15.	❏	❏	❏	❏	48.	❏	❏	❏	❏
16.	❏	❏	❏	❏	49.	❏	❏	❏	❏
17.	❏	❏	❏	❏	50.	❏	❏	❏	❏
18.	❏	❏	❏	❏	51.	❏	❏	❏	❏
19.	❏	❏	❏	❏	52.	❏	❏	❏	❏
20.	❏	❏	❏	❏	53.	❏	❏	❏	❏
21.	❏	❏	❏	❏	54.	❏	❏	❏	❏
22.	❏	❏	❏	❏	55.	❏	❏	❏	❏
23.	❏	❏	❏	❏	56.	❏	❏	❏	❏
24.	❏	❏	❏	❏	57.	❏	❏	❏	❏
25.	❏	❏	❏	❏	58.	❏	❏	❏	❏
26.	❏	❏	❏	❏	59.	❏	❏	❏	❏
27.	❏	❏	❏	❏	60.	❏	❏	❏	❏
28.	❏	❏	❏	❏	61.	❏	❏	❏	❏
29.	❏	❏	❏	❏	62.	❏	❏	❏	❏
30.	❏	❏	❏	❏	63.	❏	❏	❏	❏
31.	❏	❏	❏	❏	64.	❏	❏	❏	❏
32.	❏	❏	❏	❏	65.	❏	❏	❏	❏
33.	❏	❏	❏	❏	66.	❏	❏	❏	❏

Exam #36 Answer Form

	A	B	C	D			A	B	C	D
67.	❏	❏	❏	❏		87.	❏	❏	❏	❏
68.	❏	❏	❏	❏		88.	❏	❏	❏	❏
69.	❏	❏	❏	❏		89.	❏	❏	❏	❏
70.	❏	❏	❏	❏		90.	❏	❏	❏	❏
71.	❏	❏	❏	❏		91.	❏	❏	❏	❏
72.	❏	❏	❏	❏		92.	❏	❏	❏	❏
73.	❏	❏	❏	❏		93.	❏	❏	❏	❏
74.	❏	❏	❏	❏		94.	❏	❏	❏	❏
75.	❏	❏	❏	❏		95.	❏	❏	❏	❏
76.	❏	❏	❏	❏		96.	❏	❏	❏	❏
77.	❏	❏	❏	❏		97.	❏	❏	❏	❏
78.	❏	❏	❏	❏		98.	❏	❏	❏	❏
79.	❏	❏	❏	❏		99.	❏	❏	❏	❏
80.	❏	❏	❏	❏		100.	❏	❏	❏	❏
81.	❏	❏	❏	❏		101.	❏	❏	❏	❏
82.	❏	❏	❏	❏		102.	❏	❏	❏	❏
83.	❏	❏	❏	❏		103.	❏	❏	❏	❏
84.	❏	❏	❏	❏		104.	❏	❏	❏	❏
85.	❏	❏	❏	❏		105.	❏	❏	❏	❏
86.	❏	❏	❏	❏						

Chest Trauma

1. Chest injuries are the _____ leading cause of trauma deaths each year in the United States.
    a. primary
    b. second
    c. third
    d. fifth

2. Thoracic trauma can impair ventilation in many ways, such as:
    a. collapsing of alveoli.
    b. bruising of lung tissue.
    c. laceration of the trachea.
    d. disruption of the bellows' action.

3. The major problem with the injury to the mediastinum is:
    a. tearing of a great vessel.
    b. contusion of the heart.
    c. esophageal spasm.
    d. aortic seizure.

4. An esophageal injury such as a _____ may occur to the esophagus when the throat or upper chest is perforated.
    a. spasm
    b. tear
    c. flare-up
    d. fracture

5. When an explosion occurs within a confined space, the pressure injures the lung tissue, causing:
    a. necrosis.
    b. petechial impressions.
    c. massive lung contusions.
    d. tears.

6. The presence of subcutaneous emphysema on the closed anterior chest of a patient, as a result of a significant MOI, is suggestive of what type of internal injury?
    a. aortic rupture
    b. ruptured diaphragm
    c. perforated lung tissue
    d. perforated esophagus

7. Which of the following is not a muscle of the thorax?
    a. external intercostals
    b. mesotendons
    c. internal intercostals
    d. trapezius

8. _____ is a major muscle that moves the head and is also an accessory muscle of breathing, as it helps to lift the chest cage.
    a. Sternocleidomastoid
    b. Rhomboid
    c. Pectoralis major
    d. Latissimus dorsi

9. The muscle that originates in the occipital bone and inserts into the clavicle, with its function being to raise and lower the shoulders, is called the:
    a. rhomboid.
    b. trapezius.
    c. external costals.
    d. sternocleidomastoid.

10. The trachea extends from the anterior throat into the chest cavity and then bifurcates at the carina into the:
    a. parenchyma.
    b. anterior rhomboid major.
    c. distal rhomboid minor.
    d. mainstem bronchi.

11. _____ is the lung tissue itself rather than all the supporting connective tissues.
    a. Parenchyma
    b. Bronchi
    c. Alveoli
    d. Pleura

12. The _____ returns blood to the right atrium of the heart.
    a. aorta
    b. internal mammary artery
    c. carotid artery
    d. inferior vena cava

13. Which of the following is not a major vein of the chest?
    a. aorta
    b. internal jugular
    c. external jugular
    d. subclavian

14. The _____ is(are) located in the mediastinum, or center of the chest.
    a. diaphragm
    b. trachea
    c. abdominal aorta
    d. lungs

15. Police are on scene with a male in his 20s who has been stabbed in the chest. He is conscious, complaining of difficulty breathing, and is bleeding from the anterior chest under the right clavicle. The breath sounds are diminished on the left and absent on the right. At this point, you suspect the patient has a:
    a. ruptured aorta.
    b. simple pneumothorax.
    c. tension pneumothorax.
    d. pulmonary contusion.

16. (Continuing with the previous question) You learn that the patient was stabbed 10 minutes prior to you arriving at the scene. The patient's vital signs are respiratory rate 28 and labored, pulse rate 132 and regular, and BP is 118/98 mm Hg. What additional assessment finding would help you confirm your suspicion about the patient's condition?
    a. SpO_2 reading
    b. absence or presence of dysrythmias
    c. absence or presence of hyperresonance
    d. absence or presence of a flail segment

17. Any injury that affects the diaphragm, intercostal muscles, or _____ can severely affect the mechanics of ventilation.
    a. vagus nerve
    b. accessory muscles
    c. aortic arch
    d. sacral spine

18. Chemoreceptors, located in the aortic arch and _____, measure carbon dioxide levels in the blood.
    a. capillary beds
    b. carotid sinus
    c. parenchyma
    d. alveoli

19. Impairment of gas exchange as a result of chest trauma occurs in which of the following mechanisms?
    a. contusions on the lung tissue
    b. disruption of the bellows action
    c. ineffective diaphragmatic contraction
    d. disassociation of the alveoli from the parenchyma

20. _____ is sudden cardiac arrest with ventricular fibrillation triggered by a non-penetrating blow to the chest.
    a. Myocardial contusion
    b. Commodio cordis
    c. Brugada syndrome
    d. Long QT syndrome

21. Fractures of the left-lower ribs are often associated with:
    a. splenic rupture.
    b. pneumothorax.
    c. renal contusions.
    d. perforated bowels.

22. When managing a patient with suspected rib fractures, it is important to encourage the patient to cough and take frequent deep breaths in order to:
    a. expand all of the air sacs.
    b. assess the effectiveness of the splint.
    c. fully evaluate the patient's level of discomfort.
    d. prevent the patient from developing hypotension.

23. Ribs _____ are most often fractured because they are thin and poorly protected.
    a. one to three
    b. four to nine
    c. eight to twelve
    d. ten to twelve

24. Fractures of the first and second ribs indicate _____ and may also involve a rupture of the aorta, tracheobronchial tree injury, or a vascular injury.
    a. mild trauma
    b. moderate trauma
    c. severe trauma
    d. spinal cord injury

25. A flail segment is a very serious chest injury and has mortality rates of _____% because of the associated injuries and impact on ventilations.
    a. 5–10
    b. 10–20
    c. 20–40
    d. 40–50

26. Which of the following statements about the pathology of a flail segment is incorrect?
    a. If the flail segment is small, the paradoxical movement is minimal because of muscle spasm.
    b. Pain is a contributing factor to the severity of this injury.
    c. Pain can reduce thoracic expansion and decrease ventilation.
    d. The arterial blood flow is impaired, resulting in a ventilation–perfusion mismatch.

27. Which of the following is the most common associated complication of a flail segment?
    a. pulmonary contusion
    b. subcutaneous emphysema
    c. pericardial effusion
    d. pulmonary edema

28. The most common cause of a sternal fracture is a(n) _____ injury caused by an MVC.
    a. penetrating
    b. dislocation
    c. acceleration
    d. deceleration compression

29. The main reason why a sternal fracture has such a high mortality rate is:
    a. the high incidence of vomiting.
    b. that nearly all of these patients lose consciousness.
    c. the associated injuries.
    d. that these patients are often given too much fluid prehospitally.

30. When assessing the patient with a simple pneumothorax, the patient may have decreased chest wall movement and slight pleuritic chest pain, which may be referred to the:
    a. shoulder or arm on the unaffected side.
    b. shoulder or arm on the affected side.
    c. abdomen and upper thighs.
    d. neck.

31. A patient with an open pneumothorax can develop a ventilation–perfusion mismatch as a result of:
    a. spinal shock.
    b. hyperventilation.
    c. hypoventilation.
    d. subcutaneous emphysema.

32. When dealing with a developing open pneumothorax, if the resistance to air flow through the respiratory tract is greater than resistance through the open hole, the:
    a. respiratory effort is effective.
    b. respiratory effort is ineffective.
    c. one-way flap will develop over the opening.
    d. mediastinum will move in the direction of the injured lung.

33. The pathophysiology of a tension pneumothorax includes:
    a. lung collapse with mediastinal shift to the injured side.
    b. fluid backup in the unaffected lung as a result of shunting.
    c. collapse of the lung and causes left-to-right intra-pulmonary shunting and hypercarbia.
    d. a serious reduction in cardiac output caused by deformation of the vena cava, reducing preload.

34. Which of the following assessment findings will most likely be atypical in a patient with a tension pneumothorax?
    a. unilateral decreased or absent breath sounds
    b. hyporesonance and mediastinal shift to the ipsi-lateral side
    c. tachypnea, cyanosis, and extreme anxiety
    d. narrow pulse pressure and JVD

35. Following a traumatic injury to the chest, an intercostal artery could bleed as much as _____ cc per minute.
    a. 10
    b. 20
    c. 40
    d. 50

36. Bleeding from a pulmonary contusion generally causes 1,000–1,500 cc of blood loss, although the chest cavity can hold some _____ cc of blood.
    a. 2,000–3,000
    b. 3,000–4,000
    c. 4,000–5,000
    d. 5,000–6,000

37. Intrapulmonary hemorrhage occurs in either the bronchus or the:
    a. alveoli.
    b. aorta.
    c. parenchyma.
    d. pleural space.

38. When evaluating the patient with a developing hemothorax, you can expect to find the signs and symptoms of shock as well as:
    a. subcutaneous emphysema.
    b. respiratory distress.
    c. hyperresonance.
    d. spinal cord injury.

39. The out-of-hospital management of a hemopneumothorax includes:
    a. the use of vasopressors.
    b. positive pressure ventilation.
    c. aggressive fluid replacement.
    d. aggressive fluid evacuation by chest decompression.

40. Pulmonary contusions are very common with blunt thoracic trauma, but are often missed on evaluation because:

   a. the patient has normal vital signs.

   b. there is no change in the skin color.

   c. associated injuries are more dramatic.

   d. of failure to fully expose the patient's torso.

41. Which of the following assessment findings is atypical of a patient who has a lung contusion?

   a. decreased SpO_2

   b. tachypnea and dyspnea

   c. coughing and hemoptysis

   d. cyanosis to the face and neck

42. Patients with pulmonary contusions tend to have other severe thoracic and _____ injuries, so always assume multiple potential injuries are present.

   a. head

   b. neck

   c. spinal cord

   d. abdominal

43. The purpose of the pericardium is to anchor the heart and restrict excess movement, as well as:

   a. prevent the kinking of the great vessels.

   b. facilitate right-to-left pulmonary shunting.

   c. link the lymphatic system.

   d. conduct electrical impulses.

44. The major problem in pericardial tamponade is the impairment of _____ , which significantly decreases the amount of blood the heart is able to pump out.

   a. pulmonic systolic filling

   b. ventricular diastolic filling

   c. pulmonic diastolic emptying

   d. ventricular diastolic emptying

45. You suspect that a patient is in cardiac tamponade, but there is too much ambient noise to hear the classic "muffled heart sounds" that you are supposed to listen for. Instead, you look for other clues, such as:

   a. a cough and hemoptysis.

   b. subcutaneous emphysema.

   c. JVD and narrow pulse pressure.

   d. retrosternal and interscapular pain.

46. A victim of an assault states that he was struck in the chest with a pipe. Your physical exam reveals sternal crepitus, and crepitus over the left fifth and -sixth ribs and the sternum. His lung sounds are clear, but he is guarded and says it hurts to take a breath. His pulse rate is 118/regular, BP is 134/80 mm Hg, and skin CTC is pale, warm, and dry, with no JVD. In addition to the fractures, what internal injury is the patient likely to have?

   a. aortic dissection

   b. myocardial contusion

   c. tension pneumothorax

   d. pericardial tamponade

47. Many patients with myocardial contusion are relatively asymptomatic initially in the absence of associated injuries. Helpful signs include ECG changes, if present, and persistent:

   a. sinus tachycardia without obvious hypovolemia.

   b. right bundle branch block.

   c. narrow pulse pressure.

   d. widened pulse pressure.

48. You are treating the driver of a vehicle involved in a high-speed crash. The patient struck his chest on the steering wheel. He is alert and complains of dyspnea, chest pain, and tenderness, which increases when taking a deep breath. Vital signs are respiratory rate 22, pulse rate 118/irregular, and BP 136/90 mm Hg. His ECG is sinus tachycardia with PVCs. In addition to high-flow oxygen and starting an IV, what treatment is appropriate for this patient?

   a. administration of 2-liter fluid bolus

   b. rapid transport and observation of the patient

   c. rapid sequence intubation and pain management

   d. pain management and considering of antidysrhythmics

49. The management of a trauma patient with a myocardial rupture includes supportive care of the ABCs and observing for:

   a. respiratory alkalosis.

   b. abdominal distention.

   c. CHF or pulmonary edema.

   d. neurologic deficits.

50. The primary causes of aortic dissection/rupture are MVCs and:

   a. GSWs.

   b. falls.

   c. rib fractures.

   d. associated diaphragmatic rupture.

51. Aortic dissection/rupture is a very critical injury where _____% of the patients die instantaneously.
    a. 10–20
    b. 40–60
    c. 60–80
    d. 85–95

52. When examining a patient who has a complaint of chest pain with an acute and intense onset of pain, what other sign or symptom would make you suspect the patient is having an aortic dissection/rupture rather than an MI?
    a. The patient has a history of angina and takes nitro.
    b. The patient described the pain as a "tearing" sensation.
    c. The patient has no history of hypertension but feels dizzy.
    d. The patient states the pain can also be felt in the abdomen.

53. Which of the following treatment options should be avoided in the patient with a suspected ruptured diaphragm who is experiencing respiratory distress?
    a. IV fluids
    b. antiemetics
    c. Trendelenburg position
    d. positive pressure ventilation

54. Upon examination of the patient with an esophageal injury, the paramedic may find that the patient is having symptoms and signs of a:
    a. cardiac event.
    b. CVA.
    c. seizure.
    d. tension pneumothorax.

55. Traumatic asphyxia is produced by a sudden increase in venous pressure from direct pressure on the:
    a. head.
    b. pelvis.
    c. chest.
    d. vagus nerve.

56. The management of the patient with traumatic asphyxia includes:
    a. IV fluids for hypotension.
    b. needle decompression prior to the release of compression.
    c. needle decompression after the release of compression.
    d. MAST/PASG.

57. Tracheobronchial injury is rare and occurs in:
    a. blunt chest trauma.
    b. penetrating chest trauma.
    c. both blunt and penetrating chest trauma.
    d. high incidents in COPD patients.

58. Which of the following is an atypical assessment finding in a patient with a tracheobronchial injury?
    a. the patient is difficult to intubate
    b. signs of tension pneumothorax that do not respond to needle decompression
    c. dyspnea and hemoptysis
    d. tachy-brady dysrhythmias

59. The most frequent cause of an esophageal injury is from:
    a. a Mallory-Weiss tear.
    b. blunt trauma.
    c. penetrating trauma.
    d. acceleration forces.

60. You are assessing a 33-year-old female who was the driver of a vehicle involved in a moderate-speed rear-end MVC. She is complaining of increased difficulty breathing, and pain in the lower chest and upper abdomen. She has the presence of a scaffold abdomen, there are bowel sounds in the lower-right chest, and the area is dull to percussion. You suspect:
    a. diaphragmatic injury.
    b. tension pneumothorax.
    c. ectopic pregnancy.
    d. aortic dissection.

Exam #37 Answer Form

	A	B	C	D			A	B	C	D
1.	❏	❏	❏	❏		31.	❏	❏	❏	❏
2.	❏	❏	❏	❏		32.	❏	❏	❏	❏
3.	❏	❏	❏	❏		33.	❏	❏	❏	❏
4.	❏	❏	❏	❏		34.	❏	❏	❏	❏
5.	❏	❏	❏	❏		35.	❏	❏	❏	❏
6.	❏	❏	❏	❏		36.	❏	❏	❏	❏
7.	❏	❏	❏	❏		37.	❏	❏	❏	❏
8.	❏	❏	❏	❏		38.	❏	❏	❏	❏
9.	❏	❏	❏	❏		39.	❏	❏	❏	❏
10.	❏	❏	❏	❏		40.	❏	❏	❏	❏
11.	❏	❏	❏	❏		41.	❏	❏	❏	❏
12.	❏	❏	❏	❏		42.	❏	❏	❏	❏
13.	❏	❏	❏	❏		43.	❏	❏	❏	❏
14.	❏	❏	❏	❏		44.	❏	❏	❏	❏
15.	❏	❏	❏	❏		45.	❏	❏	❏	❏
16.	❏	❏	❏	❏		46.	❏	❏	❏	❏
17.	❏	❏	❏	❏		47.	❏	❏	❏	❏
18.	❏	❏	❏	❏		48.	❏	❏	❏	❏
19.	❏	❏	❏	❏		49.	❏	❏	❏	❏
20.	❏	❏	❏	❏		50.	❏	❏	❏	❏
21.	❏	❏	❏	❏		51.	❏	❏	❏	❏
22.	❏	❏	❏	❏		52.	❏	❏	❏	❏
23.	❏	❏	❏	❏		53.	❏	❏	❏	❏
24.	❏	❏	❏	❏		54.	❏	❏	❏	❏
25.	❏	❏	❏	❏		55.	❏	❏	❏	❏
26.	❏	❏	❏	❏		56.	❏	❏	❏	❏
27.	❏	❏	❏	❏		57.	❏	❏	❏	❏
28.	❏	❏	❏	❏		58.	❏	❏	❏	❏
29.	❏	❏	❏	❏		59.	❏	❏	❏	❏
30.	❏	❏	❏	❏		60.	❏	❏	❏	❏

Nervous System and Head, Facial, Neck, and Spine Trauma

1. The primary problem for paramedics managing a patient with blunt force trauma to the face or head is:
   a. spinal shock.
   b. blowout fractures.
   c. airway compromise.
   d. traumatic brain injury (TBI).

2. Common MOIs for penetrating injuries to the face or head include:
   a. MVCs.
   b. sticks or clubs.
   c. body-to-body contact.
   d. GSWs.

3. A patient who has suffered blunt force trauma to the face and head is most likely to have which of the following associated injuries?
   a. blindness
   b. hearing loss
   c. hoarseness
   d. cervical spine injury

4. Injuries to the throat can be fatal when:
   a. the patient has a very short neck.
   b. the patient is very young or elderly.
   c. there is an associated cervical spine injury.
   d. there is an associated injury to the major blood vessels.

5. A _____ is a hemorrhage in the anterior chamber of the eye.
   a. conjunctival hemorrhage
   b. detached retina
   c. blowout fracture
   d. hyphema

6. When traumatic pressure is transmitted through the eyeball to the relatively thin bone in the medial and inferior portions of the orbit, causing it to break, this is called a:
   a. posterior chamber divide.
   b. detached retina.
   c. blowout fracture.
   d. hyphema.

7. Isolated injuries to the mouth, such as from a _____, are very common, accounting for as much as 50% of facial trauma.
   a. punch
   b. MVC
   c. penetrating trauma
   d. fishhook

8. The LeFort classification categorizes facial fractures into three types. The higher the number, the more significant the damage, and the more potential there is for a:
   a. complicated airway.
   b. brain injury.
   c. spinal cord injury.
   d. vision disturbance.

9. LeFort fractures are based on:
   a. clinical impression.
   b. history of MOI.
   c. X-ray or CT scan findings.
   d. a combination of all of these.

10. The critical structures in the neck include all of the following, except:
    a. larynx and trachea.
    b. carotid arteries.
    c. vertebral arteries.
    d. cranial nerves one to five.

11. The _____ ear canal is considered a mucous membrane that secretes wax for protection.
    a. pinna
    b. outer
    c. external
    d. inner

12. The middle ear is separated from the external canal by the:
    a. pinna.
    b. eardrum.
    c. cartilage.
    d. inner ear.

13. Light receptors to color vision, which are located in the posterior chamber of the eye, are called:
    a. optic nerves.
    b. retinas.
    c. rods.
    d. cones.

14. The _____ is the transparent covering of the iris and pupil, which admits light into the eye.
    a. conjunctiva
    b. lens
    c. sclera
    d. cornea

15. _____ provide(s) protection for the eye and help(s) to lubricate the surface.
    a. Lens
    b. Eyelids
    c. Lacrimal apparatus
    d. Conjunctiva

16. The _____ are responsible for peripheral vision and low-light, night sight conditions.
    a. pupils
    b. rods
    c. cones
    d. retinas

17. Which of the following is not a major muscle of the mouth?
    a. hypoglossal
    b. tongue
    c. orbicular oris
    d. masseter muscle

18. The bones of the mouth include the palate, jawbone, and:
    a. hyoid.
    b. teeth.
    c. zygomatic.
    d. mastoid process.

19. When the paramedic examines the patient's face and the jaws, and notes that the teeth do not meet as they should, this is called:
    a. diplopia.
    b. malocclusion.
    c. a depressed zygoma.
    d. tetany.

20. When a patient has sustained an eye injury, often the recommendation is to cover both eyes to limit or prevent:
    a. the onset of dysconjugate gaze in the unaffected eye.
    b. the onset of dysconjugate gaze in the affected eye.
    c. movement from conjugate gaze of the uninjured eye.
    d. movement from conjugate gaze of the injured eye.

21. In the United States, approximately four _____ people sustain a head injury each year.
    a. out of a thousand
    b. thousand
    c. million
    d. billion

22. The highest risk of head injury occurs in _____ between _____ years of age.
    a. males; 2 and 12
    b. males; 15 and 24
    c. females; 15 and 24
    d. females; 65 and 85

23. The most common cause of head trauma and subdural hematoma is:
    a. MVC.
    b. falls in the elderly.
    c. sports.
    d. falls in the presence of alcohol abuse.

24. The scalp has an important freely moveable sheet of connective tissue called the _____ that helps to deflect blows.
    a. parietal fold
    b. mastoid sheath
    c. emissary
    d. galea

25. The actual bones that comprise the skull are double-layered with a spongy middle layer, allowing them to:
    a. facilitate drainage in the event of a hemorrhage.
    b. aerate the meninges.
    c. be strong yet light in weight.
    d. recycle cerebrospinal fluid.

26. Trauma to the _____ may cause disruption of the voluntary skeletal movement and may result in extremity paralysis, paresthesia, or weakness.
    a. medulla
    b. cerebrum
    c. brain stem
    d. occiput

27. When a person is struck in the _____ lobe, it may cause the patient to see "stars," have blurred vision, or experience other visual disturbances.
    a. temporal
    b. parietal
    c. occipital
    d. frontal

28. The cranial nerves (CN) that can be affected in head injury are the oculomotor nerve CN _____ and the vagus nerve CN _____.
    a. II; X
    b. III; V
    c. III; X
    d. IV; XII

29. The _____ controls the degree of activity of the central nervous system (e.g., maintaining sleep and wakefulness).
    a. vagus nerve
    b. hypothalamus
    c. foramen magnum
    d. reticular activating system

30. The arachnoid membrane, which appears to look like a web of blood vessels, is actually composed of:
    a. venous blood vessels that reabsorb CSF.
    b. venous blood vessels that drain the cerebral sinuses.
    c. arteries that stimulate cerebral function.
    d. arteries that manufacture CSF.

31. The brain has a very high metabolic rate and consumes _____% of the body's oxygen supply.
    a. 5
    b. 10
    c. 20
    d. 50

32. A mechanism called _____ is responsible for regulating the body's blood pressure to maintain the cerebral perfusion pressure (CPP).
    a. intercerebral pressure
    b. intracerebral pressure
    c. autoregulation
    d. mean arterial force

33. A 20-year-old male fell off a ladder at work. He landed on his back, struck his head, and experienced a brief loss of consciousness. Upon awakening, he is confused and does not remember how he fell. He remains conscious for the entire time you are attending to him. What type of head injury has this patient experienced?
    a. coup
    b. contra coup
    c. linear skull fracture
    d. basilar skull fracture

34. (Continuing with question 33) What type of brain injury has the patient most likely experienced?
    a. contusion
    b. concussion
    c. epidural hematoma
    d. subarachnoid hematoma

35. Cerebral contusion, intracranial hemorrhage, and epidural hematoma are all examples of _____ brain injuries.
    a. peripheral
    b. focal
    c. subarachnoid
    d. diffuse axonal

36. _____ is the effect of acceleration or deceleration on the brain.
    a. Coup
    b. Contra coup
    c. Focal
    d. Diffuse axonal injury

37. A(n) _____ is a mild diffuse axonal injury, which results in a transient episode of neuronal dysfunction with rapid return to normal neurologic activity.
    a. subarachnoid injury
    b. concussion
    c. epidural hematoma
    d. contusion

38. Which of the following is not a type of skull fracture that can be determined by an X-ray?
    a. linear
    b. depressed
    c. Battle's sign
    d. basilar

39. The most common type of skull fracture, which may or may not result in leaking of CSF, is a _____ fracture.
    a. linear
    b. depressed
    c. basilar
    d. penetrating

40. _____ hematomas are bleeds that are more common in elderly and alcoholic patients who fall down and hit their heads often.
    a. Acute subdural
    b. Chronic subdural
    c. Acute epidural
    d. Chronic epidural

41. When intracranial pressure (ICP) in the brain rises due to a hemorrhage, it can cause the brain to shift downward, resulting in any of the following assessment findings, except:
    a. vomiting.
    b. tachycardia.
    c. irregular respirations.
    d. unequal or nonreactive pupils.

42. The "Cushing" response in brain herniation with hypotension and bradycardia is a late response and usually precedes death by only _____ minutes.
    a. 4–6
    b. 10
    c. 15
    d. 20

43. Which of the following assessment findings will initially be present when a patient experiences a loss of cerebral autoregulation?
    a. seizures
    b. Cushing's reflex
    c. a drop in blood pressure
    d. elevated blood pressure

44. You are transporting an unconscious patient with a massive head injury as a result of a serious MVC. You have intubated her and have two IVs in place. The patient's initial GCS was 6, and her vital signs were: respiratory 16/irregular; pulse 50/regular; and BP 170/100 mm Hg. Her pupils are still reactive, and she withdraws with flexion to pain stimuli. What part of the brain is the increasing ICP impacting at this point?
    a. lower brain stem
    b. middle brain stem
    c. upper brain stem
    d. cerebral cortex and upper brain stem

45. Which of the following statements is incorrect regarding the impact of increasing ICP on the lower brain stem or medulla?
    a. Vegetative functions are temporarily impaired because of the pressure.
    b. The patient's injury is not considered survivable.
    c. The respirations are ataxic or absent.
    d. The ECG will have QRS, ST segment, and T wave changes.

46. With GCS being an objective measure of eye opening, verbal response, and motor response in a numerical score, a moderate head injury would be:
    a. 13–15.
    b. 8–12.
    c. 5–8.
    d. < 8.

47. Intracranial bleeding from a(n) _____ hematoma results in the presence of blood in the CSF.
    a. epidural
    b. subdural
    c. subarachnoid
    d. intracerebral

48. When assessing a patient's head for possible depressed and open skull fractures, the paramedic should be careful to use the _____ to palpate and not "poke" into the fracture site.
    a. pads of the fingers
    b. flat side of a tongue depressor
    c. stethoscope with a sterile gauze
    d. palm of the hand

49. Which of the following signs and symptoms are atypical for a patient with an expanding intracranial hematoma?
    a. nausea and vomiting
    b. changes in mental status
    c. tachycardia and tachypnea
    d. headache with increasing severity

50. You are interviewing a medical patient who had a seizure. When you inquire about his past medical history, he tells you that 2 years ago he suffered a traumatic brain injury. As a result of the injury, he experienced changes in his personality as well as seizures. What part of his brain did he injure?
    a. frontal lobe
    b. parietal lobe
    c. occipital lobe
    d. temporal lobe

51. The appropriate management of a head injury by the paramedic includes all of the following, except:
    a. assuring an adequate airway, ventilation, and oxygenation.
    b. aggressive hyperventilation.
    c. assuring adequate circulation.
    d. conducting serial neurologic assessments.

52. If hypotension develops in the patient with a head injury, it is most likely caused by bleeding from:
    a. another organ or injuries besides the brain.
    b. the middle meningeal artery.
    c. a subarachnoid hemorrhage.
    d. the circle of Willis.

53. Studies have shown that _____ improves outcomes in combative head trauma patients.
    a. the use of steroids
    b. osmotic diuretic given in the field
    c. aggressive hyperventilation
    d. paralysis prior to intubation

54. In the patient with a head injury, the use of glucose is recommended:
    a. after intubation of a combative patient.
    b. only when hypoglycemia is confirmed.
    c. only when given simultaneously with steroids.
    d. prior to sedation for intubation.

55. When treating a patient with signs and symptoms of increasing ICP, the paramedic should first:
    a. paralyze then intubate the patient.
    b. assure adequate tidal volume.
    c. hyperventilate the patient.
    d. administer an osmotic diuretic.

56. In the management of a head injury patient, the paramedic should assure that the cerebral perfusion pressure is maintained by making sure to keep the _____ BP over _____ mm Hg.
    a. systolic; 70
    b. systolic; 100
    c. diastolic; 50
    d. diastolic; 70

57. While assuring a patent airway in the patient with head trauma, the paramedic should avoid _____ as it may increase the ICP.
    a. inserting an OPA
    b. using a water-soluble jelly
    c. nasal intubation
    d. oral-tracheal intubation

58. When assessing a patient suspected of having an expanding intracranial hematoma, which of the following is the most important finding?
    a. the history of the MOI
    b. the past medical history
    c. the patient's current medications
    d. when the patient ate last

59. An unconscious patient with an open head injury has nonreactive pupils and shows abnormal flexion when pain is applied. What is this patient's GCS?
    a. 3
    b. 4
    c. 5
    d. 6

60. Which of the following types of skull fractures is easily missed in the absence of symptoms developing from an underlying hematoma?
    a. linear
    b. depressed
    c. Battle's sign
    d. basilar

61. Which age group has the highest incidence of spinal cord injury?
    a. men, 31–50
    b. men, 16–30
    c. women, 31–50
    d. women, 16–30

62. It is estimated that _____% of spinal cord injury is caused by improper handling of the patient.
    a. 5
    b. 10
    c. 25
    d. 35

63. The spine consists of interconnected bone and:
    a. ligaments.
    b. muscles.
    c. tendons.
    d. all of the above.

64. The ligament that prevents hyperflexion in the spine is the:
    a. anterior longitudinal.
    b. posterior longitudinal.
    c. cruciform.
    d. atlantoaxial.

65. A ligament that is shaped like a cross and supports the atlas vertebrae is the:
    a. anterior longitudinal.
    b. posterior longitudinal.
    c. cruciform.
    d. atlantoaxial.

66. The second cervical vertebrae is also called the:
    a. cribriform
    b. atlas.
    c. axis.
    d. pivotal.

67. The ligament that serves to hold the odontoid process close to the anterior arch is the:
    a. anterior longitudinal.
    b. transverse.
    c. cruciform.
    d. atlantoaxial.

68. The atlas pivots on the _____ or odontoid process of the axis, which permits rotation of the head.
    a. dens
    b. cribiform
    c. foramen
    d. cruciform

69. The area of the spine that is the most protected from injury is the:
    a. cervical.
    b. thoracic.
    c. lumbar.
    d. abdominal.

70. There are _____ pair of spinal nerves that are responsible for the sensory and motor function of the body below the head.
    a. 24
    b. 27
    c. 31
    d. 38

71. The _____, which is a fusion of three to five bones, is commonly referred to as the tailbone.
    a. coccyx
    b. sacrum
    c. cauda equina
    d. spinous process

72. The vertebrae consist of the body, the vertebral arch, and the:
    a. foramen magnum.
    b. transverse process.
    c. spina bifida.
    d. spinous foramen.

73. The posterior aspect of the vertebrae that projects back from the junction of two lamina is called the:
    a. vertebral arch.
    b. spinous process.
    c. intercerebral disk.
    d. transverse process.

74. The relatively soft, gel-like internal portion of the disk is called the:
    a. annulus fibrosis.
    b. lamina.
    c. odontoid.
    d. nucleus pulposus.

75. Where does the spinal cord end?
    a. C-6
    b. T-5
    c. L-2
    d. L-6

76. Where does cerebral spinal fluid come from?
    a. It comes from the intervertebral disks.
    b. It is manufactured in the ventricles of the brain.
    c. It is manufactured in the pancreas.
    d. It is stored in the bile duct.

77. The material that is located in the anatomical spinal tracts is called:
    a. white matter.
    b. melanin.
    c. myelin sheath.
    d. gray matter.

78. The _____ carries/carry impulses from body parts and sensory information to the brain.
    a. sensory system
    b. ascending nerve tracts
    c. descending nerve tracts
    d. parasympathetic nervous system

79. Corticospinal and reticulospinal are two types of:
    a. sensory system nerves.
    b. ascending nerve tracts.
    c. descending nerve tracts.
    d. parasympathetic NS.

80. What is a funiculus?
    a. a group of nerve fibers with a similar function
    b. a ligament found in the spinal column
    c. the key to the corticospinal tract
    d. the center of the reticulospinal tract

81. The lateral spinothalamic tracts:
    a. conduct sensory impulses of touch and pressure to the brain.
    b. send muscular impulses from the brain to muscle.
    c. conduct impulses of pain and temperature to the brain.
    d. coordinate impulses necessary for muscular movements.

82. A particular area where the spinal nerve provides either motor stimulation, sensations, or both is called a(n):
    a. ganglion.
    b. dermatome.
    c. axon.
    d. nerve band.

83. Following a significant MOI, a patient experiences loss of motor and sensory function from the nipple line, down. What is the highest level of the spine that has been affected?
    a. C-3
    b. C-5
    c. C-7
    d. T-4

84. Following a significant MOI, a patient experiences loss of movement of the diaphragm and loss of sensory function below the shoulder. What is the highest level of the spine that may have been affected?
    a. C-3
    b. C-4
    c. C-5
    d. C-6

85. One of the few exceptions for immobilizing a patient's neck in the position discovered, rather than the normal anatomical position is:
    a. level of consciousness.
    b. resistance to movement.
    c. uncontrolled bleeding from the scalp.
    d. the need to manage the airway with an advanced airway.

86. Your patient has experienced a significant MOI, which you believe requires spinal immobilization. The patient is not willing to have a rigid collar placed on her neck because it will make her feel restricted. She is, however, willing to lie down on a backboard. What is the most appropriate way to proceed with this patient?
    a. Do nothing but transport the patient.
    b. Insist on the rigid collar and immobilize the patient.
    c. Refuse to transport the patient unless she cooperates fully.
    d. Have the patient sign a refusal for the collar, and immobilize her without it.

87. You are assessing a female who was a passenger involved in an MVC. She is complaining of neck, back, and chest pain. When you are listening for breathing sounds, you see that she has lipstick on her shirt as if someone kissed her upper chest. You also see that she is wearing the same color lipstick. How does this finding relate to the MOI?
    a. The patient suffered a rotational MOI.
    b. The patient experienced hyperflexion.
    c. The patient experienced hyperextension.
    d. The MOI was severe enough to have caused a loss of consciousness.

88. When the spinal cord is transected at the _____ level, the result is permanent paraplegia.
    a. cervical
    b. thoracic
    c. sacral
    d. coccyx

89. Which of the following statements about spinal injuries is most correct?
    a. Spinal cord injuries always have accompanying soft tissue injuries.
    b. All spinal cord injuries can be detected by X-ray, MRI, or CT scan.
    c. The spinal cord may be injured without accompanying bone or soft tissue injury.
    d. The patient with a spinal cord injury has sharp pain over the injury site, with or without palpation.

90. When is partial spinal immobilization used in the field?
    a. when the distance a patient fell is < 30 feet
    b. when the MOI is not severe
    c. if the patient prefers not to lie down
    d. it should not be used at all

91. You are treating a toddler who fell out of a shopping cart and lacerated his head. He was initially unconscious, but now is crying and covered with blood. How should he be managed?
    a. cervical collar application and hemorrhage control
    b. full spinal immobilization with the parent providing support
    c. hemorrhage control and transport in a child car seat
    d. backboard and manual head stabilization by the parent

92. Your adult patient is refusing spinal immobilization following a minor MVC, even though she has new tenderness in her neck, shoulders, and lower back. You are making the decision as to whether the patient is reliable to refuse treatment or not. What factor is most significant in making this determination?
    a. the patient's age
    b. vital signs
    c. mental status
    d. positive pain on palpation of the spine

93. If a patient with an "uncertain MOI" complains of having some minor neck pain upon moving his head, you should:
    a. determine the range of motion.
    b. continue your assessment and document the complaint.
    c. fully immobilize the spine.
    d. call medical control for permission to clear the C-spine.

94. Why should you palpate the spinous process if you suspect a neck injury?

a. This will rule out neck injury.

b. Tender areas may not hurt unless palpated.

c. Patients appreciate the extra care.

d. The vertebrae may be dislocated even though there is still movement.

95. You have assessed a patient's upper and lower extremities before and after immobilizing her to a long backboard. Which of the following findings is most significant?

a. pain in both arms before and after immobilization

b. parethesia in the left leg after, not before, immobilization

c. weakness in the right arm before, not after, immobilization

d. weakness in the right arm before and after immobilization

96. You are treating a construction worker who did not have a helmet on while he was walking under a platform and was struck on the head by a large falling brick. Which of the following MOIs most likely occurred?

a. vertical compression of the spine

b. hyperflexion of the head and neck

c. hyperextension of the head and neck

d. distraction of the neck

97. You and your partner are immobilizing a patient who attempted to hang himself. Which of the following injuries do you associate with a hanging?

a. rotational neck injury

b. flexion of the neck

c. vertical compression of the neck

d. distraction of the neck

98. You arrive at the scene of a vehicle that was T-boned in an intersection. The EMTs are short-boarding the driver who is complaining of neck and back pain. Which of the following injuries do you suspect?

a. rotational neck injury

b. flexion of the neck

c. vertical compression of the neck

d. distraction of the neck

99. The type of spinal cord injury that is characterized by a temporary disruption of cord-mediated functions is a cord:

a. concussion.

b. contusion.

c. compression.

d. transection.

100. The type of spinal cord injury that is characterized by hypotension and vasodilation, loss of bladder and bowel control, and priapism in male patients is:

a. spinal hemorrhage.

b. spinal shock.

c. neurogenic shock.

d. cord laceration.

101. You are called to assist a patient who has fallen but has no complaint of injury. The patient has a preexisting spinal cord injury, which has left him with a loss of motor function and pain sensation, but only on the left side of his body. Which of the following conditions does this patient have?

a. anterior cord syndrome

b. central cord syndrome

c. incomplete spinal cord transection

d. Brown-Sequard syndrome

102. Degenerative disc disease is caused by a narrowing of the intervertebral disc, which results in:

a. epidural abscess.

b. spinal cord tumors.

c. variable segment instability.

d. a structural defect in the lamina or vertebral arch.

103. It is estimated that _____% of the population experience some degree of low-back pain during their lifetime.

a. 20–30

b. 40–50

c. 60–90

d. 80–100

104. When making a decision about immobilizing a patient wearing a helmet, which of the following criteria would be a reason to remove the helmet?

a. The helmet is the proper size.

b. The head moves around inside the helmet.

c. The helmet does not interfere with airway management.

d. The helmet interferes with the application of a cervical collar.

105. In which of the following spinal disorders is heredity considered to be a significant factor?

a. degenerative disc

b. spondylolysis

c. low-back pain syndrome

d. spinal cord tumors

106. What is the primary management of a patient with severe low-back pain?

a. palliative care

b. full spinal immobilization

c. partial spinal immobilization

d. rapid transport to an ED

107. What is the most common cause of spinal cord tumors?
   a. trauma
   b. heredity
   c. metastasis
   d. PCBs

108. The diameter of the spinal cord is approximately _____ mm, and the diameter of the spinal column is approximately _____ mm.
   a. 5; 10
   b. 10; 15
   c. 15; 20
   d. 20; 25

109. Which of the following statements is not correct about rigid cervical collars?
   a. They are also referred to as extrication collars.
   b. They limit movement of the neck.
   c. They totally eliminate neck movement.
   d. They are the standard for cervical immobilization.

110. Which of the following is the primary reason for removing a helmet from a patient with a suspected SCI?
   a. the paramedic is trained to do it
   b. airway management
   c. the patient needs to be immobilized
   d. ED staff does not have sufficient training to do it

111. Which of the following is not an indication for rapid extrication?
   a. compensating shock
   b. decompensating shock
   c. penetrating chest wound
   d. penetrating abdominal wound

112. For which of the following adult ambulatory patients is a standing takedown indicated?
   a. fall from a standing position with two possible fractured wrists, and no LOC
   b. female who tripped and fell, breaking her nose, yet she denies pain on palpation of her neck and back
   c. passenger involved in a high-speed MVC complaining of a headache after the collision
   d. driver with an MOI that involved airbag deployment, seat belt use, no LOC, and no complaint of injury

113. When should a child be removed from a car seat to immobilize the spine?
   a. when the child is crying
   b. when the parents are distressed
   c. when it is necessary for the patient to be supine
   d. when you cannot palpate the child's back

114. Patients are immobilized in the neutral, in-line anatomic position for all of the following reasons, except that this:
   a. position allows for the most space for the cord.
   b. position is the most comfortable for the patient.
   c. is the most stable position for the spinal column.
   d. position will help to reduce cord hypoxia.

115. Which of the following is a principle of spinal immobilization?
   a. The goal is to prevent further injury.
   b. Fifteen percent of secondary spinal injuries are preventable with immobilization.
   c. Spinal immobilization should begin after the initial assessment.
   d. Spinal immobilization should be applied to any patient with back pain.

116. Patients with herniated intervertebral disks are commonly affected in which two areas of the spine?
   a. cervical and thoracic
   b. thoracic and lumbar
   c. lumbar and sacral
   d. lumbar and cervical

117. What is the preferred method for assessing a patient for spinal tenderness?
   a. Palpate over each of the spinal processes.
   b. Palpate over each of the vertebral bodies.
   c. Ask the patient to move all four extremities.
   d. Ask the patient if he has any back pain.

118. The evaluation of motor function of the lower extremities includes assessment of plantar flexion and:
   a. great toe flexion.
   b. foot dorsiflexion.
   c. Babinski's reflex.
   d. plantar reflex.

119. The causes of traumatic spinal cord injury include direct trauma, excessive movement, and:
   a. directions of force.
   b. degeneration.
   c. Achilles' heel.
   d. blight reflexes.

120. You are assessing a conscious 20-year-old male who was removed from a pool on a backboard by lifeguards on the scene. Your assessment findings include hypotension, bradycardia, and skin that is pink and warm. He is flaccid from the waist down. What do you suspect with these findings?
   a. spinal shock
   b. neurogenic shock
   c. spinal cord compression
   d. head injury

Exam #38 Answer Form

	A	B	C	D			A	B	C	D
1.	❏	❏	❏	❏		31.	❏	❏	❏	❏
2.	❏	❏	❏	❏		32.	❏	❏	❏	❏
3.	❏	❏	❏	❏		33.	❏	❏	❏	❏
4.	❏	❏	❏	❏		34.	❏	❏	❏	❏
5.	❏	❏	❏	❏		35.	❏	❏	❏	❏
6.	❏	❏	❏	❏		36.	❏	❏	❏	❏
7.	❏	❏	❏	❏		37.	❏	❏	❏	❏
8.	❏	❏	❏	❏		38.	❏	❏	❏	❏
9.	❏	❏	❏	❏		39.	❏	❏	❏	❏
10.	❏	❏	❏	❏		40.	❏	❏	❏	❏
11.	❏	❏	❏	❏		41.	❏	❏	❏	❏
12.	❏	❏	❏	❏		42.	❏	❏	❏	❏
13.	❏	❏	❏	❏		43.	❏	❏	❏	❏
14.	❏	❏	❏	❏		44.	❏	❏	❏	❏
15.	❏	❏	❏	❏		45.	❏	❏	❏	❏
16.	❏	❏	❏	❏		46.	❏	❏	❏	❏
17.	❏	❏	❏	❏		47.	❏	❏	❏	❏
18.	❏	❏	❏	❏		48.	❏	❏	❏	❏
19.	❏	❏	❏	❏		49.	❏	❏	❏	❏
20.	❏	❏	❏	❏		50.	❏	❏	❏	❏
21.	❏	❏	❏	❏		51.	❏	❏	❏	❏
22.	❏	❏	❏	❏		52.	❏	❏	❏	❏
23.	❏	❏	❏	❏		53.	❏	❏	❏	❏
24.	❏	❏	❏	❏		54.	❏	❏	❏	❏
25.	❏	❏	❏	❏		55.	❏	❏	❏	❏
26.	❏	❏	❏	❏		56.	❏	❏	❏	❏
27.	❏	❏	❏	❏		57.	❏	❏	❏	❏
28.	❏	❏	❏	❏		58.	❏	❏	❏	❏
29.	❏	❏	❏	❏		59.	❏	❏	❏	❏
30.	❏	❏	❏	❏		60.	❏	❏	❏	❏

Exam #38 Answer Form

	A	B	C	D		A	B	C	D
61.	❏	❏	❏	❏	86.	❏	❏	❏	❏
62.	❏	❏	❏	❏	87.	❏	❏	❏	❏
63.	❏	❏	❏	❏	88.	❏	❏	❏	❏
64.	❏	❏	❏	❏	89.	❏	❏	❏	❏
65.	❏	❏	❏	❏	90.	❏	❏	❏	❏
66.	❏	❏	❏	❏	91.	❏	❏	❏	❏
67.	❏	❏	❏	❏	92.	❏	❏	❏	❏
68.	❏	❏	❏	❏	93.	❏	❏	❏	❏
69.	❏	❏	❏	❏	94.	❏	❏	❏	❏
70.	❏	❏	❏	❏	95.	❏	❏	❏	❏
71.	❏	❏	❏	❏	96.	❏	❏	❏	❏
72.	❏	❏	❏	❏	97.	❏	❏	❏	❏
73.	❏	❏	❏	❏	98.	❏	❏	❏	❏
74.	❏	❏	❏	❏	99.	❏	❏	❏	❏
75.	❏	❏	❏	❏	100.	❏	❏	❏	❏
76.	❏	❏	❏	❏	111.	❏	❏	❏	❏
77.	❏	❏	❏	❏	112.	❏	❏	❏	❏
78.	❏	❏	❏	❏	113.	❏	❏	❏	❏
79.	❏	❏	❏	❏	114.	❏	❏	❏	❏
80.	❏	❏	❏	❏	115.	❏	❏	❏	❏
81.	❏	❏	❏	❏	116.	❏	❏	❏	❏
82.	❏	❏	❏	❏	117.	❏	❏	❏	❏
83.	❏	❏	❏	❏	118.	❏	❏	❏	❏
84.	❏	❏	❏	❏	119.	❏	❏	❏	❏
85.	❏	❏	❏	❏	120.	❏	❏	❏	❏

CHAPTER
39

Abdominal and Genitourinary Trauma

1. Abdominal trauma is the _____ leading cause of preventable trauma death.
   a. second
   b. third
   c. fourth
   d. fifth

2. The abdominal cavity can hide significant blood loss. As much as _____ liter(s) can be lost before any signs of distention are apparent.
   a. 1
   b. 1.5
   c. 2
   d. 2.5

3. Immediate concerns, after the ABCs, in the management of the patient with abdominal trauma are hemorrhage, major organ damage, and:
   a. the possibility of peritonitis.
   b. the possible use of vasopressors.
   c. IV fluid replacement.
   d. associated chest injuries.

4. Abdominal trauma often goes unrecognized because the _____ is(are) often unrecognized.
   a. signs of shock
   b. golden hour
   c. MOI
   d. platinum ten minutes

5. Motor vehicle crashes often involve _____ forces that compress internal organs and cause shearing of organs that are suspended by ligaments.
   a. rapid acceleration
   b. twisting
   c. rapid deceleration
   d. subluxation

6. The _____ is the section of the small intestine that is approximately 8 feet in length, absorbing the majority of the food we eat.
   a. duodenum
   b. jejunum
   c. ileum
   d. colon

7. The _____ is the last section of the small intestine and varies in length from 15 to 25 feet.
   a. duodenum
   b. jejunum
   c. ileum
   d. colon

8. You are assessing the abdomen of a young adult male with a complaint of abdominal pain. You see that he has an old scar in the midline and ask him about it. He tells you that he had a hernioplasty 2 years ago. What procedure did he have?
   a. aortic graph
   b. hernia repair
   c. removal of the spleen
   d. removal of the appendix

9. The _____ is the largest organ in the body and often sustains injuries during rapid deceleration forces.
   a. liver
   b. kidney
   c. heart
   d. lung

10. _____ pain is caused by irritation of the peritoneum and is more commonly described as diffuse rather than localized.
    a. Visceral
    b. Somatic
    c. Obstructive
    d. Muscle spasm

11. You have just finished a light palpation of all four quadrants of a patient with an MOI suggestive of possible internal injury. You discovered that the patient had pain on palpation in the ULQ without rebound tenderness. What type of pain does the examination reflect?

a. somatic

b. visceral

c. guarded

d. obstructive

12. What organ(s) may be injured in the patient described in question 11?

a. appendix and small intestine

b. liver and stomach

c. stomach and spleen

d. liver and gallbladder

13. Kehr's sign is an assessment finding of pain in the abdomen that radiates to the left shoulder. This finding indicates:

a. acute bowel obstruction.

b. intraperitoneal bleeding and/or irritation.

c. aortic aneurysm.

d. ileus.

14. When a patient has ecchymosis in the umbilical area caused by peritoneal bleeding, this is known as:

a. Cullen's sign.

b. Grey Turner's sign.

c. periumbilical guarding.

d. peritoneals sign.

15. You and your crew have been dispatched to a football game at a local high school for a traumatic injury. Upon arrival, you find a diaphoretic 29-year-old male who is doubled over in severe pain. He tells you that suddenly, without warning, while he was sitting on the bench, he started having excruciating pain in his left testicle. He also says he feels like he is going to vomit. What do you suspect is the cause of his pain?

a. kidney stone

b. renal colic

c. testicular torsion

d. intra-abdominal bleeding

16. (Continuing with question 15) What is the most appropriate initial management plan for this patient?

a. Provide oxygen by cannula and administer IM morphine.

b. Secure the patient to a long spine board with legs flexed.

c. Move the patient into his position of comfort, and then administer analgesia and an antiemetic.

d. Administer high-flow oxygen, start two large bore IVs, and give a fluid bolus.

17. How would you treat the patient described in question 15?

a. Treat for shock and begin a rapid transport.

b. Administer oxygen and transport on a backboard.

c. Manage his pain and transport gently.

d. Apply ice and place him in the Trendelenburg position.

18. The definitive treatment for the patient described in question 15 in most cases would be:

a. prompt surgery.

b. pain management and bed rest.

c. manual repositioning in the ED.

d. rest, abundant hydration, and pain management.

19. After arriving on the scene of a possible assault, you find a 26-year-old male who denies being assaulted but confesses that he has a large foreign body stuck in his anus. He is bleeding from the rectum, has acute abdominal pain, and is tachycardic. The immediate complications associated with this type of emergency include:

a. perforations and hemorrhage.

b. traumatic peristalsis.

c. alimentary spasms.

d. hematuria.

20. What do you suspect is the cause of the abdominal pain and tachycardia in the patient described in question 19?

a. the patient is unable to pass gas

b. contamination from fecal matter

c. peritonitis from blood loss

d. ischemia from bowel strangulation

21. What is your management plan for the patient described in question 19?

a. Keep the patient in a position of comfort.

b. Attempt to remove the foreign object and control bleeding.

c. Keep the patient supine with knees flexed.

d. Apply ice and elevate the legs.

22. Associated signs and symptoms that should be anticipated by the paramedic for the patient described in question 19 include:

a. dysrhythmias.

b. narrowed pulse pressure.

c. widening pulse pressure.

d. nausea and vomiting.

23. You are on the scene of an MVC and find that the 45-year-old male driver was apparently ejected from the vehicle after it crashed into a guardrail. The patient is unconscious and has no outward signs of trauma. His breathing is shallow, clear, and equal at 16 bpm; pulse is 130 and weak; BP is 76/24 mm Hg. The most likely cause of his hypotension is:

a. head injury.

b. aortic aneurysm.

c. intra-abdominal bleeding.

d. spinal cord injury.

24. Initial treatment for the patient in question 23 includes all of the following, except:

a. airway management.

b. spinal immobilization.

c. IV fluid replacement.

d. rapid transport to a trauma center.

25. Primary traumatic injuries associated with consensual sex include all of the following, except:

a. restraint injuries.

b. tears from body jewelry.

c. fractured penis.

d. peritonitis.

26. You are assessing a 22-year-old female who states she is in her third trimester of pregnancy and that she was the driver of the vehicle in the MVC. Since this was a moderate-speed collision, you recall that the patient can lose up to _____% of her blood volume before signs of shock are evident.

a. 15

b. 25

c. 35

d. 45

27. Direct trauma to the abdomen of a 35-year-old pregnant woman may result in all of the following conditions, except:

a. uterine inversion.

b. premature labor.

c. abruptio placentae.

d. uterine rupture.

28. During the assessment of a 45-year-old male who has pain from irritation of the diaphragm, to what area would you expect his pain to radiate?

a. back

b. shoulder

c. lower abdomen

d. it will not radiate anywhere

29. Besides the kidneys and spleen, which of the following organs is partially located within the retroperitoneal cavity?

a. liver

b. gallbladder

c. pancreas

d. duodenum

30. _____ is the term for decreased motility of the intestine.

a. Alimentary

b. Viscus

c. Excursion

d. Ileus

31. You are on the scene of a call where a 19-year-old male was in a fight and his abdomen was slashed with a knife. He is alert and in a lot of pain. Some of his bowel is protruding through the wound and he has significant bleeding. What is this type of injury called?

a. aortic aneurism

b. evisceration

c. avulsion

d. penetration

32. From a management perspective what is the highest priority for the treatment of the patient described in question 31?

a. administering pain medication

b. ventilatory assistance

c. treating for shock

d. carefully replacing the loop of bowel

33. The treatment of the actual wound found in the patient in question 31 should involve:

a. applying plenty of ice to the wound.

b. pouring plenty of sterile saline into the opening in his belly.

c. simply covering the area with a clean sheet.

d. applying an occlusive dressing to the wound.

34. On reassessment of the patient in question 31, you note his vitals are respiration of 24 and shallow, pulse of 120 weak and thready, BP of 112/68 mm Hg, and SPO$_2$ of 95. How would you prioritize his condition at this point?

a. low priority and compensating well

b. low priority but needing to be watched closely

c. high priority as he is having difficulty compensating

d. high priority as he is in irreversible shock

35. Definitive care for the patient in question will need to be provided in the:

a. local ED.

b. physician's office.

c. back of your ambulance.

d. OR of the trauma center.

Exam #39 Answer Form

	A	B	C	D		A	B	C	D
1.	❏	❏	❏	❏	19.	❏	❏	❏	❏
2.	❏	❏	❏	❏	20.	❏	❏	❏	❏
3.	❏	❏	❏	❏	21.	❏	❏	❏	❏
4.	❏	❏	❏	❏	22.	❏	❏	❏	❏
5.	❏	❏	❏	❏	23.	❏	❏	❏	❏
6.	❏	❏	❏	❏	24.	❏	❏	❏	❏
7.	❏	❏	❏	❏	25.	❏	❏	❏	❏
8.	❏	❏	❏	❏	26.	❏	❏	❏	❏
9.	❏	❏	❏	❏	27.	❏	❏	❏	❏
10.	❏	❏	❏	❏	28.	❏	❏	❏	❏
11.	❏	❏	❏	❏	29.	❏	❏	❏	❏
12.	❏	❏	❏	❏	30.	❏	❏	❏	❏
13.	❏	❏	❏	❏	31.	❏	❏	❏	❏
14.	❏	❏	❏	❏	32.	❏	❏	❏	❏
15.	❏	❏	❏	❏	33.	❏	❏	❏	❏
16.	❏	❏	❏	❏	34.	❏	❏	❏	❏
17.	❏	❏	❏	❏	35.	❏	❏	❏	❏
18.	❏	❏	❏	❏					

CHAPTER

40

Orthopedic Trauma

1. As we get older, our bones become more prone to fracture because they:
   a. become denser.
   b. become more porous.
   c. are subjected to more stress.
   d. can no longer utilize calcium.

2. The axial skeleton consists of the skull, vertebral column, and:
   a. bony thorax.
   b. pelvis.
   c. rhomboids.
   d. soleus.

3. The pectoral girdle is composed of the:
   a. scapula and manubrium.
   b. latissimus dorsi.
   c. pubis.
   d. clavicle and scapula.

4. When muscles contract, they pull the _____, which then cause(s) the bones to move at the joints.
   a. tendons
   b. ligaments
   c. marrow
   d. Haversian canals

5. The three structural classifications of joints are:
   a. fusion, synovial, and skeletal.
   b. fibrous, cartilaginous, and synovial.
   c. named for the specific location in the body.
   d. named for the bones that make up the joint.

6. In addition to providing support and protection for internal organs, bones are also responsible for:
   a. homeostasis.
   b. range of motion.
   c. fighting infection.
   d. producing red blood cells.

7. The diaphysis, epiphysis, and periosteum are specific:
   a. parts of a long bone.
   b. types of smooth muscle.
   c. injuries associated with fractures.
   d. causes of pathological fractures.

8. _____ is the area between the epiphysis and diaphysis.
   a. Metaphysis
   b. Periosteum
   c. Haversian canals
   d. Bone marrow sheds

9. Which of the following is not a part of the humerus?
   a. the neck and shaft
   b. medial and lateral condyle
   c. the olecranon
   d. the elbow

10. The _____ is located on the little finger side of the lower arm and is part of the wrist joint.
    a. radius head
    b. radius shaft
    c. ulna head
    d. ulna shaft

11. You have been called to transport a football player who has separated his shoulder. This injury is actually a dislocation of the:
    a. acromioclavicular joint.
    b. sternoclavicular joint.
    c. metaphysis.
    d. olecranon.

12. A patient with a _____ fracture can easily go into decompensated shock from the 2,000 cc blood loss that can occur over the first 2 hours following the fracture.
    a. femur
    b. pelvis
    c. spinal
    d. tibula

13. Of the following components, which is not part of the pelvis?
    a. ilium
    b. ischium
    c. acetabulum
    d. femur

14. A _____ is a rounded protuberance at the articulation of a bone, similar to a knuckle.
    a. trochanter
    b. condyle
    c. phalange
    d. fossa

15. The tibia, located in the _____ lower leg, is made up of the tibia plateau, the shaft, and the _____.
    a. anterior; medial malleolus
    b. anterior; lateral condyle
    c. posterior; medial malleolus
    d. posterior; lateral condyle

16. When assessing a child with a deformity of a bone, the paramedic must:
    a. consider that pediatric bones break very easily.
    b. consider that pediatrics have high pain tolerance.
    c. suspect significant amount of energy caused the injury.
    d. suspect the injury might be associated with physical abuse.

17. The fibula, which is located in the _____ leg, is made up of the head, the shaft, and the _____ malleolus.
    a. upper; medial
    b. lower; lateral
    c. anterior; medial
    d. posterior; lateral

18. Which of the following is not a type of muscle?
    a. smooth
    b. skeletal
    c. axial
    d. cardiac

19. _____ muscle is found in the lower airways, blood vessels, and intestines.
    a. Smooth
    b. Skeletal
    c. Axial
    d. Cardiac

20. Connective tissue covering the epiphysis, which acts as a surface for articulation, is called:
    a. tendon.
    b. cartilage.
    c. ligament.
    d. muscle.

21. _____ is(are) connective tissue that supports the joints and allow(s) for range of motion.
    a. Tendons
    b. Cartilage
    c. Ligaments
    d. Muscles

22. _____ can relax or contract to alter the inner lumen diameter of vessels.
    a. Gomphoses
    b. Smooth muscle
    c. Tendons
    d. Cardiac muscle

23. Bones articulate at joints where they are:
    a. opposed.
    b. unopposed.
    c. padded by cartilage.
    d. at a diagonal direction from one another.

24. The attribute of a muscle being able to generate an impulse is referred to as:
    a. automaticity.
    b. excitability.
    c. conduction.
    d. rhythm.

25. _____ muscle is under conscious control, includes the major muscle mass of the body, and allows for mobility.
    a. Smooth
    b. Skeletal
    c. Cardiac
    d. Neonate

26. The two major hinged joints in the body are the:
    a. jaw and digits.
    b. elbow and wrist.
    c. elbow and knee.
    d. hip and shoulder.

27. A _____ is a line of fusion between two bones that are separate in early development.
    a. symphysis
    b. gomphosis
    c. syndesmosis
    d. condyloid

28. Immovable joints, where one bone is fitted into a socket of another that is not intended for movement, such as a tooth, are:
    a. symphyses.
    b. gomphoses.
    c. syndesmoses.
    d. condyloids.

29. _____ are articulations in which the bones are united by ligaments.
    a. Fusions
    b. Cartilage
    c. Syndesmoses
    d. Condyloids

30. A _____ joint is a joint filled with fluid, which lubricates the articulated surfaces.
    a. cartilaginous
    b. synchondrosis
    c. symphysis
    d. synovial

31. A(n) _____ fracture is a fracture that tears away the outer covering of the bone, often involving most of the length of the bone.
    a. spiral
    b. comminuted
    c. greenstick
    d. oblique

32. Flexion, extension, abduction, and circumduction are all movements allowed by what type of joint?
    a. synchondrosis
    b. gomphosis
    c. transverse
    d. synovial

33. A fracture where the break is at a right angle to the axis of the long bone is called a(n) _____ fracture.
    a. epiphyseal
    b. transverse
    c. oblique
    d. comminuted

34. An uncomplicated tibia/fibula fracture can bleed about _____ cc over the first 2 hours.
    a. 500
    b. 1,000
    c. 1,500
    d. 2,000

35. A partial dislocation of a joint is called a:
    a. subluxation.
    b. luxation.
    c. sprain.
    d. stress fracture.

36. A complete disruption of the integrity of a joint is called a:
    a. sprain.
    b. dislocation.
    c. fracture.
    d. subluxation.

37. A 56-year-old male was playing in his recreational basketball league when he twisted his ankle. He tells you that he felt a snap and then a severe pain above his heel. There is deformity, swelling at the site, and pain when you stabilize the injury. What type of injury do you suspect?
    a. sprain/strain
    b. Achilles rupture
    c. medial malleolar fracture
    d. posterior malleolar fracture

38. The knee dislocation can completely disrupt the blood supply to the lower leg when the _____ is displaced to the _____, compressing the posterior tibial artery.
    a. tibia; anterior
    b. tibia; posterior
    c. fibula; anterior
    d. fibula; posterior

39. The elbow, when dislocated, is very serious and can threaten the:
    a. brachial plexus, causing paralysis.
    b. radial plexus, causing paralysis.
    c. brachial artery and blood supply to the arm.
    d. radial artery and blood supply to the arm.

40. A 20-year-old volleyball player injured her knee during a game. She attempted to bear weight but was not able to walk, so she sat down on the court. When you examine the knee, she is unable to extend the knee. She has pain and swelling on and around the patella. What type of injury do you suspect?
    a. knee dislocation
    b. patellar dislocation
    c. fractured patella
    d. patellar tendon rupture

41. Non-traumatic causes of inflammation and degeneration of the joints include:
    a. diabetes and stress.
    b. bursitis and gouty arthritis.
    c. obesity and Crohn's disease.
    d. stroke and coronary artery disease.

42. The principal use of a traction splint on a femur fracture is to:
    a. keep the patient from moving the injured extremity.
    b. provide complete pain relief.
    c. prevent swelling and blood loss.
    d. relieve the muscle spasms that can worsen the injury.

43. Realignment of dislocations should be considered if distal circulation is impaired or:
    a. if the patient is in pain.
    b. when the deformity is gross.
    c. when the patient signs a release first.
    d. transportation is long or delayed.

44. The difference between a knee dislocation and a patella dislocation is that:
    a. a knee dislocation involves the tibia popping out of the knee joint.
    b. a patella dislocation is much more dangerous than a knee dislocation.
    c. the knee dislocation requires surgery and the patella dislocation does not.
    d. the patella dislocation should never be manipulated in the field.

45. The combination of a long board and PASG/MAST may be used for a _____ fracture, because of the normal blood loss accompanying this type of fracture.
    a. pelvic
    b. mid-shaft femur
    c. proximal femur
    d. tibia/fibula

46. Prior to splinting a patient who had dislocated his left shoulder, you assessed positive distal pulse, motor, and sensation in the extremity. After the application of a sling and swathe, the patient complains of paresthesia and numbness in the arm and fingers. What action should you now take?
    a. Apply ice and administer morphine IM or IV.
    b. Loosen the sling and swathe, and reassess.
    c. Remove the splint and pull traction on the arm, and resplint.
    d. Give early notification to the ED that the patient has a new deficit.

47. In compartment syndrome, edema of the muscle cells develops and increases the capillary hydrostatic pressure and if left untreated will result in:
    a. electrolyte loss.
    b. tissue hypoxia and anoxia.
    c. fluid shifts.
    d. muscle contractions and pain.

48. A Colles' fracture is a common fracture of the:
    a. shoulder.
    b. hand.
    c. wrist.
    d. forearm.

49. The key objective in the management of a closed long bone fracture is to carefully splint the long bone in a straight position without:
    a. causing the patient any pain.
    b. the use of analgesics.
    c. allowing the bone to protrude through the skin.
    d. forgetting to assess for DCAP-BTLS.

50. Which of the following conditions has the potential for developing into compartment syndrome?
    a. traumatic amputation
    b. inhalation injury
    c. fracture of the radius or ulna
    d. exposure to gamma radiation

Exam #40 Answer Form

	A	B	C	D			A	B	C	D
1.	❑	❑	❑	❑		26.	❑	❑	❑	❑
2.	❑	❑	❑	❑		27.	❑	❑	❑	❑
3.	❑	❑	❑	❑		28.	❑	❑	❑	❑
4.	❑	❑	❑	❑		29.	❑	❑	❑	❑
5.	❑	❑	❑	❑		30.	❑	❑	❑	❑
6.	❑	❑	❑	❑		31.	❑	❑	❑	❑
7.	❑	❑	❑	❑		32.	❑	❑	❑	❑
8.	❑	❑	❑	❑		33.	❑	❑	❑	❑
9.	❑	❑	❑	❑		34.	❑	❑	❑	❑
10.	❑	❑	❑	❑		35.	❑	❑	❑	❑
11.	❑	❑	❑	❑		36.	❑	❑	❑	❑
12.	❑	❑	❑	❑		37.	❑	❑	❑	❑
13.	❑	❑	❑	❑		38.	❑	❑	❑	❑
14.	❑	❑	❑	❑		39.	❑	❑	❑	❑
15.	❑	❑	❑	❑		40.	❑	❑	❑	❑
16.	❑	❑	❑	❑		41.	❑	❑	❑	❑
17.	❑	❑	❑	❑		42.	❑	❑	❑	❑
18.	❑	❑	❑	❑		43.	❑	❑	❑	❑
19.	❑	❑	❑	❑		44.	❑	❑	❑	❑
20.	❑	❑	❑	❑		45.	❑	❑	❑	❑
21.	❑	❑	❑	❑		46.	❑	❑	❑	❑
22.	❑	❑	❑	❑		47.	❑	❑	❑	❑
23.	❑	❑	❑	❑		48.	❑	❑	❑	❑
24.	❑	❑	❑	❑		49.	❑	❑	❑	❑
25.	❑	❑	❑	❑		50.	❑	❑	❑	❑

Environmental Trauma

1. An environmental emergency is a medical condition caused or exacerbated by weather, terrain, or:
   a. age.
   b. health.
   c. medications.
   d. atmospheric pressure.

2. Which of the following age groups is at greater risk for environmental emergencies than others?
   a. teens and geriatrics
   b. middle age and geriatrics
   c. small children and geriatrics
   d. early adult and geriatrics

3. Which of the following general health issues makes a person more susceptible to environmental influences?
   a. obesity
   b. smoking
   c. cancer
   d. hypertension

4. Which of the following medical conditions is a risk factor that predisposes an individual to environmental emergencies?
   a. obesity
   b. diabetes
   c. hypertension
   d. hyperthyroidism

5. Which of the following medications results in an impaired ability to sweat and dissipate heat?
   a. tricyclic antidepressants
   b. antidiabetics
   c. aspirin
   d. diuretics

6. An example of an environmental challenge that involves atmospheric pressure is a _____ accident.
   a. free-falling
   b. diving
   c. caving
   d. skiing

7. When the _____ detect(s) that the body temperature is getting too low, it prompts the skeletal muscles to quickly contract and expand (shiver).
   a. brain
   b. baroreceptors
   c. hypothalamus
   d. chemoreceptors

8. Some people frequently feel cold when others around them do not. A slow metabolism due to _____ is often the reason.
   a. heat exhaustion
   b. an overactive thyroid
   c. an underactive thyroid
   d. a depressed immune system

9. Body heat is generated as a side effect of normal _____ processes.
   a. systemic
   b. cell-mediated
   c. metabolic
   d. neural

10. _____ refers to normal body means of heat loss and gain.
   a. Thermoregulation
   b. Radiation
   c. Conduction
   d. Homeostasis

11. Body heat is gained or dissipated by which of the following mechanisms?
   a. convection
   b. homeostasis
   c. metabolysis
   d. electrolyte balance

12. When a person lies on a cold surface, such as a cold floor, heat is lost from the body by means of:
    a. radiation.
    b. conduction.
    c. convection.
    d. evaporation.

13. When the body is exposed to very high temperatures, _____ becomes the only effective method of heat dissipation.
    a. radiation
    b. conduction
    c. convection
    d. evaporation

14. With heat cramping and heat exhaustion, the underlying problem involves:
    a. dehydration.
    b. exposure.
    c. localized injury.
    d. inadequate thermogenesis.

15. Signs of thermolysis include:
    a. shivering and loss of coordination.
    b. diaphoresis and flushing.
    c. tachypnea and chest pain.
    d. slurred speech and ataxia.

16. A person who is properly acclimatized to warm temperatures is less likely to:
    a. sweat.
    b. disrupt sodium concentrations.
    c. vasodilate.
    d. maintain adequate fluid intake.

17. The primary causes of hypothermia are cold-water immersion, cold weather exposure, and _____ hypothermia.
    a. urban
    b. acute
    c. subacute
    d. chronic

18. You are evaluating a 55-year-old female who was outside watching her grandson play ball. She has a c/o of dizziness when she stands up, and a headache. Her clothing is wet with perspiration, but her skin temperature feels normal. Which of the following heat syndromes do you suspect she is experiencing?
    a. cramps
    b. exhaustion
    c. stroke
    d. exertional heat stroke

19. Your management plan for the patient described in question 18 is to cool her off in your ambulance and:
    a. treat for dehydration.
    b. provide high-flow oxygen.
    c. apply ice or ice packs.
    d. administer salt tablets.

20. Severe infection (sepsis) may actually result in _____ when the body's fever-production centers are overwhelmed.
    a. heat exhaustion
    b. heat stroke
    c. hypothermia
    d. exposure

21. The use of which of the following medications can predispose a person to environmental emergencies?
    a. nitrates
    b. estrogens
    c. antihistamines
    d. ACE inhibitors

22. A high incidence of heat exhaustion emergencies occurs in individuals who:
    a. take diuretics.
    b. work outside.
    c. exercise routinely.
    d. drink alcohol excessively.

23. Fever is a normal response to the release of chemicals called _____ and usually results from an infection.
    a. pyrogens
    b. pyrexia
    c. pylorus
    d. purines

24. In _____ the body temperature continues to rise without coming under control and leads to multi-organ damage.
    a. fever
    b. heat stroke
    c. hyperthyroidism
    d. hypothyroidsim

25. With the exception of _____, wet clothing loses approximately 90% of its insulating value.
    a. wool
    b. polyester
    c. denim
    d. cotton

26. Malignant hyperthermia is a severe reaction to _____, which causes a high fever, tachycardia rhabdomyolysis, and acidosis.
    a. the sun
    b. high humidity
    c. sun blocking lotions
    d. anesthetic medications

27. Which of the following conditions is not usually a predisposing factor for hypothermia?
    a. acute stroke
    b. intoxication
    c. shock
    d. acute MI

28. The severity of hypothermia is determined by the core body temperature (CBT) and the presence of:
    a. frostbite.
    b. signs and symptoms.
    c. frost nip.
    d. cold diuresis

29. When coming upon a patient who was knocked out by an electric shock:
    a. most often the patient will be in cardiac arrest.
    b. it is impossible to tell how much current passed through vital organs.
    c. the paramedic must determine the amount of direct current the patient received.
    d. the paramedic must identify both entry and exit points before treating the patient.

30. A person who has been hiking for several hours in the winter would most likely be at risk for _____ hypothermia.
    a. acute
    b. subacute
    c. chronic
    d. urban

31. An elderly stroke victim who has fallen and is unable to move off a tile floor would most likely be at risk for _____ hypothermia.
    a. acute
    b. subacute
    c. chronic
    d. urban

32. Sometimes hypothermia is a sign of another disease, such as:
    a. stroke.
    b. hypoglycemia.
    c. hyperthyroidism.
    d. hyperplasia.

33. Which of the following cardiac dysrhythmias/disturbances is more common during the rewarming phase rather than the development of hypothermia?
    a. atrial fibrillation (a-fib)
    b. ventricular fibrillation (V-fib)
    c. J waves
    d. long QT

34. Which of the following considerations is most accurate regarding the treatment of severe hypothermia patients?
    a. Cold may affect the potency of first-line cardiac drugs.
    b. The risk of V-fib increases with orotracheal intubation.
    c. The risk of V-fib increases with nasotracheal intubation.
    d. The hypothermic heart is never resistant to defibrillation.

35. The most common dysrhythmias in hypothermia-associated cardiac arrest are:
    a. bradycardia and heart blocks.
    b. V-fib and asystole.
    c. v-tach and a-fib.
    d. bradycardia and asystole.

36. In the management of a cardiac arrest patient with severe hypothermia, the risk of inducing ventricular fibrillation increases when:
    a. the patient is orally intubated.
    b. the patient is nasally intubated.
    c. CPR is administered prior to defibrillation.
    d. the patient is handled roughly during care and transport.

37. During the management of the submersion patient, the paramedic should assume that the patient is _____ until proven otherwise.
    a. brain-dead
    b. hypothermic
    c. in V-fib
    d. experiencing laryngospasm

38. For the paramedic managing the hypothermic patient, the first priority after airway, breathing, and circulation is to:
    a. administer a prophylactic antidysrhythmic.
    b. dress and protect frostbitten extremities.
    c. start an IV lifeline.
    d. stop ongoing heat loss.

39. Frostbite is the formation of _____ within the tissues affected.
    a. hematomas
    b. blood clots
    c. ice crystals
    d. cellulitis

40. The paramedic can differentiate between superficial frostbite and deep frostbite in the following way:
    a. Deep frostbitten skin has a white, waxy appearance.
    b. Superficial frostbite feels hard to palpation.
    c. Superficial frostbite only affects small children and the elderly.
    d. Deep frostbite has a temporary decreased loss of sensation.

41. Often, when a frostbitten area is rewarmed, the patient complains of the area feeling numb. This feeling is caused by:
    a. the formation of acute cellulitis.
    b. a lack of oxygen.
    c. the presence of small hematomas.
    d. the formation of blisters.

42. When treating a drowning (submersion) victim, the paramedic should consider the single most important factor in adult drowning, which is:
    a. the use of alcohol and mind-altering drugs.
    b. associated hypothermia.
    c. that an acute medical problem may have precipitated the drowning.
    d. that a suicide attempt may have been the cause.

43. When examining victims of submersion, it is important to realize that:
    a. they may appear normal and unaffected.
    b. they are initially going to require hyperventilation.
    c. they must be positioned head down (Trendelenburg position) to facilitate drainage of the lungs.
    d. they may require the Heimlich maneuver, as ingested water may become a foreign-body airway obstruction.

44. Aspiration of either seawater or freshwater decreases pulmonary compliance and results in:
    a. tension pneumothorax.
    b. hypoxia.
    c. pneumonia.
    d. upper respiratory infection.

45. The endpoints in a submersion incident involving saltwater are pulmonary edema, aspiration injuries, and:
    a. metabolic acidosis.
    b. respiratory acidosis.
    c. metabolic alkalosis.
    d. respiratory alkalosis.

46. The three types of drowning include dry, wet, and:
    a. primary.
    b. secondary.
    c. tertiary.
    d. central.

47. While scuba diving, pressure underwater causes _____ to dissolve in the body, which can lead to problems when the diver stays under too long or surfaces too quickly.
    a. oxygen
    b. carbon dioxide
    c. helium
    d. nitrogen

48. The best predictor of the severity of neurologic deficit following a submersion is the:
    a. type of water the patient aspirated.
    b. time to the first spontaneous gasp following removal from the water.
    c. presence of preexisting medical conditions.
    d. temperature of the water.

49. _____ drowning is defined as the recurrence of respiratory distress after successful recovery from the initial drowning incident and can occur within a few minutes or up to 4 days later.
    a. Wet
    b. Primary
    c. Secondary
    d. Central

50. SCUBA is an acronym for:
    a. sealed and condensed underwater breathing apparatus.
    b. self-compressed underwater breathing aperture.
    c. self-contained underwater breathing apparatus.
    d. solid-compact underwater breathing aperture.

51. _____ law states that, in a mixture of gases, the total pressure is equal to the sum of the partial pressures of each gas.
    a. Boyle's
    b. Henry's
    c. Dalton's
    d. George's

52. _____ law states that, at a constant temperature, the volume of a gas varies inversely with the absolute pressure.
    a. Boyle's
    b. Henry's
    c. Dalton's
    d. George's

53. When a diver ascends but forgets to exhale on the way up, the pressure will _____ with ascent, and the volume of gas trapped in the lungs will _____.
    a. decrease; expand
    b. decrease; shrink
    c. increase; expand
    d. increase; shrink

54. Which of the following injuries will the diver in question 53 most likely experience if the condition persists?
    a. stroke
    b. pericardial tamponade
    c. pneumothorax
    d. loss of consciousness

55. Decompression sickness is an illness that occurs during or after a diving ascent, secondary to rapid release of _____ in the blood.
    a. an air embolus
    b. nitrogen bubbles
    c. hydrogen bubbles
    d. subcutaneous air

56. A patient is c/o pain in the legs and shoulders 2 days after a dive. These symptoms are associated with the:
    a. bends.
    b. staggers.
    c. chokes.
    d. itches.

57. Divers can experience nitrogen narcosis at various depths because of the narcotic effect of dissolved nitrogen in the body. The effect is analogous to excessive ethanol levels, and the cause is attributed to _____ law.
    a. Boyle's
    b. Henry's
    c. Dalton's
    d. George's

58. _____ is a preexisting condition that can predispose some divers to the possibility of air embolism during or after a dive.
    a. Age
    b. Asthma
    c. Sinus infection
    d. Being of African American descent

59. Your patient is a 33-year-old male diver who is lying on the pier. He is experiencing stroke-like symptoms immediately after surfacing from an 80-foot dive. He has left-sided motor deficit and is c/o of left-sided numbness and vertigo. Which of the following conditions do you suspect?
    a. air embolism
    b. decompression sickness
    c. nitrogen narcosis
    d. ARDS

60. After managing and supporting the ABCs, how would you manage the patient described in question 59?
    a. Complete a thrombolic checklist.
    b. Consider pain management therapy.
    c. Consider decompression therapy.
    d. Treat for stroke only.

61. A diver surfaced with blood coming from his left ear. He has severe pain in the left ear and denies any injury occurring before or during the dive and he was not injured getting out of the water. What is the most likely cause of the bleeding?
    a. arterial gas embolism
    b. decompression sickness
    c. the patient is having a stroke
    d. ruptured eardrum from barotrauma

62. Hyperbaric oxygen is beneficial in both _____ and decompression sickness.
    a. pneumothorax
    b. tamponade
    c. DVT
    d. air embolism

63. Long delays are common for the treatment of decompression sickness in the sport diver group because:
    a. of the lack of recognition of symptoms.
    b. of the distance to hyperbaric treatment areas.
    c. all diving sites are in foreign countries.
    d. the dive boats rarely have radios.

64. The most common cause of scuba diving accidents is:
    a. not getting enough air.
    b. decompression sickness.
    c. bites and stings.
    d. abrasions and lacerations.

65. During which phase of a dive do squeeze syndromes, involving the ears, most commonly occur?
    a. predive surface
    b. descent
    c. bottom
    d. postdive surface

66. Three days into a planned week-long mountain climbing trip to heights reaching 8,000 feet, one of the climbers develops shortness of breath, tachypnea, and cyanosis. What condition is he most likely experiencing?
   a. AMS
   b. ACS
   c. HACE
   d. HAPE

67. High-altitude illness occurs as a result of decreased atmospheric pressure, resulting in:
   a. hypercarbia.
   b. hypoxia.
   c. vertigo.
   d. dehydration.

68. Which of the following is a highly unlikely cause of altitude sickness?
   a. skydiving
   b. mountain climbing
   c. scuba dives at high altitudes
   d. flying in an unpressurized aircraft

69. Your patient is a mountain climber who has been sick for 2 days following an ascent of a mountain in excess of 8,000 feet. He is c/o dizziness, headache, irritability, and exertional SOB. Which of the following conditions do you suspect he has?
   a. acute mountain sickness (AMS)
   b. high-altitude pulmonary edema (HAPE)
   c. high-altitude cerebral edema (HACE)
   d. acute flying sickness (AFS)

70. The most important treatment the paramedic can provide for the patient described in question 69 is to:
   a. administer high-flow oxygen.
   b. administer a diuretic.
   c. transport to a hyperbaric therapy center.
   d. administer nifedipine.

71. An employee was working with helium, transferring the liquid from one container to another, when his hand came into contact with the chemical. What type of injury did he receive?
   a. frostbite
   b. first-degree burn
   c. second-degree burn
   d. third-degree burn

72. The body part most likely to be affected by an unexpected exposure to ultraviolet radiation is the:
   a. eyes.
   b. lungs.
   c. hands.
   d. arms.

73. A diver has experienced *squeeze* during his last dive. Which body areas can be affected by squeeze?
   a. thighs and calves
   b. feet and mouth
   c. ears and sinuses
   d. hands and shoulders

74. For the last 2 hours, a rescue crew has been carrying a hiker out of the woods. The hiker lost his footing on ice and fractured his femur. The patient is very cold and, within the last 10 minutes, has stopped shivering. Why has his shivering stopped?
   a. He has gone into shock.
   b. His core temperature has reached 92°F.
   c. His glucose stores are depleted.
   d. He has acute mountain sickness.

75. A diver is experiencing nitrogen narcosis. What is the primary danger for this diver?
   a. impaired thinking
   b. barotrauma
   c. air embolism
   d. hypoxia

76. When working in high humidity climates, it is important to recall that sweating becomes ineffective if the relative humidity exceeds _____%.
   a. 15
   b. 35
   c. 55
   d. 75

77. A patient who has generalized hypothermia has been removed from the cold environment. If he is alert, has an open airway, and no nausea, he should be allowed to:
   a. refuse medical attention.
   b. drink warm fluids.
   c. walk around to help warm the body.
   d. smoke a cigarette.

78. On the scene at a private residence, you arrive at the backyard to find a small crowd standing around two people doing CPR. The patient is a teenage male who was pulled from the pool. A witness saw the male dive into the pool and then float to the surface, face down. What is the primary concern for this patient?
   a. drainage of the lungs
   b. correcting hypothermia
   c. providing high-quality CPR
   d. immobilizing the patient

79. You and your crew take over CPR and continue resuscitative efforts for the patient described in question 78. Initially the patient was easy to ventilate, but now lung compliance is getting hard to bag. What do you suspect is the cause of the increased resistance in ventilation?

    a. gastric distention
    b. laryngospasm
    c. pneumothorax
    d. hypercarbia

80. To correct the problem of increased resistance in ventilation of the patient as described in the previous questions, the paramedic would:

    a. decompress the stomach.
    b. hyperventilate the patient.
    c. decompress the chest.
    d. intubate the patient.

Exam #41 Answer Form

	A	B	C	D			A	B	C	D
1.	❏	❏	❏	❏		31.	❏	❏	❏	❏
2.	❏	❏	❏	❏		32.	❏	❏	❏	❏
3.	❏	❏	❏	❏		33.	❏	❏	❏	❏
4.	❏	❏	❏	❏		34.	❏	❏	❏	❏
5.	❏	❏	❏	❏		35.	❏	❏	❏	❏
6.	❏	❏	❏	❏		36.	❏	❏	❏	❏
7.	❏	❏	❏	❏		37.	❏	❏	❏	❏
8.	❏	❏	❏	❏		38.	❏	❏	❏	❏
9.	❏	❏	❏	❏		39.	❏	❏	❏	❏
10.	❏	❏	❏	❏		40.	❏	❏	❏	❏
11.	❏	❏	❏	❏		41.	❏	❏	❏	❏
12.	❏	❏	❏	❏		42.	❏	❏	❏	❏
13.	❏	❏	❏	❏		43.	❏	❏	❏	❏
14.	❏	❏	❏	❏		44.	❏	❏	❏	❏
15.	❏	❏	❏	❏		45.	❏	❏	❏	❏
16.	❏	❏	❏	❏		46.	❏	❏	❏	❏
17.	❏	❏	❏	❏		47.	❏	❏	❏	❏
18.	❏	❏	❏	❏		48.	❏	❏	❏	❏
19.	❏	❏	❏	❏		49.	❏	❏	❏	❏
20.	❏	❏	❏	❏		50.	❏	❏	❏	❏
21.	❏	❏	❏	❏		51.	❏	❏	❏	❏
22.	❏	❏	❏	❏		52.	❏	❏	❏	❏
23.	❏	❏	❏	❏		53.	❏	❏	❏	❏
24.	❏	❏	❏	❏		54.	❏	❏	❏	❏
25.	❏	❏	❏	❏		55.	❏	❏	❏	❏
26.	❏	❏	❏	❏		56.	❏	❏	❏	❏
27.	❏	❏	❏	❏		57.	❏	❏	❏	❏
28.	❏	❏	❏	❏		58.	❏	❏	❏	❏
29.	❏	❏	❏	❏		59.	❏	❏	❏	❏
30.	❏	❏	❏	❏		60.	❏	❏	❏	❏

Exam #41 Answer Form

	A	B	C	D		A	B	C	D
61.	❏	❏	❏	❏	71.	❏	❏	❏	❏
62.	❏	❏	❏	❏	72.	❏	❏	❏	❏
63.	❏	❏	❏	❏	73.	❏	❏	❏	❏
64.	❏	❏	❏	❏	74.	❏	❏	❏	❏
65.	❏	❏	❏	❏	75.	❏	❏	❏	❏
66.	❏	❏	❏	❏	76.	❏	❏	❏	❏
67.	❏	❏	❏	❏	77.	❏	❏	❏	❏
68.	❏	❏	❏	❏	78.	❏	❏	❏	❏
69.	❏	❏	❏	❏	79.	❏	❏	❏	❏
70.	❏	❏	❏	❏	80.	❏	❏	❏	❏

CHAPTER

Special Consideration in Trauma and Multisystem Trauma

1. Looking at a trauma scene and attempting to determine what injuries might have resulted is examining the:
   a. kinematics of trauma.
   b. nature of the illness.
   c. force of impact.
   d. details of destruction.

2. The _____ of an item/patient and its speed contribute to the kinetic energy at a trauma call.
   a. age
   b. past medical history
   c. weight
   d. velocity

3. Another term for the speed at which a projectile was traveling that needs to be taken into consideration when determining the potential injury is the:
   a. caliper.
   b. velocity.
   c. cavitation.
   d. fragmentation.

4. Penetrating trauma, in which a projectile causes bones to break and secondary injuries, is referred to as:
   a. deceleration.
   b. cavitation.
   c. MOI.
   d. fragmentation.

5. The momentary acceleration of tissue away from the tract of the projectile is known as:
   a. rapid acceleration effect.
   b. cavitation.
   c. kinetic energy.
   d. subluxation.

6. When a patient has a penetrating injury that was caused by a stabbing with a steak knife, this was most likely _____ trauma.
   a. low-energy
   b. medium-energy
   c. high-energy
   d. fatal

7. When a patient sustains penetrating trauma from a military (rifle) weapon, it is most likely:
   a. low-energy trauma.
   b. medium-energy trauma.
   c. high-energy trauma.
   d. always fatal.

8. Which of the following types of collisions has the greatest potential for occupant ejection if unrestrained?
   a. side impact
   b. roll-over
   c. rotational impact
   d. rear impact

9. The _____ collision often presents with patient injuries such as fractured humerus, rib injuries, and hip injuries.
   a. frontal impact
   b. side impact
   c. roll-over
   d. rear impact

10. An impact where the vehicle spins around the point of impact and the injuries of the unrestrained occupant are unpredictable is called a _____ impact.
    a. low-energy
    b. high-energy
    c. rotational
    d. frontal

11. Your patient was the driver of a frontal collision and was not restrained. Most likely if the windshield is cracked he may have sustained injuries to his:

a. knees.

b. hips.

c. chest.

d. femur.

12. When a patient sustains multisystem trauma from an automobile crash, the paramedic should consider each of the following, except:

a. the need to bandage all the soft tissue injuries.

b. spinal immobilization.

c. the appropriate transportation destination.

d. the mechanism of injury and kinematics.

13. Why is it important to consider transporting the multisystem trauma patient to the trauma center?

a. All prehospital protocols require transport to the trauma center.

b. A team of surgeons is needed to treat the multisystem trauma patient.

c. Those hospitals usually have a morgue.

d. Teaching hospitals need the caseload.

14. Aside from a motor vehicle crash, a good example of a mechanism that has significant potential to produce multisystem trauma would be a: _____ injury.

a. head

b. slashing

c. blast

d. frostbite

15. Your 25-year-old male patient was inside his hotel room when a passerby threw an explosive device through the window and there was an explosion. He is alive but has sustained multisystem trauma and is in critical condition. Each of the following is a consideration in the extent of the injuries to the patient, except the:

a. total body surface area.

b. blast wave damage.

c. blast winds damage.

d. heat generated and ground shock.

Exam #42 Answer Form

	A	B	C	D
1.	❑	❑	❑	❑
2.	❑	❑	❑	❑
3.	❑	❑	❑	❑
4.	❑	❑	❑	❑
5.	❑	❑	❑	❑
6.	❑	❑	❑	❑
7.	❑	❑	❑	❑
8.	❑	❑	❑	❑

	A	B	C	D
9.	❑	❑	❑	❑
10.	❑	❑	❑	❑
11.	❑	❑	❑	❑
12.	❑	❑	❑	❑
13.	❑	❑	❑	❑
14.	❑	❑	❑	❑
15.	❑	❑	❑	❑

CHAPTER

43

Obstetrics

1. A developing child in utero under 8 weeks' gestation is called a(n):
   a. fetus.
   b. embryo.
   c. ova.
   d. oocyte.

2. The umbilical vein is responsible for:
   a. the production of amniotic fluid.
   b. carrying fetal blood to the placenta.
   c. returning oxygenated blood from the fetus to the placenta.
   d. returning oxygenated blood from the placenta to the fetus.

3. Fertilization is the union of the egg and sperm, which forms the:
   a. zygote.
   b. ovum.
   c. fetus.
   d. corpus luteum.

4. Amenorrhea in the adult female is considered abnormal in which of the following circumstances?
   a. pregnancy
   b. malnutrition
   c. syphilis infection
   d. extreme and prolonged exercise

5. You are assessing a 26-year-old female who is 24 weeks pregnant. She is complaining of acute abdominal pain that is constant and severe. The pregnancy has been normal, and she has prenatal care. She feels the baby moving. However, she is having a small amount of bloody discharge that just began. You suspect which of the following?
   a. ectopic pregnancy
   b. abruptio placentae
   c. placenta previa
   d. spontaneous abortion

6. How do you manage the patient described in the previous question?
   a. Administer high-flow oxygen and begin transport.
   b. Treat for shock and begin transport.
   c. Have the patient call her gynecologist, because delivery is imminent.
   d. Prepare the patient mentally for a spontaneous abortion.

7. Pregnant women with a negative Rh factor may become sensitized if the fetus has a positive Rh factor. If a fetus in any subsequent pregnancies has a positive Rh factor, Rh antibodies may cross the placenta and:
   a. suppress the immune response.
   b. destroy fetal cells.
   c. cause gestational diabetes.
   d. precipitate preeclampsia.

8. You are dispatched to a call for respiratory distress. Upon arrival, you find a 36-year-old female who is 38 weeks pregnant. She is having severe difficulty breathing that began 1 hour ago and is getting progressively worse. She has no history of asthma, COPD, or cardiac problems, and her pregnancy has been normal with regular prenatal care. What do you suspect is the problem?
   a. heart attack
   b. hyperventilation
   c. pulmonary embolism
   d. pneumothorax

9. Your management plan for the patient in question 8 includes:
   a. nitrates and Lasix.
   b. nebulized albuterol treatment.
   c. assisted breathing with CPAP.
   d. rapid transport for a life-threatening condition.

10. Which of the following is an abnormal condition during pregnancy that needs to be managed promptly?
    a. hypertension
    b. increased cardiac output
    c. increased resting heart rate
    d. decreased blood pressure during second trimester

11. When an ectopic pregnancy occurs, the fertilized egg cannot survive and the mother's life may be threatened because
    a. local infection becomes systemic.
    b. inflammation blocks the fallopian tube.
    c. developing blood clots can become an embolism.
    d. growing tissue may destroy maternal structures.

12. Back labor is back pain caused by the fetus pressing against the _____ during labor.
    a. spine
    b. kidneys
    c. bladder
    d. vena cava

13. The hormone _____ secreted by the pituitary gland stimulates the uterus to produce stronger contractions.
    a. estrogen
    b. progesterone
    c. oxytocin
    d. epinephrine

14. In which of the following cases would it be appropriate not to start an IV on a woman in active labor?
    a. Contractions are abnormal.
    b. Labor is 2 weeks early, but the mother is mentally competent and refuses.
    c. Postpartum hemorrhage began before delivery of the placenta.
    d. The mother is full term with twins.

15. While assisting the mother during delivery, the paramedic prepares to prevent an explosive delivery by:
    a. coaching the mother to breathe deeply.
    b. coaching the mother to pant during contractions.
    c. having the mother raise her hips when the head delivers.
    d. holding one hand on the baby's head while the mother is pushing.

16. Once the baby's head delivers, the paramedic should:
    a. inspect the head for trauma.
    b. inspect for a nuchal cord.
    c. perform the first APGAR score.
    d. dry the head and face.

17. Once the baby's head is out, the natural progression is for the baby's face to turn:
    a. laterally.
    b. superiorly.
    c. purple.
    d. inferiorly.

18. The APGAR score is a well-accepted assessment score chart for evaluating newborn infants by rating the muscle tone, heart rate, respirations, and:
    a. reflex and color.
    b. color and weight.
    c. BP and reflex.
    d. BP and color.

19. In the field, the primary reason to cut the cord soon after the birth is that:
    a. the baby will suckle quicker.
    b. stage III of labor will progress quicker.
    c. the baby will be easier to manage and assess.
    d. the mother will not tear the cord.

20. When the cord is not cut immediately, the infant should be placed _____ to prevent placental transfusion.
    a. at a higher level than the placenta
    b. at a lower level than the placenta
    c. in an incubator
    d. in an infant swaddler

21. When access for medication is needed in the newborn, which of the following is preferred?
    a. IO
    b. ET
    c. umbilical vein cannulation
    d. umbilical artery cannulation

22. You have arrived at the scene of a serious MVC and find an unconscious young woman, who is obviously pregnant, behind the wheel. She is breathing agonal gasps as you approach. You assist her ventilations while your crew quickly extricates her from the vehicle. You advise your crew to position her on a long board with:
    a. her legs elevated.
    b. her head elevated.
    c. the right side of the board elevated slightly.
    d. the left side of the board elevated slightly.

23. You continue to aggressively treat the patient in question 23 by intubating her, while your crew obtains vital signs. Her pulse is 110, and BP is 80/40 mm Hg. Your management plan en route includes:

    a. aggressive fluid replacement.

    b. the application of MAST/PASG.

    c. the use of vasopressors.

    d. rapid transport to the nearest ED.

24. Listening for fetal heart tones is the standard of care:

    a. for distressed fetuses in the prehospital setting.

    b. only when a Doppler is available.

    c. only in third trimester pregnancies.

    d. in the clinical setting and not in the field.

25. The primary impact on the fetus from a state of shock in the mother includes:

    a. increased risk of hypothermia.

    b. hypoglycemic environment for the fetus.

    c. decreased liver function for the fetus.

    d. shunting of blood from the fetus.

26. You have been called to a multiparous woman who is having contractions and is at 34 weeks gestation. She tells you that the baby has not yet moved into a head-down position. Her labor is very active, and she feels like the baby is coming. You move the patient to your stretcher and prepare for transport. What is your management plan for this patient?

    a. Begin rapid transport to the hospital.

    b. Prepare for imminent delivery.

    c. Administer Pitocin®, as the fetus is premature.

    d. Position the mother in the Trendelenburg position.

27. How would you assess the woman in question 26 for signs of imminent delivery?

    a. Measure the height of her fundus.

    b. Count her contractions.

    c. Observe the birth canal for crowning.

    d. Palpate the fundus for strength of contractions.

28. You are dispatched to a residence for postpartum hemorrhage. You arrive and find that a 32-year-old woman has given birth to a healthy baby with the help of a certified midwife. The pregnancy and birth were normal; however, after the delivery of the placenta, the patient has had heavy blood loss, despite uterine massage. What is your management plan for this patient?

    a. Assist the midwife with direct pressure on the uterus.

    b. Treat for shock and begin transport.

    c. Encourage the mother to have the baby nurse during transport.

    d. Insert trauma dressings in the birth canal, apply MAST/PASG, and begin transport.

29. After assisting with the normal delivery of a healthy baby, the patient suddenly complains of severe lower abdominal pain. She does not deliver the placenta but begins heavy bleeding, and the uterus is presenting from the vagina. You immediately recognize this as uterine inversion. Your management plan for this patient is to:

    a. attempt to deliver the placenta to control the bleeding.

    b. cover the protruding tissue with moist, sterile dressings.

    c. prepare to intubate the patient, as she will probably develop a pulmonary embolus.

    d. start an IV, apply MAST/PASG, and begin a rapid transport.

30. You are assisting in the emergency delivery of an infant during the mother's 36th week of gestation. Your partner opens the OB kit while you examine the mother for crowning. You note the presenting part is both feet.

    a. Ask the patient to stop pushing.

    b. Quickly move her into the ambulance before the head delivers.

    c. Allow the cord to deliver and support the body.

    d. Place a gloved hand in the birth canal to hold the fetus.

Exam #43 Answer Form

	A	B	C	D			A	B	C	D
1.	❏	❏	❏	❏		16.	❏	❏	❏	❏
2.	❏	❏	❏	❏		17.	❏	❏	❏	❏
3.	❏	❏	❏	❏		18.	❏	❏	❏	❏
4.	❏	❏	❏	❏		19.	❏	❏	❏	❏
5.	❏	❏	❏	❏		20.	❏	❏	❏	❏
6.	❏	❏	❏	❏		21.	❏	❏	❏	❏
7.	❏	❏	❏	❏		22.	❏	❏	❏	❏
8.	❏	❏	❏	❏		23.	❏	❏	❏	❏
9.	❏	❏	❏	❏		24.	❏	❏	❏	❏
10.	❏	❏	❏	❏		25.	❏	❏	❏	❏
11.	❏	❏	❏	❏		26.	❏	❏	❏	❏
12.	❏	❏	❏	❏		27.	❏	❏	❏	❏
13.	❏	❏	❏	❏		28.	❏	❏	❏	❏
14.	❏	❏	❏	❏		29.	❏	❏	❏	❏
15.	❏	❏	❏	❏		30.	❏	❏	❏	❏

CHAPTER

Neonatal Care and Pediatrics

1. The _____ leads from the placenta to the fetus and carries oxygenated blood, rather than deoxygenated blood.
   a. umbilical vein
   b. umbilical artery
   c. ductus ovale
   d. ductus arteriosus

2. After birth, fetal circulation changes and the _____ turn(s) into a fibrous cord that serves as a ligament.
   a. umbilical arteries
   b. umbilical vein
   c. ductus venosus
   d. ductus arteriosus

3. After the baby takes its first breath, the _____ closes and shunts blood to the lungs.
   a. ductus ovale
   b. ductus venosus
   c. ductus arteriosus
   d. ductus arteriosus

4. Newborns are very sensitive to hypoxia, and, if they experience hypoxia or severe acidosis, a serious condition called _____ may occur.
   a. persistent fetal circulation
   b. hypoxic apnea
   c. neonatal pulmonary syndrome
   d. hypoxic drive syndrome

5. The condition described in question 4 can be corrected or avoided by:
   a. performing CPR as needed.
   b. intubating the newborn after birth.
   c. stimulating the newborn to breathe.
   d. administering epinephrine.

6. When apnea occurs in infants that were born full term, where no cause for the apnea can be determined, this condition is called:
   a. primary apnea.
   b. secondary apnea.
   c. apparent life-threatening event (ALTE).
   d. apnea of infancy.

7. When evaluating an infant with frequent and severe apnea, the paramedic will find the parents utilize a sleep apnea monitor and the infant is given a drug such as _____, which stimulates the respiratory centers.
   a. caffeine
   b. dexamethasone
   c. tegretol
   d. Solu-Medrol®

8. The most common cause of Down syndrome occurs when a baby is born with _____ rather than two copies of chromosome 21.
   a. one
   b. three
   c. four
   d. five

9. The paramedic can recognize a newborn that is born with Down syndrome by which of the following characteristics?
   a. large ears with an abnormal shape
   b. overall muscle tone that is rigid and spastic
   c. small tongue in relation to the size of the mouth
   d. flat facial profile with a small nose and depressed nasal bridge

10. Other distinguishing characteristics of Down syndrome include:
    a. joint contraction.
    b. excessively large fontanels.
    c. a downward slant of the eyes.
    d. an excessive space between the large and second toe.

11. The paramedic can recognize a newborn that is born with the birth defect spina bifida because the infant will have:

    a. overall weak body muscle tone.

    b. exposed spinal structures.

    c. excessively large fontanels.

    d. curvature of the spine.

12. Of the following, which is an avoidable antepartum factor that can affect childbirth?

    a. multiple fetuses

    b. no prenatal care

    c. gestational diabetes

    d. hypertension syndromes

13. Of the following, which is a significant antepartum factor that classifies the newborn as "high risk"?

    a. pyloric stenosis

    b. prolonged labor

    c. lactose intolerance

    d. feeding problems

14. _____ account(s) for 20% of infant deaths, more than from any other single cause.

    a. Birth defects

    b. Premature labor

    c. Meconium aspiration

    d. Placenta previa

15. _____ is a factor associated with low birth weights.

    a. Prolonged labor

    b. Multiple fetuses

    c. Gestational diabetes

    d. The mother's use of folic acid

16. The paramedic is assisting in the delivery of a high-risk infant. She should anticipate the initial stabilization of the infant will be to provide warmth, position, clear the airway, and:

    a. dry and stimulate.

    b. provide high-flow oxygen.

    c. provide high-quality chest compressions.

    d. intubate and gain vascular access.

17. A pregnant woman who is using crack/cocaine is creating which of the following risk factors?

    a. placenta previa

    b. infant feeding problems

    c. advanced development of motor skills

    d. high birth weight

18. Immediately after birth, the paramedic evaluates:

    a. for aspiration syndrome.

    b. approximate weight and length.

    c. for meconium staining and nuchal cord.

    d. respiratory effort, pulse rate, and skin color.

19. At 1 minute after birth, the paramedic evaluates and scores:

    a. birth weight and length.

    b. best eye opening, verbal, and motor response.

    c. appearance, pulse, grimace, activity, and reflex.

    d. blood pressure, pulse oximetry, and blood glucose.

20. In the clinical setting, newborns are screened for genetic and _____ disorders, shortly after birth.

    a. teratogenic

    b. cardiovascular

    c. infectious

    d. metabolic

21. When a baby is born without enough thyroid hormone (congenital hypothyroidism), this condition can lead to:

    a. myxedema.

    b. poor growth and mental retardation.

    c. abnormal protrusion of the eyes.

    d. goiter.

22. The newborn that is born with fetal alcohol syndrome (FAS) can be distinguished by which of the following characteristics?

    a. low birth weight, small head, and small eye openings

    b. low birth weight, large head, and thick upper lip

    c. upward slant of eyes and small head

    d. protruding upper jaw and thinned lips

23. Children born with FAS may have abnormal facial features, growth problems, and _____.

    a. long fingers and toes.

    b. connective tissue problems.

    c. large and disproportionate tongues.

    d. central nervous system problems.

24. Your patient is a 23-year-old female who is in custody of the police. She is in active labor. The police state that she is high on heroin. Which of the following complications can you expect with this delivery?

    a. prolonged labor and fetal distress

    b. prolapsed cord

    c. decreased mental status of the newborn

    d. breech presentation and delivery

25. How would you manage the delivery for the patient described in question 24?
    a. Monitor, transport, and consider administration of Pitocin®.
    b. Attempt to prevent delivery and begin a rapid transport.
    c. Administer oxygen, assist ventilations, and administer Narcan®.
    d. Assist with the delivery of the breech baby.

26. During the delivery of twins, the paramedic can tell if the babies are fraternal or identical because fraternal twins:
    a. develop from the same zygote.
    b. always have their own placenta.
    c. (one) will present as a breech.
    d. have their own umbilical cords.

27. Which of the following birth-related injuries is associated with shoulder dystocia?
    a. spinal cord injury
    b. fractured clavicle
    c. brachial plexus injury
    d. hypothermia

28. Your partner has just assisted with the delivery of a 38-week gestation newborn. You have assessed the infant after 1 minute and have determined that the infant's heart rate is 60 bpm even after you have warmed, dried, stimulated, and provided blow-by oxygen. What would you do next?
    a. Suction for meconium.
    b. Assist with ventilations by bag mask.
    c. Intubate the newborn.
    d. Start CPR.

29. (Continuing with the care of the newborn in question 28) After 30 seconds you assess the heart rate, which has not increased from 60 bpm. What would you do next?
    a. Administer high-flow oxygen.
    b. Assist with ventilations by bag mask.
    c. Intubate the newborn.
    d. Start CPR.

30. The initial steps of postarrest stabilization for the neonate include:
    a. keeping the baby warm and continuing oxygen delivery.
    b. starting an IV drip of amiodarone.
    c. administering an epinephrine bolus every 5 minutes.
    d. placing a nasogastric tube.

31. Besides airway problems, _____ problems are the most common potentially life-threatening disorder that affects neonates.
    a. hypoglycemia
    b. hypothermia
    c. fluid imbalance
    d. congenital heart

32. The out-of-hospital delivery puts the premature infant at an increased risk for problems associated with:
    a. hypoxia.
    b. vomiting.
    c. jaundice.
    d. hyperglycemia.

33. The most common type of hernia associated with neonates is a(n) _____ hernia.
    a. diaphragmatic
    b. inguinal
    c. umbilical
    d. hiatal

34. The common causes of neonatal seizures are hypoxia, fever, infection, and:
    a. hypoglycemia.
    b. alcohol.
    c. drugs.
    d. genetic disorders.

35. Any fever in neonates is serious and requires evaluation because of their:
    a. immature lungs.
    b. immature thermoregulatory system.
    c. high risk of seizures from fever.
    d. high risk of aspiration.

36. The neonate can develop infection from the mother _____ birth.
    a. before and during
    b. during
    c. during and after
    d. before, during, and after

37. Jaundice occurs when a baby's immature liver cannot dispose of excess:
    a. insulin.
    b. glycogen.
    c. bilirubin.
    d. urine.

38. Approximately 60% of full-term infants and 80% of premature infants develop jaundice in the first _____ of life.
    a. 2–3 minutes
    b. 2–3 hours
    c. 2–3 days
    d. 2–3 weeks

39. The most common causes of vomiting in the neonate include infections, increased ICP, and:
    a. drug withdrawal.
    b. genetic disorders.
    c. metabolic disorders.
    d. pyloric stenosis.

40. Complications from vomiting in the neonate include aspiration, dehydration, and:
    a. seizures.
    b. lactose intolerance.
    c. increased ICP.
    d. electrolyte imbalance.

41. Diarrhea in neonates is difficult to assess because:
    a. of residual meconium.
    b. all stools are loose.
    c. diapers can change stool consistency.
    d. of the large amount of bile excretion.

42. Neonates are prone to abdominal distention because of gastric and fluid distention caused by immature digestive systems. Other causes of distention include:
    a. drug or alcohol withdrawal.
    b. hernias.
    c. hypoglycemia.
    d. neurologic abnormalities.

43. ALS transport has been requested for a 20-day-old baby, from a pediatrician's office to the hospital. The baby is crying persistently and the transport is for severe distention of the abdomen caused by a possible bowel obstruction. Your primary concern during the transport is to:
    a. prevent infectious exposure.
    b. watch the baby's airway.
    c. stop the baby's crying.
    d. infuse at least 20 cc saline per kg.

44. Because of the child's stage of emotional development in the _____ age group, this group is the most difficult to evaluate.
    a. neonate
    b. infant
    c. toddler
    d. adolescent

45. In the _____ age group, feelings of guilt and fear of pain often dominate the thinking of these children.
    a. infant
    b. toddler
    c. preschool
    d. school-age

46. Children in the _____ age group are extremely concerned about modesty and are terrified of disfigurement and death.
    a. toddler
    b. preschool
    c. school-age
    d. adolescent

47. Infants are obligate nose breathers until _____ months of age, and they might not open their mouths to breathe even when their nose becomes obstructed from a cold, creating periods of apnea.
    a. 3
    b. 6
    c. 9
    d. 12

48. In the infant, the fontanels are used as a diagnostic aid in assessing for shock, dehydration, and:
    a. head injury.
    b. hypoglycemia.
    c. hyperthermia.
    d. hypothermia.

49. Which of the following is a unique characteristic of an infant's chest?
    a. Sternal retractions are normal in this age group.
    b. Abdominal or "belly breathing" is normal in this age group.
    c. The respiratory muscles are exceptionally well developed.
    d. Infants have the ability to compensate for long periods of time when in respiratory distress.

50. Which of the following is correct about the infant's thermoregulatory system?
    a. Infants do not have the ability to shiver to create body heat.
    b. Skin color is a poor indicator of hyperthermia.
    c. Skin color is a poor indicator of hypothermia.
    d. Full-term infants are born with a mature temperature regulation.

51. _____ is the number one cause of death in children over 1 year of age.
    a. Sudden infant death syndrome (SIDS)
    b. Abuse
    c. Infection
    d. Trauma

52. Which of the following is the immediate concern for the paramedic when treating a child who has a poisoning or drug overdose?
    a. respiratory depression
    b. anaphylaxis
    c. vomiting and aspiration
    d. shock

53. Which of the following statements about pediatric trauma is most correct?
    a. Pneumothorax and hemothorax are injuries that do not occur in small children.
    b. Injuries to the head, face, and neck occur with more frequency in children than in adults.
    c. Pediatric trauma care for EMS providers is more intensive than adult trauma care.
    d. Injuries to the chest and abdomen occur infrequently and are of little concern for the paramedic.

54. The greatest incidence of SIDS occurs:
    a. during the winter months.
    b. more often with females.
    c. during the summer months.
    d. when the infant sleeps on its back.

55. The most common triggers of asthma in children are:
    a. seizures.
    b. viral infections.
    c. cold temperatures.
    d. very warm temperatures.

56. Physical complaints associated with depression in children include:
    a. headache and muscle ache.
    b. nausea and vomiting.
    c. dizziness.
    d. delay in puberty.

57. A child abuse or neglect injury can be physical, sexual, or _____ in nature.
    a. emotional
    b. financial
    c. self-destructive
    d. congenital

58. When a paramedic notes the presence of multiple bruises of various ages on a child during a physical examination, she should document the findings by noting:
    a. the estimated age of each bruise.
    b. the location and color of each bruise.
    c. who she suspects caused the bruising.
    d. the detailed story behind every bruise.

59. Which of the following is an example of child neglect?
    a. burns on the genitalia
    b. signs of malnourishment
    c. signs of shaken baby syndrome
    d. a central nervous system injury

60. Shaken baby syndrome is a group of signs and symptoms associated with:
    a. severe head trauma.
    b. paralyzing spinal injury.
    c. a long history of child abuse.
    d. intra-abdominal hemorrhage.

61. Evidence shows that most children with shaken baby syndrome are:
    a. also victims of sexual abuse.
    b. under 1 year old when trauma is inflicted.
    c. between the ages of 18 months and 2 years.
    d. predominantly from homes in the middle to upper class.

62. Signs and symptoms of stroke are _____ in a child as in an adult.
    a. the same
    b. less severe
    c. more severe
    d. completely different

63. Which one of the following childhood infectious diseases is still not preventable?
    a. tetanus
    b. rubeola
    c. meningitis
    d. poliomyelitis

64. Your patient is a 7-year-old with Coxsackie virus (hand, foot, and mouth syndrome). You are aware that this condition is highly contagious, so you don gloves and avoid contact with:
    a. rashes and feces.
    b. discharge from the eyes.
    c. cuts or open wounds.
    d. respiratory secretions.

65. Dispatched to a local high school, you have been asked to transport a teenager with infectious mononucleosis. The nurse tells you that this condition is mildly contagious, and to wear gloves and avoid contact with:

   a. urine or feces.

   b. discharge from blisters.

   c. saliva or blood.

   d. rash or hives.

66. Which of the following conditions requires isolation technique for PPE?

   a. whooping cough (pertussis)

   b. viral meningitis

   c. meningococcemia meningitis

   d. impetigo

67. Which of the following statements about febrile seizures is most correct?

   a. Febrile seizures typically have no lasting neurological effects.

   b. Febrile seizures are associated with physical abuse.

   c. Febrile seizures often have lasting neurological effects.

   d. Most febrile seizures are focal and last several minutes.

68. _____ is(are) the number one reason for children missing school and the number one reason for pediatric ED visits caused by chronic illness.

   a. Allergies

   b. Diabetes

   c. Croup

   d. Asthma

69. Your patient is a 5-year-old male with symptoms of an upper respiratory infection, nausea, vomiting, and confusion. The parents tell you that the child has been sick with the flu, but the confusion is new. The child's medications include nebulized albuterol as needed for the last week and over-the-counter Bayer® children's aspirin as needed for fevers. You suspect the child:

   a. is developing pneumonia.

   b. is presenting with Reye's syndrome.

   c. is having an AMS caused by dehydration.

   d. may have had a seizure.

70. Your management of the patient discussed in question 68 will include support and care of the ABCs and:

   a. administration of Ventolin and Solu-Medrol®.

   b. IV fluids and seizure precautions.

   c. considering the use of acetaminophen.

   d. administration of prophylactic rectal diazepam.

71. When asthma is triggered, changes in the airways occur. Which of the following is the correct sequence of airway changes?

   a. bronchoconstriction, inflammation, and excess mucus production

   b. wheezing, excess mucus production, and bronchoconstriction

   c. inflammation, excess mucus production, and bronchoconstriction

   d. mucus production, wheezing, and bronchoconstriction

72. _____ is a condition characterized by infections of the bronchioles that results in swelling of the lower airways and tachypnea, retractions, and cyanosis.

   a. Epiglottitis

   b. Croup

   c. Bronchiolitis

   d. Pneumonia

73. Your patient is a 5-year-old who is having difficulty breathing. The patient has difficulty exhaling, the SpO_2 is 94% with oxygen, and there are decreased breath sounds bilaterally with no wheezing. Which of the following conditions do you suspect?

   a. allergic reaction

   b. bronchiolitis

   c. foreign body airway obstruction

   d. asthma attack

74. Your management plan for the patient discussed in question 73 includes continued oxygenation and:

   a. supportive care and reassessment.

   b. gentle transport with a parent close by.

   c. nebulized Ventolin®.

   d. epinephrine and Benadryl®.

75. _____ is a condition precipitated by a viral or bacterial infection and is characterized by fever, tachypnea, rales, consolidation in one or more lobes, and cough.

   a. Asthma

   b. Croup

   c. Bronchiolitis

   d. Pneumonia

76. Why does the prevalence of asthma decrease as children get older?

   a. As the immune system matures, some children outgrow the condition.

   b. Some children outgrow the condition with the use of steroids.

   c. Natural antibodies develop with the use of steroids.

   d. As airways enlarge, some children outgrow the condition.

77. The most prominent indicator of respiratory failure in children is:
   a. increased use of accessory muscles.
   b. low SpO_2 levels.
   c. decreased level of consciousness.
   d. decreased capillary filling.

78. Besides cool or cold temperatures, hypothermia in children can be caused by:
   a. prolonged infection.
   b. diarrhea.
   c. vomiting.
   d. seizures.

79. Children who are diagnosed with a new onset of diabetes mellitus will usually present to the paramedic as being:
   a. hyperactive.
   b. hypothermic.
   c. hyperglycemic.
   d. hypoglycemic.

80. Congenital heart defects are deformities of the structures of the heart that occur:
   a. after the first month of life.
   b. after 6 months of life.
   c. only when the mother has used drugs during pregnancy.
   d. while the fetus is developing in utero.

81. The primary problem associated with heart defects is that they:
   a. disrupt normal blood flow.
   b. cause murmurs.
   c. cause dysrhythmias.
   d. cause arrhythmias.

82. A defect of the heart that is characterized by valves that are absent, too small, or do not close completely is called:
   a. stenosis.
   b. coarctation.
   c. truncus.
   d. valvulitis.

83. The most common cardiac dysrhythmias seen in children are tachycardias, bradycardias, and:
   a. ventricular fibrillation.
   b. bundle branch blocks.
   c. heart blocks.
   d. asystole.

84. Always consider _____ to be the underlying cause of cardiac dysrhythmias in children until proven otherwise.
   a. hypoglycemia
   b. hypothermia
   c. hypoxia
   d. heredity

85. A highly contagious bacterial or viral disease in children that is characterized by discharge from the eyes is:
   a. impetigo.
   b. conjunctivitis.
   c. Lyme disease.
   d. German measles.

86. The pediatric patient who presents with sunken eyes, recent weight loss, and tachycardia should be evaluated to rule out:
   a. polio.
   b. pertussis.
   c. anaphylaxis.
   d. dehydration.

87. You are transporting an infant to the ED for evaluation of a URI. The child has been sick with fever, decreased PO intake, and vomiting. During the transport, the child experiences what you suspect is a febrile seizure. Which of the following is the most appropriate treatment for the child?
   a. Apply ice packs to the torso and head.
   b. Administer IV fluids.
   c. Administer Valium®.
   d. Use gentle cooling measures.

88. You are dispatched at 3:00 A.M. for a 4-year-old sick child. Upon arrival at the residence, the parents tell you that the child has been sick with a cold, but tonight it suddenly got worse when the child spiked a temperature. The child is having difficulty breathing, and has a sore throat and difficulty swallowing. You suspect the child has:
   a. croup.
   b. bronchiolitis.
   c. epiglottitis.
   d. a partial obstruction.

89. Which of the following is inappropriate management for the patient discussed in question 88?
   a. Keep a parent with the child at all times.
   b. Visualize the airway for an obstruction.
   c. Permit the child to sit up.
   d. Minimize handling and examining to prevent agitation.

90. While attempting to apply an oxygen mask to the patient discussed in question 88, the child resists. How should you proceed next?
    a. Consider the use of blow-by oxygen.
    b. Insist that the parent hold the mask in place.
    c. Turn up the liter flow so it feels like a fan.
    d. Consider RSI.

91. Transportation considerations for the patient discussed in question 88 should include:
    a. immediate, but calm, transport.
    b. rapid transport with lights only.
    c. laying the child down on the stretcher with the parent nearby.
    d. strapping the parent to the stretcher with the child in his lap.

92. Police have called you to care for a teenager who has overdosed on methadone. The 14-year-old is unconscious with shallow respirations and no signs of outward trauma. After managing the ABCs, your primary concern is:
    a. to begin a rapid transport.
    b. the patient's mental status.
    c. to be prepared for seizures.
    d. to administer IV fluids.

93. Appropriate ALS management for the patient described in question 92 includes administering:
    a. 4 mg naloxone.
    b. 2–4 ml/kg D-50 W.
    c. 0.1 mg/kg naloxone.
    d. atropine 0.5–1.0 mg.

94. You arrive at the scene of a motor vehicle collision to find an unconscious 6-year-old male lying supine on the pavement. A witness tells you the child ran out in front of a moving car and was struck. What type of injuries do you suspect?
    a. head, chest, and upper extremities
    b. head, chest, and lower extremities
    c. chest, abdomen, and upper extremities
    d. chest, abdomen, and lower extremities

95. The injury pattern for the patient described in question 94 is common and is also described as:
    a. Cushing's triad.
    b. Waddell's triad.
    c. Hendrick's triage.
    d. greenstick pattern.

96. Hydrocephalus is an excess accumulation of serous fluid within the cranium that is treated with surgical placement of an endoscopic third ventriculostomy (ETV) or:
    a. ostomy.
    b. diuretics.
    c. antidiuretics.
    d. a shunt that drains into the abdomen.

97. The most common complications associated with hydrocephalus include infection, sudden closure of ETV, and:
    a. clogged tubing.
    b. allergic reaction to medications.
    c. medications that are no longer effective.
    d. shunt malfunction.

98. _____ is a viral disease of the lungs and the leading cause of lower respiratory tract infections in infants and young children.
    a. Pneumonia
    b. Tuberculosis
    c. Bronchiolitis
    d. Respiratory syncytial virus (RSV)

99. Cystic fibrosis affects the normal function of the epithelial cells that line passageways inside the lungs and:
    a. heart.
    b. brain.
    c. digestive system.
    d. sympathetic nervous system.

100. Children with cystic fibrosis have higher incidents of respiratory infection because:
    a. their lungs have gotten tired from overuse.
    b. the lungs become stiff, making coughing difficult.
    c. there is inflammation in the lining of the lungs.
    d. bronchoconstriction traps bacteria and viruses.

Exam #44 Answer Form

	A	B	C	D			A	B	C	D
1.	❏	❏	❏	❏		34.	❏	❏	❏	❏
2.	❏	❏	❏	❏		35.	❏	❏	❏	❏
3.	❏	❏	❏	❏		36.	❏	❏	❏	❏
4.	❏	❏	❏	❏		37.	❏	❏	❏	❏
5.	❏	❏	❏	❏		38.	❏	❏	❏	❏
6.	❏	❏	❏	❏		39.	❏	❏	❏	❏
7.	❏	❏	❏	❏		40.	❏	❏	❏	❏
8.	❏	❏	❏	❏		41.	❏	❏	❏	❏
9.	❏	❏	❏	❏		42.	❏	❏	❏	❏
10.	❏	❏	❏	❏		43.	❏	❏	❏	❏
11.	❏	❏	❏	❏		44.	❏	❏	❏	❏
12.	❏	❏	❏	❏		45.	❏	❏	❏	❏
13.	❏	❏	❏	❏		46.	❏	❏	❏	❏
14.	❏	❏	❏	❏		47.	❏	❏	❏	❏
15.	❏	❏	❏	❏		48.	❏	❏	❏	❏
16.	❏	❏	❏	❏		49.	❏	❏	❏	❏
17.	❏	❏	❏	❏		50.	❏	❏	❏	❏
18.	❏	❏	❏	❏		51.	❏	❏	❏	❏
19.	❏	❏	❏	❏		52.	❏	❏	❏	❏
20.	❏	❏	❏	❏		53.	❏	❏	❏	❏
21.	❏	❏	❏	❏		54.	❏	❏	❏	❏
22.	❏	❏	❏	❏		55.	❏	❏	❏	❏
23.	❏	❏	❏	❏		56.	❏	❏	❏	❏
24.	❏	❏	❏	❏		57.	❏	❏	❏	❏
25.	❏	❏	❏	❏		58.	❏	❏	❏	❏
26.	❏	❏	❏	❏		59.	❏	❏	❏	❏
27.	❏	❏	❏	❏		60.	❏	❏	❏	❏
28.	❏	❏	❏	❏		61.	❏	❏	❏	❏
29.	❏	❏	❏	❏		62.	❏	❏	❏	❏
30.	❏	❏	❏	❏		63.	❏	❏	❏	❏
31.	❏	❏	❏	❏		64.	❏	❏	❏	❏
32.	❏	❏	❏	❏		65.	❏	❏	❏	❏
33.	❏	❏	❏	❏		66.	❏	❏	❏	❏

Exam #44 Answer Form

	A	B	C	D
67.	❑	❑	❑	❑
68.	❑	❑	❑	❑
69.	❑	❑	❑	❑
70.	❑	❑	❑	❑
71.	❑	❑	❑	❑
72.	❑	❑	❑	❑
73.	❑	❑	❑	❑
74.	❑	❑	❑	❑
75.	❑	❑	❑	❑
76.	❑	❑	❑	❑
77.	❑	❑	❑	❑
78.	❑	❑	❑	❑
79.	❑	❑	❑	❑
80.	❑	❑	❑	❑
81.	❑	❑	❑	❑
82.	❑	❑	❑	❑
83.	❑	❑	❑	❑

	A	B	C	D
84.	❑	❑	❑	❑
85.	❑	❑	❑	❑
86.	❑	❑	❑	❑
87.	❑	❑	❑	❑
88.	❑	❑	❑	❑
89.	❑	❑	❑	❑
90.	❑	❑	❑	❑
91.	❑	❑	❑	❑
92.	❑	❑	❑	❑
93.	❑	❑	❑	❑
94.	❑	❑	❑	❑
95.	❑	❑	❑	❑
96.	❑	❑	❑	❑
97.	❑	❑	❑	❑
98.	❑	❑	❑	❑
99.	❑	❑	❑	❑
100.	❑	❑	❑	❑

CHAPTER

45

Geriatrics

1. _____ is the study of the problems of all aspects of aging.
   a. Oldentology
   b. Agentology
   c. Genealogy
   d. Gerontology

2. As the body ages, the skin begins to sag and wrinkles develop because of the:
   a. increased vascularity in the skin.
   b. loss of elastic fiber.
   c. loss of T-cell function.
   d. loss of sebaceous glands.

3. With aging, the musculoskeletal system is affected by:
   a. the forming of opacities.
   b. decreased muscle and bone mass.
   c. hypertrophy of muscles.
   d. increasing bone marrow production.

4. Changes in the respiratory system caused by the effects of aging include:
   a. increased sensitivity of the gag reflex.
   b. lung capacity increases with increased elasticity.
   c. the chest wall becomes stiff and rigid, increasing the risk for fractures.
   d. increased cilia predispose the elderly to sleep apnea.

5. With aging comes a decreased _____ response, which affects the ability to increase the heart rate in response to stress and exercise.
   a. estrogen
   b. catecholamine
   c. androgen
   d. progesterone

6. Which of the following is a psychological change associated with aging?
   a. loss of support system
   b. increased isolation
   c. increased depression
   d. decreased depression

7. The changes in the endocrine system caused by aging include decreased reproductive functions and:
   a. decrease in thyroid function.
   b. atrophy of hormone receptors.
   c. surgical removal of the pancreas.
   d. excessive sympathetic stimulation.

8. During perimenopause (the years before menopause), about 90% of women experience irregular menses and begin to experience the symptoms of menopause. This is caused by:
   a. excessive hormone production.
   b. the drop in sexual hormone levels.
   c. increased release of catecholamines.
   d. decreased release of catecholamines.

9. In addition to the classic symptoms of hot flashes and irregular menstrual periods, nearly 80% of menopausal women experience other symptoms that are collectively called:
   a. postmaternal pattern.
   b. menacing disorder.
   c. menopausal syndrome.
   d. PMS.

10. In the year 2030, it is projected that one in _____ people will be age 65 or older in the United States.
    a. three
    b. five
    c. ten
    d. twenty-five

11. _____ is an example of an inflammatory disease in which the body's immune system attacks the body's joints causing pain and deformity.

   a. Gout

   b. Bursitis

   c. Osteoarthritis

   d. Rheumatoid arthritis

12. As the baby boomers grow older, it is estimated that treating psychiatric illnesses will become a crisis in the United States, with the numbers of mentally ill seniors expected to _____ by the year 2030.

   a. double

   b. triple

   c. quadruple

   d. increase tenfold

13. The actual number of people dying from _____ has risen 37% since 1950 and remains the number one cause of death in the United States.

   a. heart disease

   b. cancer

   c. COPD

   d. diabetes

14. The elderly are highly susceptible to head injuries from falling because:

   a. the size of the brain increases with age.

   b. the risk of blood clots forming increases with age.

   c. thinning hair does not protect the scalp as well as thick hair.

   d. the brain and vessels tear on the sharp, bony edges inside the skull.

15. What is the difference in the pathology of cardiovascular emergencies in older adults compared to that of younger adults?

   a. The catecholamine response in cardiac emergencies increases with age.

   b. Younger adults tend to die from ACS rather than heart failure.

   c. Coronary artery disease predisposes the elderly to superior outcomes.

   d. There is really no difference when an older or younger adult experiences an ACS.

16. The elderly patient often has atypical cardiac pain, which may be as subtle as a new onset of weakness or dyspnea. One of the reasons this occurs is:

   a. diminished pain perception.

   b. depression of the central nervous system.

   c. suppression of the inflammatory response.

   d. changes experienced during menopause.

17. Currently the single greatest health problem in the United States, it is estimated that nearly 55% of all Americans will have _____ by age 60.

   a. a stroke

   b. diabetes

   c. hypertension

   d. cancer

18. You are assessing a 64-year-old female with a chief complaint of difficulty breathing, which has been getting worse over the past 2 days. She is overweight and has a history of congestive heart failure. She does not move much from her recliner except to use the bathroom. She also has new pleuritic chest pain and describes chronic pain in her lower left leg. Which of the following conditions should you suspect first?

   a. pneumonia

   b. emphysema

   c. chronic bronchitis

   d. pulmonary embolism

19. (Continuing with the patient in question 18) Your partner administers oxygen and obtains vital signs while you obtain a 12-lead ECG. Her vital signs are: skin is warm, moist, and pale; respirations 28/shallow and lung sounds clear; pulse 70/irregular; BP 168/110 mm Hg; and ECG is controlled atrial fibrillation. Your treatment plan now includes:

   a. IV access only.

   b. nitrates and Lasix.

   c. IV fluids and analgesia.

   d. nebulized bronchodilators.

20. Emergencies with Alzheimer's patients fall into three categories. Which of the following is not one of those categories?

   a. behavioral

   b. psychiatric

   c. metabolic

   d. neurologic

21. A common emergency that occurs with patients who have Parkinson's is:

   a. hypoglycemia.

   b. injuries from falling.

   c. transient ischemic attack (TIA).

   d. recurrent thoughts of death.

22. _____ is a chronic and progressive neurologic condition that robs memory and intellect.

   a. Parkinson's

   b. Alzheimer's

   c. Hypothyroidism

   d. Hyperthyroidism

23. _____ is(are) (an) important indicator(s) of the general well-being and mental health of older Americans.
    a. Age and gender
    b. Height and weight
    c. Depressive symptoms
    d. The use of multiple medications

24. Thyroid disease, such as hypothyroidism, in elders can predispose them to risks such as:
    a. hypothermia.
    b. cholecystitis.
    c. diverticulitis.
    d. malnutrition.

25. _____ is a general term for decreased mental intellect and cognitive function that is reversible when treated in a timely manner.
    a. Senility
    b. Bipolar
    c. Dementia
    d. Encephalitis

26. The most common causes of minor GI bleeds in the elderly are:
    a. peptic ulcer and angiodysplasia.
    b. diverticular diseases.
    c. hemorrhoids and colorectal cancer.
    d. bowel obstructions.

27. Common GI problems in the elderly, such as _____, are most often caused by cancer, adhesions, or hernias.
    a. bowel obstructions
    b. hemorrhoids
    c. gastritis
    d. peptic ulcers

28. You are dispatched to the residence of a patient with abdominal pain. The patient is an 84-year-old female who is alert and complaining of abdominal pain of 8/10. She has had the pain for nearly 4 hours and describes it as "cramping." She also has nausea and has vomited twice. The patient denies dyspnea, chest pain, or weakness. Vital signs are: skin is warm and dry, with good color; respiratory rate 22/nonlabored; pulse rate 70/regular; and BP 140/100 mm Hg. What is your first impression of this patient?
    a. unstable with a GI bleed
    b. stable with a bowel obstruction
    c. stable with a urinary tract infection
    d. unstable with a possible cardiac event

29. (Continuing with the patient in question 28) The patient's ECG is sinus with a first-degree AV block, SpO_2 is 98%, and blood sugar is 110 mg/dL. She is taking atenolol for hypertension, Nexium for her stomach, miacalcin for osteoporosis, and hydrocodone for back pain. The patient's last bowel movement was 2 days ago, and she feels distended. Which of the patient's medications is most likely contributing to her chief complaint?
    a. atenolol
    b. Miacalcin®
    c. Nexium®
    d. hydrocodone

30. _____ is a chronic inflammatory disease of the bones that results in thickening, softening, and eventual bowing of the bone.
    a. Osteoporosis
    b. Paget's disease
    c. Osteoarthritis
    d. Gout

31. You are obtaining a focused history from a 76-year-old female with a new GI bleed. Which of her medications could be the cause of the GI bleed?
    a. Colace®
    b. codeine
    c. ibuprofen
    d. oxycodone

32. Elderly patients with slowed metabolism can get increased amounts of medications in the body from normal doses that can reach lethal levels. This is commonly referred to as:
    a. concurrent disease overdose.
    b. altered hepatic function.
    c. depressed renal function.
    d. drug toxicity.

33. Which of the following is not a type of nursing home regulated by state and federal standards?
    a. intermediate care facilities
    b. residential care facilities
    c. skilled nursing facilities
    d. senior retirement facilities

34. Independent living with limited nursing care, social, recreation, and rehabilitation activities is an example of a(n) _____ nursing home.
    a. intermediate care facility
    b. residential care facility
    c. skilled nursing facility
    d. senior retirement facility

35. A 64-year-old woman with a complaint of chest pain called 9-1-1 from her home. Upon exam, the patient has pain severity of 10 out of 10 and what appears to be a raised rash on the left side of her chest. She has had the pain for 3 days and today the pain is worse and the rash is new. She denied dyspnea, nausea, or loss of consciousness. What do you suspect is her problem?
    a. angina
    b. shingles
    c. psoriatic arthritis
    d. cellulitis

36. Affective disorders increase the risk of injury in the elderly by interfering with:
    a. thermoregulation.
    b. the tasks of daily living.
    c. the immune response.
    d. cardiac output.

37. Because the elderly are susceptible to problems with metabolizing medications, the paramedic should assume that the patient's medications could be contributing to nearly any health problem. Which type of medication requires frequent monitoring by testing the levels in the blood?
    a. digitalis
    b. ramipril
    c. amoxicillin
    d. furosemide

38. _____ is(are) ischemic and sometimes necrotic damage to the skin, subcutaneous tissue, and often muscle caused by prolonged periods of immobilization.
    a. Folliculitis
    b. Ulcers
    c. Pressure sores
    d. Abscesses

39. Your patient's nephew called EMS because, when he stopped in to check on his uncle as he does each day, he found him acting confused. He describes finding his uncle sitting in a very warm room, wearing several layers of clothing, but still shivering and cold to the touch. When there is no obvious environmental explanation, the paramedic should assume that hypothermia in the elderly is caused by:
    a. hypoglycemia.
    b. hypothyroidism.
    c. severe infection.
    d. adverse medication reaction.

40. Any older person can become a victim of abuse, with the most common abusers being:
    a. landlords.
    b. neighbors.
    c. friends.
    d. family members.

41. Herpes zoster is a highly contagious disease that can be spread:
    a. only to infants.
    b. by sexual contact.
    c. only to immunosuppressed patients.
    d. and once infected the victim will develop chickenpox.

42. Physiologic changes in the respiratory system that occur with aging include a decrease in airway cilia and diminished cough and gag reflexes. These changes increase the risk of:
    a. sustaining rib fractures with coughing.
    b. obtaining infectious pulmonary diseases.
    c. diminishing the inflammatory response.
    d. lung shrinkage (atrophy) and compliance.

43. During the physical examination, the older patient must be handled gently so as not to:
    a. cause any additional injury.
    b. confuse the patient with your specialized equipment.
    c. overwhelm the caretaker with your techniques.
    d. force the patient to receive unwanted care.

44. The son of an 86-year-old female called 9-1-1 when he discovered his mother was suddenly acting confused. She does not appear to be injured and when you question her she seems disoriented, but does deny having pain, dyspnea, or recent illness. When you assess her you find clear lung sounds, very warm skin, and normal range vital signs. Her SpO_2 is 98%, blood sugar is 102 mg/dL, and ECG is normal sinus rhythm. The son confirms no recent changes in medications and tells you that his mother does not go out much and but likes to watch TV. What do you suspect is the cause of her acute change in mental status?
    a. aspiration pneumonia
    b. vitamin deficiency
    c. urinary tract infection
    d. medication overdose

45. The most common complications that result from osteoporosis include hip fractures and:

    a. sepsis.

    b. vertebral fractures.

    c. deep vein thrombosis.

    d. pulmonary embolism.

46. Select the physiologic change that is abnormal or inconsistent with the aging process.

    a. developing dementia

    b. decreased brain mass

    c. altered pain perception

    d. conduction system abnormalities

47. When formulating a field impression for the patient with diseases of the nervous system, the paramedic should always consider _____ early on, as a potential cause of AMS.

    a. hypothyroidism

    b. hypothermia

    c. hypoglycemia

    d. dementia

48. The granddaughter of an 82-year-old male called 9-1-1 when he suddenly started having difficulty breathing. He is tachypneic, cyanotic, and diaphoretic. Your assessment reveals that the patient has a vascular access device in place because he has cancer and is receiving chemotherapy. Which of the following conditions is likely the cause of the acute onset of respiratory distress?

    a. embolism

    b. stroke

    c. infection

    d. sepsis

49. (Continuing with the previous question) You administer high-flow oxygen and continue care by providing:

    a. nitro, aspirin, and morphine.

    b. nitro, furosemide, and rapid transport.

    c. an IV fluid bolus, aspirin, and morphine.

    d. ventilatory support as needed and rapid transport.

50. _____ is the leading cause of new-onset blindness and end-stage renal disease in the elderly.

    a. Stroke

    b. Diabetes

    c. Hypertension

    d. Adverse medication reaction

Exam #45 Answer Form

	A	B	C	D			A	B	C	D
1.	❏	❏	❏	❏		26.	❏	❏	❏	❏
2.	❏	❏	❏	❏		27.	❏	❏	❏	❏
3.	❏	❏	❏	❏		28.	❏	❏	❏	❏
4.	❏	❏	❏	❏		29.	❏	❏	❏	❏
5.	❏	❏	❏	❏		30.	❏	❏	❏	❏
6.	❏	❏	❏	❏		31.	❏	❏	❏	❏
7.	❏	❏	❏	❏		32.	❏	❏	❏	❏
8.	❏	❏	❏	❏		33.	❏	❏	❏	❏
9.	❏	❏	❏	❏		34.	❏	❏	❏	❏
10.	❏	❏	❏	❏		35.	❏	❏	❏	❏
11.	❏	❏	❏	❏		36.	❏	❏	❏	❏
12.	❏	❏	❏	❏		37.	❏	❏	❏	❏
13.	❏	❏	❏	❏		38.	❏	❏	❏	❏
14.	❏	❏	❏	❏		39.	❏	❏	❏	❏
15.	❏	❏	❏	❏		40.	❏	❏	❏	❏
16.	❏	❏	❏	❏		41.	❏	❏	❏	❏
17.	❏	❏	❏	❏		42.	❏	❏	❏	❏
18.	❏	❏	❏	❏		43.	❏	❏	❏	❏
19.	❏	❏	❏	❏		44.	❏	❏	❏	❏
20.	❏	❏	❏	❏		45.	❏	❏	❏	❏
21.	❏	❏	❏	❏		46.	❏	❏	❏	❏
22.	❏	❏	❏	❏		47.	❏	❏	❏	❏
23.	❏	❏	❏	❏		48.	❏	❏	❏	❏
24.	❏	❏	❏	❏		49.	❏	❏	❏	❏
25.	❏	❏	❏	❏		50.	❏	❏	❏	❏

Patients with Special Challenges

1. You are assessing a patient who has a hearing impairment. The patient tells you that he lost part of his hearing when he had meningitis as a child. What type of deafness do you suspect he has?
   a. conductive
   b. pagetoid
   c. sensorineural
   d. paradoxic

2. One clue that a patient has a hearing impairment is a patient's inability to respond to verbal communication:
   a. even when you shout.
   b. even when you are extra nice.
   c. unless you are direct and forceful.
   d. unless you are making direct eye contact.

3. Which of the following actions is inappropriate when communicating with a deaf patient who reads lips?
   a. making eye contact prior to speaking
   b. speaking slowly with exaggerated lip movement
   c. speaking slowly without exaggerated lip movement
   d. speaking normally without exaggerated lip movement

4. Acute causes of visual impairment include:
   a. optic neuritis or neurosis.
   b. cataracts and glaucoma.
   c. strokes and CNS infections.
   d. diabetic retinopathy or MS.

5. Which of the following conditions may result in a transient blindness for the patient?
   a. acute head injury
   b. near drowning
   c. TIA
   d. acute hypothermia

6. Stuttering is a(n) _____ disorder, which is one of the four types of speech impairments.
   a. fluency
   b. language
   c. articulation
   d. voice production

7. The group of speech disorders that affects understanding of language, forming language, or expressing language is collectively referred to as:
   a. aphasia.
   b. dysarthria.
   c. fluency disorders.
   d. amentia.

8. When a patient is able to understand language and form speech patterns but is unable to express them properly because of physical impairment of the speech pathways, the condition is called:
   a. aphasia.
   b. dysarthria.
   c. fluency disorder.
   d. amentia.

9. Patients with a(n) _____ disorder may exhibit hoarseness, an inappropriate pitch, or an abnormal nasal resonance.
   a. fluency
   b. language
   c. articulation
   d. voice production

10. Which of the following is the most significant finding of a speech impairment for a patient in the emergency setting?
    a. hearing loss with an acute onset
    b. hearing loss with a slow onset
    c. a possible associated psychiatric disorder
    d. chronic slurred speech

11. Etiologies of obesity in humans have been associated with:
    a. a low metabolic rate.
    b. a high basal metabolic rate.
    c. decreased insulin production.
    d. the use of stimulant agents.

12. The patient you are assessing states that he is hearing voices, and his caretaker confirms that the patient has no concept of reality. Which of the following conditions does the patient have?
    a. hyalosis
    b. telepathy
    c. psychoses
    d. neuroses

13. When dealing with a patient who is experiencing hallucinations, the best management is to gently calm and reassure the patient that everything is all right using a technique called "_____ down."
    a. stand
    b. talk
    c. take
    d. show

14. Developmental disability refers to an impaired or insufficient development of
    a. speech.
    b. the brain.
    c. sensory function.
    d. motor coordination.

15. Most incidents of elder abuse and neglect:
    a. are fabricated.
    b. occur in the victim's home.
    c. are not detected until the victim dies.
    d. occur in long-term-care nursing facilities.

16. Psychoses are often associated with an underlying biochemical brain disease, such as:
    a. brainwashing.
    b. TIA.
    c. stroke.
    d. deficiency of neurotransmitters.

17. The more practical and current term for emotional or mental impairment is:
    a. maladaptive behavior.
    b. misunderstood manners.
    c. cerebrally challenged.
    d. comprehension deficit.

18. When treating a patient with a history of chronic arthritis, the paramedic may have to accommodate the patient in which of the following ways?
    a. Decreased range of motion may limit the physical exam.
    b. Speak slowly, because the patient may not understand everything you say.
    c. Paralysis of respiratory muscles may require ventilatory support.
    d. Obtaining a complete list of medications may be challenging and take more time than usual.

19. While performing a physical examination on a cancer patient, it would not be uncommon to find:
    a. transdermal pain medications.
    b. a medical alert tag with cancer information.
    c. spastic paralysis of extremities.
    d. multiple lesions on the torso.

20. When caring for a patient with cerebral palsy, the paramedic should anticipate that the patient:
    a. will be unable to ambulate.
    b. may require respiratory support.
    c. will understand everything you say and do.
    d. will typically have mild to severe retardation.

21. When caring for a patient with multiple sclerosis, it is not uncommon for the patient to be unpleasant, angry, hostile, or mean. This is normal and occurs because the patient:
    a. is seeking attention.
    b. is prone to mood disorders.
    c. has an expressive speech disorder.
    d. is taking medications that produce these emotions.

22. You are assessing a patient who is hypertensive and complaining of weakness. The patient has a history of myasthenia gravis, so you contact medical control before administering medication because:
    a. many common medications may worsen an exacerbation.
    b. the patient will probably refuse any treatment.
    c. these symptoms require treatment that is different from other patients.
    d. you may have to give the patient additional doses of her own medication.

23. A patient with spina bifida may require special attention to _____, which are often present with these patients.
    a. catheters
    b. open sores
    c. contractures
    d. muscle spasms

24. For the paramedic, the phrase "terminally ill" typically means that the patient has a condition that will result in his or her death within the next:
    a. 6–12 months.
    b. 12–18 months.
    c. 1–2 years.
    d. 5 years.

25. When caring for the patient with a terminal illness such as cancer, a major issue for the paramedic is:
    a. DNR status.
    b. which hospital to transport to.
    c. "end of life" priorities.
    d. living will status.

26. The patient you are caring for is competent but very sick. He states that he is going to refuse transport because he cannot afford to pay. To get him to go to the hospital, you should:
    a. tell him that the care will be free this time.
    b. tell him that his bill will be reduced.
    c. try to convince him that his health should be the first priority.
    d. tell him that he will die if he does not come with you.

27. If the patient described in question 26 still refuses to go to the hospital despite all of your efforts, what should you do next?
    a. Call the police and ask for restraints.
    b. Acknowledge that the competent patient has a right to refuse care.
    c. Force him to go anyway.
    d. Call medical control for consent to restrain the patient.

28. A neighbor of an elderly woman called 9-1-1 when she heard screaming coming from the elderly woman's home. Police arrived first and called EMS to come and evaluate the woman. The daughter of a 77-year-old woman is at the residence and states her mother has a hearing deficit and she has no other concerns. The patient appears frail, thin, unbathed, and smells of urine. What do you suspect is a major concern for the patient?
    a. The neighbor is a busybody.
    b. There are signs of neglect.
    c. She is being abused by her daughter.
    d. She is unable to hear what her daughter says.

29. Approximately 80% of hearing loss is related to the loss of _____ sounds.
    a. low-pitched
    b. high-pitched
    c. distant
    d. isolated

30. Which of the following is an example of a degenerative disease that causes chronic progressive vision loss?
    a. stroke
    b. multiple sclerosis
    c. congenital cataracts
    d. central nervous system infection

31. A nursing home resident requires transport for evaluation of a possible UTI. You observe that the patient's extremities are grossly contracted and that she will not fit on your stretcher like most patients. Which of the following would be appropriate for this patient?
    a. Only force the extremities to move enough to fit the patient on the stretcher.
    b. Refuse to transport the patient.
    c. Pad the contractures and use extra care during the move.
    d. Consider administering a muscle relaxant prior to moving the patient.

32. Transport of the patient with cystic fibrosis may require which of the following accommodations by the paramedic?
    a. respiratory support
    b. management of catheters
    c. padding of contractures
    d. medical consent by a caregiver

33. Cultural differences in patients vary. The paramedic should be aware of each patient's private/personal space needs. Assessment is best initiated by:
    a. examining the patient with no one else present.
    b. pointing to an area of the body before touching it.
    c. asking the patient's spouse for permission to examine.
    d. only performing the physical exam while in the ambulance.

34. When caring for patients with cultural backgrounds that differ from your own, the most important concept for the paramedic is that:
    a. language barriers will never compound cultural differences.
    b. cultural differences will limit the paramedic's judgment.
    c. patients with cultural differences have different needs and wants.
    d. culture-based preferences may conflict with a paramedic's learned medical practice.

35. You have just completed a call in which you transported a child from his home. While at the home, you observed conditions that make you suspect the child is being neglected. Which action by you is most appropriate in this case?

a. Do nothing at this time.

b. Make out a police report.

c. Notify the nurse you report to.

d. Keep good personal notes in case you get another call for the same residence.

36. When caring for an obese patient, additional manpower may be required as well as:

a. specialized assessment skills.

b. extra PPE for unique physical ailments.

c. specialized management skills.

d. appropriately sized diagnostic devices.

37. Responding to calls for patients that are living on the streets can be challenging for the paramedic because the patient:

a. is typically uncooperative and soiled.

b. has concurrent multiple health problems.

c. chooses transport to hospitals that will not accept patients who cannot pay.

d. is intoxicated and has poor hygiene.

38. When caring for a patient with a visual impairment, to lessen the patient's fear or anxiety the paramedic should:

a. describe everything she is going to do before actually doing it.

b. not ask the patient about her visual impairment.

c. leave her leader dogs at the residence, because the ambulance is unsafe.

d. avoid explaining what care may be in store for her.

39. Which of the following services provides palliative and support services under medical supervision for the terminally ill patient?

a. HMOs

b. hospice programs

c. church organizations

d. long-term-care nursing facilities

40. When the paramedic is assessing a patient with autism who has a significant illness or injury, she should consider that the patient:

a. may not exhibit the normal pain response.

b. will never allow a stranger to physically assess them.

c. can only be transported with someone who he/she is familiar with.

d. must be transported to a facility equipped for developmentally delayed patients.

41. Which of the following situations with airway devices in the home would EMS most likely be called to assist?

a. discontinued use

b. obstructed tubing

c. replacing existing tubing

d. routine suctioning

42 Special accommodations for the care of a patient with a preexisting quadriplegia include:

a. involving the alert and oriented patient in any decisions regarding movement and transport.

b. obtaining consent for treatment from the patient's caregiver.

c. full spinal immobilization.

d. complete neurologic assessment and documentation.

43. Which of the following patients is most likely to develop hyperactivity or become dangerous while in the care of EMS?

a. psychotic person

b. neurotic person

c. homeless person

d. financially impaired person

44. Obesity is defined as being _____ above ideal body weight.

a. 5–10%

b. 10–20%

c. 20–30%

d. 30–40%

45. Hospice care emphasizes comfort measures and counseling to provide for physical, spiritual, social, and _____ needs.

a. financial

b. long-distance

c. long-term

d. economic

46. Which of the following is considered noninvasive ventilation?

a. ETT

b. EOA

c. BiPAP

d. PEEP

47. A home monitoring device that detects changes in thoracic or abdominal movement and heart rate is called a(n):

a. apnea monitor.

b. nebulizer.

c. ventilator.

d. pulmonary function meter.

48. Classic signs and symptoms of myasthenia gravis include:
    a. chest pain and shortness of breath.
    b. drooping eyelids and difficulty swallowing.
    c. headache and hypertension.
    d. memory loss and cognitive dysfunction.

49. In most cases, prehospital care of the patient with myasthenia gravis will include:
    a. oxygen and nitroglycerin.
    b. supportive care and transport.
    c. oxygen and Lopressor.
    d. reorientation to time and place.

50. When caring for a patient with a previous head injury that resulted in a permanent cognitive deficit, which of the following pieces of information from the family or caretaker is the most significant to you?
    a. The patient also has motor and neurologic deficits.
    b. The patient functions in the upper range of retardation.
    c. There has been a recent change in the patient's behavior.
    d. The patient is not legally able to sign for treatment or billing.

51. The primary reasons patients are sent home with urinary catheters include:
    a. trauma and paralysis.
    b. UTI and urinary retention.
    c. immobilization and sedation.
    d. pregnancy and postoperative care.

52. When a patient in the home care setting experiences failure of a GU device, the paramedic is likely to find which problem associated with the failure of that device during her assessment?
    a. hematuria
    b. dark urine
    c. leaking catheter
    d. full bladder bag

53. The terminally ill patient has several rights, one of which includes the right to:
    a. free institutional care.
    b. home health care with charge.
    c. choose the place to die and time of death.
    d. unlimited resources for pain management.

54. There are _____ stages a dying person typically goes through, much like the stages in the grieving process following a death.
    a. four
    b. five
    c. six
    d. seven

55. During the first stage of dying, a person experiences "shock and disbelief" and moves through several stages before the final stage of acceptance. This first stage can take moments or months before moving on to the second stage, which is:
    a. bargaining.
    b. anger.
    c. depression.
    d. detachment.

56. The general term for an operation in which an artificial opening in the body is formed is:
    a. incisure.
    b. ostomy.
    c. ectomy.
    d. intomy.

57. When assessing a patient in the home care setting who receives dialysis regularly, which of the following devices would you expect to find?
    a. VAD
    b. feeding tube
    c. pulmonary function meter
    d. suprapubic catheter

58. A home health aide has called you to transport a home resident with chronic MS who has a urostomy and a feeding tube. The patient is tachypneic, febrile, and tachycardic. The aide tells you the urine output is decreased and the feeding schedule has been normal. Which of the following complications do you suspect first?
    a. local infection of the urostomy
    b. local infection of the feeding tube
    c. systemic infection
    d. respiratory infection

59. The paramedic should respectfully interact with family members of the home care patient when present, because:
    a. they often know more about the patient's special needs than anyone else.
    b. they have the patient's advanced directives.
    c. most often they will not let the patient speak for herself.
    d. you are required to do so.

60. You have been called to a residence for a respiratory distress call. Upon arrival, the family tells you that the patient does not want to be transported because the patient has an end-stage terminal illness. They allow you in to assess, but state, "Hospice is on the way and we made a mistake by calling EMS." What would be appropriate management for this patient?
    a. Wait for hospice to arrive and then leave.
    b. Insist to the family that the patient should be transported.
    c. Call for police assistance.
    d. Offer assistance to the patient and then insist on transport.

Exam #46 Answer Form

	A	B	C	D			A	B	C	D
1.	❑	❑	❑	❑		31.	❑	❑	❑	❑
2.	❑	❑	❑	❑		32.	❑	❑	❑	❑
3.	❑	❑	❑	❑		33.	❑	❑	❑	❑
4.	❑	❑	❑	❑		34.	❑	❑	❑	❑
5.	❑	❑	❑	❑		35.	❑	❑	❑	❑
6.	❑	❑	❑	❑		36.	❑	❑	❑	❑
7.	❑	❑	❑	❑		37.	❑	❑	❑	❑
8.	❑	❑	❑	❑		38.	❑	❑	❑	❑
9.	❑	❑	❑	❑		39.	❑	❑	❑	❑
10.	❑	❑	❑	❑		40.	❑	❑	❑	❑
11.	❑	❑	❑	❑		41.	❑	❑	❑	❑
12.	❑	❑	❑	❑		42.	❑	❑	❑	❑
13.	❑	❑	❑	❑		43.	❑	❑	❑	❑
14.	❑	❑	❑	❑		44.	❑	❑	❑	❑
15.	❑	❑	❑	❑		45.	❑	❑	❑	❑
16.	❑	❑	❑	❑		46.	❑	❑	❑	❑
17.	❑	❑	❑	❑		47.	❑	❑	❑	❑
18.	❑	❑	❑	❑		48.	❑	❑	❑	❑
19.	❑	❑	❑	❑		49.	❑	❑	❑	❑
20.	❑	❑	❑	❑		50.	❑	❑	❑	❑
21.	❑	❑	❑	❑		51.	❑	❑	❑	❑
22.	❑	❑	❑	❑		52.	❑	❑	❑	❑
23.	❑	❑	❑	❑		53.	❑	❑	❑	❑
24.	❑	❑	❑	❑		54.	❑	❑	❑	❑
25.	❑	❑	❑	❑		55.	❑	❑	❑	❑
26.	❑	❑	❑	❑		56.	❑	❑	❑	❑
27.	❑	❑	❑	❑		57.	❑	❑	❑	❑
28.	❑	❑	❑	❑		58.	❑	❑	❑	❑
29.	❑	❑	❑	❑		59.	❑	❑	❑	❑
30.	❑	❑	❑	❑		60.	❑	❑	❑	❑

Principles of Safety: Operating an Ambulance and Air Medical

1. _____ standards are the minimum standards for ambulance operations and are not considered the "gold standards."
   a. National
   b. State
   c. Local
   d. Regional

2. The U.S. General Services Administration's Automotive Commodity Center issues the federal regulations specifying:
   a. the required response times for high-rise buildings.
   b. BLS equipment that is mandatory on all ambulances.
   c. ALS equipment that is required on ambulances.
   d. ambulance design and manufacturing requirements.

3. Documented check sheets for ambulances are mandatory both for good practice and:
   a. for OSHA.
   b. for NIOSH.
   c. as a risk management tool.
   d. for professional services only.

4. You are transporting your partner and a patient when another vehicle crashes into your ambulance at an intersection. As the driver of the ambulance you must:
   a. continue to the ED if the patient is critical or unstable.
   b. continue, but notify the police through the dispatcher.
   c. stop to assess damage, render aid, and exchange information.
   d. stop to assess damage; if there is none, continue to the ED.

5. Special considerations for EMS providers who carry medications on their vehicles include:
   a. routinely checking expiration dates.
   b. having the junior EMS provider restock.
   c. getting the medical director to authorize medication purchases.
   d. billing the patients to recoup the cost of the medications.

6. OSHA requires that the ambulance be properly disinfected:
   a. once every 24 hours.
   b. on a weekly basis, even if there were no transports that week.
   c. after the transport of any patient with a potentially communicable disease.
   d. after the transport of any patient.

7. Each service is required, by OSHA or the state equivalent of OSHA, to have an exposure control plan that specifies:
   a. which mask to place on a patient with TB.
   b. cleaning requirements.
   c. when to open vents in the ambulance.
   d. how to transfer potentially communicable patients.

8. The strategy used by an EMS agency to maneuver its ambulances and crews in an effort to reduce response times is referred to as:
   a. line of response.
   b. ambulance deployment.
   c. ambulance stratagem.
   d. zoning.

9. _____ is the ability to muster additional crews, should all the regularly staffed ambulances be on calls or a multiple casualty incident overtaxes the system's resources.
   a. Standards of reliability
   b. System status management
   c. Peak-load backup
   d. Reserve capacity

10. A computerized personnel and ambulance deployment system designed to meet service demands with fewer resources and to ensure appropriate response time and vehicle locations is called:
   a. standards of reliability.
   b. system status management.
   c. peak-load backup.
   d. reserve capacity.

11. Appropriate response time has to be determined by each community based on:
   a. its resources.
   b. ACLS standards.
   c. American Heart Association standards.
   d. national standards.

12. You need to clean equipment that became contaminated on your last call. The product you are using to clean equipment states on the label that it will kill most bacteria, some viruses, and some fungi, but not *Mycobacterium tuberculosis* or bacterial spores. This level of cleaning is:
   a. sterilization.
   b. low-level disinfection.
   c. high-level disinfection.
   d. intermediate-level disinfection.

13. The process that kills all forms of microbial life on medical instruments is:
   a. sterilization.
   b. low-level cleaning.
   c. high-level disinfection.
   d. intermediate-level disinfection.

14. One concept that appears in most laws in statutes that deal with emergency vehicle operation is the concept of:
   a. *res ipsa loquitur.*
   b. negligence.
   c. due regard.
   d. causation.

15. The language described in the concept in question 14 sets up a _____ standard for the operator of an emergency vehicle than for any other driver on the road.
   a. safer
   b. higher
   c. lower
   d. liberal

16. Typical state laws allow the operator of an ambulance, while in emergency operation, to be exempt from:
   a. passing over railroad crossings with the gates down.
   b. passing a school bus operator with the blinking red lights on.
   c. the posted parking regulations.
   d. impeding a U.S. mail carrier's vehicle.

17. Studies have shown that most other motorists do not see or hear your ambulance until it is within _____ feet of their vehicles.
   a. 10–25
   b. 25–50
   c. 50–100
   d. 100–200

18. Air medical transport has been requested to the scene of a serious MVC with multiple patients. A minivan with a family slid off the road and struck a tree on a curve at night. The driver and front seat passenger are dead. A second-row passenger in his early 20s has a head injury with altered mental status. One passenger who was ejected is in cardiac arrest, with CPR in progress. A toddler is in a car seat and appears uninjured and also there is a 12-year-old with a possible fractured forearm and ankle. Which patient has the highest priority for air medical transport?
   a. toddler
   b. cardiac arrest
   c. head injury with AMS
   d. 12-year-old with extremity injuries

19. Whenever the ambulance is on the road, day or night, the headlights should be turned on to:
   a. increase its visibility.
   b. comply with insurance stipulations.
   c. receive lower insurance premiums.
   d. annoy other motorists.

20. When your ambulance is the first to arrive at the scene of a highway incident and no potential hazards are apparent, you should park your emergency vehicle at least _____ the wreckage.
    a. 50 feet in front of
    b. 100 feet in front of
    c. 50 feet behind
    d. 100 feet behind

21. In 1969, R. Adams Cowley, MD, convinced the _____ state legislature to fund the first statewide state police "medevac" program.
    a. New York
    b. California
    c. Florida
    d. Maryland

22. Each corner of the ambulance should have flashers that are large and blinking in tandem or unison to help oncoming vehicles:
    a. identify the name of the EMS service.
    b. identify the location and size of the ambulance.
    c. know where the EMS personnel are going to place the cones.
    d. anticipate the placement of flares.

23. While working at the scene of a highway incident, beware that the _____ of the ambulance often obstruct(s) the view of the warning lights to other motorists.
    a. lighted flares
    b. reflector tape
    c. open rear doors
    d. inexperienced driver

24. Fixed-wing aircraft are used as the primary means of emergency transport in:
    a. remote regions, such as parts of Alaska.
    b. missions under 50 miles from a hospital facility.
    c. search and rescue missions.
    d. access to remote areas.

25. Special consideration for aeromedical transport includes the need to intubate the patient prior to flight because of:
    a. the pressure changes during ascent and decent.
    b. limited treatment area in the aircraft.
    c. the temperature changes during the flight.
    d. the various altitudes that the helicopter flies.

26. A helicopter requires a landing zone of approximately _____ feet on relatively level ground.
    a. 50 × 50
    b. 50 × 100
    c. 100 × 100
    d. 100 × 200

27. Which of the following is a special treatment consideration if a patient is going to be transported by helicopter?
    a. Convert IV bags to pressure infuser bags.
    b. Stay clear of the tail rotor wash only when moving the patient.
    c. Allow the flight crew to direct and maintain a safe landing zone.
    d. Keep all traffic and vehicles 100 feet or more from the helicopter.

28. The Commission of Accreditation of Air Medical Services (CAAMS) was developed as a voluntary process for aeromedical services to:
    a. enforce the FAA standards for air travel.
    b. enforce standards for worker safety.
    c. help communities obtain funding for aeromedical programs.
    d. strengthen the safety of the aviation transport environment.

29. One major disadvantage of aeromedical evacuation is:
    a. cabin size.
    b. the need for special fuel.
    c. rapid access to remote areas.
    d. the need for technical training.

30. You and your partner are preparing your ambulance to go back into service after completing a call. The steps you are taking for the next response are:
    a. required by OSHA.
    b. key to the safety and health of you and your crew.
    c. necessary for the safety and health of your patient.
    d. vital for the safety and health of you, your crew, and the patient.

Exam #47 Answer Form

	A	B	C	D		A	B	C	D
1.	❏	❏	❏	❏	16.	❏	❏	❏	❏
2.	❏	❏	❏	❏	17.	❏	❏	❏	❏
3.	❏	❏	❏	❏	18.	❏	❏	❏	❏
4.	❏	❏	❏	❏	19.	❏	❏	❏	❏
5.	❏	❏	❏	❏	20.	❏	❏	❏	❏
6.	❏	❏	❏	❏	21.	❏	❏	❏	❏
7.	❏	❏	❏	❏	22.	❏	❏	❏	❏
8.	❏	❏	❏	❏	23.	❏	❏	❏	❏
9.	❏	❏	❏	❏	24.	❏	❏	❏	❏
10.	❏	❏	❏	❏	25.	❏	❏	❏	❏
11.	❏	❏	❏	❏	26.	❏	❏	❏	❏
12.	❏	❏	❏	❏	27.	❏	❏	❏	❏
13.	❏	❏	❏	❏	28.	❏	❏	❏	❏
14.	❏	❏	❏	❏	29.	❏	❏	❏	❏
15.	❏	❏	❏	❏	30.	❏	❏	❏	❏

CHAPTER

Incident Management, Multiple Casualty Incidents

1. An MCI is a _____, which results in casualties severely burdening or exceeding the normal EMS resources of an agency in whose area the event occurs.
   a. mass casualty incident
   b. multiple casualty incident
   c. many citizens injured
   d. mixed community incident

2. When you are the first to arrive at the scene of an MCI, the first size-up radio report to the dispatcher is very important and should include:
   a. specific location of the incident.
   b. location of the triage sector.
   c. the time of arrival.
   d. the exact number of patients.

3. A _____ incident is one where the patients need rescue or extrication to gain access to them.
   a. dangerous
   b. safe
   c. continued
   d. closed

4. Though originally developed for fire services, the incident command system (ICS) has been adopted to serve all emergency response disciplines and consists of procedures for controlling:
   a. the media.
   b. equipment and facilities.
   c. critical incident stress.
   d. post-incident stress.

5. ICS is designed to begin developing from the time an incident occurs until:
   a. all victims are safely away from the incident.
   b. the fire or hazard is extinguished or contained.
   c. the requirement for management and operations no longer exists.
   d. all emergency medical responders are safely away.

6. _____ is the functional component of an IMS, which is responsible for obtaining information about the use of technical specialists.
   a. Operations
   b. Planning
   c. Logistics
   d. Finance

7. A key component of ICS is _____, which is the desired number of subordinates that one supervisor can manage effectively at an incident.
   a. consolidated action plan
   b. span of control
   c. singular command
   d. unified command

8. The incident commander is the individual with overall responsibility for managing the incident, which includes:
   a. prioritizing training efforts.
   b. assessing overhaul costs.
   c. designating hospital bed priorities.
   d. developing the incident action plan.

9. While working in an MCI, the use of bibs and vests serves a value in:
   a. making it easy to identify the command officers.
   b. making the command officers safer, with better visibility.
   c. keeping order and avoiding chaos.
   d. identifying the priority of the patients.

10. It is not uncommon for physicians and nurses to stop at the scene of an MCI and offer assistance. Besides utilizing them in the treatment sector, what other area may be appropriate for their expertise?
    a. safety
    b. communications
    c. triage
    d. rescue

11. A very useful aspect to the use of triage tags at an MCI is that:
    a. patients can fill them out themselves.
    b. they are so easy to use.
    c. they are inexpensive.
    d. they help to eliminate the need to reassess each patient over and over again.

12. Performing a post-incident critique is commonly done after an MCI because:
    a. it serves the same function as a CISD.
    b. every incident has something to teach.
    c. it may involve media coverage.
    d. commanders can critique without the fear of offending anyone.

13. Because there may be units from many different jurisdictions at an MCI, it is easier to use simple sector titles based on:
    a. preference of the incident commander.
    b. geographic location.
    c. available resources.
    d. the function they serve.

14. What is the role of the EMS command or medical command at an MCI?
    a. to be involved in drilling
    b. to be involved in planning and education
    c. to work cooperatively with other emergency commanders
    d. to establish a command post and designate another to stay there

15. An incident involving a residential house fire where all the patients are out on the front lawn of the home is an example of a(n) _____ incident.
    a. open
    b. closed
    c. continuing
    d. dangerous

16. The _____ section at an MCI is responsible for providing services and materials, such as the communications unit, medical unit, or food unit, for the incident.
    a. operations
    b. planning
    c. logistics
    d. command

17. When all of the involved agencies at an MCI contribute to the command process by determining the overall goals and objects, and use joint planning for tactical activities, they are working under:
    a. OHSA CFR 29.
    b. NFPA standard 1500.
    c. singular command.
    d. unified command.

18. During an MCI, a consolidated action plan should be developed at the:
    a. dispatch center.
    b. unified command post.
    c. first arriving emergency vehicle.
    d. discretion of the incident commander.

19. START is an acronym for:
    a. simple triage and rapid transport.
    b. standardized triage on rapid timetable.
    c. short triage, alert by radio, and treat.
    d. stage, triage, assess, rate, and transport.

20. At an MCI, triage is done on all patients in an effort to assure that:
    a. the most serious patients are treated and transported first.
    b. all the critical patients go to the best hospitals.
    c. the most important patients get the ALS care.
    d. all low-priority patients receive a different standard of care.

21. One of the most helpful tips that can smooth out operations at an MCI is:
    a. to never let the driver, keys, or stretcher get separated from their ambulance.
    b. to use multiple radios with multiple channels to avoid confusion at the scene.
    c. to drive directly into the incident and look around to see where you are needed.
    d. to talk to the media and keep them advised of the evolving events.

22. Your unit is the first to arrive at the scene where several employees are outside of a building. They have red and watery eyes and are coughing. They tell you that another employee is inside and trapped under a container containing a hazardous material. You complete a scene size-up, notify dispatch, and:
    a. create a safe perimeter.
    b. attempt to contain the substance involved.
    c. go inside to evaluate the patient who is trapped.
    d. rapidly get any victims who can walk out of the area.

23. When working at the scene of a large incident with numerous patients and with enough resources, the incident commander can utilize up to four components, which include:
    a. fire, police, media, and mutual aid.
    b. treatment, transport, logistics, and finance.
    c. operations, planning, logistics, and finance.
    d. operations, logistics, treatment, and transport.

24. EMS and fire are dispatched for a fire alarm at a produce warehouse. When you arrive, there is a crowd standing outside the building and the police and fire departments are on the scene. The warehouse manager reports that a flood light over the dock started smoking and set off the fire alarm. An elementary class on a field trip visiting the warehouse became panicked by the alarm and a few of the students were injured while exiting the building. You grab your triage tags and begin to get a count of the number of patients, and you start sorting them to determine which ones will need immediate emergency care. After an initial triage, which of the following patients can be considered a P-3, green, or categorized with minor injuries?
    a. 8-year-old female having difficulty breathing from an asthma attack
    b. 9-year-old female complaining of headache, nausea, and vomiting
    c. 44-year-old female with a nosebleed and a possible fractured nose
    d. 28-year-old female with a swollen and deformed ankle and abrasions on both hands

25. (Continuing with the previous question) Which patient is most in need of immediate emergency care?
    a. 8-year-old female with dyspnea due to asthma
    b. 9-year-old female complaining of headache, nausea, and vomiting
    c. 44-year-old female with a nosebleed and a possible fractured nose
    d. 28-year-old male with a swollen and deformed ankle and abrasions on both hands

Exam #48 Answer Form

	A	B	C	D		A	B	C	D
1.	❏	❏	❏	❏	14.	❏	❏	❏	❏
2.	❏	❏	❏	❏	15.	❏	❏	❏	❏
3.	❏	❏	❏	❏	16.	❏	❏	❏	❏
4.	❏	❏	❏	❏	17.	❏	❏	❏	❏
5.	❏	❏	❏	❏	18.	❏	❏	❏	❏
6.	❏	❏	❏	❏	19.	❏	❏	❏	❏
7.	❏	❏	❏	❏	20.	❏	❏	❏	❏
8.	❏	❏	❏	❏	21.	❏	❏	❏	❏
9.	❏	❏	❏	❏	22.	❏	❏	❏	❏
10.	❏	❏	❏	❏	23.	❏	❏	❏	❏
11.	❏	❏	❏	❏	24.	❏	❏	❏	❏
12.	❏	❏	❏	❏	25.	❏	❏	❏	❏
13.	❏	❏	❏	❏					

CHAPTER

49

Vehicle Extrication

1. The level of rescue training that all paramedics should be trained in is the _____ level.
   a. technical
   b. command
   c. awareness
   d. operations

2. What should set the priority of each rescue?
   a. The time police are able to hold back traffic.
   b. The abilities of the heavy rescue team.
   c. The patient's medical condition.
   d. The EMS providers' need to return to service.

3. It is essential that the paramedic know:
   a. when to enter an unstable situation.
   b. when it is or is not safe to gain access.
   c. how to stabilize a toxic atmosphere.
   d. how to enter a below-grade rescue.

4. What minimal personal protective equipment (PPE) should be immediately available to paramedics in a rescue situation?
   a. helmets and eye protection
   b. turnout gear and lights
   c. SCBA
   d. back-country survival gear

5. Why are construction hard hats inappropriate for rescue work?
   a. Their duckbill brim is removable.
   b. They do not withstand severe impact.
   c. They are not warm enough.
   d. They have no ANSI rating.

6. Eye protection should be approved by:
   a. ANSI.
   b. EPA.
   c. NFPA.
   d. EDNA.

7. Eye protection is best provided by:
   a. regular glasses.
   b. a fire helmet face shield.
   c. contact lenses.
   d. industrial safety glasses.

8. The best gloves for rescue work performed by paramedics are:
   a. latex.
   b. rubber.
   c. leather work gloves.
   d. heavy gauntlet-style firefighting gloves.

9. Nomex®, PBI®, or flame-retardant cotton may be utilized by EMS providers as part of their turnout gear because these materials:
   a. provide limited flash protection.
   b. provide complete flash protection.
   c. are inexpensive and readily available.
   d. provide protection against sharp, jagged metal or glass.

10. What is the best type of blanket to use for patient protection from heat and glass dust?
    a. inexpensive vinyl tarps
    b. aluminized rescue blankets
    c. wool blankets
    d. plastic sheeting

11. What is the best choice to use for shielding the patient from sharp-edged objects or glass during a rescue?
    a. plastic sheeting
    b. sheets
    c. backboards
    d. vinyl tarps

12. What type of respiratory protection is considered adequate for most rescues?
    a. N-95
    b. HEPA mask
    c. surgical mask
    d. non-rebreather mask

13. Another name for written safety procedures used by rescue teams is:
    a. protocols.
    b. regulations.
    c. standard operating procedures (SOPs).
    d. bylaws.

14. The first three phases of a rescue operation are:
    a. hazard control, disentanglement, and gaining access.
    b. hazard control, gaining access, and medical treatment.
    c. arrival and size-up, gaining access, and disentanglement.
    d. arrival and size-up, hazard control, and gaining access.

15. The person responsible for making the "go/no-go" decision for a rescue operation is called the:
    a. incident commander.
    b. lead medic.
    c. team leader.
    d. safety officer.

16. For the patient who is entrapped for a considerable amount of time, the paramedic must be prepared to:
    a. rise above swift running waters.
    b. provide appropriate psychological support.
    c. overcome life-threatening atmospheres.
    d. develop the plan for, and lead in, the disentanglement.

17. What is the value of a rescue plan?
    a. It describes how to respond to every incident.
    b. It improves personnel safety and operational success.
    c. Fewer rescuers are needed at incidents.
    d. The location to which units respond is specified.

18. Upon arrival at the rescue incident, the EMS crew should:
    a. conduct a scene size-up.
    b. determine the hospital destination.
    c. disentangle the patient.
    d. set out flares on the roadway.

19. Examples of on-scene hazards that need to be controlled by the paramedic upon arrival at the scene include:
    a. a car fire.
    b. chemical spills.
    c. creating a safe perimeter.
    d. downed electrical wires.

20. _____ in an example of a safety precaution to be taken at every rescue.
    a. Utilizing triage tags
    b. Establishing EMS command
    c. Wearing the appropriate PPE
    d. Performing an initial assessment on each patient

21. When a vehicle rescue situation involves a hidden patient, possibly from an ejection, the paramedic should consider requesting:
    a. a surgeon to the scene.
    b. a helicopter to the scene.
    c. an on-scene search-and-rescue specialist.
    d. medical control to the scene.

22. In what phase of a rescue is the first patient contact typically made by EMS?
    a. after gaining access
    b. arrival and size-up
    c. after hazard control
    d. after disentanglement

23. Paramedics should not enter an area to provide patient care unless they are:
    a. trained in all aspects of rescue.
    b. authorized by medical control to do so.
    c. protected from hazards with PPE.
    d. responding in a two-medic unit.

24. The rescue term that means to remove the debris or parts of the vehicle from around the patient(s) so the patient may be freed for removal is:
    a. evacuation.
    b. extrication.
    c. disentanglement.
    d. gaining access.

25. Typically the most technical and time-consuming part of a rescue is the _____ phase.
    a. hazard control
    b. extrication
    c. disentanglement
    d. removal

26. The patient packaging should take into consideration the:
    a. distance the ambulance will travel to the hospital.
    b. means of egress.
    c. duration of disentanglement.
    d. age of the patient.

27. What is the greatest hazard when working a highway operation?
   a. broken glass
   b. crowds
   c. fire hazards
   d. traffic

28. When working at the scene of a highway rescue that involves a vehicle with an alternative fuel source, one potential danger is:
   a. the risk of fire or explosion.
   b. not being able to turn off the vehicle.
   c. not being able to stabilize the vehicle.
   d. not being able to disconnect the battery.

29. The ambulance loading area at a highway operation should:
   a. be used as a point to congregate.
   b. not be directly exposed to traffic.
   c. rely on the rear blinking lights to stop cars.
   d. be off the side of the road.

30. When parked at the scene of a highway operation, the ambulance should:
   a. shut off all the lights.
   b. turn on only a minimum of warning lights.
   c. keep on the alternating headlights.
   d. turn on all the emergency lights.

31. When using flares at a highway operation, they should:
   a. direct the flow of traffic away from emergency workers.
   b. only be placed by law enforcement personnel.
   c. be used when the ground is wet.
   d. not be used if there is snow on the road.

32. Why should the paramedic be especially concerned when a vehicle has gone off the road into tall grass?
   a. The potential for a fire hazard is increased.
   b. It will be difficult to find the vehicle.
   c. The potential for an electric hazard is greater.
   d. Patients may wander away from the scene.

33. How can an energy-absorbing bumper be a hazard to EMS personnel?
   a. The fluid they leak is highly toxic.
   b. If loaded, they may release when unexpected.
   c. They can hide the true damage to the vehicle.
   d. They have been known to explode.

34. A supplemental restraint system may be a potential hazard to rescue personnel because:
   a. the straps can get in the way.
   b. the straps are difficult to cut.
   c. it can be difficult to remove from the patient.
   d. it can inflate when not expected.

35. If, upon arrival at the scene of a car crash, the vehicle is on its side, off the road on an embankment, it will be necessary to rapidly:
   a. gain access.
   b. stabilize the vehicle.
   c. disentangle the patient.
   d. extricate the patient.

36. After assuring that the vehicle's ignition has been turned off, what can the paramedic do to prepare to gain access?
   a. Tell the patient to try to crawl out.
   b. Attempt to climb up on the car and open the door.
   c. Stabilize the vehicle with cribbing.
   d. Break both the front and rear windows.

37. The part of an auto's anatomy that separates the engine compartment from the occupant compartment is called the:
   a. rocker panel.
   b. firewall.
   c. Nader pin.
   d. "A" post.

38. The reason why the doors do not fly open when a car is involved in a collision is because of the:
   a. firewall.
   b. tempered glass.
   c. Nader pin.
   d. roof support posts.

39. The windshield in vehicles is made of _____ glass.
   a. unbreakable
   b. safety
   c. tempered
   d. plastic

40. The easiest way to break the _____ glass in the rear window is with a _____ object.
   a. tempered; sharp
   b. safety; sharp
   c. tempered; blunt
   d. safety; blunt

41. Unless the hydraulic spreader is used for accessing a crushed car door, the _____ must be disengaged prior to manually prying the door open.
    a. key
    b. door reinforcement bar
    c. battery cable
    d. Nader pin

42. The first step in accessing a car with a crushed door that has no safety hazards and is stabilized is to:
    a. break the glass in the rear window.
    b. remove the Nader pin.
    c. remove the roof.
    d. try to open all four doors first.

43. After taking the first step as described in the previous question, the paramedic should next consider the need to:
    a. cut off the door at the hinges.
    b. pull the steering wheel through the windshield.
    c. gain access through the window farthest away from the patient.
    d. remove the roof of the vehicle.

44. The area at a collision scene where the rescue takes place is called the:
    a. outer circle.
    b. inner circle.
    c. command post.
    d. hot zone.

45. A vehicle went off the road down a steep slope in good weather. The rescuers are capable of walking down and back up without using their hands to hold on to anything. This type of rescue approach is called:
    a. high angle.
    b. low angle.
    c. uneven terrain.
    d. limited access terrain.

46. You have extricated a patient from her vehicle and packaged her on a long backboard. You will need to transport her over rough terrain. What type of stretcher should be used?
    a. folding
    b. Stokes®
    c. wheeled
    d. limited access

47. The strongest basket stretchers are made of:
    a. wire and tubular metal.
    b. aluminum and plastic.
    c. enduro-plastic.
    d. polycarbonate.

48. A team of rescuers to carry a patient on a Stokes® over rough terrain consists of _____ rescuers and extra teams if the personnel are available.
    a. four
    b. five
    c. six
    d. eight

49. At the scene of a motor vehicle crash that went off the road down a very steep embankment, the fire department is close to freeing the patient from his vehicle. Even though you may not be trained in high-angle rescue, there will be a need for you to assist in the rescue by:
    a. hauling on the lines as instructed.
    b. rappelling down to the patient.
    c. setting up the rigging.
    d. coiling the rope.

50. A patient, whose vehicle went over a cliff, and is still alive and will need a lengthy litter carryout. This patient could benefit from a paramedic being trained to:
    a. cleanse wounds.
    b. reposition dislocations.
    c. manage hyperthermia.
    d. assess a 12-lead ECG.

Exam #49 Answer Form

	A	B	C	D			A	B	C	D
1.	❏	❏	❏	❏		26.	❏	❏	❏	❏
2.	❏	❏	❏	❏		27.	❏	❏	❏	❏
3.	❏	❏	❏	❏		28.	❏	❏	❏	❏
4.	❏	❏	❏	❏		29.	❏	❏	❏	❏
5.	❏	❏	❏	❏		30.	❏	❏	❏	❏
6.	❏	❏	❏	❏		31.	❏	❏	❏	❏
7.	❏	❏	❏	❏		32.	❏	❏	❏	❏
8.	❏	❏	❏	❏		33.	❏	❏	❏	❏
9.	❏	❏	❏	❏		34.	❏	❏	❏	❏
10.	❏	❏	❏	❏		35.	❏	❏	❏	❏
11.	❏	❏	❏	❏		36.	❏	❏	❏	❏
12.	❏	❏	❏	❏		37.	❏	❏	❏	❏
13.	❏	❏	❏	❏		38.	❏	❏	❏	❏
14.	❏	❏	❏	❏		39.	❏	❏	❏	❏
15.	❏	❏	❏	❏		40.	❏	❏	❏	❏
16.	❏	❏	❏	❏		41.	❏	❏	❏	❏
17.	❏	❏	❏	❏		42.	❏	❏	❏	❏
18.	❏	❏	❏	❏		43.	❏	❏	❏	❏
19.	❏	❏	❏	❏		44.	❏	❏	❏	❏
20.	❏	❏	❏	❏		45.	❏	❏	❏	❏
21.	❏	❏	❏	❏		46.	❏	❏	❏	❏
22.	❏	❏	❏	❏		47.	❏	❏	❏	❏
23.	❏	❏	❏	❏		48.	❏	❏	❏	❏
24.	❏	❏	❏	❏		49.	❏	❏	❏	❏
25.	❏	❏	❏	❏		50.	❏	❏	❏	❏

CHAPTER

50

Hazardous Material Awareness

1. The first standard to guide hazardous material (hazmat) operations specifically for EMS workers was NFPA:
   a. 472.
   b. 473.
   c. 704.
   d. 1500.

2. NFPA standard _____ established a system of placarding and labeling fixed facilities for hazardous materials.
   a. 472
   b. 473
   c. 704
   d. 1500

3. _____ is the minimal level of hazmat training at which the responder can perform risk assessment procedures and conduct basic control, containment, and confinement operations.
   a. First responder awareness
   b. First responder operations
   c. Hazardous material technician
   d. Hazardous material specialist

4. The role of the paramedic at the scene of a hazmat incident is determined by:
   a. the safety officer.
   b. the type of chemical involved.
   c. how many patients are contaminated.
   d. the level of training the paramedic has and the local hazmat plan.

5. There are _____ levels of hazmat training required by the Occupational Safety and Health Administration (OSHA) regulations.
   a. four
   b. five
   c. six
   d. ten

6. The _____ provides written information about the name of substances, UN numbers, placard facsimiles, emergency action guides, and evacuation and isolation information.
   a. *Emergency Response Guidebook*
   b. MSDS
   c. CHEMTREC
   d. bill of lading

7. DOT placards classify gases into the following categories: corrosive, flammable, poison A, and:
   a. poison B.
   b. combustible.
   c. noncorrosive.
   d. nonflammable.

8. _____ are used throughout the industry as a means of identifying chemicals and complying with the employee's Right to Know.
   a. Shipping papers
   b. Bills of lading
   c. MSDS
   d. Waybills

9. You and your crew have responded to a residence where three people are outside attempting to help a male in his forties. They are using a garden hose to spray him. One of them tells you that the patient was accidentally splashed with antifreeze. It went in his face, eye, mouth, and nose and is on his clothing. One of the first things you did was to direct the patient to remove his clothing and continuing pouring water on himself. This step is referred to as _____ decontamination.
   a. gross
   b. primary
   c. secondary
   d. controlled

10. _____ is(are) how and what a poison does to the body.
    a. Poison actions
    b. Poison adaptations
    c. Degradation
    d. Absorption

11. Decontamination is the physical or _____ process of removing hazardous material from exposed persons or equipment.
    a. mechanical
    b. chemical
    c. filtration
    d. biodegradable

12. The procedure for the decontamination (decon) of a critical patient is a _____ step process.
    a. two
    b. four
    c. seven
    d. eight

13. The decon corridor, which consists of _____ stages, is the method used for decontamination of noncritical patients and rescuers.
    a. five
    b. six
    c. seven
    d. eight

14. Water is a universal decon solution that dilutes and reduces _____ absorption.
    a. metabolic
    b. topical
    c. enteral
    d. parenteral

15. Which of the following is not a common solution used by EMS providers for decon?
    a. tincture of green soap
    b. isopropyl alcohol
    c. vegetable oil
    d. milk

16. The properties of potential hazards of chemical substances, which are listed on 704 placards and other references, include flammability, health hazards, and:
    a. reliability.
    b. toxicity.
    c. relativity.
    d. reactivity.

17. Prior to working at an incident where hazmat is present, _____ is(are) established to prevent injury and unnecessary exposure to the substance.
    a. officers
    b. zones
    c. quarters
    d. precedence

18. A paramedic with first responder awareness training can take which of the following actions at the scene of a hazmat exposure?
    a. Don level 1 and 2 PPE.
    b. Participate in containment.
    c. Collect a sample of the material for the ED.
    d. Instruct the patient to remove contaminated shoes and clothing.

19. _____ is how much substance it takes to cause a physiologic response.
    a. Dose response
    b. Route of exposure
    c. Synergistic effect
    d. Toxicity

20. One factor that can make field decontamination of a patient difficult is:
    a. having an MSDS available.
    b. unlimited level of training.
    c. wearing PPE that is compatible with all chemicals.
    d. critical patient condition.

21. The maximum concentration to which a healthy adult can be exposed to a hazardous material without risk of injury is called the:
    a. ceiling level.
    b. flash point.
    c. permissible exposure limit.
    d. threshold limit value-ceiling.

22. _____ is a time-weighted average concentration that must not be exceeded during any 8-hour work shift or 40-hour workweek.
    a. Ceiling level
    b. Short-term exposure limit
    c. Permissible exposure limit
    d. Threshold limit value

23. After responding to a residence for a sick person, you discover that there are other family members in the home with the same symptoms, which include nausea, headache, and weakness. They have been sick for the last 12–18 hours and now you suspect possible poisoning by inhalation due to carbon monoxide. The next action you take is to:
    a. open all the windows.
    b. get everyone out of the residence.
    c. establish a perimeter and safety zones.
    d. attempt to find the source carbon monoxide.

24. The Occupational Health and Safety Administration (OSHA) regulations are published in the:
    a. product packaging labels.
    b. MSDS.
    c. *Emergency Response Guidebook.*
    d. Code of Federal Regulations (CFR).

25. CHEMTREC is an information resource service operated by the _____ and is available by an 800 phone number for detailed information on the chemicals involved and the manufacturer of the chemical.
    a. Centers for Disease Control (CDC)
    b. Federal Regulatory Commission
    c. DOT
    d. Chemical Manufacturers Association

26. In an effort to minimize contaminating EMS equipment at the scene of a hazmat incident the paramedic should:
    a. use only disposable items.
    b. use only the equipment from the hazmat team.
    c. avoid using any EMS equipment until the patient has been decontaminated.
    d. stage equipment in the cold zone of the operation.

27. You are attempting to look up information about the flammability of a hazmat. The resource guide you are using indicates which of the following warnings?
    a. the size of the safety zones needed
    b. the type of decontamination required
    c. the product may be fatal when inhaled
    d. the product may ignite other combustible materials

28. When transporting a patient who was exposed to hazardous chemicals, the paramedic should anticipate that many emergency departments will _____ prior to accepting the patient.
    a. ask you to repeat decon on the patient
    b. contact the hazmat incident commander
    c. take the patient through their own decon procedures
    d. have the local FD respond to decon the patient again

29. Many communities preplan and train for incidents involving hazmats, multiple patients, natural disasters, and weapons of mass destruction. These plans use a tool called _____ , which manages personnel and resources during such events.
    a. Homeland Security (HLS)
    b. disaster and rescue operations
    c. incident management system (IMS)
    d. environmental disaster management

30. The fire department, local hazmat team, and your ambulance have been dispatched for a 55-year-old male with a possible exposure to a hazardous material. Your unit is the closest and will arrive first. As you perform a scene size-up, your first priority is to:
    a. determine the need for additional resources.
    b. avoid any exposure to yourself and your crew.
    c. assess the risk of primary contamination of other responders.
    d. assess the risk of secondary contamination of the patient.

Exam #50 Answer Form

	A	B	C	D			A	B	C	D
1.	❏	❏	❏	❏		16.	❏	❏	❏	❏
2.	❏	❏	❏	❏		17.	❏	❏	❏	❏
3.	❏	❏	❏	❏		18.	❏	❏	❏	❏
4.	❏	❏	❏	❏		19.	❏	❏	❏	❏
5.	❏	❏	❏	❏		20.	❏	❏	❏	❏
6.	❏	❏	❏	❏		21.	❏	❏	❏	❏
7.	❏	❏	❏	❏		22.	❏	❏	❏	❏
8.	❏	❏	❏	❏		23.	❏	❏	❏	❏
9.	❏	❏	❏	❏		24.	❏	❏	❏	❏
10.	❏	❏	❏	❏		25.	❏	❏	❏	❏
11.	❏	❏	❏	❏		26.	❏	❏	❏	❏
12.	❏	❏	❏	❏		27.	❏	❏	❏	❏
13.	❏	❏	❏	❏		28.	❏	❏	❏	❏
14.	❏	❏	❏	❏		29.	❏	❏	❏	❏
15.	❏	❏	❏	❏		30.	❏	❏	❏	❏

CHAPTER

51

Terrorism and Disasters

1. _____ is one type of violence that threatens citizens and government.
   a. Suicide
   b. Homicide
   c. Terrorism
   d. Domestic violence

2. Classifications of chemical agents that may be used at a terrorism incident include:
   a. viral agents, bacterial agents, and toxins.
   b. nerve agents, blister agents, and blood agents.
   c. explosive and incendiary agents.
   d. alpha and beta particles.

3. As part of the hazard awareness in the scene size-up, the paramedic's safety concerns begin:
   a. in the classroom.
   b. with information obtained from dispatch.
   c. as soon as you enter the neighborhood.
   d. when you arrive at the call address.

4. If, while on the scene, the paramedic becomes aware of a potential threat, weapons, or any violent or abusive action toward him, the paramedic should:
   a. look for a second exit.
   b. retreat right away.
   c. intercede with pepper spray.
   d. wait for police before further intervention.
   e. Any of the above could cause the paramedic to be mistaken for law enforcement.

5. When the paramedic finds one or more patients exhibiting acute signs and symptoms of salivation, lacrimation, urination, defecation, GI upset, emesis, or muscle twitching (SLUDGEM), he should consider that there was a possible exposure to:
   a. radiation.
   b. explosives.
   c. a nerve agent.
   d. a blister agent.

6. When dispatched to a scene with known or potential terrorism, the paramedic should stage the vehicle:
   a. at least 50 feet from the scene.
   b. at least 100 feet from the scene.
   c. out of sight of the scene.
   d. directly behind a police vehicle.

7. When approaching a suspicious address one strategy to use, in an effort to avoid injury to yourself and your crew, is to:
   a. stand to the side of the door before ringing or knocking.
   b. backlight your partner while he rings or knocks on the front door.
   c. broadcast your approach with lights and sirens, right up to the residence.
   d. announce your presence, then knock or ring, and listen for signs of danger.

8. Once the paramedic has credible information of the presence of chemical, biological, radiological, nuclear, or explosive (CBRNE) material, his next action is to:
   a. evacuate the area.
   b. establish EMS command.
   c. notify neighboring communities of the threat.
   d. attempt to identify signs of specific agent exposure.

9. Before getting out of the ambulance to approach a stopped vehicle on the highway, it is a good idea to notify the dispatcher of the situation and the:
   a. exact location.
   b. color of the vehicle.
   c. number of occupants.
   d. lack of activity where activity is likely.

10. The paramedic should initially approach the stopped vehicle from the passenger side because the:
    a. posts of the vehicle will keep the paramedic safe from a gunshot.
    b. driver would normally expect the police to approach on the driver's side.
    c. paramedic will have a better view of a dangerous situation.
    d. traffic side is usually inaccessible.

11. While approaching a vehicle on the highway, one partner initially remains in the ambulance to watch for hazards, while the other paramedic who is going to approach the vehicle should:
    a. chock the wheels of the vehicle.
    b. copy the license plate number and state.
    c. have a portable radio in hand.
    d. set up a safety zone.

12. Upon arriving at an incident involving a weapon of mass destruction (WMD), the paramedic's role includes:
    a. establishing command and performing a scene size-up.
    b. reporting to command and then to an assigned sector (group).
    c. providing the initial scene report to dispatch and requesting additional resources.
    d. identifying yourself and your level of training to the transportation sector officer.

13. You are caring for a patient with acute radiation sickness (ARS). The immediate signs and symptoms will include:
    a. seizures.
    b. internal bleeding.
    c. nausea and vomiting.
    d. destruction of bone marrow.

14. Paramedics may be called to respond to a clandestine drug lab for:
    a. injuries from an explosion.
    b. monitoring suspicious patients.
    c. assisting the DEA with moving chemicals.
    d. assisting in breaking down the cookers.

15. When working at a scene where radiation is a factor, which of the following ways is the easiest method for the paramedic to protect herself from radiation exposure?
    a. frequent hand washing
    b. decon as soon as possible
    c. decreasing the distance from the radiation source
    d. decreasing the amount of time spent near the source

16. It is not uncommon for _____ in or near a clandestine drug lab to warn the criminals of the approach of intruders.
    a. undercover FBI to be
    b. snipers to be staged
    c. booby traps to be set
    d. children

17. The presence of a street gang in a community increases the:
    a. value of the properties.
    b. awareness for graffiti.
    c. potential for street violence.
    d. Good Samaritan effort.

18. Street gangs often have unique clothing that they call their _____, which are an identifier of the group and may represent the member's status within the group.
    a. leathers
    b. rags
    c. colors
    d. stripes

19. If you believe that you have arrived at the scene of a clandestine drug lab, the safest action for you is to:
    a. not move, but call for police.
    b. act as if you do not know that it is a drug lab.
    c. care for the patient but watch out for chemical exposure.
    d. leave immediately and call law enforcement.

20. Who is considered the best personnel to manage an incident at a clandestine drug lab?
    a. the fire department
    b. the DEA
    c. a chemical specialist from the nearest college
    d. the hazmat team

21. When caring for a victim with an exposure to biological agents used as weapons, the paramedic should consider that symptoms typically appear within:
    a. seconds.
    b. minutes.
    c. an hour.
    d. hours to days.

22. A primary safety concern for paramedics and other emergency responders responding to and working at the scene of an explosive incident is:
    a. fallout from the debris.
    b. exposure to bleeding patients.
    c. the potential for a secondary device.
    d. an unsecured perimeter.

23. Which of the following actions should the paramedic avoid if she suspects domestic violence?

a. Treat the patient.

b. Provide a phone number for a domestic violence hotline or shelter.

c. Protect the victim by getting between the victim and the abuser.

d. Do not be judgmental.

24. One of the rules of tactical safety that the paramedic must follow on all calls is:

a. wait to enter the scene with the police.

b. avoid danger by never entering the scene.

c. avoidance is always preferable to confrontation.

d. if you are not sure of a potential danger, call dispatch before entering the scene.

25. If you have to retreat from a dangerous scene, be sure to:

a. document that you did not abandon the patient.

b. make sure the dispatcher does not send any further EMS units directly into the scene.

c. bring the patient with you.

d. bring cover with you.

26. Which of the following is most correct about concealment for the paramedic?

a. Concealment is positioning the paramedic or crew behind an object that hides them from the view of others.

b. Concealment offers ballistic protection if the perpetrator begins to fire a weapon.

c. An example of concealment is hiding behind a wooden picket fence.

d. Concealment should be used when approaching a residence.

27. What can the paramedics do if an aggressor seems to be chasing them?

a. Strike before the aggressor strikes you.

b. Do not try to anticipate the moves of the aggressor.

c. Use pepper spray or mace to slow the aggressor.

d. Throw the equipment to slow or trip the aggressor.

28. When making the determination of what type of personal protective equipment to don at the scene of an incident of terrorism, the paramedic must consider:

a. how readily available the equipment is.

b. that too much protection can create additional hazards.

c. how many patients are symptomatic and asymptomatic.

d. how many patients have wandered away from the incident.

29. In some cities, a limited number of EMS providers are trained in special tactics to accompany the police on high-risk operations. This program is called:

a. CONTOMS.

b. rescue EMS.

c. tactical EMS.

d. Superhero EMS.

30. The _____ program, started in 1989, was designed to meet the specialized medical training to support law enforcement operations and was funded by the Department of Defense.

a. CONTOMS

b. LEA/SWAT team

c. SWAT—Medic

d. TEMS

31. When removing clothing from a patient at a crime scene that is stained in blood or body fluids, the paramedic should avoid:

a. cutting along the seam of the clothing.

b. cutting through a knife or bullet hole.

c. having law enforcement assist.

d. placing items separately.

32. After removing the clothing from a patient at a crime scene, the paramedic should place the clothing in:

a. a paper bag.

b. a zip-lock bag.

c. a towel.

d. the patient's bathtub.

33. The Mark 1 Kit includes a single injector containing two antidote drugs, which is used for _____ exposure.

a. anthrax

b. nerve agent

c. toxin

d. mustard gas

34. Wearing gloves while working at the scene of a crime may prevent the paramedic from leaving fingerprints, but it does not prevent:

a. leaving the moisture from her skin at the scene.

b. leaving the oil from her skin at the scene.

c. destroying or "smudging" the perpetrator's prints.

d. the spread of bloodborne disease.

35. The paramedic can minimize risks when working in a potentially dangerous situation by:

a. not wearing a clip-on tie.

b. keeping hands in his pockets to appear non threatening.

c. keeping a safe stance with feet apart, ready to react.

d. keeping a stethoscope around the neck to look like a doctor.

36. An early-morning small engine plane crash in an apartment complex has 66 residents out on the street watching their homes being destroyed. Many of the residents were asleep when the fire started, and nearly half of them are coughing or complaining of a burning sensation in the throat. Until proven otherwise, EMS should suspect that:
    a. there may still be residents in the building.
    b. the pilot may still be alive and needs rescue.
    c. there is a possibility of carbon monoxide poisoning in all the victims of this fire.
    d. many of these victims may have seizures within an hour.

37. Your unit is one of several dispatched to stand by at a railroad accident, which has resulted in a major tire fire. You have been staged a quarter-mile away. From there you can see that the fire is significant and that black smoke is rising in extremely large clouds. With residential housing surrounding three sides of the junkyard, which of the following environmental factors could create an immediate hazard for these residents?
    a. rain
    b. snow
    c. lightning
    d. wind direction

38. At the scene of an unexpected, vacant building collapse, emergency responders have learned that there may be victims hidden in the rubble. Which of the following resources should be requested to the scene?
    a. a surgeon
    b. a helicopter
    c. medical control
    d. search-and-rescue specialists

39. The paramedic can better understand what his role may be in disaster operations by:
    a. becoming involved in preplanning and training.
    b. realizing that there is really no way to prepare for major disasters.
    c. obtaining the highest level of medical training affordable.
    d. talking to as many people as possible who have been in disasters.

40. A flooding incident has become large enough to require the resources of agencies outside of the community. Communication among all the resources will:
    a. work best when plain English is used.
    b. be designated by the incident commander.
    c. use the common "disaster system" terminology.
    d. use the code system of the originating jurisdiction.

Exam #51 Answer Form

	A	B	C	D			A	B	C	D
1.	❏	❏	❏	❏		21.	❏	❏	❏	❏
2.	❏	❏	❏	❏		22.	❏	❏	❏	❏
3.	❏	❏	❏	❏		23.	❏	❏	❏	❏
4.	❏	❏	❏	❏		24.	❏	❏	❏	❏
5.	❏	❏	❏	❏		25.	❏	❏	❏	❏
6.	❏	❏	❏	❏		26.	❏	❏	❏	❏
7.	❏	❏	❏	❏		27.	❏	❏	❏	❏
8.	❏	❏	❏	❏		28.	❏	❏	❏	❏
9.	❏	❏	❏	❏		29.	❏	❏	❏	❏
10.	❏	❏	❏	❏		30.	❏	❏	❏	❏
11.	❏	❏	❏	❏		31.	❏	❏	❏	❏
12.	❏	❏	❏	❏		32.	❏	❏	❏	❏
13.	❏	❏	❏	❏		33.	❏	❏	❏	❏
14.	❏	❏	❏	❏		34.	❏	❏	❏	❏
15.	❏	❏	❏	❏		35.	❏	❏	❏	❏
16.	❏	❏	❏	❏		36.	❏	❏	❏	❏
17.	❏	❏	❏	❏		37.	❏	❏	❏	❏
18.	❏	❏	❏	❏		38.	❏	❏	❏	❏
19.	❏	❏	❏	❏		39.	❏	❏	❏	❏
20.	❏	❏	❏	❏		40.	❏	❏	❏	❏

CHAPTER

52

Basic and Advanced Cardiac Life Support Review

1. The care provided in the first few minutes of a life-threatening emergency is called:
   a. CPR.
   b. secondary assessment.
   c. basic life support.
   d. reassessment.

2. One of the major changes in the Guidelines 2005, which was again reinforced in Guidelines 2010, was to improve the effectiveness of the delivery chest compressions by:
   a. emphasizing that all rescuers should push hard and fast.
   b. allowing more time between compressions for better chest recoil.
   c. increasing the compression rate and omitting ventilations for the lay rescuer.
   d. adding voice prompts in AEDs and defibrillators, which remind the rescuer to maintain the correct compression rate.

3. The general term that is used to describe the spectrum of disease from acute angina to myocardial infarction is:
   a. heart attack.
   b. acute coronary syndrome (ACS).
   c. unstable angina.
   d. coronary illness.

4. In an effort to maintain the most effective delivery of chest compressions during a sudden cardiac arrest (SCA), it is recommended that the rescuers performing compressions switch positions every _____ minutes.
   a. 2
   b. 3
   c. 4
   d. 5

5. For the adult patient who is not breathing, each rescue breath should be provided:
   a. one second per breath.
   b. over 2 seconds.
   c. every 6–8 seconds.
   d. every 30 seconds.

6. The recommendation for one-rescuer CPR is for a compression ventilation ratio of:
   a. 30:2 for all rescuers.
   b. 30:2 for lay rescuers only.
   c. 15:2 for health care providers only.
   d. 30:2 for health care providers only.

7. The goal of the Guidelines 2010 was to develop widely accepted international resuscitation guidelines that were:
   a. based on a majority vote.
   b. based on the least cost to implement.
   c. based on scientific evidence.
   d. easy to read and explain.

8. Guidelines that are supported by very good evidence of effectiveness and safety in humans are class:
   a. I.
   b. IIa.
   c. IIb.
   d. III.

9. Guidelines supported by fair to good evidence of effectiveness and safety in humans with evidence of harm are class:
   a. I.
   b. IIa.
   c. IIb.
   d. III.

10. Actions or interventions with insufficient evidence to support a final recommendation for clinical use are placed in class:
    a. IIa.
    b. IIb.
    c. III.
    d. Indeterminate.

11. The Guidelines 2010 recommend that when attempting defibrillation:
    a. all rescuers deliver one shock followed by immediate CPR for 2 minutes.
    b. lay rescuers deliver one shock followed by immediate CPR for 5 minutes.
    c. using an AED, on children 1–8 years old, the dose is the same as an adult.
    d. health care providers deliver three shocks followed by immediate CPR for 1 minute.

12. Terminating the code on a non-traumatic cardiac arrest victim, after an adequate trial of BLS and ALS has been done, to support the survivors would be an example of a class _____ guideline.
    a. I
    b. IIa
    c. IIb
    d. III

13. All health care providers with a duty to perform CPR should be trained, equipped, and authorized to perform defibrillation is a class _____ guideline.
    a. I
    b. IIa
    c. IIb
    d. III

14. For the infant or child patient who is not breathing, each rescue breath should be provided:
    a. over 2 seconds.
    b. every 1–2 seconds.
    c. every 3–5 seconds.
    d. every 6–8 seconds.

15. The recommendation for interruptions in CPR for pulse checks should:
    a. occur once every minute.
    b. take less than 5 seconds.
    c. take less than 10 seconds.
    d. not occur more than once every 5 minutes.

16. When the rescuer performing the chest compressions allows the chest to recoil after each compression, this action:
    a. allows the heart to fill with blood.
    b. allows each ventilation to fill the lungs.
    c. reduces the amount of compressions delivered each minute.
    d. increases the amount of compressions delivered each minute.

17. When providing ventilations without an advanced airway in the patient experiencing cardiac arrest, the rescuer should avoid overventilation because it:
    a. impedes blood return to the heart.
    b. increases the venous capacity of the heart.
    c. reduces the threshold for cardioversion.
    d. reduces the ventricular fibrillation threshold.

18. When an individual executes his right of self-determination and declares he does not want to be resuscitated if he becomes unresponsive, this is referred to as a(n):
    a. unrecognized determination.
    b. DNAR order.
    c. termination order.
    d. final rite.

19. The Guidelines 2010 are considered:
    a. the legal standard of care.
    b. national regulations.
    c. consensus standards.
    d. international law.

20. The initial dose for shocking ventricular fibrillation using a monophasic waveform for treatment is:
    a. 120 J.
    b. 200 J.
    c. 300 J.
    d. 360 J.

21. After the initial dose, subsequent shocks using monophasic waveform for treatment of ventricular fibrillation are:
    a. 150 J.
    b. 200 J.
    c. 300 J.
    d. 360 J.

22. If a patient received an adequate trial of ALS in the field, in which circumstance should you continue the arrest and transport to the local ED?
    a. a lengthy downtime
    b. the patient has a mortal injury
    c. a low body temperature
    d. rigor mortis is apparent

23. In the out-of-hospital setting, the 5-year-old child who collapses from sudden cardiac arrest should first receive _____.
    a. 1 minute of CPR
    b. 2 minutes of CPR
    c. ten cycles of CPR
    d. defibrillation with an AED

24. Of all the interventions available to the cardiac arrest patient, which has the most scientific evidence in its favor?
    a. CPR
    b. defibrillation
    c. compressions
    d. high-dose epinephrine

25. The use of the AED is encouraged for all patients over the age of:
    a. 50.
    b. 15.
    c. 8.
    d. 1.

26. Where is the best "bang for the buck" in saving cardiac arrest patients?
    a. adding more ALS units
    b. expanding the use of fibrinolytics
    c. removing barriers to implementing PAD
    d. training EMTs to intubate

27. In the Guidelines 2010, updates in health care provider training for CPR on a "child" applies to:
    a. opening the airway.
    b. patients between 1 and 8 years old.
    c. patients from 1 year old to the onset of puberty.
    d. two-rescuer, two-thumb-encircling-hands technique.

28. In what situation should you phone first instead of phone fast?
    a. a child with previous MI
    b. a child who may have drowned
    c. a child with a possible airway obstruction
    d. when you are not near a phone

29. In adults, when should the rescuer consider phoning fast instead of phoning first?
    a. cardiac arrest caused by electrical shock
    b. preexisting MI
    c. poisoning or drug overdose
    d. patients over 60 years old

30. When using a bag mask, the rescuer should:
    a. enlist a second rescuer to help squeeze the bag.
    b. use the "C"/"E" clamp hand position.
    c. provide breaths over 1 second.
    d. all of the above.

31. Which is the best position for the ventilator when using a bag mask on a supine patient?
    a. at the patient's side
    b. about 18" above the head of the patient
    c. straddling the patient
    d. lying flat on your stomach

32. Which statement is incorrect?
    a. Proper use of the bag mask requires practice.
    b. The jaw thrust can be used with one-rescuer technique on a trauma patient.
    c. Tidal volumes of 400–600 ml can be given over 1 second.
    d. The bag mask should be attached to 100% oxygen.

33. When smaller tidal volumes are used with the bag mask, the:
    a. patient should be hyperventilated.
    b. breaths need to be given faster.
    c. breaths need to be more forceful.
    d. chest should rise visibly.

34. When a victim suddenly collapses and has no signs of circulation, the rescuer should first provide _____.
    a. two rescue breaths
    b. defibrillation with an AED
    c. one cycle of thirty compressions
    d. five cycles of thirty compressions followed by two rescue breaths

35. What evidence helped researchers recommend dropping the pulse check step for laypersons?
    a. No one checks it anyway.
    b. The patient often still has a faint pulse.
    c. It takes too much time to teach.
    d. They were frequently wrong in their assessment.

36. When biphasic waveform defibrillation is used on an adult in sudden cardiac arrest, the initial shock dose is:
    a. 150 J.
    b. 200 J.
    c. 300 J.
    d. 360 J.

37. If a foreign body airway obstruction is suspected in an adult patient, the health care provider should:
    a. call for the defibrillator.
    b. reposition the neck and reattempt to ventilate.
    c. simply give chest compressions.
    d. perform a blind finger sweep.

38. The initial shock dose for a child in ventricular fibrillation using a monophasic or biphasic manual defibrillator is:
    a. 1 J/kg.
    b. 2 J/kg.
    c. 3 J/kg.
    d. 4 J/kg.

39. If a person has a foreign body airway obstruction (FBAO) and is an adult:
    a. do not do chest compressions.
    b. chest compression may be helpful.
    c. reach down his throat to remove the object.
    d. ventilate twice as fast.

40. Where are the hands placed to do CPR compressions on an adult?
    a. on the bottom of the breastbone
    b. at the top of the breastbone
    c. on the seventh intercostal space
    d. in the center of the chest, between the nipples

41. At what rate should the chest be compressed for an adult patient in sudden cardiac arrest?
    a. 60 per minute
    b. 80 per minute
    c. 90 per minute
    d. at least 100 per minute

42. The compression-to-ventilation ratio for infants and children older than 1 year, when performed by two health care providers, is:
    a. 5:1.
    b. 15:2.
    c. 30:1.
    d. 30:2.

43. When providing chest compressions on a child in sudden cardiac arrest, the rescuer should use:
    a. the heel of only one hand to compress the lower half of the sternum.
    b. the heel of one or two hands to compress the lower half of the sternum.
    c. one hand to compress to a depth of one-quarter of the chest diameter.
    d. both hands to compress to a depth of one-quarter of the chest diameter.

44. The first choice technique for chest compression in an infant when there are two rescuers is to do the:
    a. two-thumb-encircling-hands chest technique.
    b. two fingers at the center of the chest.
    c. one-handed technique.
    d. two-handed technique.

45. Under certain clinical conditions, evidence shows that:
    a. the LMA is superior to an ET tube.
    b. the LMA and Combitube® are better than a bag mask.
    c. the Combitube® is a dangerous device.
    d. all EMTs should be trained in the use of the Combitube®.

46. Who should decide if EMTs are trained to use the LMA?
    a. the training officer
    b. the International Resuscitation Committee
    c. the AHA
    d. the agency's director

47. The principles of _____ medicine classify interventions into one of five categories.
    a. diagnostic
    b. evidence-based
    c. homeopathic
    d. osteopathic

48. While performing CPR with an advanced airway in place, the rescuer delivering the ventilations should provide _____ ventilation(s) every _____ seconds.
    a. one; 6–8
    b. one; 5–6
    c. two; 15
    d. two; 30

49. The Guidelines require training in the use of a(n) _____ by all health care providers.
    a. bag mask
    b. LMA
    c. Combitube®
    d. ET tube

50. The preferred method of medication administration during a cardiac arrest is through:
    a. an IV or IO.
    b. a synchronized IV drip.
    c. the endotracheal tube at normal dose.
    d. the endotracheal tube at double dose.

51. CPR is in progress on an adult when you arrive with a defibrillator. You quickly analyze the rhythm, detect pulseless ventricular tachycardia, and administer one shock. The next step is to:
    a. check the pulse, reanalyze the rhythm, and resume CPR for 2 minutes.
    b. reanalyze the rhythm, check the pulse, and resume CPR for 2 minutes.
    c. resume CPR for five cycles, then reanalyze the rhythm and check the pulse.
    d. reanalyze the rhythm, resume CPR for five cycles, and then check the pulse.

52. Which of the following devices provides a continuous visual display of the level of expired CO_2?
    a. capnometer
    b. capnography
    c. colorimetric device
    d. pulse oximetry

53. Which of the following is incorrect about the Combitube® airway device?
    a. The Combitube® is an advanced airway.
    b. This device is inserted blindly.
    c. It is placed orally and inserted past the hypopharyngeal space.
    d. This device requires extensive training to use.

54. During a cardiac arrest resuscitation emergency, cardiac drugs should be administered:
    a. after every shock.
    b. every 2 minutes during CPR.
    c. every 3 minutes during the rhythm check.
    d. during CPR, as soon as possible after rhythm checks.

55. _____ is a vasopressor that may be given to replace the first or second dose of epinephrine in cardiac arrest.
    a. Dopamine
    b. Vasopressin
    c. Dobutamine
    d. Isoproterenol

56. Pediatric post-resuscitation interventions that may improve the neurologic outcome include:
    a. avoiding hyperventilation.
    b. maintaining normal blood sugar levels.
    c. treating hyperthermia and allowing a mild hypothermia to exist.
    d. all of the above.

57. The use of high-dose epinephrine in pediatric cardiac arrest has been de-emphasized for all of the following reasons, except that it:
    a. is very difficult to accurately dose to the patient's weight.
    b. can increase myocardial oxygen demand.
    c. can cause tachycardia and hypertension.
    d. can cause myocardial necrosis.

58. _____ is the preferred antiarrhythmic in the management of potentially fatal pediatric dysrhythmias.
    a. Epinephrine
    b. Amiodarone
    c. Vasopressin
    d. Cardizem

59. One major change in neonatal resuscitation and the management of meconium staining is:
    a. routine suctioning is no longer recommended.
    b. endotracheal suctioning is a class III treatment.
    c. aggressive suction must be started as soon as possible.
    d. endotracheal suctioning should be used first and exclusively.

60. You are treating a 45-year-old patient who is complaining of chest and left arm pain, nausea, and sweating. While you begin treatment and complete your assessment, you also consider whether or not the patient is a candidate for fibrinolytic therapy. For which of the following factors may this type of therapy be a contraindication in the patient you are treating?
    a. the patient's age
    b. the patient takes metoprolol
    c. the patient takes warfarin
    d. the patient's heart rate is 56

61. _____ has been shown to be effective for VF or pulseless VT, torsades de pointes, and dysrhythmias with known hypomagnesemia.
    a. Sodium bicarbonate
    b. Amiodarone
    c. Vasopressin
    d. Magnesium sulfate

62. _____ is an agent that appears to be as effective as epinephrine in cardiac arrest and lasts between 10 and 20 minutes, so only one dose is recommended.
    a. Lidocaine
    b. Amiodarone
    c. Vasopressin
    d. Procainamide

63. You have responded to the home of a patient found in cardiac arrest. The patient's initial rhythm is asystole, and he was last seen alive 30 minutes ago. The patient is 70 years old and has a cardiac history. The patient's wife is asking you to do anything you can to save her husband, and more family members are arriving. What action is appropriate to take next?
    a. Ask the family if the patient has a health care proxy or any advanced directives.
    b. Offer the wife and family members the choice to observe the attempt at resuscitation.
    c. Begin resuscitation and assign a team member to remain with the family and answer questions.
    d. All of the actions listed above are appropriate and should be done.

64. Acute MI and unstable angina are now recognized as part of a spectrum of disease known as:
    a. acute coronary syndromes (ACS).
    b. advanced coronary syndromes.
    c. ACLS disorders.
    d. acute cardiac disorders.

65. Cardiac patients who are not eligible for fibrinolytic therapy because of exclusionary criteria should be considered for transport or transfer to a hospital with _____ facilities.
    a. outpatient placement
    b. hyperbaric oxygen therapy
    c. primary angioplasty and intra-aortic balloon placement.
    d. primary beta-blocking central line

66. Intravenous fibrinolytics have been shown to improve neurologic outcome in stroke patients who meet the criteria, provided they are administered within:
    a. the first 72 hours after symptoms start to resolve.
    b. 2 hours after the symptoms start to resolve.
    c. 3 hours of the onset of stroke symptoms.
    d. 3–6 hours of the onset of stroke symptoms.

67. The treatment of choice for an overdose of tricyclic antidepressants is the induction of:
    a. systemic alkalosis.
    b. an antidysrhythmic agent like lidocaine.
    c. procainamide.
    d. beta-blocker.

68. Cocaine overdose has been shown to be associated with serious:
    a. ventricular dysrhythmias.
    b. atrial dysrhythmias.
    c. hypomagnesium.
    d. hypothermia.

69. The Guidelines recommend all of the following for cocaine overdose, except:
    a. nitrates as a first-line therapy.
    b. benzodiazepines as a first-line therapy.
    c. alpha-adrenergic blocking agents as a second-line therapy when the first-line treatment fails.
    d. beta-blocking agents as a second-line therapy when the first-line treatment fails.

70. Recommended prehospital medications for all patients with ACS include _____ in the absence of contraindications.
    a. aspirin
    b. nitroglycerin
    c. beta-blockers
    d. none of the above

Exam #52 Answer Form

	A	B	C	D			A	B	C	D
1.	❏	❏	❏	❏		36.	❏	❏	❏	❏
2.	❏	❏	❏	❏		37.	❏	❏	❏	❏
3.	❏	❏	❏	❏		38.	❏	❏	❏	❏
4.	❏	❏	❏	❏		39.	❏	❏	❏	❏
5.	❏	❏	❏	❏		40.	❏	❏	❏	❏
6.	❏	❏	❏	❏		41.	❏	❏	❏	❏
7.	❏	❏	❏	❏		42.	❏	❏	❏	❏
8.	❏	❏	❏	❏		43.	❏	❏	❏	❏
9.	❏	❏	❏	❏		44.	❏	❏	❏	❏
10.	❏	❏	❏	❏		45.	❏	❏	❏	❏
11.	❏	❏	❏	❏		46.	❏	❏	❏	❏
12.	❏	❏	❏	❏		47.	❏	❏	❏	❏
13.	❏	❏	❏	❏		48.	❏	❏	❏	❏
14.	❏	❏	❏	❏		49.	❏	❏	❏	❏
15.	❏	❏	❏	❏		50.	❏	❏	❏	❏
16.	❏	❏	❏	❏		51.	❏	❏	❏	❏
17.	❏	❏	❏	❏		52.	❏	❏	❏	❏
18.	❏	❏	❏	❏		53.	❏	❏	❏	❏
19.	❏	❏	❏	❏		54.	❏	❏	❏	❏
20.	❏	❏	❏	❏		55.	❏	❏	❏	❏
21.	❏	❏	❏	❏		56.	❏	❏	❏	❏
22.	❏	❏	❏	❏		57.	❏	❏	❏	❏
23.	❏	❏	❏	❏		58.	❏	❏	❏	❏
24.	❏	❏	❏	❏		59.	❏	❏	❏	❏
25.	❏	❏	❏	❏		60.	❏	❏	❏	❏
26.	❏	❏	❏	❏		61.	❏	❏	❏	❏
27.	❏	❏	❏	❏		62.	❏	❏	❏	❏
28.	❏	❏	❏	❏		63.	❏	❏	❏	❏
29.	❏	❏	❏	❏		64.	❏	❏	❏	❏
30.	❏	❏	❏	❏		65.	❏	❏	❏	❏
31.	❏	❏	❏	❏		66.	❏	❏	❏	❏
32.	❏	❏	❏	❏		67.	❏	❏	❏	❏
33.	❏	❏	❏	❏		68.	❏	❏	❏	❏
34.	❏	❏	❏	❏		69.	❏	❏	❏	❏
35.	❏	❏	❏	❏		70.	❏	❏	❏	❏

Appendix A:
Answers and Rationale for Questions

Chapter 1: Workforce Safety & Wellness

1. a. Health—Defined by the World Health Organization as not merely the absence of disease or infirmity; it is a state of complete physical, mental, and social well-being.

2. c. mental and emotional health.—The components of wellness include physical well-being and proper nutrition, as well as mental and emotional health.

3. d. weight control.—The principles of weight control (e.g., eating in moderation, limiting fat consumption, and exercise) must be understood and included in proper nutrition.

4. d. two-thirds—Eating too much animal food, fat, oil, and sugar, while eating too few complex carbohydrates, such as fresh vegetable and fruits, whole grains, and legumes, contributes to the development of degenerative diseases. These include the major killers like heart disease, diabetes, cancer, stroke, and obesity.

5. c. diabetes.—Poor diet and nutrition contribute to the development of degenerative diseases such as diabetes, hypertension, heart disease, and stroke.

6. a. limited access to choices of food types.—When you are only able to get meals on the run, and are limited to fast food choices, the choices are typically not the healthiest.

7. c. stopping for fast food when you are hungry and did not bring a meal.—Typical fast food is loaded with fat and calories. Stopping for good food fast is a better approach. Many fast-food restaurants now have menus that include some items for those conscious of diet, nutrition, and their waistline.

8. b. making small changes with a slow transition—Extreme changes in diet tend to lead to failure in sticking to the diet. Look closely at the label for both fat and calorie content. Experts say it takes 20 minutes to feel full once you have started eating. Drink water before and during a meal to achieve that feeling to avoid overeating.

9. d. Snacks can fill the voids between meals and should be a part of your food plan.—Healthy snacks can help fill the void between meals, will decrease your appetite for the next meal, and can help to avoid overeating. High-fiber snacks are better for dental health, so include healthy snacks in your food plan.

10. a. attitude.—The elements of physical fitness include a positive attitude, strength, endurance, and aerobic conditioning. It is great to have a personal trainer and heart rate monitor, but not necessary. Running is not physically possible for many people. There are many other options for aerobic conditioning.

11. a. a physician will identify any specific limitations to consider.—This precaution is routinely given for those who are looking to begin a new exercise plan, or for other good reasons. The physician can make recommendations that will help to avoid injuries or excess stress on the body, based on age, past medical history, current weight, and general physical condition.

12. c. Lyme disease.—Hepatitis B, rubella, tetanus, and diphtheria are required immunizations. Paramedic students are required to have these prior to entering most colleges and clinical settings.

13. c. improved personal appearance and self-image.—Additional benefits include increased resistance to injury and illness; decreased blood pressure and resting heart rate; increased muscle mass and metabolism.

14. d. physical endurance.—Aerobic conditioning trains the heart to eject a larger volume with each stroke and does not need to pump as often. The oxygen-carrying capacity of red blood cells increases with improved physical endurance.

15. b. circadian rhythms—These biological cycles include hormonal and body temperature fluctuations, appetite and sleep cycles, and other bodily processes.

16. a. fatigued night-shift workers.—Three Mile Island and the Chernobyl nuclear plant accidents can also be attributed in part to fatigued night-shift workers.

17. c. blood pressure.—Increased blood pressure may have serious long-term effects on the entire body. Additional considerations should include: cardiovascular endurance, total cholesterol, triglycerides, estrogen use, and stress.

18. c. high-level disinfection.—A product that is designed to kill all forms of microbial life, except high numbers of bacterial spores, is a high-level disinfection.

19. a. bending at the hips—The recommendation for safe lifting is to keep the back straight. Use the stronger muscles of the legs rather than the muscles of the back to lift. Bending at the waist when lifting can place the spine at risk for serious and permanent injury.

20. c. Leave yourself an exit and be prepared to retreat.—Safety should come first for you and your crew. This patient has an altered mental status (confused) with an obvious injury that needs medical care. Stay with her at a safe distance until further help arrives.

21. a. daytime, on clear, dry roads.—Ambulance collisions occur with high frequency in daytime hours on clear, dry roads, often in intersections.

22. b. there are limitations with these devices.—These emergency devices do not guarantee the right of way. The operator has the responsibility to drive with due regard while using these devices and is held to a higher standard than other drivers.

23. d. driving with due regard for the safety of other drivers—In most states, the emergency vehicle operator is held to a higher standard with regard to all others. Escorts increase the chance of a chain reaction collision, and are not recommended. Emergency lights and sirens should only be used on high-priority emergency calls.

24. c. Test all drivers on their knowledge of standard operating procedures (SOPs).—Other strategies to consider include: providing hands-on training; checking driver's license and qualifications; assuring familiarity with ambulance size, weight, use of mirrors, braking distances, steering and turning radius, and speed controls.

25. a. what to do when a collision occurs—Additional topics that should be included in SOPs include: how the agency qualifies drivers, who is not allowed to operate the ambulances, a policy on prudent speed, how to approach an intersection, and using a spotter when backing up the ambulance.

26. d. all of the above.—Depending on the type of collision, the safety equipment a paramedic may use will range from eye protection and helmet to full turnout gear.

27. c. The blood pressure decreases.—Cigarette smoking causes the heart rate and blood pressure to increase. It also causes blood vessels to constrict, decreasing peripheral circulation.

28. c. one-half—According to the American Lung Association, many benefits of smoking cessation occur at different time intervals following your last cigarette.

29. b. For long-time smokers, stopping is not of any benefit.—Even heavy smokers show potentially significant improvement in both cardiac and pulmonary function after quitting.

30. a. nicotine has no effect on nerve cells—During the day, nerve cells become desensitized to nicotine.

31. b. addiction—A persistent, compulsive use of a substance, such as nicotine or heroin. A stimulant excites.

32. a. Stress is associated with positive events.—Stress is defined as a factor that induces bodily or mental tension. Stress is associated with both positive (eustress) and negative (distress) events.

33. c. alarm, resistance, and exhaustion.—The process and development of human stress is equated with the three stages: alarm reaction, stage of resistance, and stage of exhaustion.

34. a. level of resistance in the resistance phase.—During this stage, the body continues to adapt by actively using its homeostatic resources to maintain its physiologic integrity and resist the changes imposed on it.

35. d. susceptibility to physical and psychological ailments.—When one or more organ systems fail or become exhausted (stage of exhaustion) under the stress of adaptation, the organism can develop a disease of adaptation. Such diseases are also referred to as stress-related diseases (e.g., heart attack, gastric ulcer, stroke, or diabetes).

36. b. disorientation—Additional cognitive signs and symptoms of stress include: memory problems, poor concentration, and difficulty making decisions.

37. b. panic reaction.—Additional emotional signs and symptoms of stress include: fear, anger, denial, or feeling overwhelmed.

38. a. nausea and vomiting—Additional physical signs and symptoms of stress may include: difficulty breathing, chest pain, profuse sweating, flushed skin, sleep disturbances, or aching muscles and joints.

39. d. behavioral—Additional behavioral signs and symptoms of stress may include: crying spells, depression, changes in eating and sleep patterns, and increased alcohol consumption.

40. d. All of the above—Environmental stress is often caused by: siren noise, inclement weather, confined work spaces, rapid scene response, or life-and-death decision making.

41. a. a conflict with a supervisor or coworker.—Additional causes of psychosocial stress may include: stressed family relationships, a spouse or significant other who doesn't understand what EMS work or training involves, or abusive patients or their family members.

42. a. feelings of guilt.—Additional causes of personality and emotional stress in paramedics may include: response to the death or injury of a child or coworker, personal expectations, feelings of anxiety or incompetence, or the need to be liked.

43. b. Coping—During this process, information is gathered and used to change or adjust to a new situation.

44. b. Controlled breathing—Examples of techniques used to manage stress include: reframing, controlled breathing, progressive relaxation, and guided imagery. Extensive information is available on each of these techniques in the "self-help" section in bookstores and libraries.

45. d. Critical incident stress management (CISM)—This process involves a network of peers and mental health professionals who support EMS providers who have been involved in a critical incident.

46. c. signs of gastrointestinal distress.—Signs of crisis-induced stress will vary for the individual and may include: headache, nausea, vomiting, anxiety, excessive humor or crying spells, or increased smoking, drinking, or drug use. The other answers listed are techniques used for reducing stress.

47. c. line-of-duty death or serious injury.—Crisis-induced stress reactions are also associated with disaster situations, emergency worker suicides, death of an infant or child, extreme threats to emergency workers, and death or injury of a civilian caused by the EMS provider.

48. c. increasing cigarette smoking.—Smoking increases heart rate and blood pressure, and impairs circulation.

49. a. allow them to express their feelings as best as you can.—Do not take this action personally or argue with the person. Avoid expressing any opinions or judgments.

50. b. 6–9 years old—At this age, children are beginning to understand the finality of death. They will seek out detailed explanations for the death and want to understand the difference between a fatal illness and just being sick.

51. b. Tell the truth and be straightforward when talking about the death of a loved one.—This can be very

difficult. Do not distort reality by saying that the person who has died has "gone to sleep" or "God took him." These phrases can lead to unnecessary fears.

52. b. shock.—There is no timetable on how long it generally takes for someone to go through the steps. The steps in order of occurrence are: shock, denial, anger, bargaining, depression, and acceptance.

53. d. sterilizing all ambulance equipment on a regular basis.—This is not practical or necessary. Sterilizing certain non-disposable items, such as laryngoscope blades, is appropriate.

54. a. exposure—An example of an exposure would be respiratory secretions sprayed into the face of the EMS provider.

55. c. completing the required medical follow-up.—Also included in the procedure for an exposure are properly reporting and documenting the situation in which the exposure occurred, and cooperating with the investigation.

56. c. actions taken to reduce chances of infection.—This may include: washing the affected area as soon as possible, seeking immediate medical attention when appropriate, and complying with recommended prophylaxis by your medical director or infection control expert.

57. b. Disinfection—There are three levels of disinfection: low, intermediate, and high.

58. d. prevent contact with body substances such as blood and urine.—Standard precautions is a series of practices designed to prevent contact with body substances such as blood, urine, fecal material, vomitus, and so forth.

59. b. biofeedback.—A technique used for managing stress that uses mental control to manipulate the heartbeat or brain waves.

60. b. vaccination—Vaccinations are utilized for preventing diseases.

Chapter 2: EMS Systems, Roles and Responsibilities of the Paramedic

1. b. Cincinnati—A few years later, ambulance service was provided by the New York City Department of Health from Bellevue Hospital.

2. b. 1928—The first rescue squad was launched in Roanoke, VA by Julien Stanley Wise.

3. b. mouth-to-mouth resuscitation.—Doctors Safar and Elan demonstrated the effectiveness of mouth-to-mouth ventilation in humans.

4. d. portable defibrillator—Developed at the Johns Hopkins Hospital in 1959 as a treatment for cardiac arrest patients.

5. b. Highway Safety Act—This act also required the secretary of the DOT, through their newly created EMS program, to develop a series of training programs to respond to the needs of patients injured on the highways.

6. a. The television show *Emergency*—Portrayed rescue workers and paramedics working in the streets of Los Angles, CA.

7. c. Ambulance Specifications—Published in 1974 by the DOT and referred to as the KKK-A-1822 Ambulance Design Specifications.

8. c. Nancy Caroline, MD and the University of Pittsburgh, PA—In 1975, the development of the first EMT-Paramedic National Standard Curriculum was given to Nancy Caroline, MD and the University of Pittsburgh, PA.

9. c. 1995—The last revision of the EMT-B curriculum included the application of the AED skills for EMTs.

10. c. EMS system—The components of the emergency medical services system (EMSS) have evolved over the past 30 years from fifteen essential components (EMSS Act of 1973) to ten standard components (NHTSA Technical Assistance Program 1988).

11. b. licensure.—Examples of licenses include: a medical license or fishing license and, in some states, a paramedic license.

12. a. certification—This is usually used to refer to an action of a nongovernmental entity granting authority to an individual who has met predetermined qualifications to participate in an activity.

13. c. critical care technician—The four levels of prehospital training recognized by the National Registry of Emergency Medical Technicians (NREMTs) are: emergency medical responder, EMT, advanced EMT, and paramedic.

14. a. emergency medical responder.—The role of the EMR is initial and basic stabilization, and to interact with the EMS system. An EMR could be a part of a responding team firefighter, police officer, or part of a responsive team at a work site.

15. d. all of the above—Each level of EMS responder has the role and responsibility of providing safety, primary assessment and treatment, and portraying a professional and positive appearance.

16. b. contributing to the development of professional standards.—The National Registry is also responsible for verifying competency, developing and administering practical and written examinations, simplifying the process of reciprocity or credentialing, and spreading the costs of exam development and validation across a larger user base than most states.

17. c. The current paramedic curriculum does not contain recertification curricula.—This is true. NHTSA, however, issued a lengthy position paper emphasizing the need for states to move toward recertification by using continuing education and adhering to a form similar to that used by the National Registry.

18. c. Reciprocity—The process of issuing credentials based on prior training in another state.

19. d. refreshes knowledge and skills, and introduces new material.—Attending CE also increases the paramedic's knowledge base and understanding of relevant EMS issues.

20. a. integrity—This means honesty in all of your actions and words. This important attribute is assumed by the public to be part of the responsibility of a paramedic.

21. b. The expectations by society of health care professionals are high, both on and off duty.—EMS providers are very visible role models whose behaviors are closely observed. Image and behavior in public, both on and off duty, are extremely important.

22. b. Ethics—The principles of conduct governing an individual or group.

23. c. peer review.—A couple of examples are a coworker providing tips on how to lift a patient out of a tight spot or reviewing each other's paperwork for better ways to document what was done on the call.

24. a. integrity.—One of the most important attributes for the EMS professional is integrity. Examples of behavior demonstrating integrity are always telling the truth, never stealing, and providing complete and accurate documentation.

25. b. empathy.—Having empathy in emergency medicine means identifying with and understanding the feelings, situations, and motives of your patients.

26. a. Empathy—Examples of behavior demonstrating empathy include: showing caring and compassion, being supportive and reassuring, and demonstrating respect.

27. b. having a good understanding of your limitations.—Someone who is self-confident, but not overly confident, knows when to call for backup or consult with medical direction rather than getting in over one's head.

28. d. help to instill confidence in the patient and his or her family.—The manner in which you walk and carry yourself is important! Patients do not appreciate an EMS provider with bad breath, body odor, or too much aftershave or perfume.

29. d. is dressed appropriately and prepared to work when the shift begins.—Good patient care involves good time management skills. Examples include: prioritizing tasks during patient care; being punctual for meetings, appointments, and work shifts; and being prepared to work at the start of the shift.

30. a. careful documentation of care administered.—The ways in which errors happen include: skills-based failures, rules-based failures, and knowledge-based failures.

31. b. Diplomacy—Diplomacy is tact and skill in dealing with people and goes hand in hand with teamwork. Being a diplomat also involves saying and doing things that are considered "politically correct."

32. b. disagreeing with a coworker in public.—The patient's bedside is no place for interprofessional disagreements. Doing this in public, especially in front of a patient, is unprofessional and may negatively impact the image of you and your ambulance service.

33. d. be an advocate for your patient.—Part of your responsibility as the EMS provider is to advocate for

your patient. Sometimes this means not just delivering the patients to the busy ED, but staying with them for a few minutes to ensure that the ED staff fully understands the extent of the mechanism of injury (MOI) or nature of illness (NOI).

34. b. Telling a patient who smokes that he or she is really stupid for doing so.—Instead of scorning the patient, use this event as a teaching moment, and explain the risks associated with smoking and the benefits of cessation.

35. b. protecting the patient's confidentiality.—Protecting patient confidentiality is also a legal and ethical responsibility.

36. c. protecting the patient's furniture while moving your stretcher through the living room.—A good paramedic pays attention to details. There may be times when the details are skipped due to the patient's severity, but most calls involve enough time for you to pay attention to things like wiping your feet before entering a patient's home.

37. a. ensure quality patient care.—The primary role of the medical director is to ensure quality patient care. The responsibilities include: authority over patient care and the authority to limit patient care activities of those who deviate from established standards; involvement with the ongoing design, operation, evaluation, and revision of the EMS system; and development and implementation of medical policies and procedures.

38. c. Protocols—Most protocols involve specific medical treatments and, as such, come under the domain of medical direction.

39. a. participating in the development of continuing education.—Additional typical roles include: participating in the personnel selection process, equipment selection, participating in quality improvement and problem resolution, interfacing between EMS systems and other health care agencies, and advocating within the medical community.

40. a. the ability to obtain real-time direction and orders.—Many patients have complicated problems that do not fit into specific protocols. Being able to obtain online direction can help the paramedic to provide better patient care with expanded treatment options.

41. b. protocols.—Off-line or indirect medical control utilizes guidelines (protocols) for the management of specific patient presenting problems. The protocols have appropriate "stop lines" to allow certain treatment options before having to establish online or direct medical control.

42. d. All of the above.—Confirm that the physician is a medical doctor who is willing to come with you and the patient to the hospital. Contact medical control to advise of the situation, and have the two physicians speak with each other.

43. d. by conforming to the standards of a health care professional providing quality patient care—Having a

college degree, a lawyer on retainer, or knowing as many customers as possible in your area of response is fine, but not necessarily what one needs to be prepared to work as a paramedic.

44. a. clinical capabilities—Ideally, you would not bring a patient having a heart attack to a hospital that could not perform cardiac catherizations, or a serious burn patient to a non-trauma hospital.

45. d. replacing disposable items available from the hospital.—Restocking the ambulance with disposable items at the hospital in order to get the ambulance back in service as quickly as possible is a primary responsibility of the EMS provider.

46. a. It enhances visibility and a positive image of the paramedics and their agencies.—The primary benefits include: improving the health of the community regarding injury and illness prevention, ensuring appropriate utilization of resources by making sure the public knows when, where, and how to use EMS, improving the integration of EMS with other health care and public safety agencies, and enhancing visibility and a positive image of EMS providers and their agencies.

47. c. training to be a career paramedic/firefighter.—This is an example of a personal goal rather than an example of citizen involvement in EMS systems.

48. a. patient well-care visits.—One of the activities the EMS Agenda for the Future recognizes is the integration of health services. One example is to expand the EMS role in public health and involve EMS in community health monitoring activities.

49. b. the transportation alternatives are very costly.—When considering the system finance aspect, it is recommended that there be a collaborative effort with other health care providers and insurers to enhance patient care efficiency and develop proactive financial relations between EMS, other health care providers, and health care insurers.

50. c. integration of EMS with other health care providers to deliver quality care.—It also discusses expansion of the EMS role in public health in community health monitoring activities; being cognizant of the special needs of the entire population; and incorporation of health systems within EMS that address special needs.

51. c. develop information systems that provide linkage between various health care services.—It also speaks to the development of academic institutional commitments to EMS-related research, and the allocation of federal and state funds for major EMS system research.

52. a. authorizing and funding a lead federal EMS agency.—It also discusses establishing and funding the position of state EMS medical director in each state, and implementing laws that provide protection from liability for EMS providers when dealing with unusual situations.

53. b. Collaboration with other health care providers.—It also addresses compensating EMS on the basis of a preparedness-based mode, reducing volume-related incentives, and realizing the cost of an emergency safety net.

54. a. conducting EMS occupation health research.—It also discusses developing a system of reciprocity for EMS-provider credentials, and developing collaborative relations between EMS and academic institutions.

55. a. require appropriate credentials for all those who provide online medical directions.—Other proposals include: appointing state EMS medical directors, and formalizing relations between all EMS systems and medical direction, with the appropriate resources to do so.

56. d. bridging and transitioning EMS programs with all health professions' education.—Since many courses in health care overlap, an example of this would be a course that would provide training to allow the student to graduate as a nurse and a paramedic, or a physician's assistant and a paramedic.

57. c. exploring and evaluating public education alternatives.—Other goals include collaborating with other community resources and agencies to determine public education needs, and engaging in continuous public education programs.

58. b. assess the effectiveness of resource attributes for EMS dispatching.—This includes assessing the effectiveness of personnel and requiring that personnel have the education, experience, and resources to optimally query the caller, make a determination of the most appropriate resources to be mobilized, and implement an effective course of action.

59. d. commit to a common definition of what constitutes baseline community EMS care.—Additional goals include establishing proactive relationships between EMS and other health care providers, and subjecting EMS clinical care to ongoing evaluations to determine its impact on patient outcomes.

60. c. develop a mechanism to generate and transmit data that are valid, reliable, and accurate.—Additional goals include adopting uniform data elements and definitions, incorporating the elements into information systems, and developing systems that are able to describe an entire EMS event.

61. c. determine EMS effects for multiple outcome categories and cost-effectiveness.—Additional elements of the evaluation component include evaluating EMS effects for various medical conditions and developing valid models for EMS evaluations that incorporate consumer input.

62. b. uncover problems and provide solutions.—Specifically in the areas of medical direction, training, communication, dispatch, public information and education, mutual aide, and disaster planning.

63. c. National EMS Education Standards—The education that a paramedic should receive to become a competent entry level provider is outlined in the National EMS Education Standards.

64. b. Cardiac rescue technician—The levels of EMS providers described in the National EMS Educational Standards are: EMR, EMT, advanced EMT, and paramedic.

65. c. profession—Professions usually involve a specialized body of knowledge or expertise. They are often self-regulating through a licensure or certification process that requires competence validation.

66. a. Your image and behavior in the public's eye are not significant.—There are high expectations by society of health care professionals, both on and off duty.

67. d. patients and their families.—Certainly, empathy can be expressed in many ways to many people; however, the paramedic would typically express empathy to a patient, families of patients, or even other health care providers.

68. b. taking advantage of all learning opportunities—Self-motivation is the internal drive for excellence. Examples of this include taking the initiative to complete assignments, improve, and correct behavior, or taking advantage of as many learning opportunities as possible.

69. d. politically correct.—The paramedic job is very dynamic and, at times, includes playing the role of the diplomat, peacekeeper, negotiator, and tactician.

70. c. Most of what paramedics do involves communication skills.—Paramedics talk on radios, talk to coworkers and other emergency service providers, and, most importantly, establish a rapport with patients so a history and assessment can be obtained.

Chapter 3: Public Health and Research

1. d. Epidemiology—This is the branch of medicine that deals with the incidence, distribution, and control of disease in a population.

2. a. morbidity.—The state or incidence of a disease or injury.

3. a. heart disease—The CDC reports, for the year 2002, that disease of the heart remains the leading cause of death.

4. a. For ages 1 through 44, accidents were the leading cause of death.—This is why injury prevention is

so important and why it is sensible for EMS providers to be involved in injury and illness prevention efforts in their communities.

5. b. There are more expectations for EMS services to provide care for patients being managed in the home setting.—As the hospitals have moved toward doing more procedures on an outpatient basis and are decreasing the number of hospital stay days for the treatment of injuries and illnesses, the reliance on EMS has increased.

6. a. accidents.—When death rates of Caucasians are compared to those of African Americans, the leading causes of death are the same except in two age groups. In the 15-to 24-year-olds, the leading cause was accidents in whites and homicide in blacks.

7. d. Injury risk—The definition of injury risk is a real or potentially hazardous situation that puts individuals at risk for sustaining an injury.

8. a. prevention and control efforts.—Injury surveillance is the ongoing systematic collection, analysis, and interpretation of injury data essential to the planning, implementation, and evaluation of public health practice. Timely dissemination of this data is needed for prevention and control efforts.

9. b. Secondary—This is where EMS has a great responsibility. For example, while extricating a victim with a possible cervical injury from a significant wreck, the EMS provider must assure adequate stabilization of the spine to prevent further (secondary) injury during the process.

10. b. tertiary injury prevention.—Examples of this would be preventing infection, or making modifications to a patient's home to accommodate a disability.

11. b. pick a cause that best suits your interest.—Select an interest you have always wanted to know something about and stretch a little to learn about the cause.

12. c. Over 95% of victims of bicycle-related head injuries were not wearing helmets when injured.—The solutions to the problem include education in injury prevention, legislation requiring the use of helmets, and distribution of helmets.

13. c. Requiring personal flotation devices (PFDs) to be worn whenever children or adults who cannot swim are on or near water.—The other recommendations listed are impractical or impossible.

14. d. getting everyone in the vehicle to wear seat belts.—The evidence from data clearly shows a direct correlation between wearing seat belts and lives saved.

15. d. use of child-resistant packaging of toxic substances for in-home use.—With more than 90% of poisoning exposures to children age 5 and under occurring in the home, the strategy behind this legislation was a push to educate the parents and older children to lock up the hazardous substances and label them appropriately.

16. c. homes.—This is why legislation was enacted in 1970 (Poison Prevention Act) to require the use of child-resistant packaging for toxic substances used in and around the home.

17. a. practice family fire escape plans every 6 months.—Additional strategies are to know what to do when your clothing catches fire, to change the batteries every 6 months, and to never smoke in bed.

18. a. educating riders to always wear a helmet and protective gear.—This is the most practical and proven strategy. Wearing a helmet reduces the chance of death and serious head injury as a result of a collision.

19. b. making sure that any surface that children may fall onto is soft and padded.—The best playgrounds have surfaces with at least 6 inches of mulch chips, pea gravel, fine sand, or shredded rubber to cushion a fall.

20. c. Injuries from falls affect the very young and the elderly more severely.—Childhood falls account for an estimated two million ED visits each year, while one in every three adults age 65 or older falls each year.

21. b. Installing tiles in kitchens and baths.—Tiled surfaces can be very slippery, especially when wet.

22. c. drawstrings on curtains or blinds—Another common cause of strangulation is drawstrings on clothing (sweatshirts). They can become entangled in playground equipment, fences, and furniture, causing strangulation.

23. a. disassembling the National Rifle Association.—Some might argue that this is the best strategy for the prevention of firearm injuries and fatalities.

24. d. 50,000—Each year, approximately 82,000 pedestrians are injured in traffic crashes. This includes over 50,000 children, who often sustain a serious brain injury.

25. a. avoid drinking and walking.—Drinking and driving is known to be one of the biggest contributors to highway deaths and injuries. However, drinking and walking near traffic is unsafe too and contributes to highway death and injury.

26. b. set examples in all activities of the organization.—There are many ways EMS providers can make it acceptable and, within the mission of the organization, can be involved in prevention activities.

27. b. develop sensible policies and procedures promoting safety in all work activities.—The EMS leader also has the responsibility to provide EMS workers with appropriate personal protective equipment (PPE) and to provide all necessary safety training as required by OSHA.

28. c. extreme ambient temperatures.—The paramedic must able to recognize exposure to hazardous materials, temperature extremes, vectors, communicable disease, assault, battery, and structural risks.

29. b. child protective services.—Additional resources to be cognizant of include: access to specialty equipment or devices, counseling services, alternative health care (e.g., free clinics), rehabilitation, grief support, and immunization programs.

30. b. recognizing the teachable moments.—Try to use concepts of effective communication such as: having a sense of time, being nonjudgmental, being objective, informing individuals about the use of protective devices, and informing the patient how he or she can prevent a recurrence.

31. d. all of the above—Some agencies use a special incident report to document hazards. Documentation of safety hazards should include: primary injury information, care provided, and any other specific information required by the EMS agency.

32. a. Scene conditions—Mechanism of injury (MOI), use of protective devices, absence of protective devices, and risks overcome are additional examples of primary injury data.

33. a. higher education attainment—Data have shown that higher education attainment is associated with a lower risk of death.

34. b. of their perspective offered in out-of-hospital care.—Paramedics come into the homes of the customers and have one of the best views or perspectives of any health care provider.

35. c. Primary injury prevention—An example would be not allowing diving in the shallow end of a swimming pool in an effort to prevent spinal injury or death.

36. d. research can be influenced by biases.—Quality EMS research is beneficial to the future of EMS, and biases can hinder and spoil research.

37. d. negatively affecting patient care.—The health care provider's philosophy is to "First do no harm."

38. a. what a randomized and controlled group is.—Several basic research concepts need to be understood, such as: the value of peer review and publishing research, types of research, how to randomize and select a control group, or how to select a sample using various methods. A statistics course can be very helpful in understanding the basics of research.

39. a. Collect the funding needs for the hypothesis development.—Funding is typically associated with working the hypothesis, rather than developing it.

40. c. providing results that lead to system improvements.—For example, research may reveal that repositioning emergency response units based on the location and frequency of calls can improve the average response time.

Chapter 4: Communications: EMS Systems and Therapeutic

1. d. the code summary on a monitor-defibrillator unit.—Pulse oximeters, capnography, electronic BP, and temperature devices are other examples of electronic communication used by paramedics.

2. c. detection.—Occurrence is the first phase of communication necessary to complete a typical EMS call, and detection is the second phase.

3. b. treatment.—In the treatment phase of communication necessary to complete a typical EMS call, the paramedic may choose to contact medical control to discuss treatment options for the patient.

4. b. Receiver gives feedback.—The basic model of communication has six steps: sender has a message; sender encodes the message; sender sends the message; receiver receives the message; receiver decodes the message; receiver gives feedback to the sender.

5. c. the patient's family physician.—Although this is not required, there are times when calling the patient's physician can be helpful. For example, when the patient initially refuses transport for evaluation for a serious condition (e.g., chest pain), the physician can help persuade the patient to go to the hospital.

6. c. add an unnecessary level of complexity.—Many services that previously used special radio codes have changed to plain English to prevent confusion or the possibility of multiple interpretations.

7. c. global positioning device—Many cell phones already have a global position system, and, in the near future, all cell phones will have this technology.

8. b. semantics.—Semantics and technical terminology are two factors that tend to impede verbal communication.

9. a. avoid technical terms.—To help avoid confusion, select your words and phrases with the audience in mind.

10. b. it helps avoid cutting off the first few words.—This is called "keying the microphone."

11. a. getting angry in return—Anger and hostility is often misdirected at the caregiver. Do not get angry in return; it is nonproductive and stressful.

12. a. close proximity to computers—Sometimes, 60-cycle interference can occur when the radio is too close to a computer, fluorescent light fixture, or electronic motor.

13. b. prearrival instructions.—The emergency medical dispatcher (EMD) is trained to give prearrival instructions to the caller. These instructions may include helping the caller deliver a baby, providing bleeding control, or the compression of CPR.

14. a. direct.—With unstable and critical patients, ask questions that require a one- or two-word answer. With a patient in severe respiratory distress, ask questions that require nonverbal answers.

15. d. queue—During this time, the dispatcher determines the type of call, the most appropriate units to dispatch, and their response mode.

16. b. the scene time may be inaccurately lengthened.—On calls where it takes a while to find the patient, the scene time can be extended. This extra scene time should be explained on the PCR.

17. b. a lengthy extrication.—An extrication can take minutes or hours, depending on the type of entrapment.

18. b. Encoding—The communication process used by the EMS provider that is focused around a message. The message moves through various forms: written, verbal, nonverbal, encoding, message, decoding, receiver, and feedback.

19. b. second-party caller.—The first party is the patient calling for herself.

20. d. all of the above.—The FCC is responsible for regulating all aspects of the communication industry.

21. b. pre-arrival instructions—The emergency medical dispatchers trained using Jeff Clawson's system provide prearrival instructions that effectively create a "zero-minute" response time.

22. d. The paramedic could lose the patient's trust.—It is better to explain what is happening and what is going to happen next. If the patient perceives that you are lying, you may not get the cooperation you need.

23. c. give them time to prepare for the patient.—A verbal report over the radio or telephone helps prepare the ED for the arrival of the patient.

24. a. patient's name—The airways are public and open for all to hear. Never say anything over the radio, including divulging the patient's name, that you would be uncomfortable saying on public television.

25. a. drugs administered on standing orders.—The other choices listed are information that would normally be provided in the standard radio report.

26. a. receiver.—The message moves through various forms: written, verbal, nonverbal, encoding, message, decoding, receiver, and feedback.

27. c. say each digit for clarity when transmitting a number.—This technique is a basic principle of proper radio system usage.

28. b. digital transmitters do not require voice transmission time over the radio.—Some EMS systems have mobile data terminals that can receive a call from a dispatcher and print it out.

29. b. frequency.—Depending on the range, radio frequency may be very high (VHF) or ultra high (UHF).

30. a. call simplex.—On this system, it is not possible to transmit and receive at the same time.

31. d. repeater.—Repeaters can be used on radio towers or ambulances.

32. b. communication—The communication process used by the EMS provider is focused around a message.

33. b. FM; AM—Frequency modulation is more reliable than amplitude modulation.

34. b. analog transmission.—Analog is a voice transmission.

35. b. You don't smoke, do you?—Condescending or judgmental questions can make a patient uncomfortable, and this may cause him to lie about other information, or lead to information being withheld.

36. d. avoid the use of complicated medical terminology.—Stick to the use of lay terms as much as possible. If you are caring for a health care professional who understands medical jargon, it should become apparent quickly, and the use of medical terminology may be appropriate.

37. b. inattentiveness.—Inattentiveness can make a patient feel uncomfortable and lead to information being withheld.

38. c. Facilitation—Positive examples of facilitation include sitting close to the patient and making eye contact, while you nod or say, "I'm listening" or "Please tell me more."

39. d. reflection.—Reflection helps the patient feel that you are listening and can confirm information that is pertinent to the event.

40. a. Interpretation—An example would be to say, "It appears that when you exert yourself physically, you develop a shortness of breath."

41. a. the patient is blind—An overtalkative or symptomatic patient can be challenged when faced with limited time for interview and care, and, if the condition of the developmentally disabled patient is severe, information may be omitted.

42. c. Vial of life®.—This is an example of a commercial device available to provide medical and other emergency information about a patient to emergency medical providers.

43. a. Use positive body language while you begin care.—Ideally, the best solution is to find a translator. Otherwise, use positive body language, such as friendly facial expressions and slow movements to assess, take vital signs, and provide treatment.

44. d. ask permission to touch the patient before actually touching him or her.—This action is appropriate with most every patient, but especially with a blind person. You can avoid frightening the patient and reduce anxiety by first explaining prior to touching.

45. c. depression.—Do not hesitate to ask a patient about her feelings. Depression is associated with some psychological illnesses.

46. d. Try using direct "yes or no" questions.—Attempt to get the patient to focus on one thing at a time by having him answer questions that require a "yes or

no" answer. It may keep both of you from becoming frustrated.

47. c. Establishing a rapport with the patient—It begins from the time the call is dispatched and lasts until the patient is turned over to the ED.
48. c. MedicAlert® tags—A number of information sources are found on patients in the field. Some wear necklaces or bracelets, while others use smart cards, computer chips, or wallet cards. The most common are the necklaces and bracelets available from the MedicAlert® Foundation, which maintains a 24-hour Emergency Response Center.
49. a. ADA—The Americans with Disabilities Act includes a provision that requires the hospital to provide a sign interpreter within 30 minutes of the patient's arrival.
50. d. look to see if his hearing aid is on.—Many patients who have hearing aids do not wear them. Ask the patient if he has one, and help him to place it and turn it on.

Chapter 5: Documentation

1. b. an indication of poor assessment.—Some say the paperwork is almost as important as the care itself. Whether or not your assessment and care were optimal, poor documentation is a difficult hurdle to overcome.
2. a. Documentation serves as a legal record of the incident.—The documentation that is completed for out-of-hospital care provides a professional link between the field assessment and in-hospital management.
3. a. NHTSA—The National Highway Traffic Safety Administration, a part of the Department of Transportation, has defined the minimum data set in order to standardize and compare data from different agencies and systems.
4. c. disposition of the call—The patient data includes patient name, address, date of birth, gender, age, nature of the call, mechanism of injury, nature of illness, location of the patient, SAMPLE history, signs and symptoms, assessment findings, treatment, changes in patient condition, and disposition of the call.
5. d. level of training of the crew members—The run data includes: the date, times, service name, unit identifier, and the names and level of training of the crew members.
6. d. DNAR.—The do not attempt resuscitation order (DNAR) or DNR is prepared by the patient and his physician.
7. b. the patient's address—Patient demographic information includes the patient's name, address, age, date of birth, phone number, Social Security number, and so on.
8. c. Remove patient's name from documentation.—The patient's name must be removed or completely covered if the forms will be used for discussion with providers other than those who were present on the specific call.
9. a. Vital signs should be documented before and after a medication administration.—Vital signs are documented before and after interventions to determine the effect.
10. b. being objective, specific, and concrete.—When documenting, use objective language. Be precise by writing exactly what you see, hear, feel, or smell, and avoid making judgments.
11. b. both sides.—Circum –around; ambl/y –dim, dull, or lazy; ant –against or opposed to.
12. b. development, formation.—Dynia –a painful condition; -plasty –a surgical repair; -plegia –paralysis.
13. d. "speaks for itself."—A PCR should, by itself, provide a complete and accurate portrait of the patient's needs and the care given.
14. c. averting further legal action during the "discovery phase" of a lawsuit.—The proper documentation of patient care is one more step toward keeping clear of legal entanglements.
15. d. "The patient stated she vomited four times last night."—Remain objective and be precise by writing exactly what you see, hear, feel, or smell, and avoid making judgments.
16. d. the length and design of stylet used to facilitate the intubation—Unless there is something very unique about this piece of equipment, this information is irrelevant.
17. a. A patient struck his head in MVC and denies a loss of consciousness.—A pertinent negative is a negative response, such as the answer to a question that adds to the assessment. Pertinent negatives are valuable data that are routinely documented on PCRs.
18. a. Subjective—This information consists of symptoms or answers to questions.
19. c. Objective—This information is exactly what you read, see, hear, feel, or smell.
20. d. held in confidence.—HIPAA laws help to ensure this.
21. c. pale, diaphoretic skin—Objective findings are things you can see or measure, such as vital signs or the patient's skin CTC.

22. b. to show trends in the patient's condition.—Take vital signs every 5 minutes for critical or unstable patients and every 15 minutes for stable patients.

23. c. had something to hide.—The proper documentation of patient care is one more step toward keeping clear of legal entanglements.

24. b. dorsiflexion—bending backward; protraction—pushing forward; lateral rotation—rotating outward away from the body's midline; cephalad extension—stretching or moving in a straight line toward the head.

25. c. who adjusted the drip rate.—Unless there is an extenuating circumstance, this is extraneous information. The paramedic has oversight of this and is responsible for any amount of fluid infused.

26. b. the patient's medical insurance information—In most agencies, this information is recorded on a separate billing form or included with the PCR. Narcotic use, such as administering morphine, is documented on the PCR and often requires special documentation on another form, both of which are separate from the billing form.

27. b. triage tags—This is a form of documentation used in special situations (multiple casualty incident [MCI]).

28. b. follow your state and local guidelines.—Each state has its own guidelines for mandatory reporting of suspected child abuse or neglect.

29. d. Erase the entry.—Erasing an entry may appear as if the record is being altered.

30. c. Radio failure delayed contact with medical control and subsequent medical orders.—Any unusual occurrence during the call that affects the patient should be documented on the PCR. In addition, a special incident report may be needed depending on the service's standard operating procedures.

31. a. Adequacy of the neurovascular supply before and after immobilization.—Excellent documentation of pre- and post-splinting (or immobilization) findings may be vital when defending your care.

32. b. document the statement in "quotes."—Examples of statements to quote include a dying statement, admission of guilt to a crime, or a threat of suicide.

33. c. standardized and professional.—Many agencies and regions have approved lists of terms or abbreviations to use or avoid in documentation.

34. b. q.i.d.—This information may be found on prescription drug bottles or in a patient's medical records. When discovered by the paramedic, this information must be passed on to the next health care provider.

35. c. patient's marital status.—The information may be included in the narrative by the paramedic in a statement such as "The patient's wife reported. . . ."

36. c. compare data from different agencies.—The National Highway Traffic Safety Administration has defined the minimum data set in order to standardize and compare data from different agencies and systems.

37. a. The record contains everything it should in a clear, legible, and concise fashion.—When the PCR "stands on its own," you or anyone else should be able to refer to it in the future and be perfectly clear about what happened.

38. a. SOAP and CHART.—CUPS and AVPU are used for level of consciousness and to assess mental status. SAMPLE, OPQRST, and PMHX are used to obtain a focused history, and APGAR is used for assessing the newborns.

39. c. professional responsibilities—Often, decisions about the patient's care are made based on PCR documentation. The PCR must accurately reflect what the paramedic found and what was done for the patient.

40. c. a police officer who is a friend of the patient—Patient's have a legal right to have their medical information held in confidence, and breaching that right may cause harm or embarrassment to the patient and her family.

41. d. all of the above—Documenting special situations may require additional forms or may need to be cleared through the supervisor or another superior. There are correct and incorrect methods of correcting documentation errors.

42. a. The specific recommendation for care and transport, and consequences of refusing care.—Document the competency of the patient and avoid nonprofessional statements.

43. c. at the ED, after transfer of the patient to a bed.—Ideally, the PCR should be completed while the information is fresh in your mind. Then a copy of the record should be left at the hospital as part of the patient's permanent record.

44. a. narrative.—The administrative and demographics sections are usually in a format that requires filling in or checking boxes.

45. d. all findings should be recorded—Each finding is important and should be documented. Often, decisions about the patient's care are made based on PCR documentation. The PCR must accurately reflect what the paramedic found and what was done for the patient.

46. d. Libel—Slander is false or malicious statements in the form of spoken words.

47. a. All personnel and resources involved in the call should be recorded.—This is called covering yourself. Be sure to include duty supervisors also.

48. d. superficial—The other terms have different relationships to the body.

49. a. Stasis—stomy –a surgical opening; scopy –to see; plasty –surgical repair.

50. a. nephr/o—Hepat/o –relates to the liver; ganglio –a knot; dacry/o –a tear.

Chapter 6: Medical/Legal and Ethics

1. c. legislative—Legislative law is made up of statutes that are voted on and passed by the legislature. An example of legislative law is a state's EMS Act.

2. a. legislative—Legislative law is made up of statutes that are voted on and passed by the legislature, be it the city council, county board, state legislature, or Congress.

3. c. "jury of your peers."—A jury may be selected by either the judge or the attorneys for each side.

4. b. EMS code.—The EMS code of rules and regulations that outline the specifics of the EMS law for each state will vary.

5. c. case—Case law is often used in a court to decide pending cases.

6. b. criminal—Criminal law deals with wrongs against members of society, such as homicide and rape. Federal, state, and local governments prosecute individuals for violating these laws.

7. c. civil—In a civil case the jury determines damages, such as money, for compensation, but the judge may modify the award. When there is no jury, the judge takes on both roles.

8. d. defendant.—The defendant is the person required to make answer in a legal action or suit.

9. b. hearing.—A hearing is a session in which testimony is taken from witnesses.

10. b. jury—In a court of law, a jury is comprised of persons legally sworn to give a verdict on some matter submitted to them according to the evidence.

11. b. may be appealed to a higher court.—An appellate court decision can uphold the decision of the trial court, overrule it, or send it back (remand) to the lower court for various reasons.

12. c. grand jury—An example of a case that may go to the grand jury is one involving allegations of wrongdoing during an ambulance collision. It is often the grand jury that decides if the DA will charge the driver of the ambulance for actions that may have caused injury, death, or property damages.

13. b. negligence.—This is also called malpractice when speaking of a failure to exercise an acceptable degree of professional skill or competence.

14. c. civil court.—In civil court cases, the jury determines damages, such as money, for compensation, but the judge may modify the award. When there is no jury, the judge takes on both roles.

15. b. breach of duty.—A breach of duty occurs if you have an established duty to act and do not comply with that duty (e.g., receiving an EMS call and refusing to respond).

16. a. nonfeasance.—Nonfeasance is the failure to perform a required duty or act.

17. a. proximate cause.—Proximate cause means that the damages to the patient were directly caused by the paramedic's act of omission or commission.

18. a. proximate cause.—Proximate cause means that the damages to the patient were directly caused by the paramedic's act of omission or commission.

19. b. gross negligence.—Gross negligence involves willful, wanton, intentional, or reckless actions, such as passing an endotracheal tube down the esophagus to see how long it takes for the pulse oximeter to drop below 80%.

20. d. abandonment.—An example of abandonment is delivering a patient to a busy ED, placing the patient onto a stretcher in the hall, and leaving without giving a report to the ED physician.

21. b. false imprisonment.—This is one of the major reasons why it is so important to get consent before taking the patient to the hospital.

22. c. slander.—Rumors or malicious spoken words about another person can hurt the reputation of that person.

23. a. libel.—Examples of libel might be written graffiti or anonymous notes.

24. b. delegation.—Delegation of authority is the granting of medical privileges by a physician, either online or off-line, to an EMS provider to perform skills or procedures within the EMS provider's scope of practice.

25. a. scope of practice.—The scope of practice is usually set by state law or regulation and by local medical authorities.

26. c. *res ipsaloquitur*—This term is used in reference to malpractice in which the cause of the damages does not require any special expertise to detect; the negligence is evident to a layperson.

27. c. negligence per se.—Negligence per se is the unexcused violation of a statute. An example of this would be an ambulance traveling through a red light at an excessive speed and injuring a pedestrian while doing so.

28. d. contributory negligence.—Contributory negligence arises when the actions of the plaintiff contribute to his own injury. As a result, the damages awarded the plaintiff may be reduced.

29. b. an investigation.—After an incident occurs, the plaintiff's representative investigates to see what facts can be uncovered. With the information discovered from the investigation, the plaintiff's representative will then decide whether to file a complaint and serve the defendant.

30. b. discovery.—Discovery may involve releasing documents such as dispatch tapes, patient records, and PCRs.

31. a. settlement.—At any time while the case is pending, an agreement may be made between the parties to settle the case.

32. a. interrogatories.—Obtaining interrogatories occurs during the discovery phase and allows the opposing sides to formulate their theories of the case and how they will present them, and to prevent surprise at trial.

33. c. liability.—Something for which someone is responsible.

34. b. statute of limitations.—The applicable time limits differ from state to state and are also dependent upon the cause of action.

35. b. strengthen and validate our own inner value system.—It also serves to give direction to our moral compass and becomes the foundation upon which we can commit.

36. a. expressed—Expressed consent is when the patient directly agrees, either verbally or nonverbally, to receive care.

37. d. informed—Informed consent is given after full disclosure, or explanation, of information is provided to the patient.

38. b. emergency doctrine.—This type of consent applies to emergency intervention given to a patient who is physically or mentally unable to provide expressed consent.

39. a. no—This means that a parent or guardian must be contacted if the minor is involved in a medical emergency.

40. b. acting in the patient's best interest.—Be careful not to fall into the trap of making a value judgment; always act in the patient's best interest.

41. d. full disclosure was provided to an alert patient.—A refusal of medical assistance (RMA) is considered legal if it is obtained in a proper manner with full disclosure to the patient of assessment findings, treatment recommendations, and the implications of refusal.

42. c. consult medical control.—It may be helpful in some instances to put the patient on the phone with the physician.

43. c. No, persons with an altered mental status are not usually able to make a competent decision.—As most EMS providers do not receive formal training to make the judgment about the level of intoxication and do not carry equipment to measure the percentage of alcohol in the blood, the police should be utilized in these cases.

44. a. Not without additional training.—As most EMS providers do not receive formal training to make the judgment about the level of intoxication and do not carry equipment to measure the percentage of alcohol in the blood, the police should be utilized in these cases.

45. b. Yes, under the emergency doctrine.—Emergency doctrine or implied consent is the type of consent that applies to emergency intervention given for a patient who is physically or mentally unable to provide expressed consent.

46. b. A mental health officer.—Involuntary commitment requirements and procedures vary from state to state. Speak with your agency's attorney to learn what your state's laws are in this area.

47. b. protective custody.—The police can, in most jurisdictions, take a person into protective custody for a limited period of time if they feel the person may have a serious condition that could pose a life-threat without the appropriate emergency care.

48. b. Involve the police for some assistance.—EMS providers are often put in a difficult position by family members who would like them to take the patient away against his will.

49. b. Civil Rights Act.—Services that employ EMS providers are responsible for complying with the Civil Rights Act (Title VII) of 1964, which is the federal law prohibiting discrimination based on race, color, religion, sex, or national origin.

50. d. all of the above.—A durable power of attorney or health care proxy allows a person to designate another person (agent) to act in cases where the person is unable to make decisions for him- or herself.

51. b. health care proxy—This is also referred to as a Healthcare Power of Attorney.

52. a. when a third party requires the information for billing—Release of patient information requires written permission from the patient or legal guardian, except when: a third party requires the information for billing, mandatory reporting by law (e.g., child abuse), in response to a subpoena, or to other health care providers who need to know how to provide care to the patient.

53. a. Humane restraints—The use of padded leather restraints or sheets are more acceptable to reduce the potential harm to the patient. Handcuffs are not considered humane restraints.

54. b. ethical—Typically there is no legal responsibility, but the paramedic does have an ethical responsibility to resuscitate all potential organ donors so that others may benefit from the organs.

55. c. the information has to be quickly available for billing.—The PCR is an important part of the patient's record, and a copy needs to go to the ED in the patient's chart. It should be completed while information is fresh in the paramedic's mind. It also must be a record made "in the course of business" and not completed later.

56. a. her harmful actions.—Not all states allow plaintiffs to seek punitive damages. If awarded, these are usually not covered by malpractice insurance.

57. d. receiving a direct (online) order that is medically acceptable but morally wrong.—Occasionally, the paramedic is given a physician order that he believes is contraindicated, medically acceptable but

not in the patient's best interest, or medically acceptable but morally wrong.

58. b. plaintiff—The plaintiff brings the suit, so the burden of proof is on the plaintiff.

59. a. Scope of practice—Scope is the range of skills and knowledge in which the EMS provider is trained. The standard of care is based on national standards, national curricula, national testing standards, and the recognized treatment for patients in similar circumstances.

60. c. Freedom of Information Act—Sometimes called the Freedom of Information Law, or FOIL. The agency that is being requested to provide the information may charge a minimal fee for the duplication or preparation of the information, and must provide the information within a reasonable time of its request.

61. d. "borrowed servant"—If the paramedic is acting as a preceptor or in a supervisory capacity, he may be held liable for the actions of that intern.

62. c. false imprisonment.—The imprisonment of someone that is contrary to the law.

63. a. Was the signal that was given audible and/or visible to motorists and pedestrians?—Points that are considered include: was the signaling equipment actually used, was the signal that was given audible or visible to motorists and pedestrians, and was it reasonably necessary under all of the circumstances to use the signaling equipment?

64. c. creating laws protecting patient's rights.—In addition, the preplans, such as wills and advanced directives, are used to make patient wishes known.

65. a. certificate—A certification is the act of certifying or the state of being certified.

66. b. The operator of the emergency vehicle assumes the extra burden of driving with due regard for others.—The operator has the added responsibility of ensuring that no one is injured and that no property becomes damaged because of his driving.

67. c. has hearing impairment—A qualified individual is one who has a disability that limits one or more major life activities. Temporary disabilities and illegal drug use are not covered under the ADA.

68. b. witnessing a coworker do something unethical and saying nothing.—This is a personal decision that you should think through before it occurs!

69. b. FLSA—Fair Labor Standards Act is the federal law that regulates minimum wages and overtime in the workplace. In EMS, the law has an impact on issues such as on-call pay, compensatory time, long shifts, and overtime pay.

70. b. encourage the improvement of existing safety and health programs.—The purpose of OSHA is to develop standards and guidelines for employers and employees that reduce the incidence of deaths, injuries, and illnesses, and develop an enforcement procedure for safety and health standards. Those who are exempt from OSHA regulations are self-employed

people, farms where only family members are employed, and those employed by federal agencies.

71. d. patients have a right to know who you are and your level of training.—The paramedic should always wear an ID tag or patch indicating level of training and name. It is a good practice to introduce yourself to your patient by name and level of training.

72. b. online and off-line supervision.—The medical director's liability for out-of-hospital care falls into two categories: online (direct) and off-line (indirect) supervision.

73. d. all of the above.—Even if you provide the correct care to your patient, you can still be sued.

74. c. protect himself and the crew.—Safety is always the first and foremost priority at any scene.

75. d. observations made of the patient's residence—This varies from state to state, but typically paramedics are required to make a report or personally notify a mandated reporter in the receiving facility of cases that may involve: child abuse or neglect, elder or spousal abuse, sexual assault, gunshot and stab wounds, animal bites, and communicable diseases.

76. a. treatment protocols.—Also used are prospective and retrospective reviews of medical decisions.

77. a. a system of principles governing moral conduct.—Socrates defined ethics as how one should live. Actually, ethics comes from the Greek word "ethos," which means moral custom.

78. d. societal; personal—Morals relate to societal standards and ethics relate to personal standards. Acting in a lewd or crude manner might be considered immoral, whereas cheating on an examination is considered unethical.

79. d. "What is in the patient's best interest?"—Deciding what the patient wants should incorporate what the patient has said, what the patient has written, and family input.

80. c. Ethics can affect the extent to which you should persuade a patient to receive treatment.—The extent to which you attempt to persuade a patient to receive treatment or transport can be vague and may involve an ethical decision.

81. a. liability—This immunity from liability does not extend to a willful, wanton, or malicious disregard for the wishes of the patient.

82. b. use language/terms the patient can understand.— The best approach is to be honest and help the patient understand the ramifications of his decision in terms that are easily understood.

83. d. preplanned wills—A will is a legal instrument that attorneys deal with. The paramedic deals with "do not attempt resuscitation" orders (DNARs), living wills, and health care proxies.

84. d. make decisions on health care.—This is a fundamental element of the patient–physician relationship and is stated in the American Medical Association Code of Medical Ethics.

85. a. implied consent—When in doubt, always act in the patient's best interest.
86. a. capabilities of the hospital—The paramedic has a significant influence on the patient's decision about where to be transported. Consider this in all cases. "What would I do if this was my parent or child needing care for this presenting problem?"
87. c. Deciding whether or not to stop to render assistance when not on duty.—Deciding whether you should act as a Good Samaritan and stop to render assistance when not on duty can involve an ethical decision for some.
88. b. Ethics involve larger issues than a paramedic's practice.—Ethics have been described as "how one should live."
89. a. true parity.—True parity is comparing what is fair for everyone. It is one of the criteria used in allocating scarce EMS resources.
90. a. True parity—True parity is comparing what is fair for everyone. It is one of the criteria used in allocating scarce EMS resources.
91. b. the patient's advanced directives.—The paramedic is accountable to the patient and the medical director, and to fulfilling the standard of care.
92. b. good faith—Avoid any emotional decisions, and use reason, morals, and good faith when considering your answer to an ethical question.
93. a. the patient's statements—For the alert patient who is unimpaired, the patient's wishes must be considered first and foremost. The best approach is to be honest and help the patient understand the ramifications of his decision in terms that are easily understood.
94. d. When in doubt, resuscitate.—Sometimes it becomes an ethical decision whether or not to resuscitate when considering the patient's wishes and the presence or absence of an advance directive, and the family members do not agree. When in doubt, resuscitate.
95. b. Integrity—Integrity is derived from a combination of the words "integritas" and "integer." It refers to the putting on of armor; of building a completeness, a wholeness in character.

Chapter 7: Anatomy and Physiology and Medical Terminology

1. b. physiology.—The study of the function of the body is called physiology.
2. a. anatomy.—The study of the components of the body is called the anatomy.
3. c. pathophysiology.—The study of how a disease develops and progresses is covered best in pathophysiology.
4. d. homeostasis.—The functions of the body which attempt to keep metabolism functioning within normal ranges of temperature and pH is referred to as homeostasis.
5. b. axillary.—When preparing a report and giving a report, a paramedic should refer to the patient's "armpit" as their axillary.
6. b. brachial.—An artery found in the upper arm which is used for obtaining a blood pressure is called the brachial.
7. c. lumbar.—The area of the spine which is posterior to the abdomen is most-likely the lumbar spine.
8. a. in describing a route of medication administration.
9. c. cardiac—A condition that effects the heart of the patient is referred to as a cardiac condition.
10. d. pectoral.—The muscles on the anterior surface of the patient's chest wall are referred to as pectoral.
11. c. plantar.—Of the terms listed, the term plantar does not refer to the head.
12. b. renal—The term for the major artery in the kidneys is renal.
13. b. umbilical—The term for the artery that supplies oxygen to a growing fetus is the umbilical artery.
14. c. popliteal—Of the terms listed, the popliteal artery is the only one in the extremity.
15. a. inguinal.—Pain caused by an injury to the ligament between the abdomen and the pelvis is said to be inguinal.
16. c. gluteal.—The larger quantities of IM injections are given in the gluteal muscle.
17. b. temporal.—A batter's helmet is designed to protect the temporal region of the brain.
18. c. cross-section—The plane that shows the bone in the middle and the nerves, artery, veins, and lymphatic vessel surrounding the bone is the cross-section.
19. b. skeleton—The bones are a component of the skeleton system.
20. c. integumentary system—The integumentary system takes up the largest space of those listed.
21. d. respiratory—The alveoli are a component of the respiratory organ system.
22. c. digestive—The alimentary canal is a part of the digestive organ system.
23. a. spinal—The spinal cavity is considered a dorsal cavity.

24. b. lymphatic—Immune cells are found in the lymphatic organ system.
25. c. triglycerides.—Triglycerides are not considered carbohydrates.
26. c. lipid.—A steroid is a chemical form of a lipid.
27. b. polypeptides—Polypeptides are not considered nucleic acids.
28. b. synovial—The specialized extracellular fluid found in the joints is called synovial fluid.
29. c. phagocytosis.—When cells surround and engulf a foreign substance, this is referred to as phagocytosis.
30. c. connective—Areola is a form of connective tissue.
31. a. simple cuboidal—Simple cuboidal is not considered a specialized connective tissue.
32. b. epithelial—Simple cuboidal, simple columnar, and transitional are types of epithelial tissue.
33. a. elastic is not a type of muscle tissue.
34. a. synovial.—Synovial is not a type of membrane.
35. c. cartilage.—The connective tissue at the tip of your nose and ears is made of cartilage.
36. d. appendicular.—The skeleton has two major subdivisions, the axial and the appendicular.
37. a. manubrium and xiphoid process.—The rib cage consists of 12 pairs of ribs and the manubrium and xiphoid process.
38. c. metatarsals.—When a patient falls on an outstretched arm, he may injure the radius, the ulna, or the humerus. The metatarsals are in your foot.
39. b. patella.—When a patient falls onto his knees, it is likely he may injure his patella.
40. b. hinge joint—The knee is a hinge joint.
41. a. cholinesterase.—The sources for muscle contraction include creatinine phosphate and each of the following, except cholinesterase.
42. b. visceral pleura.—The membrane that surrounds the lung is called the visceral pleura.

43. d. prothrombin.—Each of the following is a type of leukocyte, except prothrombin.
44. c. cochlea.—The inner ear contains the bony labyrinth, perilymph, and the cochlea.
45. d. skin.—The sebaceous, ceruminous, and eccrine glands are all found in the skin.
46. a. calcitonin.—Calcitonin is not found in the anterior pituitary gland.
47. c. Addison's disease.—Diseases of the adrenal cortex include Cushing's syndrome and Addison's disease.
48. b. cortisol.—In addition to parathyroid hormone, each of the following is a hormone that affects kidney function, except cortisol.
49. b. aldosterone—Angiotensin II is responsible for stimulating the secretion of the hormone aldosterone, which acts on the kidney to increase the reabsorption of sodium into the blood.
50. d. toward the head.—The term *cephalad* means toward the head.
51. a. transverse plane.—The imaginary plane that passes through the body and divides it into the upper and lower sections is called the transverse plane.
52. c. ambi-—The prefix ambi- means "with both sides."
53. b. endo-—The prefix endo- means "within."
54. c. brady-.—The prefix that means "slow" is brady-.
55. a. pachy-.—The prefix that means "thicken" is pachy-.
56. b. -genic.—The suffix that means "giving rise to" is -genic.
57. c. -opsy.—The suffix that means "a viewing" is -opsy.
58. d. hypertension.—The term for blood pressure that is excessive or beyond normal is *hypertension*.
59. c. electrolysis.—The term for destruction by passage of an electric current would be *electrolysis*.
60. a. urethritis.—The term used to describe an inflammation of the tube where urine exits the body is *urethritis*.

Chapter 8: Pathophysiology

1. d. the study of how normal physiological processes are altered by disease.—The functional changes that accompany a particular disease or syndrome.
2. b. etiology.—The causes of disease or abnormal conditions.
3. c. exacerbation.—To cause a disease or its symptoms to become more severe.
4. d. the actions of a health care provider.—Iatrogenic disease requires a specific action or lack of action.
5. c. syndrome.—A commonly known syndrome is Down syndrome, a combination of a specific physical appearance and some degree of mental impairment.
6. a. atrophy.—The actual number of cells remains unchanged. An example is a leg that has been in a cast

for 6 weeks or more. When the cast is removed, the muscle is typically atrophied.
7. c. cellular adaptation.—When cells are exposed to adverse conditions, they go through a process of adaptation. In some situations, the cells change permanently; in others, they change their structure and function temporarily.
8. d. hyperplasia.—This excess growth often causes tumors that may be malignant or benign.
9. a. dysplasia.—The growth may be normal or abnormal, as in a developing tumor.
10. a. neoplasia.—Neoplasia is a generic term for the growth of a new type of cell. These cells may be either benign or malignant.
11. d. virulence.—Virulence measures the disease-causing ability of a microorganism.

12. c. protect it from ingestion and destruction by phagocytes.—Not all bacteria are encapsulated, but they can still resist destruction.

13. b. septic shock.—Endotoxins are lipopolysaccharides that are part of the cell wall of gram-negative bacteria.

14. d. fever to develop.—Pyrogens act by affecting the hypothalamic thermoregulatory center.

15. b. viruses do not produce exotoxins or endotoxins.—Bacteria produce toxins, which are usually referred to as exotoxins or endotoxins.

16. a. inflammation.—White blood cells (WBCs) release endogenous pyrogens that cause a fever to develop.

17. c. Down syndrome.—In Down syndrome, the child is born with an extra chromosome, usually number 21.

18. b. It helps the cells in fighting off diseases.—Good nutrition is required to maintain good health and assist the cells in fighting off diseases.

19. b. changes in cell distribution with aging.—The cellular environment includes: the distribution of cells throughout the body; changes in cell distribution with aging and disease; the movement of water, sodium, and chloride in and out of cells; and acid–base balance in the cells and surrounding tissues.

20. c. 50–70%—The body consists primarily of water. About 50–70% of the total body weight is fluid.

21. b. intracellular fluids—Most (63%) of the body's fluid is in the cells and is called intracellular fluid (ICF).

22. b. 2,500 ml—The average adult takes in about 2,500 ml of water a day. Most is taken in by drinking, some comes from the water in foods, and the remaining is a byproduct of cellular metabolism.

23. a. sodium.—Sodium, the major extracellular cation, is often lost along with large amounts of fluid. The loss may affect nerve and muscle function, as well as extracellular fluid (ECF) volume.

24. c. extracellular—Extracellular fluid is broken down into the fluid that is between the cells (interstitial fluid), fluid inside the blood vessels (intravascular fluid), lymph, and transcellular fluid.

25. d. diffusion.—The movement of a substance from an area of higher concentration to an area of lower concentration.

26. c. endocytosis.—Endocytosis is one of several cell-specific ingestion processes.

27. d. phagocytosis.—Phagocytosis is one of several cell-specific ingestion processes.

28. b. osmotic—Water moves between intracellular fluid (ICF) and extracellular fluid (ECF) by osmosis. This is also referred to as osmotic pressure.

29. b. 18–40 years—The distribution of body fluids changes with age and varies with gender. Women of this age group have approximately 51% body fluid weight, whereas the men have approximately 61%.

30. b. hypotonic—The solution with a lower solute concentration has a lower osmotic pressure and is referred to as hypotonic.

31. a. facilitated diffusion.—Facilitated diffusion is a form of passive transport and one of two general methods of water and dissolved particle movement.

32. a. albumin—Albumin is in blood plasma, muscle, egg whites, milk, and other substances, and in many plant tissues and fluids.

33. d. capillary colloidal osmotic pressure.—This is osmotic pressure generated by dissolved proteins in the plasma that are too large to penetrate the capillary membrane.

34. c. capillary hydrostatic pressure.—Because the pressure is higher on the arterial end than the venous end, more water is pushed out of the capillaries on the arterial end and more is reabsorbed on the venous end.

35. a. edema.—An abnormal excess accumulation of serous fluid in connective tissue or in a serous cavity.

36. a. ascites.—Accumulation of serous fluid in the spaces between tissues and organs in the abdominal cavity.

37. d. all of the above.—The clinical manifestations of edema may be local at an injury site or generalized.

38. b. decreased colloidal osmotic pressure.—Extensive burns cause an increased loss of plasma proteins, resulting in decreased colloidal osmotic pressure.

39. b. pitting edema.—Pitting edema can be significant in the patient with chronic heart failure.

40. c. to exchange three sodium ions for every two potassium ions.—If the pump is impaired due to insufficient potassium in the body, sodium accumulates and causes the cells to swell.

41. a. tonicity.—Changes in water content can cause a cell to shrink or swell. Tonicity refers to the tension exerted on cell size due to water movement across the cell membrane.

42. c. have the same osmolarity as intracellular fluid.—Solutions that body cells are exposed to are classified as isotonic, hypotonic, or hypertonic. When the cell neither shrinks nor swells, it is isotonic.

43. d. hypertonic; pulled out of—When the osmolarity of a solution is greater than the ICF, it is hypertonic.

44. b. lower; swell—When the osmolarity of a solution is less than the ICF, it is hypotonic.

45. c. sodium.—The average adult has 60 mEq of sodium for each kilogram of body weight. Most of the body's sodium is found in the ECF.

46. b. 500 mg.—Sodium is taken in with foods. As little as 500 mg/day meets the body's needs.

47. c. stimulating sodium reabsorption.—Angiotensin II is responsible for stimulating sodium reabsorption by the renal tubules. It also constricts the renal blood vessels, slowing kidney blood flow and decreasing the glomerular filtration rate.

48. a. renin.—Renin is a protein enzyme that is released by the kidney into the bloodstream in response to changes in blood pressure, blood flow, the amount of sodium in the tubular fluids, and the glomerular filtration rate.

49. b. aldosterone—Besides angiotensin II, three other factors stimulate aldosterone release: increased extracellular potassium levels, decreased extracellular sodium levels, and release of adrenocorticotropic hormone (ACTH).

50. b. hypernatremic.—Hypernatremia is defined as a serum sodium level that is above 148 mEq/L.

51. b. seizures and coma.—Any alteration of mental status is considered severe.

52. c. vomiting and diarrhea—Causes may include excess sweating from hot environments or exercise and GI losses through vomiting, diarrhea, or diuresis.

53. c. hyponatremia.—During prolonged or extreme periods of extreme exercise or hot environments, excessive sodium loss can cause symptoms associated with hyponatremia: weight gain, headache, confusion, weakness, abdominal cramps, nausea, vomiting, diarrhea, stupor, or coma.

54. b. potassium.—Potassium is necessary for neuromuscular control, regulation of the three types of muscles, acid–base balance, intracellular enzyme reactions, and maintenance of intracellular osmolality.

55. a. excessive vomiting or diarrhea.—Hypokalemia is defined as a decreased serum potassium level and can be caused by numerous conditions related to fluid imbalance.

56. c. low T wave and sagging ST segment.—Peaked T waves, depressed ST segments, depressed P wave, and widening QRS complex are associated with hyperkalemia.

57. c. renal failure.—A common cause of hyperkalemia is renal failure.

58. a. paresthesia and intestinal colic.—Potassium is necessary for neuromuscular control, regulation of the three types of muscles, acid–base balance, intracellular enzyme reactions, and maintenance of intracellular osmolality.

59. c. widened QRS.—Peaked T waves, depressed ST segments, depressed P wave, and widening QRS complex are associated with hyperkalemia.

60. d. bones—The vast majority (99%) of the body's calcium is found in the bones.

61. a. strength and stability to bones.—The purpose of calcium is to provide strength and stability for the collagen and ground substance that forms the matrix of the skeletal system.

62. c. through the GI tract—Calcium enters the body through the GI tract and is absorbed from the intestine by vitamin D.

63. a. renal failure.—Some of the causes of hypocalcemia include: hypoparathyroidism, hypomagnesemia,

vitamin D deficiency, impaired ability to activate vitamin D, renal failure, increased pH, increased fatty acids, and acute pancreatitis.

64. b. rapid transfusion of citrated blood.—Other causes include liver and kidney disease, hyperphosphatemia, and rapid transfusion of citrated blood.

65. a. skeletal muscle cramps.—The manifestations of hypocalcemia include: paresthesia, skeletal muscle cramps, abdominal spasms and cramps, hyperactive reflexes, carpopedal spasm, tetany, laryngeal spasms, hypotension, bone pain, deformities, and fractures.

66. b. calcium.—A decreased serum calcium level (hypocalcemia) may cause symptoms of skeletal muscle cramps, abdominal spasms, bone pain, deformities, and fractures.

67. d. hypocalcemia.—In addition to osteomalacia, the manifestations of hypocalcemia include: paresthesia, skeletal muscle cramps, abdominal spasms and cramps, hyperactive reflexes, carpopedal spasm, tetany, laryngeal spasms, hypotension, bone pain, deformities, and fractures.

68. b. excess calcium in the diet.—The causes of hypercalcemia include: excess vitamin D or excess calcium in the diet, excess milk or calcium containing antacids, increased levels of parathyroid hormone, malignant neoplasms, prolonged immobilization, thiazide diuretics, and lithium therapy.

69. c. hypercalcemia.—Additional manifestations of hypercalcemia include: increased thirst, nausea, vomiting, muscle weakness, atrophy, ataxia, loss of muscle tone, behavioral changes, stupor, coma, hypertension, shortening of the QT interval, and atrioventricular block.

70. a. hypercalcemia—Manifestations of hypercalcemia include: increased thirst, nausea, vomiting, muscle weakness, atrophy, ataxia, loss of muscle tone, behavioral changes, stupor, coma, hypertension, shortening of the QT interval, and atrioventricular block.

71. d. diabetic ketoacidosis.—Additional causes of hypophosphatemia include: antacids, severe diarrhea, lack of vitamin D, alkalosis, hyperparathyroidism, alcoholism, recovery from malnutrition, and renal tubular absorption defects.

72. c. hemolytic anemia.—Manifestations of hypophosphatemia include: ataxia, paresthesia, hyporeflexia, confusion, stupor, coma, seizures, muscle weakness, joint stiffness, bone pain, osteomalacia, anorexia, dysphagia, impaired WBC function, platelet dysfunction with bleeding disorders, and hemolytic anemia.

73. b. hyperphosphatemia.—Additional causes of hyperphosphatemia include: heat stroke, seizures, tumor lysis syndrome, potassium, deficiency, hypoparathyroidism, phosphate-containing laxatives, and enemas.

74. b. hypomagnesemia—The causes of hypomagnesemia include: alcoholism, malnutrition or starvation, malabsorption, small bowel bypass surgery, parenteral hyperalimentation with inadequate amounts of magnesium, and high dietary intake of calcium without concomitant amounts of magnesium.

75. a. hypomagnesemia.—Additional manifestations of hypomagnesemia include: personality change, athetoid or choreiform movements, nystagmus, tetany, tachycardia, hypertension, and cardiac dysrhythmias.

76. c. Trousseau's—Trousseau's sign is associated with hypomagnesemia.

77. c. 7.35–7.45—pH is the measurement of the hydrogen ion concentration. A blood pH greater than 7.45 is called alkalosis, and a blood pH of less than 7.35 is called acidosis.

78. b. greater; alkalosis—A blood pH greater than 7.45 is called alkalosis, and a blood pH of less than 7.35 is called acidosis.

79. b. metabolic acidosis.—Metabolic acidosis is an accumulation of abnormal acids in the blood for any of several reasons (e.g., sepsis, diabetic ketoacidosis, and salicylate poisoning).

80. a. respiratory acidosis.—Respiratory acidosis occurs when CO_2 retention leads to increased levels of pCO_2. It also occurs in situations of hypoventilation or intrinsic lung diseases.

81. c. respiratory acidosis.—Respiratory acidosis occurs when CO_2 retention leads to increased levels of pCO_2. It also occurs in situations of hypoventilation (e.g., depressed respiratory effort from a heroin overdose) or intrinsic lung diseases (e.g., asthma or COPD).

82. d. respiratory alkalosis.—Excessive "blowing off" of CO_2 with a resulting decrease in the pCO_2 causes respiratory alkalosis.

83. a. genetic histories of population.—Analyzing disease risk involves reviewing the rates of incidence, prevalence, and mortality, as well as causal and noncausal risk factors.

84. b. Parkinson's disease.—Some diseases are more prevalent in men, such as lung cancer, gout, and Parkinson's disease. Women are more likely to get osteoporosis, rheumatoid arthritis, or breast cancer.

85. d. allergy.—Allergies are an acquired hypersensitivity. First, the person is exposed or sensitized to the antigen. Repeated exposures cause a reaction by the immune system to the allergen.

86. b. rheumatic fever—Rheumatic fever develops following a streptococcal infection (e.g., strep throat) and is characterized by myocarditis and arthritis.

87. a. recent weight gain—The American Cancer Society uses the acronym "CAUTION" to list the signs:
Change in bowel or bladder habits
A sore that does not heal
Unusual bleeding or discharge
Thickening or lung development
Indigestion or difficulty swallowing
Obvious change in a wart or mole
Nagging cough or hoarseness

88. c. asthma.—Asthma is exhibited by constriction of the bronchi, wheezing, and dyspnea.

89. d. asthma.—Acute asthma is a recurring condition of completely or partially reversible acute airflow obstruction in the lower airway. Asthma is the leading cause of chronic illness in children.

90. c. lung—Lung cancer is the leading cause of cancer deaths and the second leading cause of cancer cases in males and females.

91. c. Type I requires exogenous insulin.—Type I diabetic patients are absolutely dependent on exogenously administered insulin, while type II diabetic patients typically are not.

92. b. Their digestive juices would destroy oral forms.—This is why insulin injections are necessary.

93. d. pancreas—Insulin is a hormone produced and released from the pancreas.

94. c. drug-induced anemia.—Drug-induced hemolytic anemia is a hemolytic anemia that is characterized by an increased destruction of red blood cells.

95. a. The cause is unknown.—The cause is unknown, but it has been associated with Marfan's syndrome, osteogenesis imperfecta, connective tissue disorders, cardiac, metabolic, neuroendocrine, metabolic, and psychologic disorders.

96. a. is inherited.—Hereditary prolongation of the QT interval may occur by itself or may be associated with other diseases.

97. b. hemophilia.—Hemophilia is a gender-linked hereditary bleeding disorder most commonly passed on from an asymptomatic mother to a male child.

98. b. cardiomyopathies.—There are a number of disease forms. The diseases cause the heart muscle to become thin, flabby, dilated, or enlarged.

99. d. cardiovascular disease—Almost half of all cardiovascular deaths result from coronary heart disease.

100. d. hypertension—Often referred to as the silent killer, hypertension typically has no signs or symptoms.

101. c. gout.—The disease leads to inflammation of the joints due to a metabolic problem in the breakdown of proteins.

102. b. changing the size and shape of the heart.—The myocardial geometry (shape) changes that occur with chronic hypertension cause the hypertrophied heart to work harder to maintain a given output.

103. c. Nicotine causes vasoconstriction.—Arteries become damaged due to the excessive pressure of vasoconstriction and then become weakened. The weakened areas develop blood clots and thrombosis or they rupture and hemorrhage critically.

104. b. renal calculi.—Also called renal calculus.

105. c. males; 30–50—Kidney stones are most prevalent in men between the ages of 30 and 50.

106. c. ulcerative colitis.—A nonspecific inflammatory disease of the colon with no known cause.

107. b. lactose intolerance.—Lactose intolerance is likely the most common GI abnormality known to mankind. Some studies suggest that it affects more than half of the world's population.

108. a. peptic ulcers.—Peptic ulcer disease involves erosions of either the stomach or duodenum.

109. c. gallstones.—Cholelithiasis is the production of gallstones and the condition that results from it.

110. c. gallstones.—Gallstones can block the lumen, interfering with bile flow.

111. b. hypotension.—Hypertension is a health risk associated with obesity.

112. d. respiratory function impairment.—The formation of the adipose tissue around the neck, chest, and abdomen can impair normal respiratory function and cause sleep apnea.

113. b. Huntington's disease.—The disease produces localized death of brain cells and there is no cure. Symptoms do not usually develop until patients are over 30 years of age, and by then they may have already passed the gene to their own offspring.

114. a. multiple sclerosis.—MS is a demyelinating disease of the central nervous system. It is the major cause of neurological disability in young and middle-aged adults.

115. c. impaired cognition and abstract thinking.—In stage 2 of Alzheimer's disease, judgment and cognition become impaired and social behavior becomes inappropriate.

116. c. an extensive acute myocardial infarction.—Initially the signs and symptoms are the same as seen with ACS. As the body's compensating mechanism fails and shock progresses, severe hypotension develops and organ tissues die.

117. c. Pericardial tamponade—Additional causes include: vena cava syndrome, dissecting aortic aneurysm, pulmonary embolism in the pulmonary circulation, and a ball valve thrombus in the cardiac chambers.

118. c. electrolyte loss from dehydration.—Additional causes of hypovolemic shock include: internal or external hemorrhage, plasma loss from burns or inflammation, trauma, anaphylaxis, and envenomation.

119. c. multiple organ dysfunction syndrome—MODS involves the progressive failure of two or more organ systems after severe illness or injury. The mortality rate is between 60% and 90%.

120. c. autoimmune—Autoimmunity occurs when a person's T cells or antibodies attacks the new red blood cells, causing tissue damage and organ dysfunction.

121. b. Vasodilation—The local effects of an inflammation response are vasodilation, increased capillary permeability, and the development of exudates.

122. a. fever.—The systemic responses to an acute inflammation include: fever, leukocytosis, and an increase in the circulating plasma proteins or acute phase reactants.

123. a. natural—Natural or native immunity is acquired either by getting the disease or receiving antibodies from your mother (also referred to as passive immunity).

124. c. complement.—The complement system plays a vital role in attracting WBCs to the site of the infection, as well as initially attacking bacteria. The activation of the complement system during a severe illness, though, may lead to "self-destruction" by activated components.

125. a. phagocytes—Phagocytes are one of the cellular components of inflammation, and their role is to engulf foreign matter and bacteria.

Chapter 9: Life Span Development

1. b. 3.0–3.5 kg.—The average weight of a newborn is between 3.0 and 3.5 kilograms, or 6.5 and 7.5 pounds.

2. b. 5–10—There is a normal weight loss of 5–10% during the first week of life due to the excretion of extracellular fluid present at birth.

3. c. 4–6 months—During the first month, the infant grows by approximately 30 grams per day. As a result, the infant's weight should double by 4–6 months and triple by 9–12 months.

4. d. The ductus arteriosus has closed.—The circulatory changes lead to: closing of the ductus arteriosus, closing of the ductus venosus, and closing of the foramen ovale. When these changes are complete, the infant has made the shift from fetal circulation to normal infant circulation.

5. a. four weeks—Any occlusion of the nares during this time is the functional equivalent of an upper airway obstruction.

6. d. The ribs are positioned horizontally, causing diaphragmatic breathing.—The lung tissue on an infant is fragile and more prone to barotrauma. In the infant, there are fewer alveoli and the chest wall is less rigid. The accessory muscles are also immature and susceptible to early fatigue.

7. a. three months—The posterior fontanelle closes by 3 months of age, and the anterior fontanelle closes between 9 and 18 months of age.

8. c. 9–18 months—The posterior fontanelle closes by 3 months of age, and the anterior fontanelle closes between 9 and 18 months of age.

9. c. abnormal thyroid hormone levels—Abnormal levels of thyroid hormone and growth hormone can cause abnormally fast bone growth.

10. b. 2—The rate of weight gain slows dramatically as the infant becomes a toddler. The average child gains only 2 kilograms per year during this period.

11. b. modeling—Modeling is imitation of another's behavior, dress, mannerisms, or attitudes.

12. c. school age—With each interaction, school-age children compare themselves with others. This leads to the development of self-esteem, either positive or negative.

13. b. secondary sexual development.—Secondary sexual characteristics are the external physical characteristics of sexual maturity resulting from the action of sex hormones. These include male and female patterns of body hair, fat distribution, development of external genitals, and deepening of the voice in males.

14. a. Gonadotropins released by the pituitary gland promote the production of testosterone.—These promote the production of testosterone by the testes, which contribute to further development of secondary sexual characteristics and to sexual maturity.

15. a. decrease in elasticity of the diaphragm.—In addition, a decreased muscle mass leads to relative chest wall weakness.

16. b. weakening of the chest wall.—This, combined with decreased elasticity of the diaphragm, leads to decreased respiratory function.

17. b. decrease in insulin production.—Insulin production decreases, leading to abnormalities in glucose metabolism and sometimes type II diabetes.

18. d. changes in renal function.—Nearly 50% of functioning nephrons are lost during late adulthood. As a result, decreased excretion of fluid, salts, and waste products may occur.

19. c. their muscular sphincters become less effective with age.—Muscular sphincters (e.g., esophageal and rectal) become less effective, resulting in acid reflux and stool incontinence.

20. c. Growth spurts begin with enlargement of the feet and hands.—Most adolescents experience a rapid growth spurt lasting 2–3 years. It begins distally with an enlargement of the feet and hands.

21. a. infancy—During infancy, the kidneys are unable to concentrate the urine, resulting in a specific gravity usually no greater than that of distilled water.

22. b. Osteoarthritis is the type of arthritis that affects the bone by wearing down the cushion that pads the space between bones.

23. a. 6 months—Antibodies transferred from the mother maintain passive immunity throughout the first 6 months of life. By then, the infant's own immune system has begun to provide protection, at least to some extent.

24. d. 100—Rates below 80 bpm usually require CPR.

25. b. abnormal—At birth, the respiratory rate is normally between 40 and 60 breaths per minute. It drops rapidly after the first few minutes of life (30–40 breaths per minute), and slows to 20–30 breaths per minute by the time the infant reaches her first birthday.

26. b. triple—During the first month, the infant grows by approximately 30 grams per day. As a result, the infant's weight should double by 4–6 months and triple by 9–12 months.

27. b. 5–7—The first baby teeth begin to erupt at 5–7 months of age.

28. d. expectancy.—Life expectancy is the amount of time remaining before a person is expected to die. The average life expectancy depends on many factors.

29. b. accidents—Accidents are the leading cause of death in this age group.

30. c. middle adulthood—The cardiac output decreases throughout this period, and cholesterol levels tend to increase.

31. d. As the number of cells (neurons) in the brain decreases the memory tends to become less efficient.

32. d. Life span—Life span is a retrospective measurement. It measures how long a person actually lived.

33. b. orthostatic—Postural hypotension becomes more common because of inadequate compensatory mechanisms.

34. a. arteriosclerosis.—Vessel walls thicken, often due to arteriosclerosis. This results in an increase in peripheral vascular resistance with variable reductions in organ blood flow.

35. c. less elastic.—This leads to an increased workload on the aging heart.

36. b. Sick-sinus—Patients alternate from normal sinus rhythm to supraventricular tachycardias, to bradycardia and AV block, without apparent logic.

37. b. poor nutrition and malabsorption.—As a result, low-grade anemia is relatively common (though not normal) in late adulthood.

38. c. Peristalsis throughout the entire GI tract is decreased. The result is a tendency toward bowel slow down (ileus), blockage (obstruction), and constipation.

39. d. They have a loss of normal mucous membrane linings.—As a result, inhaled air is less humidified.

40. a. aneurysms.—Atherosclerosis can produce ballooning of large vessels (aneurysms) and possible rupture of the vessels.

41. a. sleep–wake cycle.—Normal aging results in a loss of neurons and neurotransmitters. The clinical effects are variable. Generally, the sleep–wake cycle is disturbed.

42. c. osteoporosis of the spine—In late adulthood, no new growth takes place and height may decrease due to osteoporosis of the spine.

43. c. early adulthood—As a rule, all body systems are at optimal performance and a person reaches a peak in physical condition between 19 and 26 years of age.

44. b. school-age—With each interaction, school-age children compare themselves with others. This leads to the development of self-esteem. Moral development varies considerably from child to child and depends on many facts. Individuals move through moral development throughout school age and young adulthood at very different paces.

45. b. 3–4 years—Hearing reaches peak (maturity) levels by 3 and 4 years of age.

46. c. permissive–indulgent—Parents who are low in authority and high in responsiveness are typified as engaging in an indulgent style of parenting. These parents are committed to their children and are tolerant, warm, and accepting, but they do not exercise much authority and make few demands for mature behavior on the part of the child.

47. c. Growth spurts in girls typically occur before boys.—Growth begins in the limbs followed by the trunk. Growth spurts in girls typically precede menstruation by nearly 6 months.

48. d. Presbycusis—A lessening of hearing acuteness resulting from degenerative changes that occur in the ear, especially in the elderly.

49. c. a decrease in cortisol production.—Cortisol production by the adrenal glands is diminished by 25%. Because cortisol is produced during stress, the late adult is less equipped to handle bodily stresses (e.g., severe infection).

50. a. loss of normal cardiac pacemaker cells.—Degeneration of the cardiac conduction system may lead to a combination of brady- and tachy-dysrhythmias. This is often termed the "tach-brady" syndrome or "sick-sinus syndrome."

Chapter 10: Principles of Pharmacology and Medication Administration

1. b. drug.—The two terms, drug and medication, are used interchangeably, yet there is a difference. A medication is a medicinal substance used as a treatment or remedy, whereas a drug is any chemical substance that, when taken into a living organism, produces a biological response.

2. a. pharmacokinetics.—Once a drug has been introduced into the body, it goes through five distinct stages: absorption, distribution, desired effect, metabolism, and elimination.

3. a. pharmacodynamics.—Specifically, it looks at the biochemical and physiological effects on, or interactions with, the target organ(s) or tissue(s).

4. d. biotransformation.—Biotransformation or metabolism is the chemical breakdown of the drug (stage 4) as it travels through the body.

5. d. research.—Medications are administered to achieve a therapeutic effect, a prophylactic effect, or a diagnostic effect.

6. a. drug action.—The interaction between a drug and a body organ or tissue is only a physiologic modification of the organ or tissue because drugs do not produce new functions. The drug-induced physiologic change to a body function or process is known as a drug action.

7. a. agonist.—A chemical substance capable of combining with a receptor on a cell and initiating a reaction.

8. b. target organs or tissues.—There are several ways by which a drug affects a body organ or tissue. This is called the drug's mechanism of action. The major mechanism by which a drug affects the body is by joining with receptors located on the target organs or tissues.

9. d. sympathomimetic.—This group of drugs is commonly used in the out-of-hospital setting, particularly within advanced cardiac life support (ACLS).

10. a. dopamine.—In addition to being a sympathomimetic drug, dopamine, an antecedent to the formation of epinephrine, can also act as a neurotransmitter in the sympathetic nervous system.

11. d. sympathomimetics.—This group of drugs is commonly used in prehospital emergency care, particularly within ACLS.

12. c. sympatholytics.—Beta-blockers (e.g., atenolol, metoprolol, and propranolol) are included in this group of drugs.

13. a. acetylcholine.—Drugs that perform similarly to acetylcholine and mimic the parasympathetic response are referred to as cholinergic or parasympathomimetic.

14. d. atropine.—Atropine primarily blocks parasympathetic stimulation of the heart, causing the rate to increase, but it also affects other body systems.

15. a. energy produced through a chemical reaction.—Active transport is the movement of chemical substance by the expenditure of energy through a cell membrane in concentration or electrical

potential and opposite to the direction of normal diffusion.

16. d. cumulative effect.—The cumulative effect occurs when a dose is repeated before the prior dose has been metabolized.

17. a. idiosyncrasy.—Idiosyncrasy is an abnormal or unpredictable response to a drug that is peculiar to an individual rather than a general group.

18. b. blood-brain barrier.—The blood-brain barrier is a physiologic barrier that exists between circulating blood and the brain. This barrier protects brain tissue and cerebral spinal fluid from exposure to certain substances.

19. a. official—The official name is the same as the generic name and is followed by the initials USP (*U.S. Pharmacopoeia*) or NF (*National Formulary*), denoting its listing in one of these official publications.

20. b. angiotensin I from converting angiotensin II.—Angiotensin-converting enzyme (ACE) inhibitors work by affecting the renin–angiotensin–aldosterone system. This system supports the sodium and fluid balance of the body and maintains blood pressure.

21. a. ingredients.—A chemical assay is a test that determines the ingredients and their exact amounts.

22. d. label all dangerous ingredients in drug products.—In 1906, the U.S. government passed the first law to protect the public from impure or mislabeled drugs.

23. d. drug enforcement.—The Drug Enforcement Agency (DEA), in the Department of Justice, became the nation's sole drug enforcement agency in 1973.

24. b. the total body weight affects the distribution of the drug.—The total body weight and the amount of a drug given have a direct association to the distribution and concentration of a drug.

25. a. affinity.—The joining of a drug and a receptor site is called affinity, and is often compared to the connection of a lock and key. The drug is the key and the lock is the receptor.

26. d. antagonist.—When a drug inhibits a receptor, it is called an antagonist, which means "to block."

27. a. dopaminergic and adrenergic.—The two types of sympathetic receptors are adrenergic receptors and dopaminergic receptors. Adrenergic receptors are subdivided into the following four types: alpha 1 and 2, beta 1 and 2.

28. d. passive transport.—Passive transport of water and dissolved particle movement includes the following processes: diffusion, facilitated diffusion, osmosis, and filtration.

29. a. osmotic—Osmotic pressure is produced or associated with osmosis. It helps control the movement of water into or out of the cell.

30. c. drug interaction.—A drug interaction is the combined effect of drugs taken at the same time that alters the expected therapeutic effect.

31. b. potentiation—The combined effects of two drugs are better than either could have produced alone (e.g., 1 + 1 = 3 or more.)

32. a. additive—The additive synergistic effect of two agreeable drugs produces an effect that neither could alone.

33. d. antagonism.—The example described in the question is chemical antagonism. The charcoal binds with and absorbs the toxins present in the GI tract to inactivate them.

34. c. half-life—Half-life refers to the amount of time that a drug remains at a therapeutic level to produce a desired effect and the time it takes the body to metabolize or inactivate a drug's concentration by 50%.

35. a. controlled the sale of narcotics and drugs that cause dependence.—The Controlled Substance Act of 1970 superseded the Harrison Narcotic Act. This act sets forth the rules for the manufacture and distribution of drugs that have the potential for abuse.

36. d. V—Schedule V is the rating for the lowest abuse potential. Cough syrups and diarrhea medications fall into this schedule.

37. b. four—These phases include testing, approval, and marketing requirements before new drugs can reach the consumer.

38. b. The defect occurred before it left the manufacturer.—For the drug product liability to exist, the following three criteria must be met: the defect caused harm, the defect occurred before it left the manufacturer, and the product is defective or not fit for its intended reasonable uses.

39. b. therapeutic effect.—Because drugs are classified by their chemical class, mechanism of action, or therapeutic effect, looking at the medications a patient is taking can give you a lot of information about her medical history.

40. c. a quicker absorption rate than lower doses.—The dosage is a predominant factor for the absorption rate of a drug.

41. a. A loading dose is typically a single dose of a drug.—A loading dose is considered to be a single dose or the accumulation of several closely repeated single doses (boluses) used to obtain the therapeutic level to achieve a desired effect.

42. a. dehydration—Medications are often a cause of altered mental status, especially in the elderly. Improper diuretic use can lead to dehydration and electrolyte imbalances, especially with potassium. Colace is a stool softener.

43. b. decreased renal function—Impaired renal or liver function interferes with the body's ability to

metabolize and eliminate drugs. This can lead to a cumulative effect and toxicity.

44. b. *U.S. Pharmacopoeia.*—A U.S. government publication and the only official book of drug standards in the United States since 1980.

45. d. Drugs with weak acidity. —Drugs that have a weak acidity, such as barbiturates, are absorbed better in the stomach than in the intestine. Drugs that have a weaker base, such as morphine sulfate, have a better reaction if given by a route other than orally so as to avoid the high acidity of the stomach.

46. b. it may elevate diagnostic enzyme levels.—The measurement of CK-MB (creatine kinase; M, muscle; B, brain) and troponin used in cardiac enzyme testing are a couple of examples.

47. b. Wear a face mask.—Wearing a face mask will reduce the chance of inhaling aerosolized particles, including medications and infectious particles. Consider the use of a spacer with aerosolized medications to better direct the medication.

48. c. heart muscle—Most drugs are metabolized and eliminated by way of the liver, kidneys, GI tract, and lungs.

49. a. iatrogenic.—An adverse mental or physical condition inadvertently induced by a health care provider, medical treatment, or diagnostic procedure.

50. a. standardization.—Standardization is necessary because many drugs are made from plants. The strength from plant to plant may be different based on a number of variables, such as where it was grown and how it was processed.

51. b. indirect orders of medical control.—Indirect orders for medication administration are commonly used with specific circumstances such as an asthma attack or a cardiac arrest. These orders are written as standing orders and referred to as protocols.

52. a. avoid making medication administration errors.—This phrase refers to some of the universal principles of medication administration in an effort to avoid making an error when giving a patient a medication.

53. c. antiseptic.—Preventing or stopping the growth of microorganisms.

54. d. disinfectant.—A chemical agent that destroys microorganisms.

55. b. open ampule.—Sharps are any medical products that can cause a puncture or cut to anyone who handles them. An open ampule has an exposed glass edge.

56. a. local infection—The most common complication is that the patient develops a local infection at the site of injection. This is directly associated with poor (dirty) technique by the person who performed the skill.

57. c. twice a day—A Latin abbreviation (*bis in die*) used in writing prescriptions.

58. c. subcutaneous—An injection under the dermis into connective tissue or fat for slow absorption.

59. a. household—The household method is a system commonly used in the home, also called the United States system, and is based on the traditional English system.

60. c. gram.—In the metric system, the basic unit of mass (weight) is the gram; the basic unit of volume is the liter; and the basic unit of length is the meter.

61. c. either KVO or TKO.—Keep vein open or to keep open.

62. d. absorption effects are more predictable.—Drugs administered by IV have the fastest and most predictable absorption rates. Drugs administered by mouth will have many more factors that can affect the absorption rate, making this route slow and often unpredictable.

63. a. buccal—The space between the cheek and gum is the buccal area. Medications placed there dissolve through the buccal mucosa.

64. a. enteral—Because enteral routes are through the alimentary canal, which begins at the mouth and ends at the rectum, enteral drugs are taken orally (PO) or rectally (PR).

65. b. epidural.—This is a parenteral route.

66. b. 3.5 grams—$(3{,}500 \text{ mg}) \div (1{,}000) = 3.5 \text{ g}$

67. a. 0.0012 grams—First convert to milligrams $(1{,}200 \text{ mcg}) \div (1{,}000) = 1.2 \text{ mg}$. Next, convert milligrams to grams $(1.2 \text{ mg}) \div (1{,}000) = 0.0012 \text{ grams}$.

68. d. 2,500 ml—$(2.5 \text{ liters}) \times (1{,}000) = 2{,}500 \text{ ml}$

69. c. 90 kg—kilograms $= (\text{lb}) \div (2.2)$. $(198 \text{ lb}) \div (2.2 \text{ kg}) = 90 \text{ kg}$.

70. c. 145 lb—pounds $= (\text{kg}) \times (2.2)$. $(66) \times (2.2) = 145.2$. Round down to 145 lb.

71. b. 120 mg—Convert pounds to kilograms $= (176 \text{ lb}) \div (2.2) = 80 \text{ kg}$. Next, multiply $(1.5) \times (80) = 120 \text{ mg}$.

72. b. 12 ml—The drug comes packaged as 100 mg in 10 ml. Two packages will be needed; all of one and 2 ml of the second, for a total of 12 ml.

73. b. 100 gtt/min—

$$\text{Administration Rate} = \frac{(\text{volume ordered})(\text{drip set})}{\text{time}}$$

$$= \frac{(300 \text{ ml})(10 \text{ gtt})}{30 \text{ min}}$$

$$\frac{3000}{30} = 100 \text{ gtt/min.}$$

74. b. 25—D-50 comes packaged in 50 ml, or 0.5 g/ml, or 25 grams.

75. c. Dilute the D-50 by one-half, then administer.—The pediatric dose is a lesser concentration (D-25), and the neonate dose is less (D-10).

76. c. 45 gtts—First mix the 20-mg lidocaine in the 50-ml bag for a concentration of 4:1 = 4mg/ml.

$$\text{Administration Rate} = \text{gtt/min} = \frac{(\text{dose/min})(\text{drip set})}{\text{dose/ml}}$$

$$= \frac{(3\ \text{mg/min})(60\ \text{gtt/ml})}{4\ \text{mg/ml}} = 45\ \text{gtt/min}.$$

77. c. 1.5 ml—Two vials with a total of 8 mg in 4 ml or 2 mg in 0.5 ml. You administer 5 mg in 2.5 ml, and what is left is 3 mg in 1.5 ml.

78. a. 37°—Temperature conversions:
Fahrenheit = F = (9/5C) + 32
Celsius = C = 5/9 (F – 32)
Fahrenheit temperature of 98.6°, and you desire to convert it into degrees on the Celsius scale. Using the above formula, you would first subtract 32 from the Fahrenheit temperature and get 66.6 as a result. Then you multiply 66.6 by five-ninths and get the converted value of 37° Celsius.

79. b. vial.—A small, closed container for fluids.

80. d. aspirin—Enteral drugs are taken orally (PO) or rectally (PR).

81. a. The absorption rate is fast.—Medications taken orally absorb much slower than medications administered by other routes.

82. c. PR allows for rapid absorption.—The rectum is vascular, allowing for rapid absorption that does not go through biotransformation in the liver before reaching its target organs.

83. b. use a single line to mark out the error, make the change, and initial it.—Erasing or deleting information gives the appearance of hiding information. Instead, mark a single line through the error, write your initials next to it, and then write the correction.

84. d. 70–80 mmHg—This range is tight enough to occlude venous return but not restrict arterial flow.

85. b. a reaction from the bee sting.—Hypotension is not typically a side effect of Benadryl®. The patient experiencing an allergic reaction has likely become hypotensive from vasodilation as a progression to anaphylactic shock.

86. a. kilo—(k) kilo = 1,000, (c) centi= 1/100 or 0.01, milli= 1/1,000 or 0.001, and (mcg or mg) micro = 1/1,000,000 or 0.000001.

87. c. 50 gtt/min—First mix 150 mg into 50 ml = 3:1 concentration or 3 mg/ml.

$$\text{Drip rate} = \frac{(X)(10\ \text{gtt})}{3\ \text{mg/ml}} = \frac{(15\ \text{mg/min})(10\ \text{gtt/ml})}{3\ \text{mg/ml}}$$

$$= 50\ \text{gtt/min}$$

Another method:
Order is to give 50 ml over 10 min.
1 ml = 10 gtt
10 ml = 100 gtts
$$50\ \text{ml} = 500\ \text{gtts} = \frac{500\ \text{gtt}}{10\ \text{min}} = \frac{50\ \text{gtt}}{\text{min}}.$$

88. b. 25 gtt/min—First mix 2g (2,000 mg) into 50 ml = 4:1 concentration or 40 mg/ml. You need to administer 2,000 mg over 20 min = 2,000 mg/20 min = 100 mg/min.

$$\text{Drip rate} = \frac{(X)(10\ \text{gtt/ml})}{40\ \text{mg/ml}} = \frac{(100\ \text{mg/min})(10\ \text{gtt/ml})}{40\ \text{mg/ml}}$$

$$= 25\ \text{gtt/min}.$$

89. c. 25—Because D5W contains 5 grams of sugar per 100 ml of solvent, 500 ml contains five times as much, or 25 grams.

90. a. 19—1,600 mcg/ml in 250: (5 mcg) (100 kg) = 500 mcg/min.

$$\text{Drip rate} = \frac{(500\ \text{mcg/min})(60\ \text{gtt/min})}{1,600\ \text{mcg/ml}} = \frac{30,000}{1,600} = \frac{30}{1.6}.$$

$$= 18.75\ \text{round up } 19\ \text{gtt/min}.$$

91. a. 0.1 mg—First convert pounds to kilograms = 12 lb ÷ 2.2 = 5.45. Round down to 5 kg. Next (5 kg) (0.02 mg/kg) = 0.1 mg.

92. d. 100—

$$\text{Drip rate} = \frac{(50\ \text{ml})(60\ \text{gtt/min})}{30\ \text{gtt/min}} = \frac{3,000}{30} = 100\ \text{minutes}.$$

93. d. 120 ml—

$$\frac{(X\ \text{ml/min})(60\ \text{gtt/min})}{60\ \text{gtt/min}} = \frac{(20\ \text{ml/min})(60\ \text{gtt/min})}{10\ \text{gtt/min}} \quad 10$$

$$= \frac{1200}{10} = 120\ \text{ml}.$$

94. d. 23 mg—First convert pounds to kilograms = 200 lb ÷ 2.2 = 90.9. Round up to 91 kg.
Next (0.25 mg) (91 kg) = 22.75. Round up to 23 mg.

95. b. 5 cc—The package of medication has 25 mg in 5 ml, or 5 mg/ml. The dose is 23 mg, so the smallest syringe to use for one dose is a 5-cc syringe.

96. b. 15—You need to administer 150 mg over 10 min = 150 mg/10 min =15 mg/min.

97. d. 30—One quart = 2 pints. If the total volume is 12 pints, 3.5 pints is 30%. (3.5) ÷ (12) = .29166, or approximately 30%.

98. d. 42 gtts/min—

$$\text{Drip rate} = \frac{(250\ \text{ml/hr})(10\ \text{gtt/ml})}{60\ \text{min}} = 42\ \text{gtt/min}.$$

99. b. 29—350 liters at 12 lpm (350 L) ÷ (12 L/min) = 29 min.

100. b. 23-ga and 0.5-inch needle—Subcutaneous injection is made using a small size needle (23–29 gauge) (1/2 to 5/8 inch) at a 45° angle.

Chapter 11: Emergency Medications

1. c. Activated Charcoal, 200 grams—The dose of activated charcoal is 1–2 grams/Kg. This patient is 220 lbs which is 100 Kg. Therefore the appropriate dose would be 100–200 grams, provided he is alert and has a gag reflex and the substance is noncorrosive.
2. b. Adenosine, 6 mg—Administer the adenosine 6 mg as a rapid bolus followed by 20-ml saline flush. Consider an additional adenosine 12-mg rapid bolus in 2 minutes if no response.
3. c. Albuterol, 2.5 mg—The patient who would benefit from a smooth muscle relaxer focused on the bronchial tree and the peripheral vasculature should be given albuterol 2.5 mg diluted into 2.5-mL saline as a nebulizer treatment.
4. d. Amiodarone, 300 mg—The first antidysrhythmic drug that is used in a cardiac arrest is amiodarone 300 mg. If the patient is in VF or in torsades de pointes, then magnesium is considered. The Lidocaine dose is 100 mg and not 200 mg.
5. b. Aspirin, 160–325 mg (chewed)—As long as the cardiac patient does not have any allergy to aspirin, it is appropriate to administer 160–325 mg by having him chew the pills.
6. d. Atropine Sulfate, 0.5 mg—Atropine sulfate would not be appropriate to administer to the patient with a tachydysrhythmia.
7. b. They can cause GI bleeding.– GI bleeding is a common side effect of the three medications.
8. c. Diazepam, 5–10 mg—Diazepam would be the most appropriate medication to administer for status epilepticus of those listed.
9. c. Diltiazem, 0.25 mg/kg.—Diltiazem is a calcium channel blocker and antidysrhythmic used with tachydysrhythmias from the atria.
10. b. Diphenhydramine, 25 to 50 mg—In a patient having a mild to moderate allergic reaction with stable vital signs, typically diphenhydramine is administered prior to resorting to epinephrine.
11. c. Dopamine Hydrochloride, 2–20 ug/kg/min drip—Dopamine would be appropriate as long as the patient is not hypovolemic in a tachydysrhythmia or in VF.
12. c. Etomidate—Etomidate is not a sympathomimetic class drug. It is a nonbarbiturate hypnotic anesthesia induction agent.
13. b. Epinephrine, 1 mg—The patient who is experiencing a severe allergic reaction will need epinephrine.
14. c. Fentanyl citrate, 85 ug IV—The 85-kg patient with extremity fracture and severe pain can be given 1 ug/kg or 85 ug.
15. b. Furosemide, 0.5–1 mg/kg—Furosemide can be administered to CHF patients who have pedal edema and pulmonary edema to help remove water from their system.
16. d. Glucagon, 0.5–1 mg IM—Glucagon would be appropriate for the diabetic patient who does not have an immediate IV site to access.
17. a. Haloperidol Lactate, 2–5 mg IM—Haloperidol lactate would be an appropriate drug to use on this patient. The midazolam hydrochloride dose should be 2- to 2.5-mg IV.
18. c. Hydroxocobalamin, 5 grams—Hydroxocobalamin is the drug in CYANOKIT that is used for cyanide poisoning.
19. b. Meperidine Hydrochloride, 50–100 mg IM—Ipratropium is often mixed with albuterol in the nebulizer treatment of the patient with severe bronchospasm or bronchoconstriction.
20. a. Levalbuterol—Levalbuterol is a sympathomimetic bronchodilator and not an analgesic.

Chapter 12: Airway Management, Respiration, and Artificial Ventilation

1. a. alveoli—The alveoli are located within the lungs.
2. c. ring in the trachea.—The cricoid ring is the only complete ring in the trachea. In the pediatric patient, it is the narrowest portion of the trachea.
3. a. Infants and children have a more flexible trachea than adults.—The pediatric trachea is softer and more flexible than that of an adult. This is why airway positioning is critical in the unconscious pediatric patient.
4. d. They are proportionately larger and take up more space in the mouth.—Proportionately, the tongue and epiglottis are larger, softer, and more floppy than those of an adult.
5. d. ethmoid bone—The ethmoid bone is a structure in the nose.
6. a. warm, filter, and humidify the air we breathe.—It also includes the nose, which is the organ for the sense of smell.
7. c. exchange oxygen and carbon dioxide at the cellular level.—Normally, each alveolus is surrounded by a functional pulmonary capillary, where carbon dioxide passes from the blood and is eliminated

by breathing. Simultaneously, oxygen is absorbed from the alveolus into the capillary.

8. a. Ventilation; oxygenation—Ventilation refers to the movement of carbon dioxide out of the lungs during breathing. This process differs from oxygenation, the movement of oxygen into the lungs, though they are often interrelated.

9. c. 760; 100—At sea level, the atmospheric pressure, measured in torr (mmHg and torr are interchangeable terms) should add up to 760 torr and should equal 100%.

10. d. be inserted into the esophagus and seal it off.— When intubation is unsuccessful after two attempts, the paramedic may use the King Airway (LT-D) as an alternative to endotracheal intubation for advanced airway management.

11. b. the brain stem has been injured. – Specific respiratory patterns may be able to give the paramedic a clue as to what type of problem the patient is experiencing. The paramedic who can recognize specific patterns and understand the pathology may be better prepared to manage the patient.

12. b. patient's metabolic status.—Especially the acid–base balance.

13. a. medulla—The rate of respiration is controlled by the medulla and pons in the brain. The medulla is the primary involuntary respiratory center. It connects to the respiratory muscles by the vagus nerve.

14. d. apneustic—The pons take over if the medulla fails to initiate breathing.

15. c. CSF.—The analysis sends messages to the brain to increase or decrease the respiratory rate.

16. a. aortic arch.—Chemoreceptors are most plentiful in the carotid sinus and the aortic arch.

17. b. high concentration of carbon dioxide—When chemoreceptors sense the level of carbon dioxide rising, they send a message to the brain to increase the respiratory rate to rid the body of the excess carbon dioxide.

18. c. trapped or retained CO_2.—The loss of normal alveolar structure leads to a decrease in the elastic recoil, which creates resistance to expiratory airflow. Air is trapped within the lungs, resulting in poor air exchange.

19. d. This patient would most likely do well with CPAP —The patient is in respiratory distress and appears to require higher oxygen concentrations. Observe the patient carefully for changes in the mental status and respiratory rate. If the patient begins to deteriorate, apply CPAP. CPAP decreases the work of breathing for the patient allowing them to rest and improve at the same time. The use of CPAP often eliminates the need for emergency intubation.

20. b. Smoking inhibits the normal movement of mucus out of the lung.—Cigarette smoking directly inhibits the normal movement of mucus via bronchial cilia out of the lung. As a result, the lung is unable to clear pathogens (e.g., bacteria and viruses) as effectively. Allowed to remain, these infectious agents multiply, resulting in pneumonia.

21. d. hypoxia.—A deficiency of oxygen reaching the tissues of the body.

22. c. Hypoxemia—Inadequate oxygenation of the blood.

23. b. hypoventilating and hypoxemic—Neurologic emergencies (e.g., stroke, seizure, brain injury, and tumor) cause abnormal respirations; altered mental status; paralysis; and vision, speech, and motor disturbances. Carefully assess the respiratory status for signs of hypoventilation and hypoxemia.

24. c. laryngeal spasm—Laryngeal spasm is a closure of the vocal cords and surrounding muscles. A frequent cause is trauma from an overly aggressive intubation attempt.

25. a. The patient is contagious.—Consider any patient with possible pneumonia to be contagious, and act accordingly.

26. d. open the airway, assess for breathing – If the patient is not breathing, advanced life support techniques for airway obstruction include visualizing the airway with a laryngoscope and using Magill forceps to removed the obstruction.

27. c. manual suction—The bulb syringe, V-Vac®, and foot pump style suction units are operated manually and require no oxygen or electric sources to operate.

28. d. deplete your oxygen source rapidly.—Unless you have an endless supply of oxygen, this can be a significant disadvantage.

29. c. suctioning the tracheobronchial region.—Sterile suctioning, also referred to as deep suctioning or closed suctioning, is the technique used to suction the tracheobronchial region through an endotracheal tube.

30. b. tickling the back of the throat.—The gag reflex, or vagal response, can be easily stimulated by suctioning the back of the mouth and throat.

31. a. prevent the tongue from obstructing the glottis.— OPAs are airway adjuncts designed to keep the tongue from becoming an obstruction.

32. b. they do not provide a secured airway.—Nasal airways can be suctioned through, can provide a patent but not secured airway, and can be tolerated by conscious patients. Nasal airways can be safely placed blindly and do not require the mouth to be opened during insertion.

33. b. The bevel is designed to face the nasal septum.— For this reason, nasal airways are usually designed to be inserted in the right nostril. That does not mean they cannot be used in the left if there is difficulty inserting one in the right.

34. c. collect in the lung tissue, causing a chemical aspiration pneumonia.—Water-soluble products are less irritating to the tissue if a small amount should get into the lungs.

35. a. systolic; inspiration—The cause is felt to be increased intrathoracic and pericardial pressures that decrease the venous return to the heart. A change in pulse quality may also be detected during inspiration.

36. b. during an asthma attack.—The cause is felt to be increased intrathoracic and pericardial pressures that decrease the venous return to the heart.

37. c. protective reflexes used by patients to modify their respirations.—Patients may modify their respiration with any of the following protective reflexes: cough, sneeze, gag reflex, sigh, or hiccup.

38. b. Sighing—Sighing increases the opening of alveoli to prevent localized collapsed areas of non-aerated lung.

39. c. Kussmaul's—Deep, gasping respirations representing hyperventilation to blow off excess CO_2 and compensate for an abnormal accumulation of metabolic acids in the blood or metabolic acidosis (e.g., kidney failure, sepsis, aspirin poisoning, alcoholic ketoacidosis, and diabetic ketoacidosis).

40. a. helps to make it easier to breathe.—Patients may modify their respirations by positioning themselves to make it easier to breathe. Often patients are not consciously aware that they took on a "special breathing position."

41. b. airway is not properly opened.—Gastric distension is an expansion of the stomach, usually due to an excess of trapped air. Excess air enters the esophagus and, ultimately, the stomach.

42. a. creating resistance to bag mask ventilation.—The enlarging stomach places pressure on the diaphragm and limits the lung expansion.

43. a. slowly applying pressure to the epigastric region.—Gastric distention can be relieved by being prepared to suction potentially large volumes, placing the patient in the left lateral position, and then slowly applying pressure to the epigastric region, suctioning as necessary to ensure that the patient does not aspirate.

44. b. It is tolerated by conscious patients.—The use of a gastric tube does not interfere with intubation, can be tolerated well by conscious patients, and mitigates recurrent gastric distention and nausea.

45. b. heart block.—Vagus nerve stimulation may lead to bradycardia, heart block, or asystole. The risk is greatest in persons with inferior wall myocardial infarction.

46. a. Terminate the procedure.—In most cases, patients respond promptly to termination of the procedure and atropine.

47. a. administering atropine.—In most cases, patients respond promptly to termination of the procedure and atropine. Be prepared to manage a cardiac arrest with high-quality compressions!

48. d. exposure to body fluids.—The risk of infection to the paramedic is serious due to the exposure to body fluids. Protect yourself from body fluids that could spread diseases such as hepatitis, tuberculosis, meningitis, or influenza.

49. b. valve stem—The regulator can be easily damaged, but if the valve stem breaks it could send the pressurized vessel flying like a missile, injuring everything and everyone in its path.

50. b. 10—OSHA has guidelines for the proper procedures for recording and documenting hydrostat dates.

51. a. react with the oxygen and cause a fire.—The oxygen could react with the adhesive and debris and cause a fire.

52. c. A therapy regulator is designed to be attached to the cylinder stem or wall of the ambulance.—It is generally set at 50 PSI, and the actual delivery to the patient is adjustable on the flow meter in liters per minute.

53. b. 30—The maximum pressure recommended for positive-pressure ventilation should not exceed 30 cm of water pressure.

54. d. exacerbated congestive heart failure patient—The patient has to be breathing to create negative pressure on the valve. The device then administers oxygen to the patient throughout inspiration.

55. b. When ventilating a *complete* laryngectomy patient, you do not need to cover the mouth.—If the patient has a partial laryngectomy, there may still be an open pathway through the mouth as well as a stoma. In this case, when ventilating through the stoma, you have to cover the mouth so the air does not exit there.

56. c. Ventilations can exit the pop-off valve without getting air into the patient.—There have been cases when a bag mask with a pop-off valve was used to ventilate a patient, and the EMS provider did not realize that all of the volume was exiting through the pop-off valve and no air was going to the patient.

57. a. two hands provide manual inline immobilization.—Whenever the patient's head and neck is not taped down to the long board, there must always be two hands providing manual inline stabilization until the neck is cleared in the ED.

58. b. when a patient has poor tidal volume—IPPB is not indicated in noncompliant patients (breathing patients that fight the device, patients with poor tidal volume, and small children).

59. b. it reduces the risk of over inflation.—IPPB can be self-administered, and it delivers a high-volume and a high-oxygen concentration. No oxygen is wasted because it is delivered in response to the inspiratory effort.

60. a. biphasic positive airway pressure—Similar to a CPAP mask, the BiPAP device can help alleviate the need for intubation. This device can vary the degree of positive pressure during inspiration and expiration separately. The ability to vary the pres-

sure makes the system more comfortable and effective in most patients.

61. d. ATVs improve lung inflation or absent gastric inflation compared with other devices, including mouth-to-mouth, bag mask devices, and manually triggered devices.

62. d. Unconscious patients who are sedated.—ATVs are used in both intubated and unintubated patients who require extended ventilation. ATVs allow for control of the ventilation volume and rate.

63. c. Noninvasive ventilation—The first use of this technique originated in-hospital when continuous positive airway pressure (CPAP) was applied by mask to respiratory and cardiac patients.

64. a. intubation may be avoided where it may have previously been required.—The principle is that the patient constantly breathes against a small amount of positive pressure. The pressure causes previously collapsed airways to open, improving oxygenation.

65. b. atelectasis.—The term means to collapse due to inadequate aeration.

66. b. fractured ribs—Taking a large breath or sighing helps to open the small airway and prevents atelectasis. Taking a deep breath is very painful for patients with a fractured rib, and they avoid doing so. As a result, they decrease their tidal volume and their small airways collapse.

67. c. The right mainstem bronchus is straighter.—This anatomical difference in bronchial tubes is the reason for right mainstem intubation when the tube is inserted too far.

68. a. Sedate the patient.—Post intubation, sedation is the safest option for both the patient and the paramedic.

69. a. Tidal Volume: 500—The volume of gas inhaled or exhaled in respiratory cycle, during a normal regular breath. In an adult male, tidal volume is approximately 500 ml.

70. c. aspiration of vomitus—Removing an endotracheal tube often causes vomiting.

71. a. When pressure is applied improperly, airway obstruction results. This technique is still used for intubation to bring the cords into view but it is no longer recommended as a means of preventing regurgitation.

72. d. lateral edge; the cuff is inflated—It is important that this pressure be on the lateral edge of the cartilage, rather than the middle; otherwise, visualization of the glottic opening may actually be more difficult, and airway obstruction results.

73. b. has chest trauma.—The device cannot be used under high-pressure airway conditions (e.g., chest trauma, airway trauma, or restrictive COPD).

74. d. ETT—Of the three acceptable advanced airway devices, an endotracheal intubation is placed directly into the trachea. Properly inserted, it protects the airway from secretions and foreign objects.

75. a. there is a suspected cervical spine injury.—This technique is most helpful in an unconscious patient when either the larynx cannot be seen on direct laryngoscopy or there is a suspected cervical spine injury.

76. a. involves an invasive procedure beyond intubation.—Retrograde intubation involves placing a needle through the cricothyroid membrane. A guide-wire is then threaded upward toward the oropharynx. The ET tube is placed over the guide-wire into the trachea. The wire is removed when the tube is in place.

77. c. infrared—An infrared light beam measures the oxygen saturation of the blood.

78. c. Any condition that causes an altered hemoglobin molecule can cause a false reading.—The principle of pulse oximetry assumes normal capillary blood flow, normal hemoglobin concentration, and a normal hemoglobin molecule.

79. a. The hemoglobin concentration is low due to shock.—The pulse oximetry may not be reliable during shock and severe anemia. The infrared light beam measures the oxygen saturation of the hemoglobin in the blood. If the patient has a reduced hemoglobin count due to blood loss, and the few remaining are saturated, the reading will be high even though there is not enough to adequately perfuse the tissues. If the patient looks sick and the pulse oximetry reading is normal, the patient is still sick.

80. b. colorimetric—Colorimetric devices attach to the ET tube and detect exhaled CO_2 via color changes in the center of the device. This device is not used for continuous monitoring because the moisture in expired air ruins the paper filter in the device.

81. a. wash out any residual $EtCO_2$ that may be present in the esophagus.—This is especially necessary in non-perfusing patients to avoid false readings.

82. b. hypoxic drive. – This mechanism works in contract to the normal person where the blood level CO_2 stimulates respiration.

83. b. esophageal intubation detector—A few studies have questioned the reliability of this device. Always combine your clinical intuition with other methods of verification to decide on proper ET tube placement.

84. a. Verify lung sounds.—The movement associated with transport can cause the tube to become displaced. Lung sounds should be reassessed frequently on any transport.

85. a. the technique does not require the use of a laryngoscope.—Nasotracheal intubation is performed without visualization of the vocal cords. When rapid sequence induction is not available or is contraindicated, nasotracheal intubation is an ideal option for the patient with clenched teeth.

86. a. is a blind technique.—Nasotracheal intubation is performed without visualization of the vocal cords. The patient must be breathing for this procedure.

87. b. nasotracheal intubation.—These devices are specially designed to facilitate nasotracheal intubation. The BAAM is a whistle placed on the end of the endotracheal tube, which provides a whistle sound when the patient exhales through the tube. The Endotrol® has a trigger that curves the tube to the airway anatomy.

88. c. Needle cricothyrotomy—A large-bore angiocatheter is inserted through the cricothyroid membrane into the trachea to create an emergency airway.

89. a. through the cricothyroid membrane.—A means of providing ventilation through a large bore needle that is directly inserted through the cricothyroid membrane.

90. d. risk of hyperkalemia.—Succinylcholine is a safe and short-lasting neuromuscular blocking agent used in rapid sequence induction. It is contraindicated in patients with massive tissue damage (e.g., burns or severe crush injuries) due to the risk of hyperkalemia.

91. c. the cricoid cartilage narrows the trachea and serves as a functional cuff.—The smallest portion of the pediatric airway is the cricoid ring, which serves as a functional cuff. Passing a cuffed tube through this opening may be difficult and cause trauma to the area.

92. c. nasal airway—The nasopharyngeal airway is a very good airway adjunct for a patient with clenched teeth. It does not require visualization of the airway or the absence of a gag reflex.

93. b. use of a pediatric "pop-off" device that prevented adequate oxygenation of a patient—Ventilations can exit the pop-off valve without getting air into the patient. There have been cases when a bag mask with a pop-off valve was used to ventilate a patient, and the EMS provider did not realize that all of the volume was exiting through the pop-off valve and no air was going to the patient.

94. c. rapid sequence intubation – Prehospital RSI for trauma patients is a safe and effective form of airway management and can be performed with low rates of complications and without significant delay in transport.

95. a. Suction the airway and insert a nasal airway.—Manage the airway with the basic steps first and proceed to advanced techniques from there.

96. a. it has no face mask seal to maintain.—The mask fits into and shrouds the glottic opening, where it partially occludes the esophagus. The patient is ventilated with a bag mask device attached to the distal end of the tube.

97. d. Assist ventilations with bag mask device slowly and gently over 2 seconds.—It is important to allow sufficient time for exhalation when a patient is in bronchospasm. Slow and gentle ventilations can prevent barotrauma, especially in a patient with high airway pressures.

98. b. conscious, uncooperative patient in respiratory failure—An example of an ideal patient for RSI is a combative, head-injured patient. The sedative used can also reduce the anxiety level during the short period of neuromuscular paralysis.

99. d. neuromuscular blocking agents.—Succinylcholine is safe and short lasting (less than an hour), but can produce muscular tremors that are generally of no consequence in most patients. These tremors rarely lead to hyperkalemia.

100. a. LMA—The LMA cannot be used under high-pressure airway conditions (e.g., chest trauma, airway trauma, bronchospasm, or restrictive COPD). The device is designed for patients with normal airway pressures and will be ineffective or cause further complications under high-pressure airway conditions.

Chapter 13: Scene Size-Up and Primary Assessment

1. b. primary assessment.—The scene size-up is the first component, which is followed by the primary assessment, focused history, and physical exam.

2. a. make use of door stops.—One of the best ways to keep a scene safe is to keep an exit open.

3. d. trip and fall from a standing position.—Near drowning, GSW, and a fall from a height of 30 feet are all significant MOIs.

4. a. Waddell's triad.—A triad injury pattern associated with pediatric patients struck by a motor vehicle.

5. a. the look test.—The general impression is your first impression of the patient as you approach. This has been referred to for years as the "look test," a "gut reaction," or your "assessment from the doorway."

6. a. determine the patient's mental status.—AVPU represents the patient's initial mental status as being: Alert, Verbal, Painful response, and Unresponsive.

7. c. recognizing hazards and your safety.—Safety first for the responders. Recognizing that hazards are present and then avoiding them is the first priority on any call. This is a dynamic process, and responders will continuously assess hazards throughout all phases of the call.

8. b. Three out of four family members are complaining of headache.—All of the scenarios described are potentially dangerous to the responder, but when three out of four members of the same household have a complaint of headache, the paramedic

should first consider the possibility of high carbon monoxide levels and take the appropriate actions.

9. d. A potentially violent scene is safe for EMS.—Any potential hazard that can injure the responders, the bystanders, or further injure the patient makes a scene unsafe and unsecured (e.g., dangerous crowds, downed power lines, broken glass, or pets). When the actual or potential hazards are removed, the scene is considered secured.

10. a. a 3:00 a.m. response to a house that has no lights on—For an EMS call in a residential area at night, you would typically see lights on and possibly someone outside waving to the ambulance. These instructions are provided by dispatches as part of the EMD protocol.

11. b. Continue to remove the patient and do not let anyone touch the gun.—Safety first, so do not allow anyone to touch the gun. Call a police officer over to secure the weapon. The patient is critical, so continue to rapidly extricate him from the vehicle. Once outside, a pat down should be completed for any additional weapons. This can be done while moving to the ambulance.

12. a. staging area around the corner—In many systems, dispatch will advise the ambulance to "stage in the area" or give a specific location on where to stage until police or fire notifies dispatch that the scene is secure or safe to proceed into.

13. b. a patient with a productive cough—A cough may seem relatively insignificant, but it can actually be a serious hazard, especially when it is productive. Many pathogens are spread through droplets by coughing and sneezing.

14. b. engage the emergency brake on a car that has been left in neutral—Setting the emergency brake, turning off the ignition and removing the key, and letting the air out of tires are all examples of simple and quick actions the paramedic can take to make the scene safer.

15. d. working in traffic at the scene of a collision—Working in traffic is one of the most common and dangerous aspects of the job for EMS responders, firefighters, police, and so forth.

16. c. twisting of the knee.—Falling or twisting of the knee is commonly associated with these sports. These MOIs often injure the supporting structures of the knee.

17. c. attempted hanging.—There is trauma associated with hanging (MOI), even though the nature of illness (NOI) that led up to the attempt is a behavioral problem.

18. c. mechanism of injury (MOI)—When the paramedic takes the time to learn about common MOIs, he can make some predictions or be better prepared to suspect specific injury patterns.

19. b. general impression—The general impression is your first impression of the patient as you approach. This has been referred to for years as the "look test," a "gut reaction," or your "assessment from the doorway."

20. c. Complete the assignment and search for the next patient.—Each responder is expected to report in, complete assignments as directed, and report back for additional assignments. Freelancing is one of the worst things to do in an incident command situation and can result in dangerous situations for others at the scene.

21. c. painful.—The patient is not aware of you by visual or verbal stimulation. He did respond to your touch and, therefore, is not unresponsive.

22. a. withdraw from pain—A purposeful withdraw from pain is an appropriate response and a good sign. No response, flexion, or extension are all inappropriate responses and indicate a serious problem.

23. d. asking the parent or caregiver to determine if the response is normal.—This is appropriate when the infant is not unconscious. The parent or caregiver can tell you if the infant is acting normal or not. If the infant is not acting normal, they can tell you in what way the behavior is abnormal.

24. b. Level of consciousness—The level of consciousness is often used interchangeably with mental status, although they do have different meanings. The mental status is the appropriateness of the patient's thinking. The LOC is the degree of the patient's alertness, wakefulness, or arousability.

25. b. low-level—An unconscious patient who exhibits (decorticate or decerebrate) posturing is exhibiting neurological posturing. This may occur all the time or only when pain is applied. It is illustrative of low-level brain functioning.

26. b. metabolic causes.—Metabolic causes, such as severe diabetic ketoacidosis or sedative overdose, can cause neurological posturing.

27. a. broken jaw.—Fractures to the face can cause potentially serious airway problems. The paramedic must be alert to this and assess the need for airway management.

28. c. neck injury.—The MOI described has the potential to cause cervical spine injury and the paramedic must take the appropriate precautions.

29. a. Mental status—The level of consciousness is often used interchangeably with mental status, although they do have different meanings. The mental status is the appropriateness of the patient's thinking. The LOC is the degree of the patient's alertness, wakefulness, or arousability.

30. d. minute volume.—The minute volume is the amount of gas inspired or expired in a minute. An inadequate minute volume exists if the respirations are shallow and the rate is too slow.

31. b. close the airway.—When an infant's neck is hyperextended or hyperflexed, it can actually close off the airway. A neutral or slightly flexed position is best for an infant.

32. c. carotid artery—During the primary assessment, the pulse is assessed at the carotid artery for the "quick check" to determine whether the adult or child patient has a pulse. In infants, the pulse is assessed at the brachial artery.

33. a. radial; distal—When a patient has a distal (radial) pulse, this finding suggests the patient has an effective blood pressure.

34. b. color, temperature, and condition—The color, temperature, and condition (CTC) are the features that are assessed about the skin.

35. d. cyanosis—Blue, or cyanotic, skin is associated with a lack of oxygen resulting from inadequate breathing or heart function. A person with hepatic or renal failure is more likely to have skin that is jaundice (yellow) and pale. Red or flushed skin can be caused by heat exposure, hypertension, or emotional excitement in any patient.

36. d. palms or soles—The nail beds, lips, and eyes are additional areas of the skin to assess for skin color.

37. d. 3-year-old asthmatic—The usefulness of capillary refill has been downplayed in adults because there are many unreliable factors that can interfere with the capillary refill time. However, in children, circulation is much better than in adults, and capillary refill is a useful assessment finding.

38. c. to determine the need for rapid transport and definitive care at the hospital.—The paramedic must make the determination of the need for rapid transport based on the patient's condition and location, and whether or not additional assistance is needed (e.g., helicopter or critical care transport unit).

39. d. in the operating room by a surgeon—Severe trauma is not something that can be stabilized in the field. The basic rule is that the internal bleeding is stopped by the surgeon within the first hour (the golden hour) after the injury has occurred.

40. a. use of a short board immobilization device—When this step is skipped or expedited, it is called rapid extrication.

41. c. reassessment—The reassessment includes serial vital signs and checking on interventions such as administered medications, IVs, or airway adjuncts.

42. b. focused—The focused physical exam is typically directed at the patient's chief complaint or life-threatening condition discovered in the primary assessment.

43. a. condition may be changing rapidly.—The primary assessment is repeated as needed throughout the call. It may frequently be repeated in critical patients and when the patient's condition is changing rapidly.

44. b. Trending—Trending is an important tool in patient care. It is the process of obtaining a baseline assessment, repeating the assessment multiple times, and using the information to determine whether the patient is getting better, worse, or shows no change.

45. b. responsive and unresponsive.—The patient assessment algorithm for the medical patient subdivides patients into responsive and unresponsive.

46. a. significant and nonsignificant—The patient assessment algorithm for the trauma patient subdivides patients into two categories based on the MOI being significant or not.

47. c. any threat to life—Immediate threats to life are managed first in all patients.

48. d. Provide rapid transport to an OR.—The basic rule is that the internal bleeding is stopped by the surgeon; IVs can be started and maintained en route to the hospital, and should not delay transport.

49. b. sickle cell crisis—Sickle cell crisis is painful and potentially deadly. Symptoms include shortness of breath and severe abdominal pain.

50. a. patella dislocation—An isolated extremity fracture or dislocation is typically a stable condition, unless there is a loss of distal pulse, or motor or neuro function.

Chapter 14: History Taking

1. d. allow twice as much interview time.—Successful communication with patients who do not speak the same language as the paramedic will take extra time. Consider that interpretation of speech, tone of language, facial expressions, body language, and gestures all take more time between the communicants.

2. a. speak with them.—Speaking with the patient is the best way to assess the mental status. Determine the AVPU (Alert, Verbal, Painful stimuli, Unresponsive) during the primary assessment and follow up using the Glasgow Coma Scale. During the patient interview, you should be able to determine whether the patient is conversing normally, is responding reasonably to questions, and is oriented.

3. a. Active listening—This technique involves restating the patient's statements and asking frequent questions to ensure you are understanding the patient.

4. a. complete health—This includes every surgery, hospital visit, illness, injury, immunization, and psychiatric problem. It also includes all medications, allergies, family history, activities, religious beliefs, daily routines, patient outlook, relationships, sleep patterns, and other personal stress factors.

5. b. present illness.—The acronym OPQRST is used in the out-of-hospital setting to remember the set of questions to be asked in order to obtain information about the present illness or injury.

6. c. Is this event similar to any previous events?—If the answer is yes, additional information to ask about should include: How many times has an event like this happened? When was the last event? and What treatment was received?

7. d. present illness or injury.—The acronym OPQRST is used in the out-of-hospital setting to remember the set of questions to be asked in order to obtain information about the present illness or injury. It represents: Onset, Provocation, Quality, Relief (Radiation, Region, Recurrence), Severity, and Time of onset.

8. a. Mirror and matching—Adapt your vocal pitch to the patient's and match your body language as well. Pay particular attention to how loudly you are speaking.

9. d. tonsillectomy in childhood—The paramedic must quickly obtain information that is relevant to the present illness or injury.

10. a. develop a treatment plan.—The time typically spent with a patient is short. The paramedic obtains a history from the patient and/or spouse, family, or caretakers, while performing an assessment in an effort to develop and employ a treatment plan.

11. a. Showing empathy helps to obtain more cooperation from the patient.—Showing empathy is a therapeutic communication technique to help the patient with his feelings and to obtain more information.

12. b. calling the patient "honey"—Using a patient's proper name, Mr., Mrs., or Ms. Jones, shows respect. If the patient gives permission to use another name, then it is okay to use that name. It is disrespectful to use terms of endearment (e.g., "honey" or "dear") or pet names (e.g., "chief" or "doll").

13. b. Why did you call us here today?—This question will, in many cases, get a nervous or confused patient talking and focusing on the problem.

14. d. embarrassed.—Take into consideration who else is present when you are interviewing a patient. The patient may not want family, coworkers, or bystanders to know certain information about herself.

15. d. open-ended—This type of question allows the patient to answer with more than a "yes" or "no."

16. b. when specific information is required—This can be especially important when the patient is unstable or critical (e.g., respiratory distress or chest pain). Attempt to get the answer to the most important questions before the patient is unable to answer any questions.

17. c. Native Americans—Other cultures take offense to where or how they are touched or spoken to. Consider obtaining more information about this topic.

18. d. The paramedic could lose the patient's trust.—It is better to explain what is happening and what is going to happen next. If the patient perceives that

you are lying, you may not get the cooperation you need.

19. b. Do you have sharp chest pain?—If you asked, instead, "Are you having chest pain?" this would be a "yes or no" type question and not leading.

20. b. You don't smoke, do you?—Condescending or judgmental questions can make a patient uncomfortable, and this may cause him to lie about other information, or lead to information being withheld.

21. d. avoid the use of complicated medical terminology.—Stick to the use of lay terms as much as possible. If you are caring for a health care professional who understands medical jargon, it should become apparent quickly, and the use of medical terminology may be appropriate.

22. b. inattentiveness.—Inattentiveness can make a patient feel uncomfortable and lead to information being withheld.

23. c. Facilitation—Positive examples of facilitation include sitting close to the patient and making eye contact, while you nod or say, "I'm listening" or "Please tell me more."

24. d. reflection.—Reflection helps the patient feel that you are listening and can confirm information that is pertinent to the event.

25. a. Interpretation—An example would be to say, "It appears that when you exert yourself physically, you develop a shortness of breath."

26. a. a patient is blind—An over talkative or symptomatic patient can be challenged when faced with limited time for interview and care, and, if the condition of the developmentally disabled patient is severe, information may be omitted.

27. c. Vial of life®.—This is an example of a commercial device available to provide medical and other emergency information about a patient to emergency medical providers.

28. a. Use positive body language while you begin care.—Ideally, the best solution is to find a translator. Otherwise, use positive body language, such as friendly facial expressions and slow movements to assess, take vital signs, and provide treatment.

29. d. ask permission to touch the patient before actually touching him or her.—This action is appropriate with almost every patient, but especially with a blind person. You can avoid frightening the patient and reduce anxiety by first explaining prior to touching.

30. a. getting angry in return—Anger and hostility is often misdirected at the caregiver. Do not get angry in return; it is nonproductive and stressful.

31. c. depression.—Do not hesitate to ask a patient about her feelings. Depression is associated with some psychological illnesses.

32. d. Try using direct "yes or no" questions.—Attempt to get the patient to focus on one thing at a time by

having him answer questions that require a "yes or no" answer. It may keep both of you from becoming frustrated.

33. c. Establishing a rapport with the patient—It begins from the time the call is dispatched and lasts until the patient is turned over to the ED.

34. a. direct.—With unstable and critical patients, ask questions that require a one- or two-word answer. With a patient in severe respiratory distress, ask questions that require nonverbal answers.

35. d. current vital signs—The current vital signs are part of your assessment. A history of irregular vital signs, such as hypertension or an irregular heartbeat, is considered part of the health history.

36. b. focused history.—A focused history is the chronological history of the present illness or injury.

37. b. Encoding—The communication process used by the EMS provider that is focused around a mes-

sage. The message moves through various forms: written, verbal, nonverbal, encoding, message, decoding, receiver, and feedback.

38. c. MedicAlert® tags—There are a number of information sources found on patients in the field. Some wear necklaces or bracelets, while others use smart cards, computer chips, or wallet cards. The most common are the necklaces and bracelets available from the MedicAlert® Foundation, which maintains a 24-hour emergency response center.

39. a. American's with Disabilities Act (ADA)—The Americans with Disabilities Act includes a provision that requires the hospital to provide a sign interpreter within 30 minutes of the patient's arrival.

40. d. look to see if his hearing aid is on.—Many patients who have hearing aids do not wear them. Ask the patient if he has one, and help him to place it and turn it on.

Chapter 15: Secondary Assessment: Medical Patient

1. b. after the primary assessment has been completed.— The focused history often begins concurrently with the physical exam immediately after the primary assessment has been completed. When the patient is unresponsive, a rapid physical exam follows the primary assessment and management of the ABCs.

2. c. the patient's chief complaint.—With the conscious patient, the focused physical exam is typically directed toward the patient's chief complaint (e.g., for a patient with difficulty breathing, the paramedic will focus on the pulmonary, respiratory, and cardiac areas). When the patient is unresponsive, the primary assessment and management of the ABCs is started immediately. Because the patient is not able to provide a history, the rapid physical exam follows.

3. a. TIA.—The patient has described having neurologic symptoms (e.g., possible loss of consciousness, temporary loss of motor and neurologic function); therefore, the stroke/TIA should be considered first. Vitals signs, glucose reading, ECG, and a focused history and physical exam will help to rule out possible causes and narrow the differential diagnosis.

4. d. Determine if there is trauma associated with this event.—The dispatch information was for an unresponsive patient and you have found the patient lying on the floor. It is appropriate to determine if there actually was a loss of consciousness and if there are any injuries associated with a possible fall before proceeding with the other tasks.

5. c. the events that preceded this episode.—The acronym SAMPLE stands for Signs and symptoms, Allergies, Medications, Past medical history, Last meal–last similar event, and Events leading up to the current episode.

6. b. positive findings and pertinent negatives.—As part of the focused history, positive findings (such as a loss of consciousness prior to stroke symptoms) and pertinent negatives (such as the patient denying chest pain when she has difficulty breathing) are obtained by the paramedic.

7. d. difficulty breathing—The paramedic is asking about possible pertinent negative and positive findings associated with a respiratory complaint.

8. c. look for peripheral edema.—In addition to assessing the patient's work of breathing for a patient with a complaint of dyspnea, the paramedic should assess lung sounds, assess for peripheral or sacral edema, obtain vitals signs, an ECG, and pulse oximetry.

9. b. altered mental status.—AEIOU-TIPS stands for: Alcohol, Epilepsy, Infection, Overdose, Uremia, Trauma, Insulin, Psychoses, and Stroke (or shock). It is used to remember the possible causes of altered mental status.

10. c. concurrent medical problems.—Many patients, especially the elderly, have a lengthy medication list for a number of concurrent medical problems. Always consider medications as a possible cause of new or worsened symptoms in any patient.

11. a. rapid physical examination.—When the patient is unresponsive, the primary assessment and

management of the ABCs is started immediately and is followed by the rapid physical exam.

12. c. bronchodilator.—The patient's chief complaint is dyspnea. The chest pain changes with breathing, indicating a non-cardiac pain. The focused physical exam includes clear lung sounds and stable vital signs. Bronchodilator therapy is appropriate for this patient.

13. c. pertinent negative findings.—In a patient with respiratory distress, these are important pertinent negative findings, which help to differentiate the causes of the patient's distress.

14. b. good clinical judgment and experience.—The guideline for repeating the ongoing assessment is every 5 minutes for an unstable or critical patient and every 15 minutes for a stable patient. However, there are many variables to each call, which can alter treatment and ongoing assessment. Good clinical judgment and experience should prevail.

15. c. associated signs and symptoms.—These are positive associated signs and symptoms for a respiratory distress patient.

16. c. neurologic—Dizziness and nausea may be signs of vertigo. A neurologic problem and the history of a recent cold could have caused an inner ear problem.

17. c. gain trust and cooperation from the patient.—Establishing a rapport with the patient is necessary to gain consent from most patients. Gaining a patient's trust and cooperation helps to move along the physical assessment and proceed with treatment.

18. a. examining the body for urticaria.—Urticaria or hives may be present anywhere on the body but often appear on the chest, back, or axilla first.

19. c. cardiac—Weakness, dizziness, and nausea are atypical cardiac symptoms, but in the elderly patient they may be the only signs of a cardiac problem.

20. d. chief complaint; and findings in the primary assessment. PE can be a dynamic process in the out-of-hospital setting. The way the focused PE is approached is based on the patient's chief complaint, the findings from the initial assessment, the focused history, and other findings discovered along the way.

21. b. stabilize and transport.—Many of the presenting medical problems involve the same field management in the first 30–60 minutes, so it is not always necessary, or practical, to make a diagnosis in the field. Strive to assess emergent signs and symptoms, stabilize the patient to the best of your ability, and transport to the nearest appropriate facility.

22. a. cardiothoracic—Assess for the most serious potential problem first. Consider a cardiac problem first and intra-abdominal bleeding second.

23. d. obtain an ECG and pulse quality.—As the most serious possible problem may be cardiac in nature, an ECG, pulse rate, and quality should be assessed quickly.

24. a. OPQRST—The acronym OPQRST stands for: Onset, Provocation, Quality, Relief (Radiation, Region, Recurrence), Severity, and Time of onset.

25. b. neurologic—The new onset of problems affecting sensation, coordination, and bowel control are signs of a neurologic problem.

26. b. possible CO poisoning.—When two or more members of the same household have a complaint of headache, the paramedic should consider the possibility of high carbon monoxide levels first and take the appropriate actions.

27. a. skin.—The acronym DCAP-BTLS is used to remember what is assessed about the patient's skin. It stands for: Deformity, Contusion, Abrasion, Puncture/penetration, Burn, Tenderness, Laceration, and Swelling.

28. a. an unresponsive 40-year-old male—The rapid physical exam is performed on medical patients who are unresponsive or have a severely altered mental status.

29. c. a rapid assessment of the entire body.—When the patient is conscious, the interview comes first and physical exam second.

30. b. neurologic—Assessment motor function and sensation are part of the neurologic and orthopedic exams.

31. c. Intracranial pressure can stimulate the vomiting reflex.—Nausea and vomiting are associated with many disorders. Frequently, but not always, vomiting is preceded by nausea. When brought on by injury, or accompanied by severe abdominal pain or headache, nausea and vomiting may indicate a serious condition. The vomiting reflex is located in the vomiting centers in the medulla.

32. a. vertigo is a vestibular disorder.—Vertigo is often used as a synonym for dizziness or lightheadedness. True vertigo is a vestibular disorder that includes motion sickness.

33. b. cardiac—Dysuria (difficulty urinating) and back pain are signs and symptoms of a urologic/genitourinary problem.

34. a. To reduce vagal stimulation.—Cardiac patients may be put on stool softeners as to avoid straining during bowel movements. Straining can produce a vagal response, which will slow the heart rate.

35. a. internal bleeding.—Orthostatic hypotension occurs due to sudden peripheral dilation with a compensatory increase in cardiac output. This is common in the elderly as their compensatory mechanisms deteriorate. In young adults, orthostatic changes are not common without an underlying cause such as prolonged bed rest, from certain medications, or from hypovolemia with a blood loss of greater than 1,000 cc.

36. a. after the rapid physical exam.—For the unresponsive medical patient the order of assessment begins with the primary assessment, followed by the rapid physical exam, vital signs, and gathering a history from anyone who can provide one.

37. a. take C-spine precautions.—There is a lot of potential for traumatic injury in the bathroom (e.g., porcelain and tile showers, bowls, sinks, walls, and floors).

38. c. vasovagal—One of the common causes of syncope in the bathroom is a parasympathetic response from stimulation of the vagus (e.g., bearing down on the commode, shaving the neck and stimulating the carotids, or tying a tie, and pressing on the eye while manipulating contact lenses).

39. c. Vasovagal stimulation—Other non-cardiac causes of syncope include: dehydration, neurologic, hemorrhagic, pharmacologic, respiratory, and emotional.

40. a. beta-blockers.—Many drugs can cause syncope, and beta-blockers are one of the most common types of medications. Others include: diuretics, nitrate, digitalis, antihypertensives, antiarrhythmics, and narcotic analgesics.

41. d. blood pressure—Obtaining a baseline set of vital signs while getting a focused history is appropriate for this patient.

42. b. limbic system disorders.—Prolonged or frequent vomiting may produce GI bleeding as a result of the reflux of acid and bile. It may also cause Mallory–Weiss tears.

43. c. speech problems.—The neurological assessment includes the stroke exam. Assess for acute onset facial droop, speech or vision problems, unilateral weakness or paralysis, and mental status changes.

44. a. bathroom.—One of the common causes of syncope in the bathroom is a parasympathetic response from stimulation of the vagus (e.g., bearing down on the commode, shaving the neck and stimulating the carotids, or tying a tie, and pressing on the eye while manipulating contact lenses).

45. c. heart block—A heart block can be an immediate, life-threatening condition, producing a heart rate too slow to provide adequate circulation.

46. c. assess the patient from head to toe.—Assess each area of the body for signs of injury, medical ID devices or medical devices, and any other possible clue to the patient's condition.

47. a. cardiac dysrhythmias.—Cardiac dysrhythmias, such as SVT, Stokes–Adams syndrome, and sick sinus syndrome.

48. b. endocrine—Excessive thirst, generalized weakness, and excessive urination may indicate diabetes is soon to be diagnosed.

49. b. positional symptoms.—There are wide variances in "normal ranges" for orthostatic vital signs. More significant are positional symptoms, especially if associated with significant pulse and blood pressure changes.

50. c. cardiothoracic—The paramedic should complete a thorough cardiothoracic exam making a differential diagnosis of an acute coronary syndrome (ACS), pleurisy, pneumonia, pericarditis, and other conditions that provoke chest pain.

Chapter 16: Secondary Assessment: Trauma Patient

1. c. any injury that interferes with the ABCs—Life-threatening conditions include any injury that interferes with the airway, breathing, and circulation. The factor involved most often in traumatic injuries is shock.

2. b. 1 hour—Assessment-based patient care, not diagnostic-based care, provides the best chance for the survival of critical trauma patients. This is because it takes time to make a diagnosis. When you consider the golden hour, there is not enough time to diagnose injuries in the field, and often not even in the ED.

3. a. 10—For the best possible patient outcome, the EMS provider must consider the golden hour for critical trauma patients and take no longer than the "platinum ten minutes" to get the patient in the ambulance and on the way to the hospital.

4. d. rapid transport—Rapid transport is reserved for the critical trauma patient in most cases.

5. b. MOI—The most important aspect of trauma assessment is the MOI. Evaluating the MOI to understand the pathology of what happened is part of the foundation of excellent trauma patient care.

6. b. DCAP-BTLS—The acronym DCAP-BTLS is used to remember what is assessed about the patient's skin. It stands for: Deformity, Contusion, Abrasion, Puncture/penetration, Burn, Tenderness, Laceration, and Swelling.

7. c. 32-year-old female at 34 weeks' gestation complaining of abdominal cramping after falling in her home—The third-trimester pregnant patient with a traumatic injury should be considered a high priority. The secondary assessment should be done–route to avoid delay of transport. The other patients

described have non-life-threatening injuries without significant MOIs.

8. d. transportation should not be delayed while waiting for ALS to arrive—For the best possible patient outcome, the EMS provider must consider the golden hour for critical trauma patients and take no longer than the platinum ten minutes to get the patient in the ambulance and on the way to the hospital. ALS can meet the ambulance en route to the hospital without delaying transport.

9. b. primary assessment—The information obtained at this point is enough to determine the patient's condition and to make the decision to "load and go" or "stay and play."

10. a. the MOI—The most important aspect of trauma assessment is the MOI. When the patient has sustained a significant MOI, the paramedic must consider the energy impact on the body and have a high index of suspicion for specific injury patterns.

11. b. every 15 minutes—The reassessment includes reassessing vital signs and checking on interventions such as administered medications, IVs, or airway adjuncts. It is repeated every 5 minutes for critical and unstable patients and every 15 minutes for noncritical and stable patients.

12. d. IV—Level IV trauma centers are established for rural and remote communities. A level IV may be a clinic rather than a hospital. The goal is to provide initial stabilization and then transfer the patient to a level I, II, or III.

13. a. I—Most level I trauma centers have a full range of resources, services, and programs.

14. d. traumatic cardiac arrest—The reason for this is that the survival rate of a traumatic cardiac arrest is so low that the closest facility that can provide stabilization may be the patient's best chance.

15. d. the loss of consciousness—The MOI, combined with the loss of consciousness and the confusion, are appropriate criteria for aeromedical transport.

16. b. trauma score—The trauma score was developed in 1980 as a scale to be used for triage and to predict patient outcome. Howard Champion, MD, is the physician responsible for the latest version of the trauma score referred to as the revised trauma score.

17. a. fractures of the heels, ankles, and hips—When considering that the energy created by motion stays in motion from the point of impact (feet) through the entire body, the patient would also be likely to have spinal fractures.

18. a. full spinal immobilization—The long backboard serves as a splint for the entire body during the care of a critical trauma patient. Minor injuries should be attended to only after major and life-threatening injuries.

19. c. children—Trauma is the leading cause of death for people from 1–44 years of age and, more specifically, is the number one killer of children in the United States.

20. b. body fat minimizes the body's protection (padding) against traumatic injury.—Muscle and fat mass decrease with age.

21. b. Head injury—Trauma is the number one killer of children in the United States, and, more specifically, head trauma from falls is the most common cause.

22. a. falls.—Trauma is the number one killer of children in the United States, and, more specifically, head trauma from falls is the most common cause.

23. a. the presence of rib fractures is a critical finding.—Rib fractures are rare due to soft bones. When present, the risk of mortality is increased.

24. b. vomiting.—This increases the risk of aspiration as well. Always be prepared for nausea, vomiting, and airway management in the pregnant trauma patient.

25. c. 30%—During pregnancy, the mother's blood volume increases and reaches a nearly 50% increase.

26. a. aorta—An MOI that results in a rapid deceleration with a head-first impact should cause obvious damage to the cranium, as well as injury to the spine and internally producing thoracic aortic disruption. Fractured ribs, sternum, and trachea are injuries more consistent with a blow to the chest, such as a steering wheel impact.

27. c. spine, knee, and lower legs—When an unrestrained patient is found under the steering wheel, suspect knee, femur, hip, pelvis, and spine injuries.

28. c. broken steering wheel—Physical signs of the vehicle that lead you to suspect underlying injuries include: a starred or cracked windshield, a broken steering wheel, a broken dash, and intrusion into the side of the passenger compartment.

29. b. coup-contra coup—Coup injuries develop directly below the point of impact, and contracoup injuries develop on the opposite side of the point of impact. These are common when the back of the head is struck.

30. a. Waddell's triad—When struck by a vehicle, this is the injury pattern in children involving the legs, chest, and head: the legs from a direct blow, the chest from being thrown onto the car hood, and the head from being thrown clear of the vehicle when the vehicle comes to a stop.

31. d. cavitation.—Cavitation is the momentary acceleration of tissue laterally away from the projectile (bullet, knife, etc.) tract. This is like the ripple effect of a rock dropped into a pond. The tissue waves can cause damage and explain why a bullet near the spine can actually injure the spine. They

also explain why the exit wound is usually larger than the entrance wound.

32. c. 1,300—It is estimated that the chances of a spinal injury increase up to 1,300 times when not wearing a seat belt and being thrown clear of the vehicle. Of course, this is assuming you are not run over by another vehicle.

33. d. epidural hematoma—Bleeding of an artery traveling along the inner surface of the cranium will result in a hematoma above the dura mater (epidural).

34. c. chest and abdomen.—Primary injuries are typically in the head, neck, and spine. Secondary injuries involve the chest and abdomen.

35. a. long backboard—The long backboard is a splint for the entire body, which can be utilized safely and quickly.

36. b. The patient has an altered mental status.—The paramedic should consider causes other than a normally uncooperative disposition for the behavior of a victim of a serious MOI. Consider hypoxia, head injury, hypoglycemia, or shock as the possible cause of the patient's behavior.

37. a. regional protocols.—Regional protocols typically provide specific information on when and where to transport trauma patients. State guidelines provide general information, as well as national guidelines, which are listed in many EMS texts.

38. d. Children compensate for shock better than adults in early shock.—Children in shock may appear better

than they actually are because, initially, they compensate better than adults. When they begin to decompensate, it occurs quickly and is an ominous sign.

39. d. immobilize the C-spine and open the airway.—Priority with unconscious trauma patient is airway as well as spinal immobilization, so open the airway with a jaw thrust maneuver.

40. a. The medication list.—When caring for an elderly patient with a traumatic injury, the medications must be considered. For example, blood thinners may produce serious internal and external bleeding. Beta-blockers can mask the body's ability to compensate for shock.

41. c. intra-abdominal hemorrhage—Dizziness, diaphoresis, and pale skin color are signs and symptoms of shock. With the MOI, the paramedic should suspect intra-abdominal hemorrhage.

42. c. complicated airway—Airway, breathing, and circulation are the primary priorities of care in any patient.

43. d. wheezing is present with a hoarse voice—Airway, breathing, and circulation are the primary priorities of care in any patient.

44. b. level I trauma center—Examples of criteria for transport to a level I trauma center are severe burns or major trauma, especially when the patient is a pediatric, geriatric, or pregnant patient.

45. b. C3 and C4—Paralysis below the neck is associated with injury to C3 and C4 of the spine.

Chapter 17: Monitoring Devices and Vital Signs

1. c. blood sugar level.—You are assessing a 25-year-old male adult with a chief complaint of chest pain for the past 20 minutes. The blood sugar level would not be routinely a vital sign taken on this patient with this complaint.

2. b. 65–75 beats per minute—The most appropriate pulse for a 50-year-old female patient would be 65–75 beats per minute.

3. b. 18 per minute—The most appropriate respiratory rate for a 65-year-old male patient found sitting on the couch, alert and in little distress would be 18 breaths per minute.

4. c. utilize a length-based tape to determine.—If you have not memorized all the vital sign rates for each age group, a useful resource to use with small children would be to utilize a length-based tape to determine.

5. b. 99°F.—The expected body temperature of an adult male patient complaining of the chills is most likely 99°F.

6. d. tachycardia. —When a patient has a pulse rate over 100 bpm, this is called tachycardia.

7. c. hypertension.—When a patient has a systolic BP of 146 mmHg, this is referred to as hypertension.

8. d. 28 times a minute.—An alert 35-year-old male patient who is in respiratory distress is likely to have a breathing rate of 28 times a minute.

9. c. carbon dioxide; exhalation.—An EtCO$_2$ monitoring device measures, the amount of carbon dioxide during each breath at the end of exhalation.

10. b. SpO$_2$ 88% in a 4-year-old having an asthma attack.—The pulse oximetry reading would be most useful to the paramedic in a patient with SpO$_2$ 88% in a 4-year-old having an asthma attack.

11. a. ambient noise is too loud to hear pulse sounds.—The method of obtaining a blood pressure by palpation is often used by the paramedic because ambient noise is too loud to hear pulse sounds.

12. d. Korotkoff sounds.—While taking a blood pressure, the sounds heard with a stethoscope that indicate the systolic and diastolic readings are called Korotkoff sounds.

13. c. carotid.—When checking for the pulse on an unconscious patient, the paramedic should assess the carotid pulse.

14. a. radial—When checking for the pulse on an alert patient, the paramedic should assess the radial pulse.

15. c. tachypnea.—When a patient has rapid respirations, this is referred to as tachypnea.

16. b. 90 bpm.—For a child who is of preschool age (3–6 years), a normal heart rate range would include 90 bpm (range 80–140).

17. b. 100 bpm.—For a child who is of toddler age (1–3 years), a normal heart rate range would include 100 bpm (range 90–150).

18. c. 110 mm Hg.—For a child of school age (6–12 years), a normal systolic BP range would include110 mm Hg (range 80–100).

19. d. mottling.—When assessing the skin of a patient, you locate patchy skin discoloration due to vasoconstriction or vasodilatation. This is called mottling.

20. c. continuous ECG monitoring—All patients, presenting with cardiac-related signs and symptoms should have continuous ECG monitoring.

21. a. It can shorten the door-to-treatment interval for cardiac patients.—A key reason for 12 lead ECG acquisition by the paramedic in the field is that it can shorten the door-to-treatment interval for cardiac patients.

22. c. equidistant between V2 and V4.—When applying the 12 lead ECG in the field, V3 should be placed on the patient's chest equidistant between V2 and V4.

23. b. fifth intercostal space in left midclavicular line.—When applying the 12 lead ECG in the field, V4 should be placed on the patient's chest in the fifth intercostal space in the left midclavicular line.

24. c. waveform capnography device—The standard for prehospital confirmation and monitoring of endotracheal tube placement is a waveform capnography device.

25. b. 70 g/dl—The decision is made to assess the blood of a patient who has an altered mental status with a glucometer. The reading of 70 g/dl indicates the need for dextrose administration in the field.

26. d. ECG calipers.—An example of a tool that is not a monitoring device is an ECG caliper.

27. b. 12 lead ECG and glucometer—If you are assessing and managing a patient with a suspected stroke in addition to monitoring the BP, use the 12 lead ECG and glucometer.

28. c. 95°F—When assessing a patient who has been outdoors in the cold rain without the appropriate clothing, you find he is severely shivering. If you took his body temperature, it would most likely be 95°F.

29. b. less than or equal to 0.12 seconds.—On an ECG, a normal QRS complex should be less than or equal to 0.12 seconds.

30. a. 0.12–0.20 seconds.—On an ECG, a normal PR interval should be 0.12–0.20 seconds.

Chapter 18: Reassessment and Clinical Decision Making

1. c. Trending will help the paramedic identify changes in the patient's condition—The key aspects of reassessment are: trending, adapting, time constraints, manpower limitations, anticipating changes, and altering or modifying care.

2. b. improved muscular strength—The natural hormonal responses include: improved reflexes and muscular strength, enhanced visual and auditory acuity, diminished concentration and assessment abilities, and impaired critical-thinking skills.

3. b. stimulants of the "fight or flight" response for paramedics.—There are many stimulants and variants for the individual. The most common stimulants are: alarms, pagers, dispatch information, cell phones, emergency lights, sirens, traffic, and other hazards.

4. a. short transport time—With an unstable patient, managing the ABCs may take all available resources; if the transport time is short, it may alter how reassessment is completed.

5. d. The time interval for repeating the reassessment for the critical trauma patient is the same for the critical medical patient.—The reassessment of the critical patient, either trauma or medical, is repeated every 5 minutes. For the noncritical patient, it can be repeated every 15 minutes.

6. a. Trending—Trending is an important tool in patient care. Treatment is continued as is, or modified, using the information obtained from trending.

7. b. subtle changes in the patient's mental status.—An example is the head-injured patient whose condition may deteriorate quickly. The earliest indications are often subtle changes in the patient's mental status.

8. a. Isolated measurements are generally less helpful than changes over time.—This is why trending is such an important tool.

9. d. think and work under pressure.—The out-of-hospital environment is uncontrolled and dynamic.

Gathering information, evaluating, and processing information while developing and implementing appropriate patient management is different for every call.

10. b. evaluating and processing information.—The essential concepts of clinical decision making include: gathering, evaluating, and processing information, while implementing appropriate patient management.

11. c. collect more history and process the information—Getting a good history is key to formulating concepts, in turn you can interpret and process the information, apply additional treatment, reassess, and reflect.

12. b. The hospital is a relatively controlled environment.—The out-of-hospital environment is uncontrolled and dynamic.

13. c. the patient's blood pressure—Hypotension is the hallmark sign of cardiogenic shock and dopamine is used to raise the blood pressure. Blood pressure has to be monitored closely when a dopamine drip is running.

14. c. the patient's level of discomfort—For the patient presenting with cardiac chest pain, your goal is to reduce and eliminate the pain while quickly transporting the patient to the most appropriate facility.

15. d. achieving and maintaining an adequate body of medical knowledge.—As with any health care provider, this is an ongoing process, because the medical field is dynamic and continually improving.

16. a. Assess for JVD, peripheral edema, and start an IV.—The patient described is in moderate to severe respiratory distress. Listening to lung sounds and providing a treatment of nebulized bronchodilator right away is appropriate for most patients in this condition. Now complete the cardiothoracic exam by assessing for JVD, peripheral edema, and obtaining an ECG. Review the patient's medications and obtain a history using questions with yes or no answers, to allow the patient to inhale the treatment without interruption. You will need vascular access for additional medications.

17. c. Look up the correct dose in your protocol book.—Never guess, especially with medications. Take a few seconds to look up the information you need, like all other medical professionals do.

18. d. Identifying and managing medical ambiguity—Other fundamental elements of critical thinking include: gathering and organizing data, forming concepts, analyzing and comparing similar situations, differentiating between relevant and nonrelevant data, articulating and documenting decision-making reasoning, and constructing valid arguments.

19. a. clearly define performance parameters.—In addition, they provide a standard approach to patient care and speed the application of critical-care interventions, while providing structure for the EMS provider.

20. c. They can speed the application of critical interventions.—Additional benefits of using protocols and standing orders include promoting a standard approach to patient care, defining performance parameters, and providing some structure to patient care.

21. c. practice the same scenario frequently.—Practicing complex and high-stress scenarios helps the paramedic to gain experience and hone skills. By analyzing and comparing similar situations, the paramedic can better process information and formulate and apply treatment.

22. a. Collect information and formulate concepts, interpret and process information, apply treatment, reevaluate, and reflect.—The flow of the critical-thinking process should follow a logical plan that resembles this format.

23. a. Stop and think before acting.—Mental preparation tricks to use when critical thinking becomes clouded include: staying calm, anticipating and planning for the worst, reassessing frequently, and pausing to take a deep breath.

24. a. planning for the worst scenario.—Mental preparation tricks to use when critical thinking becomes clouded include: staying calm and stopping to think before acting, anticipating and planning for the worst, reassessing frequently, and pausing to take a deep breath.

25. a. an unrestrained victim of an MVC sustaining facial lacerations on the windshield.—It would be appropriate to use a teaching moment with a patient who is an alert and stable patient after experiencing injuries that could have been prevented.

26. a. CUPS—In some areas, the acronym CUPS—Critical, Unstable, Potentially unstable, and Stable—is used to describe a patient's priority after completing the primary assessment.

27. a. manage similar experiences.—For most, the more an individual is exposed to an experience, the better she is able to avoid panicking, manage similar experiences, and generally be able to overcome having a bad day.

28. b. trending mental status and vital signs.—These are repeated every 5 minutes for a critical patient and every 15 minutes for a noncritical patient.

29. a. Take a deep breath and revert back to assessing the ABCs.—Reassess the airway, breathing, and circulation. This will help you to refocus and will give you information to proceed.

30. a. consult medical control.—Standing orders and protocols provide clear performance parameters and often speed up treatment for critical patients. However, they do not fit all patient problems or patients with concurrent problems. Never hesitate to consult medical control with complex situations.

Chapter 19: Critical Thinking and Assessment-Based Management

1. b. Assessment—An assessment is the foundation of care. It is difficult to report or manage a problem that you did not find.
2. c. history.—The history should be focused toward the organ systems that are associated with the complaint.
3. b. environment—A supermarket can be a loud and busy place, making a proper field assessment difficult. Consider moving the patient to the ambulance for privacy for the patient, and a more controlled environment for you and your crew.
4. c. rule out hypoglycemia—Any patient with an altered mental status should be considered for hypoxia and hypoglycemia early in the assessment.
5. a. frequent flyer—Labeling patients is unfair, because they may not be afforded the full attention that all patients deserve.
6. a. organ systems associated with the complaint.—The history should be focused toward the organ systems that are associated with the complaint. One's knowledge of a disease and its assessment findings, as well as maintaining a degree of suspicion about a particular problem, affects the quality of a history taken from the patient.
7. b. Recognition of various injury patterns can help the paramedic be better prepared to provide the proper emergency care.—With this understanding, the paramedic can potentially make a significant difference in the patient's outcome.
8. c. equipment to conduct the primary assessment of the patient's ABCs—The "first-in" equipment should contain the following items: airway, breathing, and circulation control equipment; scissors and blanket to expose the patient; ECG monitor or AED; and pad and pen for notes.
9. b. guidelines for care.—There are both benefits and disadvantages to protocols, standing orders, and patient-care flow charts. One benefit is that they provide some structure for the EMS provider, and a major disadvantage is that they do not fit every patient.
10. a. having a bias against people who do not have a background similar to hers.—Having a biased or prejudicial "attitude," or attempting to classify patients by a social status, can cause the EMS provider to miss vital pieces of information, often short-circuiting the information-gathering process.
11. c. a biased or prejudicial "attitude"—Having a bias against people who do not have a similar background or attempting to classify patients by a social status can cause the EMS provider to miss vital pieces of information, often short-circuiting the information-gathering process. Tunnel vision or myopia can be very dangerous!
12. d. accompany the patient through definitive care.—The team leader is usually the EMS provider who will accompany the patient through definitive care. The team leader takes on many responsibilities, including: establishing a dialogue and rapport with the patient, obtaining a history, performing the physical exam, presenting the patient, completing documentation, coordinating transport, and designating tasks.
13. c. acting as the initial EMS command in an MCI.—Typically, this is the role of the team leader.
14. b. red flag.—A sign or symptom that suggests the patient may have a serious injury or medical condition is often referred to as a "red flag."
15. a. a poor assessment and care were made.—A good oral presentation suggests effective patient assessment and care; a poor presentation suggests poor assessment and care.

Chapter 20: Medical Overview

1. d. L—last meal—The last meal, last medication dose, last menses, or last similar event will help the paramedic to possibly determine why this event is occurring or how to proceed with treatment.
2. a. Proceed as if the condition is new.—In the absence of a reliable source, the paramedic must proceed as if the problem is new and begin looking for possible causes and begin care and transport.
3. a. have and practice a preplan.—You should have a preplan to avoid the appearance of confusion. Practice the preplan before you need it.
4. a. Choreography—The paramedic must learn to be proficient at choreographing the scene of a call. This includes maintaining overall patient perspective and designating tasks at all types of calls, ranging from a two-person crew to EMS command at a multiple casualty incident (MCI).
5. b. seeing a local drug abuser and immediately blaming his disorientation on the drugs rather than looking for a medical problem.—Labeling patients can be very destructive to the assessment process. Even the frequently intoxicated patient or people whom

you feel abuse your services get sick and injured once in a while.

6. d. make the appropriate management decisions.—Decisions are only as good as the information they are based on.

7. d. An unorganized approach can lead to important information being overlooked.—An organized approach allows for a complete and smooth assessment.

8. c. it allows for a complete and smooth assessment.—With one EMS provider, there is sequential information gathering and treatment. With two, there can be simultaneous information gathering and treatment, which is more efficient. When multiple responders are present, the team leader should designate to avoid confusing the patient or missing answers to questions asked by different responders.

9. b. existing treatment protocols.—Treatment decisions involve a combination of information obtained from the history, the physical exam, recognition of injury patterns and disease processes, the field impression, and existing BLS or ALS treatment protocols.

10. b. The paramedic's knowledge of a disease and its assessment findings.—The history should be focused toward the organ systems that are associated with the complaint. One's knowledge of a disease and its assessment findings, as well as maintaining a degree of suspicion about a particu-

lar problem, affects the quality of a history taken from the patient.

11. b. Important information can be missed by performing a cursory physical exam.—For most EMS responders, there are time constraints. However, you cannot benefit from the information obtained from the physical exam if you overlook some part or just do a cursory physical exam.

12. d. provide excellent customer service through good people skills.—EMS is a profession as well as a business and the patients are the paying customers.

13. a. more efficient.—With two, there can be simultaneous information gathering and treatment, which is more efficient than one. When multiple responders are present, the team leader should designate to avoid confusing the patient or missing answers to questions asked by different responders.

14. d. preplanning and practicing with her crew.—Some agencies assign critical roles or positions based on the equipment an EMS provider carries into the call. For example, the person who carries the drug box and defibrillator may be the team leader, and the person carrying the oxygen and advanced airway kit may go right to the patient's head for airway control.

15. c. watching everyone's back to make sure no one gets hurt.—The patient care provider is also responsible for gathering scene information, obtaining vital signs, performing skills as requested by the team leader, and performing triage at an MCI.

Chapter 21: Respiratory

1. d. perfusion.—The flowing of fluid through organs.

2. a. Ventilation; oxygenation—PO_2 measures oxygenation, and pCO_2 measures ventilation.

3. c. rightward; leftward—Shifts to the right or to the left affect the affinity of hemoglobin for oxygen.

4. b. does his oxygen need.—With increased body temperature, the body automatically tries to provide more oxygen to the tissues.

5. a. decreased body temperature—Decreased body temperature and alkalosis are the most common causes of a leftward shift of the curve.

6. c. 35–40—Levels over 40 mmHg can cause an increase in the blood acid level, and decreased levels result in a decreased blood acid level.

7. d. acid.—Levels over 40 mmHg can cause an increase in the blood acid level, and decreased levels result in a decreased blood acid level.

8. a. 0.1—Blood gases are very straightforward, and there is a direct relationship between pH and

pCO_2. They always move in opposite directions by a 10:0.1 ratio.

9. d. 80—Lower levels lead to hypoxia.

10. b. The only predictable and reproducible relation in blood gases is between the pH and pCO_2.—Blood gases are very straightforward, and there is a direct relationship between pH and pCO_2. They always move in opposite directions by a 10:0.1 ratio.

11. c. pCO_2.—This can also occur in situations of hypoventilation or intrinsic lung diseases (e.g., asthma or COPD).

12. a. respiratory acidosis—Respiratory acidosis occurs when CO_2 retention leads to increased levels of pCO_2.

13. a. tonsillitis—The other answers are associated with the lower airways.

14. c. clubbing of the fingers or toes—Clubbing occurs in patients with pulmonary disease, heart disease, gastrointestinal disease, inflammatory diseases and cirrhosis. The specific cause is unknown.

15. b. anemia—Other perfusion-related factors that may impair gas exchange include: hypovolemia, impaired circulatory blood flow, and chest wall pathology.

16. c. impairment of chest wall movement.— Neuromuscular diseases can impair movement of the chest wall by causing phrenic or spinal nerve dysfunction.

17. d. acute respiratory distress syndrome—With ARDS, the lungs become inflamed and filled with fluid. ARDS can affect people of any age and is life threatening.

18. c. out against a partially closed epiglottis.—In infants and toddlers, grunting is a sign of respiratory distress.

19. c. pharyngitis—Pharyngitis is often referred to as a sore throat and is rarely serious. Most cases resolve without intervention. The student cannot stay in school with a fever. Many schools have a policy of having to be without fever for 24 hours without using medication for fever.

20. b. mentation—Confusion suggests hypoxemia or hypercarbia, while lethargy or coma is a sign of severe hypoxia or hypercarbia.

21. a. a possible clue to a history of severe pulmonary disease.—More information about the previous intubation should be obtained quickly, if possible. This information can help the paramedic decide how aggressively or not to treat the patient.

22. b. beta-blockers—In addition, allergic reactions to any medication may lead to wheezing and exacerbate underlying respiratory conditions.

23. d. spontaneous pneumothorax—The sharp chest pain is often localized to the side of the lung involved. Decreased breath sounds are present on the affected side, and the respiratory rate is increased.

24. c. a congenital bleb.—A congenital bleb is an air filled sac on the surface of the lung that has been present since birth.

25. d. bradycardia—Tachycardia is a sign of hypoxemia and fear. A slowing respiratory rate in the face of an unimproved condition suggests patient exhaustion and impending respiratory failure.

26. d. Cheyne–Stokes respiration.—Can occur with emergent conditions such as brain injury (cerebral) or drug overdose.

27. a. ataxic.—This breathing pattern often precedes agonal gasps and apnea.

28. c. Kussmaul's.—A pattern of very deep, gasping respirations. This breathing pattern is associated with coma and metabolic acidosis.

29. a. right heart failure.—As a result, blood backs up into the venous system, especially the neck veins, peripheral edema, and sometimes ascites.

30. c. right-sided heart failure—Distended neck veins, peripheral edema, and ascites are the most common manifestations of right-sided congestive heart failure, whatever the underlying cause. The liver and spleen are also engorged with blood backed up through the portal circulation.

31. a. barrel chest; increased—Trapped air leads to hyperinflation of the lungs, resulting in a widening of the anterior–posterior diameter of a person's chest.

32. a. crackles.—Crackles or rales usually result from fluid in the airways, in the interstitial tissue, or in both.

33. c. Carpopedal—The change in pH from respiratory alkalosis increases the binding of calcium to albumin. This leads to a decreased level of unbound calcium in the blood. Because calcium participates in nerve transmission and muscle contraction, both are affected, leading to spasm.

34. a. sleep apnea.—CPAP may be helpful in some cases of acute pulmonary edema.

35. a. end-tidal CO_2.—pO_2 and pCO_2 are blood levels, and peak flow is the measured effectiveness of exhalation.

36. b. COPD.—COPD is sometimes subdivided into emphysema and chronic bronchitis, though many patients have clinical features of both.

37. a. Administer Versed 0.05 mg/kg.—An asthma patient who required intubation will need to stay intubated for evaluation at the ED. Post-intubation sedation is appropriate with either Versed or etomidate.

38. b. wheezing.—The transmitted sound becomes high pitched and somewhat squeaky.

39. a. irritation—People with asthma have extra-sensitive bronchial airways that are easily irritated.

40. c. Respiratory infections—This includes cold, the flu, and sinus infections. These illnesses trigger asthma attacks because they temporarily inflame and damage the lining of the air tubes, causing bronchospasm, increased mucus production, and swelling.

41. b. cold—Cold weather irritates the bronchial airways.

42. b. respiratory alkalosis—The change in pH from respiratory alkalosis increases the binding of calcium to albumin. This leads to a decreased level of unbound calcium in the blood. Because calcium participates in nerve transmission and muscle contraction, both are affected, leading to spasm.

43. c. Adult respiratory distress syndrome— Administering 100% oxygen often requires a ventilator in a hospital setting, and arterial blood gas measurements are needed to confirm a diagnosis of ARDS.

44. b. Status asthmaticus—Its onset may be sudden or insidious, and is frequently caused by a viral respiratory infection.

45. a. inadequate use of anti-inflammatory medication.— These medications include steroids and leukotriene blockers.

46. b. Chronic bronchitis—These patients have a productive cough for at least 3 months per year for 2 or more consecutive years.

47. c. Emphysema—The decrease in elastic recoil creates resistance to expiratory airflow. Air is trapped within the lungs, resulting in poor air exchange.

48. b. cigarette smoking—Industrial inhalants, air pollution, and tuberculosis also contribute to the condition.

49. d. come on relatively quickly—The patient with an acute COPD episode complains of a shortness of breath with symptoms gradually increasing over a period of days.

50. a. FBAO—Small children explore and learn by putting things in their mouths. Suspect a foreign body airway obstruction first in a child with a sudden onset of respiratory distress, with isolated wheezing or stridor.

51. b. bronchodilating—Nebulized bronchodilators, such as albuterol and epinephrine are commonly used in the out-of-hospital setting.

52. d. anti-inflammatory—Steroids are beneficial in the chronic treatment of nearly all asthmatic patients and many COPD patients.

53. b. fewer—The inhaled forms of steroids are not free of side effects. Additional oral or IV steroids underlie the successful treatment of acute obstructive airway disease.

54. a. take at least 1 or 2 hours to work.—Initiating therapy in the field can help the patient to a quicker discharge a few hours later.

55. c. Leukotrienes—Specific medications that directly attack leukotriene production or action have emerged in the past few years.

56. a. smooth muscle relaxing—It is not known exactly how magnesium sulfate helps some patients with severe bronchoconstriction. However, magnesium sulfate is a smooth muscle relaxer and this may be the action that helps.

57. c. a healthy person to breathe.—The carbon dioxide drive stimulates breathing centers in the brain when the CO_2 levels rise.

58. a. movement of mucus via bronchial cilia out of the lungs.—As a result, the lung is unable to clear pathogens as effectively. Allowed to remain, these infectious agents multiply, resulting in respiratory infection and pneumonia.

59. b. weakened immune system caused by ethanol.—In addition, drinkers are especially likely to get aspiration pneumonia during passing-out spells.

60. c. Cystic fibrosis—An inherited disease that affects many body organs. In the lungs, thick mucus accumulates and clogs alveoli. The patient has difficulty clearing the mucus and develops difficulty breathing. The mucus collects bacteria which causes infections.

61. b. The clinical approach to viral or bacterial pneumonia is the same.—In the out-of-hospital setting, it is impossible to tell whether a person has bacterial versus viral pneumonia.

62. b. hypoxic drive.—This backup mechanism can be seen in cases of COPD. If the level of oxygen in the blood goes very low, brain breathing centers are stimulated, leading to the reflex response of breathing.

63. c. nonproductive cough—A cough productive of purulent (rust colored or green) sputum is a typical finding with pneumonia.

64. b. Take standard precautions for a contagious condition.—Consider any patient with a cough and cold or flu-like symptoms to be contagious and take standard precautions.

65. a. pertussis—Also known is that whooping cough begins with symptoms of a common cold, mild fever, runny nose, and cough. In adults, the initial symptom may be just a dry cough. Within 2 weeks, coughing increases with choking attacks of coughing, with retching or vomiting afterwards, and sometimes a whoop sound as the patient attempts to catch their breath.

66. a. Ventolin—A sympathomimetic that stimulates beta-2 receptors of the bronchi, leading to bronchodilation.

67. a. viral—Influenza is an acute and highly contagious viral disease.

68. b. cultures.—In the out-of-hospital setting, it is impossible to tell whether a person has bacterial versus viral respiratory infection.

69. c. with or without antibiotics.—URI is an acute, usually self-limited infection of any part of the upper respiratory tract. Most commonly, the mouth, throat, and ears are affected. Most people have a spontaneous resolution of symptoms within 7 days. People who have underlying disease may develop more severe infections, such as pneumonia or sepsis.

70. a. Some URIs cause bronchoconstriction.—URI is used interchangeably with the "common cold," and serious complications can develop in patients with underlying diseases, such as COPD or cancer.

71. c. spleen—Patients who have had their spleen removed lose resistance to common organisms that often cause a bacterial URI. For these patients, this can become a life-threatening illness.

72. c. cigarette smoking.—Other diseases, such as coal miner's lung and asbestosis, also predispose people to lung cancer, but cigarettes often still play a role.

73. a. cardiac arrest—Altered mental status, severe cyanosis, or profound hypotension also suggest the presence of a life-threatening embolus in a proximal location.

74. a. nausea, vomiting, and weakness—The most common side effects from chemotherapy are nausea, vomiting, diarrhea, and hair loss. Some patients become significantly dehydrated following therapy.

75. c. dry cough or shortness of breath—More commonly, patients are asymptomatic but may experience dry cough. Scar tissue from radiation treatment may restrict lung expansion, leading to shortness of breath.

76. c. exposure to a contagious patient—Consider any patient with possible pneumonia to be contagious, and act accordingly.

77. d. cardiac ischemia—Sometimes people with severe CHF develop pulmonary edema. Typically, they do not.

78. c. CHF is a spectrum of conditions associated with decreases in cardiac function.—Pulmonary edema is a general term for fluid in the lung, for any of several reasons.

79. a. the recumbent position increased venous return to the heart.—The result is an increase in the preload or amount of blood that the heart must pump out.

80. c. vasodilation of both veins and arteries.—Nitroglycerin causes non-selective vasodilation of blood vessels. This may result in a drop in blood pressure.

81. c. nebulized Ventolin—Aerosolized medications help loosen mucus in the lungs. The patient's level of distress may require more aggressive ventilatory support and suctioning.

82. a. Reduces cardiac preload and afterload.—This may result in a drop in blood pressure.

83. b. the conversion of angiotensin I to angiotensin II in the lungs.—Angiotensin II is a powerful vasoconstrictor. By blocking it, vasodilation occurs, leading to a decrease in cardiac work.

84. b. increase intrathoracic pressure.—Increased airway pressure causes the expansion of previously atelectatic (collapsed) portions of the lung and improves overall ventilation. It may also increase intrathoracic pressure and counteract increased pulmonary capillary hydrostatic pressure.

85. c. spontaneous pneumothorax—The sharp chest pain is often localized to the side of the lung involved. Decreased breath sounds are present on the affected side, and the respiratory rate is increased. The reasons for the association of smoking and bleb rupture are not clear.

86. c. affect levels of natural anticoagulants in the blood.—The result is a hypercoagulable (thicker) state and increased risk of embolism.

87. a. pulmonary arterial circulation.—Usually, the obstruction is due to a piece of blood clot that has broken away from a pelvic or deep leg vein.

88. a. bronchospasm—The release of histamine from white blood cells causes bronchoconstriction and may be responsible for localized wheezing sometimes heard during the physical exam.

89. b. ACS—The patient may experience classic symptoms of an acute myocardial infarction or spontaneous pneumothorax (e.g., dyspnea, tachypnea, and chest pain).

90. a. The presence or absence of pleuritic chest pain.—Pain that is clearly worsened by breathing is more likely due to a lung or chest wall problem than myocardial ischemia.

91. d. tachycardia.—Breath sounds are usually normal, though localized wheezing is heard occasionally. SpO_2 may be normal, and, after several hours, a pleural friction rub (grating sound) may be heard.

92. c. young, tall, male smoker—These patients are the most likely to develop pneumothorax from the rupture of a congenital bleb, the most common cause of spontaneous pneumothorax.

93. a. low; increases—The change in pH results in respiratory alkalosis.

94. c. Assuming that the patient is experiencing a simple anxiety attack.—Many disease states and serious conditions cause hyperventilation (e.g., asthma attack, COPD, MI, pulmonary embolus, spontaneous pneumothorax, CHF, increased metabolism, central nervous system lesions, hypoxia, drugs, increased metabolic acids in the body, and psychogenic factors). A conservative approach demands that you assume the patient is seriously ill until proven otherwise.

95. b. Offer the patient a nasal cannula.—Putting a mask over the patient's face may make him feel like he is suffocating, which worsens the patient's anxiety and overall condition.

96. a. pulmonary embolism—Fat released from the bone marrow of a fractured long bone can cause pulmonary embolism.

97. a. fat embolus from bone marrow—Fat released from the bone marrow of a fractured long bone can cause pulmonary embolism.

98. c. spontaneous pneumothorax—These patients are the most likely to develop pneumothorax from the rupture of a congenital bleb, the most common cause of spontaneous pneumothorax. The reasons for the association of smoking and bleb rupture are not clear.

99. d. carpopedal spasm—Stress and anxiety may cause the patient to hyperventilate.

100. a. providing high-flow oxygen and watching for changes in mental status.—Many disease states and serious conditions cause hyperventilation. A conservative approach demands that you assume the patient is seriously ill until proven otherwise.

Chapter 22: Cardiovascular

1. a. pulmonic and aortic—The tricuspid and mitral valves are known as the atrioventricular valves.
2. a. stenotic.—Stenosis can occur in any or all valves and may produce a murmur.
3. b. right atrium.—The coronary sinus empties into the right atrium.
4. c. pulse deficit.—Pulse deficit is associated with atrial fibrillation.
5. a. pulsusparadoxus.—This is a symptom of various conditions (e.g., pericarditis).
6. c. mitral and tricuspid—This sound is the louder of the two normal heart sounds.
7. d. heart failure.—S3 is a soft, low-pitched sound heard about one-third of the way through diastole.
8. b. pericardial friction rub.—A pericardial friction rub sounds like a grating or scraping noise and is sometimes mistaken for a cardiac-related sound. The sound stops when the patient holds his breath.
9. c. endocardium.—Endocarditis is a potentially fatal bacterial infection of the endocardial layer of the heart, most commonly the heart valves.
10. b. 50—The abnormal collection of pericardial fluid is called pericardial effusion. The rapid accumulation of as little as 50 ml can result in pericardial tamponade and death.
11. c. endocarditis.—Endocarditis is a potentially fatal bacterial infection of the endocardial layer of the heart, most commonly the heart valves.
12. b. diastole—The passive expansion of the chambers of the heart during which they fill with blood.
13. d. Starling's law of the heart.—This refers to the preload of the heart. It is based on the fact that the greater the initial length or stretch of the cardiac muscle, the greater the degree of shortening that will occur.
14. b. decrease heart rate—Chronotropism relates to influencing the rate of the heartbeat.
15. c. increase force of muscular contractility—Inotropic is influencing the force of muscular contractility. Positive inotropy is an increase in the force.
16. d. pulmonary embolism—The clot can occlude blood flow or can break apart and become lodged elsewhere (e.g., lungs, brain).
17. c. visceral—Visceral pain impulses are carried by nerve fibers that return to the spinal cord at several levels from both sides of the body; the pain is typically perceived by the patient as being poorly localized and ill-defined.
18. b. neuropathy.—The loss of pain sensation is why patients who develop ulcers wait until they are quite advanced before seeking treatment.
19. b. diabetes—A diabetic patient may suffer atypical symptoms from myocardial ischemia due to neuropathy.
20. a. ischemia—Ischemia means lack of oxygen. Prolonged ischemia will progress to infarction (cell death).
21. b. pulmonary embolism.—They are also used to treat deep vein thrombosis, arterial thrombosis, arterial embolism, and arteriovenous cannula occlusion.
22. a. referred pain.—A patient with chest pain may also feel pain in the neck and arm because, during embryonic life, the heart, neck, and arms originate together.
23. c. history.—In a significant number of cases, it is difficult to diagnose ACS based on any one component of an examination or test. The history is a significant aspect to the diagnosis of an acute myocardial infarction (AMI).
24. d. Prinzmetal's—Chest pain may be severe and can occur at rest, similar to unstable angina. Oxygen, nitroglycerin, aspirin, and drugs that influence calcium metabolism by the myocardium are of benefit.
25. a. coronary thrombosis.—Blood clot occurs about 90% of the time.
26. b. weakness.—Weakness is not a classic symptom associated with ischemic chest pain in the young adult, but in the elderly it may be the only initial indication of cardiac ischemia.
27. b. QRS complex.—The QRS is usually composed of a group (three separate waves) of waveforms.
28. c. Sedate the patient and begin transcutaneous pacing.—The patient has symptomatic bradycardia with a third-degree heart block. The heart rate needs to be corrected. Sedation and pacing is the recommended treatment, and a dose of atropine and a fluid bolus should be considered while awaiting pacing or if pacing is ineffective. Another consideration is that the blood pressure may be too low for sedative medications.
29. c. acute pericarditis and Prinzmetal's angina.—Many things can cause ST segment elevation or depression. This is an abnormal finding, and, in most cases, you must assume that these represent ACS until proven otherwise.
30. a. nitroglycerine.—This is because, with reduced right ventricular function, the patient needs a high preload to maintain forward flow through the lungs. These patients often respond to fluid administration.
31. c. II, III, and a VF—These leads provide a view of the inferior wall and normal conduction pathway of the heart.
32. b. V_3 and V_4—These leads provide a view of the left anterior ventricle.
33. a. V_1 and V_2—These leads provide a view of the septal wall of the heart.

34. c. peripheral artery disease.—Claudication most commonly occurs in the calves, but may occur in the feet, thighs, hips, buttocks, and rarely the arms.

35. d. Adams–Stokes syndrome—Also called Stokes–Adams attack, this is a disorder found more commonly in the elderly.

36. a. reduces the chance of post-shock dysrhythmias.—Synchronization is used to avoid shocking the heart in the relative refractory phase of the conduction cycle.

37. c. external pacing.—The use of this device is a temporary measure until an invasive pacemaker can be placed in the patient.

38. d. Wolff–Parkinson–White syndrome.—This condition is also referred to as pre-excitation syndrome. These changes may be asymptomatic or may be associated with paroxysmal supraventricular tachycardia or atrial fibrillation.

39. b. kidney disease—These risk factors carry potential dangers from excessive bleeding.

40. b. automaticity.—These tissues automatically fire at a given rate under certain conditions, without external nerve stimulation.

41. a. self-excitation.—The ability of cardiac muscle to conduct impulses rapidly throughout the heart.

42. a. hypokalemia—A deficiency of potassium in the blood.

43. c. slow heart rate.—Too much potassium (hyperkalemia) or too little (hypokalemia) slows the heart rate.

44. d. calcium.—Calcium is important for initiating muscle contractions.

45. a. use of supplemental salt tablets—Too much salt (hypernatremia) slows the heart.

46. a. SA node—The sinoatrial node is the normal pacemaker for the heart.

47. d. absent or abnormal P waves.—The SA node is the primary pacemaker and if it should fail for any reason the AV node (backup pacemaker) should take over causing the complexes in the ECG to have a P wave that is absent, or very close to the QRS, either right before or right after.

48. b. lowers stroke volume—Acetylcholine also slows the heart rate.

49. b. dopamine.—The major catecholamines (hormones produced by the adrenal glands) are epinephrine, norepinephrine, and dopamine.

50. d. SA and AV nodes.—These nerves affect the heart rate and the contractility of the heart by the use of the natural chemicals acetylcholine, epinephrine, and norepinephrine.

51. c. accessory pathway.—Reentry, aberration, and accessory pathways are related to the conduction pathway of the heart.

52. a. reentry.—Reentry, aberration, and accessory pathways are related to the conduction pathway of the heart.

53. c. the preload and afterload are directly affected.—As a result, the circulation of blood does not effectively reach all areas of the body, and a backup of fluid develops in other areas.

54. d. hypertrophy.—Enlargement of the heart muscle, typically the left ventricle.

55. d. renal failure.—The kidneys become damaged and shut down.

56. b. permanent organ damage.—The organs most likely to be at risk are the brain, heart, and kidneys.

57. d. hypertension.—If cerebral autoregulation is lost, such as during a stroke or after head injury, the only way for the brain to maintain adequate perfusion is to elevate the arterial BP.

58. a. cerebral autoregulation.—This occurs with the opening and closing of sphincter muscles in the small arterioles of the brain.

59. a. phlebitis.—It can develop from intimal damage to the vein from catheters, injection of irritating substances, and the use of oral contraceptives.

60. d. spontaneous rupture of the aorta—These patients develop aneurysms that typically involve the aortic arch.

61. c. claudication—Similar to angina, it typically occurs with exertion and subsides with rest. The calf is most commonly affected.

62. c. preload.—Starling's law of the heart is based on the fact that the greater the initial stretch of the cardiac muscle, the greater the degree of shortening that will occur.

63. a. venous congestion—When the heart fails to pump effectively, blood backs up in the venous system.

64. b. sympathetic nervous system.—The system circulation is stimulated to increase the tone in the blood vessels to provide better venous blood flow to the heart.

65. d. chronic hypertension.—Often this is a cumulative problem as a result of multiple heart attacks.

66. b. shock.—Cardiogenic shock is the most severe form of pump failure resulting in inadequate cardiac output due to left ventricular malfunction. Out-of-hospital treatment begins with treating for shock.

67. a. ascites.—This occurs when blood is not pumped adequately from the system circulation into the lungs.

68. c. cardiogenic shock.—Acute MI, endocarditis, and pericardial tamponade are primary causes of carcinogenic shock. When the heart is suddenly injured or weakened to the point where it cannot pump enough blood to meet the body's demands.

69. c. hypothermia—The hypothermic heart may be resistant to defibrillation and first-line cardiac drugs.

70. b. decreasing preload.—Positioning the patient is a primary treatment step. When possible, the patient sitting upright with legs dangling assists in venous pooling and helps to decrease the preload.

71. c. ventilatory support—Assisted ventilations with bag mask, CPAP, or intubation may be necessary.

72. a. cardiogenic shock.—Cardiogenic shock greatly diminishes blood flow throughout the body; tissues deteriorate rapidly, and death ensues. The most common cause is as a result of an extensive MI.

73. d. past medical history of heart disease.—Sometimes it is really impossible to tell a difference, but past history may be helpful. Look for a history of heart disease because this tends to be consistent with APE, whereas a history of COPD is consistent with CHF. However, the patient may have both.

74. b. cardiac tamponade—This life-threatening condition quickly progresses from decreased cardiac output to cardiac failure and cardiogenic shock.

75. a. CHF versus APE.—Many providers, when in doubt, give both furosemide and an inhaled bronchodilator. This generally covers both conditions, as long as careful attention is paid to the basics of the ABCs.

76. b. ACS.—The most common cause is as a result of an extensive MI. As the body's compensating mechanism fails, shock progresses, severe hypotension develops, and organ tissues die.

77. a. chronic CHF—Peripheral edema and neck vein distension are far more common in chronic CHF than in acute pulmonary edema. Do not make the error of excluding the possibility of acute pulmonary edema simply because no peripheral edema is present.

78. b. Positioning the patient upright.—Positioning the patient is the primary treatment step. When possible, the patient sitting upright with legs dangling assists in venous pooling and helps to decrease the preload.

79. d. paroxysmal nocturnal dyspnea.—Most people sleep in a prone or near-prone position. Blood pools in the lungs, leading to pulmonary congestion and difficulty breathing. Typically, the patient wakes suddenly from sleep and is extremely diaphoretic and short of breath.

80. d. blood glucose—Two conditions that must be ruled out quickly with any patient who has an altered mental status are hypoxia and hypoglycemia. Administer oxygen and obtain a blood glucose reading quickly.

81. d. hypertensive emergency.—Hypertension is a devastating disease that affects the cardiovascular system. A hypertensive emergency is life threatening, sudden, and with severe increase in BP that can lead to serious, irreversible end-organ damage within hours if left untreated.

82. b renal failure.—The weakened areas of the blood vessels develop blood clots and thrombosis or they rupture and hemorrhage critically.

83. a. an embolism.—The clot forms in the deep veins of the legs (DVT) or pelvis, then travels to other parts of the body and blocks an artery (embolism). If an artery in the lung is affected, it is a pulmonary embolism. If an artery in the brain is blocked, a stroke occurs.

84. a. pain.—As the bulging of the sac continues to grow, the pressure it exerts on other structures often causes symptoms such as abdominal or back pain.

85. d. sudden death.—It may leak, causing pain, or grow and burst like a balloon. The significant and rapid blood loss from the rupture results in sudden death.

86. a. rapid transport.—Rapid, gentle transport and early notification to the ED is the best approach.

87. b. headache, vision disturbance, and confusion.— Backache, chest pain, and dyspnea are not typical symptoms, but may be present with concurrent emergency conditions.

88. c. heart and blood vessels.—The cardiovascular features of Marfan syndrome include aneurysm at the proximal aorta leading to aortic dissection or rupture. Within the heart, abnormalities of the mitral valve can lead to mitral valve prolapse or regurgitation.

89. a. bradycardia—Too much potassium (hyperkalemia) or too little (hypokalemia) slows the heart rate.

90. d. dissecting abdominal aortic aneurysm.—As the aneurysm grows, the pressure it exerts on other structures often causes symptoms such as abdominal or back pain. As it leaks or ruptures, the blood loss causes other symptoms, such as syncope, dyspnea, and pain or numbness in the lower extremities.

91. b. restore perfusion.—Aspirin is used to decrease the risk of vascular mortality with suspected acute MI. Aspirin produces inhibition of platelet aggregation, helping to restore perfusion.

92. b. Kussmaul's—Kussmaul's signs may be observed during the physical exam.

93. d. location of the damage.—This rather simple device has saved many people whose hearts cannot beat effectively alone.

94. c. left chest area—The site of implantation is usually the left-chest area, although it may be placed in other areas.

95. d. dysrhythmias.—Cardiac irritability from hypoxia or other causes typically produces dysrhythmias.

96. a. heart block—There are three types of heart block, first, second and third degree. The first is the least severe and rarely causes symptoms. Second-degree heart block can produce skipped beats, dizziness, or syncope. Third-degree heart block is the most severe requiring prompt treatment because it can be fatal.

97. b. relieve cardiac compression.—This is accomplished by placing a needle directly into the pericardial sac (pericardiocentesis) to remove the fluid.

98. b. external pacemaker—A complete or third-degree heart block as a result of an MI can be fatal. A temporary pacemaker (external) may be used to keep the heart beating until a permanent pacemaker can be inserted.

99. b. junctional escape—The intrinsic rate of the junctional pacemaker is 40–60. The QRS is narrower than NRS, and the P wave may be before the QRS with a short P-R interval, during, or after the QRS.

100. b. Administer nitroglycerine and aspirin.—The patient's blood pressure is more than adequate for nitroglycerin. Due to the patient's cancer, you should ask the patient if he can tolerate aspirin.

Chapter 23: Neurology

1. a. monitor internal changes of the body.—The nervous system is the most complex of the body systems. It acts as the control center of the body.

2. b. cerebrum.—Also called telencephalon, this is the location of higher cognitive abilities such as learning, analysis, memory, and language.

3. b. telencephalon—Also called cerebrum; this is the location of higher cognitive abilities such as learning, analysis, memory, and language.

4. c. basilar artery.—Brain gets its blood supply from the two internal carotid arteries and the basilar artery, which connect into a cerebral arterial circle (circle of Willis).

5. c. circle of Willis.—If for any reason blood flow gets disrupted, the circle of Willis may provide for collateral cerebral circulation, reducing the chances for serious complications.

6. b. midbrain, pons, and medulla oblongata.—These structures are critical to the maintenance of vital functions.

7. a. pineal body—It functions primarily as an endocrine organ.

8. c. cerebellum.—It is located in the back of the skull, beneath the cerebrum and surrounding the brain stem.

9. d. subarachnoid space.—SCF is produced in the ventricles of the brain and is completely replaced several times a day.

10. d. help the brain to recognize changes in CO_2 levels.—The brain monitors changes in the CSF CO_2 level and activates responses in the respiratory centers to regulate the CO_2 and pH of the body.

11. b. Hydrocephalus—Sometimes this condition results in increased pressure within the skull (increased intracranial pressure).

12. b. pia mater—The pia mater is the innermost layer of meninges.

13. c. CSF—Meningitis may be life-threatening, especially when caused by bacteria.

14. a. not covered with myelinated fibers.—White matter is the white fibers of the brain and spinal cord that are covered with myelin (myelinated). Myelin is a layer or coating that protects the axon process and increases the conduction of nerve impulses.

15. b. neuron.—Also called nerve cells, these are dependent on aerobic metabolism, meaning they require oxygen to function.

16. d. mitochondrion—Nerve cells (neurons) need an enormous amount of energy. Mitochondria use oxygen and glucose to produce most of the cell's energy.

17. c. glucose.—The brain cannot create or store either of these, so it relies heavily on the supporting cells as a source of energy.

18. a. multiple sclerosis.—Some disease processes, such as multiple sclerosis, interfere with the myelin sheath.

19. d. synapses.—The synapse (junction) is the place where impulses are transmitted to the axons and dendrites of other neurons.

20. a. reticular activating system—The RAS controls the degree of activity of the central nervous system, as in maintaining sleep and wakefulness.

21. b. peripheral—The peripheral nervous system (PNS) consists of 12 mitochodrium pairs of cranial nerves and 31 pairs of peripheral nerves exiting the spinal cord between each vertebra.

22. b. Amyotrophic lateral sclerosis (ALS) — Amyotrophic lateral sclerosis is a rapidly progressive disorder leading to atrophy of all body muscles and death.

23. c. multiple sclerosis—A demyelinating disease marked by patches of hardened tissue in the brain or the spinal cord.

24. d. hydrocephalus—This condition is caused by either a blockage or decreased reabsorption of CSF, and sometimes results in increased pressure within the skull.

25. c. ruptured aneurysm—Cerebral aneurysm is a congenital defect on the wall of a cerebral artery. This is the fourth-leading cause of cerebrovascular disorder in the United States. The loud sound the patient hears is a classic finding associated with this disorder.

26. b. atherosclerosis—Vascular dementia is caused by atrophy and death of brain cells due to decreased blood flow.

27. b. secondary—Medical research has demonstrated that all brain damage does not occur at the moment

of impact. Rather, it occurs over the next few hours and days.

28. c. concussion.—Symptoms most commonly include headache, memory loss, and irritability, which usually resolve in 2 hours but may persist for months.

29. c. Rapidly transport the patient to a trauma center.—The greatest reduction in mortality and morbidity of the head-injured patient includes: prompt resuscitation, rapid transport to a trauma center, CT scanning, prompt evacuation of significant intracranial hematomas, ICP monitoring, and treatment.

30. c. This is a chronic disorder that does not require emergency care.—The condition described is Parkinson's disease. These symptoms are associated with the chronic and slowly progressive disorder. There is no information that suggests that this patient requires emergency care.

31. c. the TIA has no lasting effect.—A TIA or mini-stroke is a temporary occlusion of an artery to the brain caused by a blood clot. It is believed to be a warning sign of future CVA.

32. b. a major stroke.—TIAs are strong predictors of stroke risk and may occur days, weeks, or months before a stroke.

33. c. seizure.—Seizures can occur in patients of all ages, though the causes of seizures vary slightly in each age group.

34. b. Cluster—Cluster headaches occur cyclically, thus the name. Cluster attacks can last a few days, weeks, or months. This is followed by remission periods during which no headaches are experienced. There is no known cause or cure, but medication can provide some relief.

35. b. complex partial—The aura with this type of seizure may include hallucinations of sounds, visuals, smells, and tastes.

36. a. brain damage can occur.—Prolonged seizures tend to present with very little or no body movement (fixed gaze only). This does not mean the patient has stopped seizing. The patient's neurons are burning out, so treat and stop the seizures.

37. c. medication.—Many common home medications may be the culprit of a syncopal event.

38. a. by speaking with the patient—Subtle changes in the patient's mental status are usually the earliest indicator of nervous system dysfunction. Talking to the patient and performing serial assessments are the best ways to pick up on the subtle changes.

39. a. performing serial assessments—Subtle changes in the patient's mental status are usually the earliest indicator of nervous system dysfunction. Talking to the patient and performing serial assessments are the best ways to pick up on the subtle changes.

40. a. Glasgow coma scale (GCS)—The Glasgow coma scale is a numerical tool used to assess and score a patient's best response to eye opening, verbal, and motor response.

41. d. apneusis.—An abnormal respiratory pattern associated with neurological emergencies.

42. c. Cheyne–Stokes respirations.—This abnormal breathing pattern occurs when the brain stem has been injured.

43. b. autisms.—When autisms are present together with an altered mental status, this may indicate the presence of a lesion in the lower brain stem.

44. c. Ataxic—This abnormal breathing pattern is also associated with lesions in the lower brain stem.

45. b. binocular vision.—Binocular vision is controlled by the forebrain. If this reflex fails, double vision occurs.

46. a. accommodation—A normal function of the eyes that allows the normal eye to focus on objects closer than 20 feet.

47. c. nystagmus.—Nystagmus may be induced by alcohol intoxication, irritation of the inner ear, blindness, and neurologic diseases.

48. d. miosis.—Miosis is seen in the early stages of meningitis, as well as in some types of drug overdose, brain lesions, and sunstroke.

49. a. anisocoria.—Always ask the patient if this finding is normal for her before assuming that it is an abnormal finding.

50. a. chorea.—This involuntary movement may be blended with voluntary movements that can hide the involuntary motions.

51. b. athetosis.—Chorea often occurs simultaneously with athetosis.

52. c. Tourette's syndrome.—This disorder begins in childhood and is three times more prevalent in boys than girls.

53. c. Assess the six cardinal positions of gaze.—As assessment of the six cardinal positions of gaze is used to evaluate cranial nerves III, IV, and VI, in order to detect midbrain and pontine dysfunction.

54. d. V—Assessment of the cranial nerves can help clue you in to the location of a brain injury or insult. Cranial nerve V is linked to speech, swallowing, chewing, and the blinking reflex.

55. b. Ataxia—The inability to coordinate voluntary muscular movements.

56. a. spinal cord injury.—When this finding is present during the exam of a patient with a suspected spinal cord injury, the paramedic should mark the level on the chest for comparison with serial assessments to follow.

57. b. heat stroke—These signs include: altered mental status, neurological dysfunction, elevated temperature, and hot and dry skin.

58. d. behavioral changes.—This occurs because the cerebral hemispheres are the most susceptible to injury.

59. a. pons.—Arm and leg extension is also referred to as decerebrate posturing.

60. c. Decorticate—Characteristics include muscle rigidity with arms flexed and held tightly to the chest,

clenched fists, and legs extended and internally rotated.

61. b. late—The three signs of rising ICP are: rising BP, changing respiratory patterns, and a decreasing pulse rate.

62. a. pyramidal—Babinski's reflex or sign is a reflex movement in which, when the sole of the foot is tickled, the great toe turns upward instead of downward.

63. a. the corpus callosum—The cerebrum is the largest part of the brain and is connected by nerve tissue called the corpus callosum.

64. b. parietal—It also controls speech and memory.

65. d. hypothalamus—It is responsible for many important functions for survival and pleasure, such as: eating, drinking, temperature regulation, and sex.

66. c. ventricles of the brain—CSF is present in the subarachnoid space, cavities, and canals of the brain and spinal cord.

67. d. thalamus and hypothalamus.—Werneiche's syndrome is caused by thiamine (B$_1$) deficiency. Thiamin helps produce energy needed to make neurons function properly. A thiamin deficiency can lead to damage or death of neurons.

68. a. venous—Arterial bleeding is associated with epidural hematoma.

69. b. Bell's palsy—It is a temporary weakness or paralysis, typically on one side of the face, caused by damage to the facial nerve (cranial nerve VII).

70. b. Dendrites—Axons carry impulses away from the cell.

71. a. myelin.—A soft, white, fatty material that forms a thick sheath.

72. b. epidural and subdural.—The two most common hematomas that may develop within the brain are epidural and subdural hematomas, named by the location in relation to the meninges.

73. c. spina bifida.—A malformation of the spinal column with an opening in the membrane that covers the vertebra.

74. a. Poliomyelitis—Also called polio.

75. b. contusion—Concussion, amnesia, and aphasia cannot be seen on a CT scan of the brain.

76. d. Retrograde—This type of amnesia presents with a loss of memory of events that occurred before an adverse event.

77. d. subarachnoid hemorrhage—Bleeding from a leading cerebral aneurysm. The patient's words "I have the worst headache of my life." are a clue to brain hemorrhage. Ask about associated symptoms: nausea, vomiting, confusion, stiff neck, and consider subarachnoid hemorrhage.

78.   results of a stroke exam—Brain bleeding and hemorrhagic stroke are interchangeable terms. Patients with hemorrhagic stroke present with similar neurological deficits but tend to be more ill than patients with ischemic stroke. The results of the stroke exam are the most valuable information with this type of patient.

79. c. uncontrolled hypertension—The blood pressure inclusion factor for the use of thrombolytics is a systolic BP between 90 and 200.

80. a. anticholinergics—Anticholinergics antagonize or block the muscarinic acetylcholine receptors in the eye, which inhibits the pupils from constricting, and the result is dilation.

81. b. dolls-eye maneuver—With the patient's eyes opened, the head is turned quickly from side to side or up and down. The normal response is for both eyes to move in conjugate gaze to the opposite side of the head turning, similar to the doll with counterweighted eyes.

82. a. 1—Another abnormal finding is a dilated pupil greater than 4 mm.

83. b. Aphasia—Aphasia is categorized as expressive or receptive.

84. c. restricting blood flow into the brain.—Cerebral blood flow must be maintained to ensure a constant delivery of oxygen and glucose as well as the removal of "waste" products. Rising intracranial pressure (ICP) can restrict flow to the brain.

85. b. mean different things to different people.—These are nonspecific antiquated terms that have different meanings to different people.

86. b. irregular breathing pattern—Additional neurological deficits to look for in the unconscious patient include: abnormal eye movement, (including pupil reaction), Babinski's reflex, muscle tone, and signs of rising ICP (early versus late).

87. b. rising ICP.—Loss of extraocular movement on the affected side is due to increased pressure on the cranial nerves.

88. a. herniated disc—Pressure on the spinal nerves (pinched nerve) may cause pain in the extremities.

89. c. Bell's palsy.—Paralysis of the facial nerve causing distortion on one side of the face.

90. d. during sleep—The patient awakens with symptoms of a stroke or is difficult to awaken.

91. a. epilepsy.—This is the patient's first seizure, which precludes epilepsy. Epilepsy is more common in children than in infants or toddlers.

92. c. tonic.—This phase typically lasts 15–20 seconds and alternates with muscle spasms (clonic) lasting up to 5 minutes.

93. c. syncopal—Fainting.

94. c. neoplasm—A new growth of tissue serving no physiological function.

95. c. hypertension—The other choices are neurologic disorders.

96. b. V—Also called trigeminal neuralgia.

97. a. heredity.—Glaucoma is a disease in which elevated pressure in the eye, due to an obstruction of the outflow of aqueous humor, damages the optic nerve and causes visual defects.

98. b. glaucoma—Symptoms may occur suddenly and are sometimes accompanied by nausea and vomiting. If

untreated, glaucoma may result in permanent blindness within a few days.

99. d. compression on the spinal cord—The spinal cord may be compressed by: bone, tumors, ruptured or herniated disk, a collection pus or hematoma or connective tissue. These patients require immedi-

ate medical attention to provide any chance of reversing or lessening the loss of function.

100. c. spinal immobilization.—The compression must be relieved immediately, typically by surgery. Carefully immobilize the spine and transport the patient to an appropriate facility.

Chapter 24: Endocrine Diseases

1. c. diabetic problems—Diabetes and related complications affect approximately 8.3% of the U.S. population.

2. a. hyperlipidemia—This is a risk factor associated with heart disease.

3. a. Diabetes—The most common of the endocrinologic emergencies is diabetic problems, which occur more frequently than all of the rest put together.

4. a. chemical—The normal secretion of hormones is tightly regulated by a feedback mechanism involving the: hypothalamus, pituitary gland, target gland, and end-organ.

5. d. nervous—The nervous system acts as the control center of the body; together with the endocrine system, the body's internal physiological balance is monitored and controlled.

6. b. Hormones—Hormones move through the body and produce specific effects on target cells and organs.

7. d. blood.—In the blood, they move through the body and produce specific effects on target cells.

8. b. a pancreas transplant.—At the current time, type I diabetes is without a cure, except for a pancreas transplant.

9. c. pituitary—The pituitary gland is associated with hormones that directly and indirectly affect most basic bodily functions.

10. a. parathyroid—Four small endocrines glands that are adjacent to the thyroid gland and secrete a hormone that regulates the metabolism of calcium and phosphorus in the body.

11. c. pancreas—The pancreas secretes the hormones insulin and glucagon as well as hormones that aid in digestion.

12. d. adrenal—Either of a pair of organs that are located on top of the kidney. The adrenal glands secrete the hormones epinephrine and norepinephrine.

13. b. Excessive hormone production—Endocrine emergencies also occur when normal hormone production fails and with failure of feedback inhibition systems.

14. b. glucagon.—The pancreas secretes the hormones insulin and glucagon.

15. a. stored.—In addition, insulin prevents the breakdown of fat tissue in the body.

16. a. Type I diabetes—Type I diabetes is an autoimmune type of disease.

17. c. many diabetics have some form of neuropathy.—Many diabetic patients (both type I and II) have an acquired dysfunction of the peripheral nervous system (neuropathy).

18. d. permanent neuronal damage.—A period of hypoglycemia is far more dangerous to the patient than an equivalent period of hyperglycemia.

19. c. dehydrated; fluids—The most important immediate problem in hyperglycemia is dehydration. Identify and correct it as soon as possible following local protocols. Always look for other sources of symptoms, especially if the patient has an altered mental status.

20. a. amino acids—Free fatty acids, amino acids, and sugar fail to enter the cells properly, resulting in hungry cells.

21. d. ketones and ketoacids—As the patient's blood sugar rises significantly and the fatty tissue breaks down, the body forms compounds called ketones and ketoacids from the fat tissue. These substances change the acid–base balance in the body, harming the patient.

22. d. total body potassium.—The elevated blood sugar level makes the patient urinate more frequently than usual, leading to dehydration and a loss of body chemicals, particularly potassium.

23. b. infection.—The stress of the infection results in an increased insulin requirement in the body. Unless the diabetic patient recognizes the need to increase the daily dose of insulin when sick, metabolism and the regulation of blood sugar level become abnormal.

24. b. Not every patient with hyperglycemia will have DKA.—Whether symptomatic or not, patients who develop hyperglycemia may not have DKA or hyperosmolar hyperglycemia nonketotic coma (HHNC).

25. c. stored fats—Free fatty acids from stored triglycerides are released and metabolized in the liver to ketones. When ketones dissolve in the blood, they form ketoacids.

26. a. blood; high—When ketones dissolve in the blood, they form ketoacids. If the level of ketones is high enough, the patient is not only ketotic but develops an acidosis. The combination is called ketoacidosis.

27. b. hyperosmolar hyperglycemic nonketotic coma.—Not all people with elevated blood sugar levels have DKA or HHNC. Many people have glucose intolerance and hyperglycemia with absolutely no symptoms.

28. a. early warning signs from the counter-regulatory hormones fail.—The production of glucagon and epinephrine in response to low blood sugar normally causes symptoms of tachycardia and diaphoresis. This early warning system may fail, and the patient remains asymptomatic until the sugar level drops low enough to result in loss of consciousness.

29. d. caffeine—Caffeine increases a person's sensitivity to hypoglycemia.

30. d. glycogenolysis.—Glycogenolysis, together with gluconeogensis (enzymes that cause the liver to manufacture more glucose), tends to raise the blood sugar.

31. c. thyrotoxicosis—Acute thyrotoxicosis, also known as thyroid storm, is a potentially life-threatening acute exacerbation of ongoing hyperthyroidism.

32. a. atrial fibrillation and fever.—Additional signs and symptoms include: flushing, sweating, tachycardia, CHF, agitation, restlessness, delirium, seizures, coma, nausea, vomiting, diarrhea, and fever out of proportion to other clinical findings.

33. b. hypothyroidism—Hypothyroidism is a clinical syndrome due to a deficiency of thyroid hormones. The group of hypothyroid symptoms is often referred to as myxedema.

34. b. myxedema coma—Myxedema coma is a life-threatening condition that results from severe untreated hypothyroidism. The lack of sufficient thyroid hormones leads to decreased metabolism in most vital organs.

35. c. sinus bradycardia—Myxedema is characterized by hypothermia, extreme weakness, altered mental status, hypoventilation, and hypoglycemia. Sinus bradycardia is the most common dysrhythmia.

36. a. Cushing's syndrome—The production of excess corticosteroids by the adrenal or pituitary glands produces an abnormal condition resulting in excess body weight and muscular weakness.

37. d. Cushing's syndrome—Rounding of the face (moon face) and dorsocervical fat pad (buffalo hump) are recognizable characteristics of this disorder.

38. d. tumors in the adrenal glands.—Others causes include oral steroid replacement therapy, and excess production of adrenocarticotropic hormone (ACTH) by the pituitary gland or other sources (e.g., tumors, hyperplsia).

39. c. Addison's disease—The condition is characterized by weight loss, extreme weakness, low blood pressure, GI disturbances, and brown pigmentation of the skin and mucous membranes.

40. b. cortisol and aldosterone—Steroid use is the most common cause of exogenous adrenal suppression.

41. a. the use of oral or inhaled steroids.—Steroid use is the most common cause of exogenous adrenal suppression.

42. b. weight loss, fatigue, and joint pain.—In addition, the patient may experience vomiting, diarrhea, anorexia, salt craving, abdominal pain, postural dizziness, and increased pigmentation (e.g., extensor surfaces, creases of the palm and oral mucosa).

43. a. hypovolemia.—The acute life threats in adrenal insufficiency are hypotension and hypoglycemia.

44. a. hyperthyroidism.—If this finding is present during thyroid storm, it is a helpful diagnostic feature. However, less than 50% of patients with acute thyrotoxicosis have visible eye changes.

45. c. stimulating the pancreas to secrete more insulin.—In general, oraldiabetic agents stimulate the pancreas to secrete more insulin soon after eating. They are taken right before or after eating, which in turn prevents the rise of blood glocose from foods.

46. c. human—Many insulin preparations are available. Made from various sources, some are faster acting than others, while some are longer lasting than others.

47. c a state of cell starvation.—Diabetic patients, whether type I or type II, lack the normal effects of insulin. As a result, sugar and other substances (e.g., amino acids, free fatty acids) fail to enter the cells properly. This results in two concurrent situations: "hungry cells" due to inadequate nutrient supply and elevated blood sugar, and sometimes triglyceride levels.

48. c. administer IV dextrose—IV administration of dextrose must be given first, as the patient is hypoglycemic. IV fluid hydration is appropriate next because of the hypotension. The patient may be experiencing acute adrenal insufficiency due to the steroid use.

49. a. acute adrenal insufficiency—The patient may be experiencing acute adrenal insufficiency due to the steroid use. The acute life threats in adrenal insufficiency are hypotension and hypoglycemia.

50. a. adrenal—The resultant excess affects carbohydrate, protein, and lipid metabolism.

51. b. hyperglycemia—Until a blood glucose reading is obtained, hypoglycemia should be suspected. However, the history and the physical findings (e.g., Kussmaul's respirations, warm and dry skin, and dehydration) suggest possible hyperglycemia.

52. c. Deep respirations are a response to increased acid levels from excess ketones.—Kussmaul's respirations are the body's response to attempts to blow off excess acid in the body.

53. d. glucagon, epinephrine, and growth hormone.—Insulin release is stimulated by glucose, amino acids, and hormones (glucagon, growth, epinephrine). Release is inhibited by hypoglycemia, somatostatin, and norepinephrine.

54. d. administer another 25 grams of dextrose—Manage the airway and breathing with BLS techniques until the patient receives additional dextrose.

55. b. diabetic emergency—For any patient with an altered mental status, the paramedic must rule out hypoxia and hypoglycemia first.

56. b. glucose reading—For any patient with an altered mental status, the paramedic must rule out hypoxia and hypoglycemia first.

57. a. Beta-blockers will conceal compensatory signs of shock.—Decreased blood sugar levels result in the production of glucagon and epinephrine in the body's attempt to raise the sugar. This causes a sympathetic response (tachycardia and diaphoresis). Beta-blockers inhibit this response and mask the signs.

58. b. the amount of glycogen reserves in the liver—Glucagon increases the sugar level in the blood by breaking down glycogen in the liver.

59. b. glucagon—Insulin and glucagon are both produced in the pancreas. Glucagon increases the sugar level in the blood by breaking down glycogen in the liver.

60. d. permanent nerve damage.—Parts of the body most affected by complications of diabetes are the nerves, (neuropathy) eyes, kidneys, blood vessels, heart, gums, and feet.

61. a. moon face—The other findings are associated with other endocrine disorders or emergencies.

62. a. typical findings—Excess growth of body hair is another classic finding.

63. b. DKA—When ketones dissolve in the blood, they form ketoacids. If the level of ketones is high enough, the patient is not only ketotic but develops an acidosis. The combination is called ketoacidosis.

64. c. pancreas—The pancreas produces the hormones insulin and glucagon, as well as hormones that aid in digestion.

65. d. pituitary—Also called vasopressin, it increases blood pressure and exerts an antidiuretic effect.

Chapter 25: Allergies and Immunology

1. c. immune response.—An immune response is a bodily response occurring when a foreign substance tries to invade the body.

2. c. allergic reaction—Damage to the tissue includes swelling and cell wall breakdown.

3. a. basophils and mast cells.—The reaction causes the release of histamines, leukotrienes, and other mediators.

4. b. angioneurotic edema.—This may occur as a result of anaphylaxis or other types of reactions (e.g., cold or drugs).

5. d. blood products.—The other examples are common allergens.

6. c. bradycardia.—A person experiencing symptoms of a severe allergic reaction would show signs of compensating shock.

7. a. skin.—The skin may have urticaria (hives) and signs of shock (pale, diaphoretic, clammy, etc.). Additional signs not so visible include itching, cramping, and nausea.

8. d. 0.3; 0.15—The epinephrine auto-injector is prescribed to patients with known allergic reactions for emergency use and may be used by trained EMS providers with permission from medical direction.

9. b. antihistamine—Benadryl® is routinely administered to counteract the effects of histamine release.

10. c. latex sap is chemically related to these fruits and vegetables.—This results in a "cross-reactivity" of antigens to IgE.

11. d. When peripheral circulation is so poor, SQ injections will be ineffective.—The peripheral circulation shuts down as shock progresses. SQ injections will not be effective in this condition, and obtaining IV access becomes more difficult as well.

12. c. markings of the animal—Distinguishing the type of bite may be difficult at best. A good history describing the markings of the animal is most helpful.

13. c. administer nebulized albuterol—The patient's vital signs are relatively stable and bronchodilator medications such as albuterol (Ventolin), ipratropium (Atrovent), and orlevalbuterol (Xopenex) are appropriate to treat wheezing.

14. a. slow histamine release.—Solu Medrol or hydrocortisone may be helpful over the first few hours following a reaction.

15. c. Cortisol—Cortisol is the natural hormone that corticosteroids mimic.

16. a. transferred from breast milk.—This is one of many reasons why experts favor breast-feeding.

17. c. competes with histamine at the receptor sites, blocking the effects of histamine.—Benadryl® is routinely administered to counteract the effects of histamine release.

18. d. anaphylaxis is a severe, whole body allergic reaction.—Anaphylaxis produces many symptoms because of all the body systems that are affected.

19. b. bronchospasm—Epinephrine is the main treatment as a bronchodilator.

20. b. increase dilation of the capillaries.—Histamine release also causes contraction of smooth muscle and stimulation of gastric acid secretion.

21. a. the airway.—Not all of the following signs and symptoms are present in every case; however, the patient may develop hoarseness, stridor, pharyngeal edema, or pharyngeal spasm in the upper airway and hypoventilation; labored accessory muscle use; abnormal retractions; prolonged expirations; wheezes; and diminished lung sounds in the lower airways.

22. c. SC epinephrine 0.01 mg/kg (1:1,000).—The pediatric dose of epinephrine for an allergic reaction is 0.01 mg/kg of 1:1,000.

23. c. epinephrine—Epinephrine is the primary treatment as a bronchodilator.

24. a. degree of sensitivity.—The severity of the reaction varies significantly from patient to patient and exposure to exposure.

25. b. Adjust the pump to stop the flow of antibiotic.—Stop the infusion of the suspected cause of the allergic reaction first! Follow local protocol.

26. b. repeat epi and give fluid boluses—All patients with any type of acute anaphylactic reaction need to be treated with epinephrine. Fluids are needed to treat for shock.

27. b. Administration of a vasopressor drip.—Vasopressors, such as Dopamine, may be helpful for hypotension not responsive to fluids alone.

28. a. blood vessels dilate and become permeable.—As a result of the vascular dilation, plasma escapes into the tissues, causing urticaria and angioedema.

29. d. Antihistamines block H_1 receptors in blood vessels.—Antihistamines do not block all of the released mediators, only histamine. Therefore, treating an anaphylactic reaction with antihistamines alone is potentially fatal.

30. c. renal and mesentery artery vasodilation—Low dosages cause renal and mesenteric vasodilation and should be avoided.

Chapter 26: Abdominal, Gastrointestinal, Genitourinary, and Renal

1. c. referred.—Referred pain is pain that originates in one area but is sensed in another area.

2. b. Somatic—An example of somatic pain is the sharply localized lower-right quadrant pain of the later phase of appendicitis.

3. a. Visceral—This type of pain is typically described as crampy, gaseous, and often intermittent.

4. b. gallbladder—There are several characteristic patterns of referred pain. Biliary pain commonly radiates around the right side to the back and angle of the scapula.

5. a. pelvic inflammatory disease (PID), diverticulitis, and ovarian cyst.—These conditions are associated with pain in both the right- and left-lower quadrants.

6. c. ruptured aneurysm.—Some patients will experience numbness in the lower extremities or a syncopal event with the rupture of an abdominal aortic aneurysm.

7. d. swallowed blood from epistaxis—The most common "false alarm" in GI bleeding calls is swallowed blood from a nosebleed that is subsequently vomited back up.

8. d. esophageal varices—The other conditions are causes of lower GI bleeding.

9. b. diverticulosis—The other conditions are causes of upper GI bleeding.

10. b. renal colic.—The pain from kidney stones is excruciating even for those with a high pain threshold.

11. a. It appeared tarry and black.—Melena is tarry, sticky black stool and may indicate upper GI bleeding or the ingestion of iron or bismuth preparations, such as antacids.

12. b. treatment for shock.—Administer fluids per your local protocol.

13. b. Cholecystitis—An inflammation of the gallbladder.

14. d. acute hepatitis—Acute hepatitis refers to an inflammation of the liver for any reason. Often jaundice and upper-right quadrant tenderness are present.

15. b. is not cancerous.—BPH can lead to serious problems when the prostates enlarges to the point of being unable to urinate and UTI is a common problem. BPH is not cancerous, but a patient can have both.

16. d. reflux esophagitis—This condition may range from asymptomatic to severe chest pain, or any degree of symptoms in between. Even if a patient has a history of heartburn, assume that chest pain is due to myocardial ischemia until proven otherwise.

17. b. history—Sudden, abrupt pain suggests an acute perforation, strangulation, torsion, or vascular accident. Inflammatory lesions and obstructive phenomena are slower in their development.

18. a. appendicitis—Typically, the pain gradually increases with appendicitis, whereas the other conditions present with acute pain.

19. a. cholecystitis—Ingestion of fatty foods may precipitate an attack of acute cholecystitis.

20. c. peritoneal inflammation—Somatic pain is caused by a stimulation of nerve fibers in the parietal peritoneum due to chemical or bacterial infection. The patient usually lies quietly with the thighs flexed to relax the peritoneum.

21. c. absence of sounds—Realistically, in the out-of-hospital setting, it is difficult to differentiate specific conditions by the presence of bowel sounds. More helpful is the total absence of bowel sounds in all four quadrants.

22. d. peritoneal irritation.—Any maneuver that jars the inflamed peritoneal cavity should result in rebound tenderness. This includes: the direct release of palpation pressure, moving the stretcher quickly, and percussion of the soles of the feet.

23. c. inguinal hernia—This type of hernia is common and occurs in males more than females. It can appear as a bulge in the groin and may go all the way down into the scrotum.

24. c. lactose intolerance.—Lactose intolerance is probably the most common GI abnormality worldwide. Some studies suggest that it affects more than half of the world's population.

25. d. irritable bowel syndrome.—Also called "spastic colon," IBS is often associated with emotional stress.

26. b. ascites.—An accumulation of serous fluid in the spaces between the tissues and organs in the abdominal cavity.

27. b. the release of digestive enzymes often worsens the condition.—Food causes the release of digestive enzymes that often worsen most abdominal conditions.

28. d. Dialysis—The most common emergency from peritoneal dialysis is an acute infection of the peritoneum.

29. c. oxygen as tolerated, IV fluids, IV Zofran, and morphine—Until the patient's nausea passes, oxygen by cannula is appropriate. The patient needs fluids, pain relief, and an antiemetic.

30. a. appendicitis—The "classic" presentation of appendicitis is periumbilical crampy pain that then localizes in the lower-right quadrant. Nearly all persons with acute appendicitis have anorexia.

31. a. avoiding taking a BP in any extremity with a fistula.—Another special consideration for the dialysis patient is to avoid the dialysis vascular access site for drawing blood or giving IV fluids.

32. b. urinary tract infection (UTI)—Clinically, a UTI is diagnosed on the symptoms described. Next to respiratory infections, uncomplicated UTIs are the most common problem encountered in EDs.

33. b. ectopic pregnancy—Acute urinary retention may be the initial presenting symptom of ectopic pregnancy.

34. a. torsion of the testicle—Testicular torsion is an acute urological emergency that threatens the male's future reproductive capabilities. The condition is usually unilateral, although cases of bilateral torsion have been reported.

35. a. cirrhosis—Cirrhosis is the condition; alcoholism and hepatitis are the causes of the condition.

36. a. to maintain proper balance between water and salts in the blood.—The renin–angiotensin–aldosterone mechanism is responsible for the kidneys' regulation of sodium, potassium, and water in the body.

37. c. oxygen and morphine—The administration of nitrates within 24 hours of a patient taking Viagra® may result in patient death. Morphine is far safer in treating acute pulmonary edema or suspected myocardial ischemia under these circumstances.

38. b. chlamydia.—Women are commonly asymptomatic, whereas men often have urethral burning, especially during urination, and a discharge.

39. b. pain management.—The pain from kidney stones is excruciating even for those with a high pain threshold.

40. b. Epididymitis—Males of any age can develop this condition, which presents with pain and swelling. It is typically caused by STD or bacterial infection from the urethra or bladder.

41. d. Bright red blood can occur with bleeding in the lower or upper GI tract.—Bright red discoloration of stool may be due to vegetables in the diet. The most immediate concern is GI bleeding.

42. a. Referred—There are several characteristic patterns of referred pain. For example, blood or pus under the diaphragm presents as aching pain in the top of the shoulder.

43. a. upper—A lower GI bleed involves bleeding located more distally to the duodenojejunal junction.

44. b. bright red blood in the stool—Hematochezia may be seen with upper GI bleeding and acute transit, or left colon, or sigmoid colon bleeding.

45. b. Pancreatitis—The primary symptom of pancreatitis is pain, which can radiate to the left shoulder blade. The patient may also have signs of shock (e.g., tachycardia, hypotension, tachypnea).

46. b. small piece of stool.—As the obstructed appendix distends, its blood supply is cut off.

47. b. bile flow.—Blockages are typically caused by gallstones. These are particles of variable size that block the lumen, interfering with bile flow.

48. c. Colitis—The most common causes of colitis are: infections, inflammatory disease, and sexually transmitted disease.

49. d. varices.—Alcoholic varices are secondary to cirrhosis caused by alcohol ingestion. Nonalcoholic cirrhosis and varices are four times as likely to bleed from varices as from peptic ulcer.

50. b. hemorrhoids.—Hemorrhoids are a common cause of lower GI bleeding and are rarely hemodynamically significant.

Chapter 27: Toxicology

1. a. the patient's home.—Over 80% of exposures occur in the home.
2. c. 35 to 44—Over 50% of poisoning fatalities occurred in 20- to 49-year-old individuals.
3. b. unattended children—Failure to supervise children properly and childproof the home are major reasons that children are at high risk for toxic exposures, especially ingestion.
4. c. the development of pulmonary edema.—Inhaled irritant gases cause pulmonary edema and severe hypoxia.
5. a. insect stinger—Needles and insect stingers may inject toxic poisons.
6. b. absorption.—Pesticides and agricultural chemicals are often absorbed this way.
7. a. the type of poison.—Some poisons affect the central nervous system, whereas others affect the peripheral and autonomic nervous systems.
8. d. sea urchin—Other sea creatures that can sting include: Portuguese man-of-war, lionfish, and jellyfish.
9. a. salivation and nausea—Nerve agents produce SLUDGEM: salivation, lacrimation, urination, defecation, GI upset, emesis, and miosis.
10. a. Toxidromes—They are useful for remembering the assessment and management of toxicological emergencies.
11. d. aspirin—Normally an antipyretic, toxic doses cause metabolic acidosis and hyperthermia.
12. b. bradycardia.—Other drugs that cause bradycardia include: beta-blockers, pesticides, clonidine, calcium channel blockers, local anesthetics, and cholinergic agents.
13. c. Anticholinergics—Mydriasis is also caused by sympathomimetics, mushrooms, and substance withdrawal.
14. d. constricted.—Narcotics and opiates cause miosis.
15. b. Botulism—Symptoms include: headache, blurred vision, and respiratory paralysis.
16. c. tricyclic antidepressants and mushrooms.—Antihistamines, anti-diarrheals, over-the-counter cold remedies, and antipsychotics are all anticholinergics.
17. b. narcotics—Opiates also cause these assessment findings.
18. a. sympathomimetics—These include: amphetamines, over-the-counter diet pills, caffeine, and cocaine.
19. c. ingestion—Deliberate ingestions often consist of more than one substance. This often results in a potentially complex variety of signs and symptoms.
20. c. ensure your own safety first.—Assure the safety of yourself and crew before attempting to care for others.
21. a. poisoning involves exposure to a substance that is generally harmful and has no beneficial effects.—Overdose suggests excessive exposure to a substance that has normal treatment uses, but taken in excess results in harm.
22. c. aspirin.—Gastric dialysis and the induction of vomiting is appropriate treatment for many substances in the ED. Follow your local protocols.
23. c. has a decreased mental status.—An altered mental status may cause aspiration.
24. a. strychnine—Other substances to avoid inducing vomiting include ingested corrosives, petroleum products, and drugs that may cause a sudden altered mental status.
25. a. activated charcoal.—Gastric dialysis is effective for many common household substances and drugs, such as phenobarbital, theophylline, tricyclic antidepressants, salicylates, and iron.
26. c. consider administering activated charcoal—Activated charcoal has been shown to absorb many different ingested toxins from the stomach.
27. a. hypoxia.—Systemic toxins such as carbon monoxide often result in severe hypoxia, shock, and death.
28. d. carbon monoxide exposure.—There are many poisonous gases to consider exposure to, following a fire (e.g., cyanide, chlorine).
29. a. seizures—Additional assessment findings associated with theophylline toxicity include: nausea, vomiting, altered mental status, and cardiac dysrhythmias.
30. a. blood thinners.—When obtaining a history from a patient, be sure to ask about the use of vitamins and herbal supplements.
31. c. diuretics.—The most common cause of digitalis toxicity is potassium depletion, which can occur with diuretic therapy.
32. d. sedative hypnotics—The risk varies by the specific drug.
33. c. Monitor her ABCs and administer oxygen.—Manage the airway, breathing, and circulation. Specific antidotes are available only for a few agents.
34. b. The substance is absorbed at the alveolar level, leading to systemic toxicity.—This is the case with carbon monoxide poisoning where the gas competes for receptor sites on the hemoglobin molecules at a rate 200 times greater than oxygen.
35. c. reversal of the respiratory depression—Narcan is administered to reverse the effects of narcotics (e.g., respiratory depression).
36. a. seizure control—The clinical use for benzodiazepines is for seizures and anxiety disorders. They depress sensory cortex, motor activity, and produce sedation and drowsiness.
37. b. atropine—Most herbicides and pesticides are nerve agents.
38. c. He had an excessive exposure to insecticides.—Most herbicides and pesticides are nerve agents.

39. b. tolerance.—When a person develops a tolerance to a substance, more and more of the substance is required to achieve the same effect. That person may accidentally take too much and develop toxicity.
40. c. dependence.—Drug dependence is a psychological problem, not a physical one.
41. a. smuggling from Colombia—Many illegal drugs are smuggled into the United States from Central and South American countries such as Colombia.
42. c. liver and kidney failure.—Long-term use of NSAIDs can produce bleeding, ulcers, heart attack, stroke, and liver and kidney failure.
43. b. tricyclic antidepressants.—These drugs block the reuptake of serotonin and norepinephrine.
44. b. alcohol.—Alcohol (ethanol) overdose decreases inhibitions, causes visual impairment, muscular incoordination, slowed reaction time, slurred speech, ataxia, hypothermia, hypoventilation, and hypotension.

45. d. tricyclic antidepressants—Beware of delayed toxicity. The patient may not appear ill at first, but then can deteriorate rapidly affecting mostly the brain and heart.
46. a. huffing.—Found in solvents and manufacturing hydrocarbons, these are highly volatile.
47. a. iron—An overdose of iron is serious and results in an initial critical state, followed by an apparent recovery phase, a relapse into metabolic acidosis, and organ failure.
48. c. a hyperbaric chamber.—Hyperbaric therapy helps to rid hemoglobin of carbon dioxide so that oxygen can bind normally.
49. c. rebound hypertension—Withdrawal syndromes can result from the sudden stoppage of several prescription medications that are not considered addictive by most criteria.
50. b. lead poisoning—The toxidrome of symptoms describe lead poisoning.

Chapter 28: Infectious Diseases

1. b. pathogen.—Bacteria that cause disease are called pathogens.
2. a. normal flora.—Normal flora is found over the entire body and on the protective coverings of the respiratory, GI, and genitourinary systems.
3. b. protozoa.—Protozoa can be found in almost every kind of habitat.
4. d. virus.—Viruses are known to cause infectious diseases.
5. c. mucous membranes.—The mouth, nares, or rectum.
6. c. are more likely to die of the infection.—Antibiotics are also known as antimicrobial drugs. Improved use of these mediations causes bacteria to be resistant. When a person is infected with antimicrobial organisms, they are going to have longer and more expensive hospital stays and increased chance of dying from the infection.
7. c. skin—The external barriers on the body are skin and normal flora.
8. b. latency—Once a host is infected, the first stage is the latency period. The duration of this stage varies by specific disease.
9. b. incubation—This is the third stage, and its duration varies by specific disease.
10. d. disease—The duration of a disease period varies by specific disease.
11. b. hospital—Health care facilities are also responsible for reporting communicable diseases seen by health care providers.
12. c. 48—Notification is made by a designated officer who acts as a liaison between the hospital and exposed EMS provider.

13. a. Federal—Other federal agencies involved in disease outbreaks include the U.S. Department of Health and Human Services, Centers for Disease Control (CDC), National Institute for Occupational Safety and Health (NIOSH), and the U.S. Department of Defense.
14. c. direct skin to skin contact.—Staph bacteria is carried on the skin and in the nose. The primary mode of transmission is through direct skin to skin contact, such as throughcuts, scrapes, and openings in dry skin.
15. a. HBV, HCV, and HIV—Pneumonia and URI are not caused by needle sticks.
16. d. hand washing.—This is still the best protection against the spread of disease.
17. c. No further titers are necessary, even after an exposure.—The whole point of the postvaccination titer is to make sure the series of shots had its desired effect of protection against HBV. If there is no response to the first series, a second series is administered. If there is no response to the second series, no further series are recommended.
18. a. rodents.—People can become infected with hantavirus through contact with infected rodents, their urine, or droppings.
19. c. hepatitis—More than 700,000 new infections occur annually, making this the most serious infectious disease in the United States.
20. c. seven—This infectious disease causes inflammation of the liver, which interferes with liver functions. There used to be seven types (A–G), but F was discredited. Only the first four are common in the United States.

21. c. complete only the third dose—This is the current recommendation.
22. a. sexual contact.—HCV may also be contracted through blood transfusions.
23. b. HCV—No vaccine or prophylactic post-exposure treatment for HCV is available currently.
24. b. oral–fecal—It is spread by direct contact with feces, usually through food or water contact by an infected person who has not washed after using the toilet.
25. a. productive cough—TB spreads through droplets from coughing and sneezing. The bacteria are inhaled and settle in the lungs. From the lungs, it is transported in the blood to other organs in the body.
26. b. rabies—An acute viral infection of the CNS.
27. d. bacteria—*Helicobacter pylori*, or *H. pylori*, is the cause of most gastric ulcers.
28. b. rabies.—Without intervention, the disease progresses rapidly and death results.
29. a. *Salmonella*—*Salmonella* are gram-negative bacteria that live in the intestinal tracts of humans and other animals. Food may also become contaminated by an infected person who has not washed his hands after using the toilet.
30. a. *salmonella*—Over 1,400 species of *salmonella* can cause mild gastroenteritis or severe and often fatal food poisoning.
31. b. respiratory and renal failure.—Serious complications of hantivirus are kidney, heart, and lung failure.
32. c. Lyme disease—Further progression of the infection leads to altered mental status, paralysis, paresthesia, stiff neck, sensitivity to light, dysrhythmias, and chest pain.
33. b. meningitis—A history of recent respiratory illness or sore throat often precedes symptoms of fever, headache, vomiting, and the classic stiff neck. Changes in mental status follow, and dehydration may lead to shock. The finding of a stiff neck was not given in the case, due to the altered mental status.
34. b. an inflammatory response.—Internal barriers work through the inflammatory and immune responses.
35. b. designated officer.—The Ryan White Act of 1990 requires that all EMS providers be notified by the hospital or health care facility if they have been exposed to infectious diseases. Notification is made by a designated officer who acts as a liaison between the hospital and exposed EMS provider.

36. d. the skin, joints, nervous system, and heart.—Lyme disease can affect different body systems. If detected early Lyme disease can be cured with antibiotics. If detected late, symptoms are treatable.
37. b. Varicella—Chicken pox vaccination.
38. a. Standard precautions—The concept is to wear gloves for all patient contact.
39. d. staph—This is why hand washing is still the best preventative measure for spreading disease.
40. c. red—The exact guidelines for decontamination and disposal of contaminated equipment should be posted or easily available for reference in every EMS agency.
41. b. puncture-proof containers—The exact guidelines for decontamination and disposal of contaminated equipment should be posted or easily available for reference in every EMS agency.
42. b. shingles—Herpes zoster, or shingles, is caused by a varicella-zoster virus, the same virus that causes chicken pox. Pain and inflammation occur on unilateral nerve tracts and may follow the path of one or more adjacent dermatomes.
43. b. titer—Titers are used to determine if adequate immunity has been achieved through immunization.
44. c. employer—The exact guidelines to follow for an exposure should be posted or easily available for reference in every EMS agency.
45. d. tuberculosis—One reason why TB is making a comeback is that more resistant strains are developing. Estimates are that nearly eight million new cases occur each year, with only one in five getting treatment.
46. c. Gastroenteritis—This condition usually is not serious in healthy individuals. Children, the elderly, and patients with chronic illness can develop complications, such as dehydration.
47. b. arbovirus—Arbovirus is a group of viruses that is transmitted to humans by mosquitoes and ticks.
48. c. Lyme disease—Signs and symptoms begin with an expanding rash around the area of the bite. Flu-like symptoms and muscle joint aches follow, with or without a rash.
49. a. pneumonic.—Plague is an acute febrile, infectious, and highly fatal disease caused by gram-positive bacteria.
50. b. Colorado.—Bubonic plague is the most prevalent type and is a primary disease found in rats and rodents.

Chapter 29: Psychiatric

1. b. emotion—A psychic and physical reaction subjectively experienced as strong feelings and physiological changes.
2. b. mental disorder.—Also called emotional disorder.

3. a. In the United States, behavioral and psychiatric disorders incapacitate more people than all other health problems combined.—Some researchers indicate that one in seven people will require

treatment for an emotional illness at some time in his or her life.

4. c. Having a mental disorder is cause for embarrassment and shame.—Though some people still feel this way, it is a result of inappropriate pressure from society rather than any scientific evidence.

5. d. lose control and become aggressive.—Impulse-control disorders involve an abnormal inability to resist a sudden and often irrational urge or action.

6. a. cognitive—Cognitive disorders affect a person's thinking and judgment.

7. b. Schizophrenia—These individuals suffer from delusions and hallucinations. They are often withdrawn from interaction with society and display disorganized thought.

8. d. bipolar.—Mood disorders include depression and mania. When these moods alternate, it is called a bipolar disorder.

9. c. anxiety—The common theme with anxiety disorders is that apprehension, fears, and worries dominate a person's life.

10. a. psychologic—Dependence is a psychological problem, not a physical one.

11. b. Somatoform—The major types of somatoform disorders are somatization syndrome and conversion disorders.

12. a. dissociative—Also called multiple personality or schizophrenia. The result is an altered state of consciousness or confusion in the patient's identity.

13. c. Personality—This large group of disorders is often broken down into three clusters: cluster A (paranoid, schizoid, schizotypal), cluster B (antisocial, borderline, histrionic, narcissistic), and cluster C (avoidant, dependent, obsessive-compulsive).

14. d. spending more time with the patient than other types of calls.—Rapid intervention is often necessary for a behavioral emergency, but intervention does not always mean rapid transport. Unless the patient is also experiencing a medical emergency that requires rapid transport, the paramedic should be prepared to spend extra time with the patient to avoid further agitation.

15. c. crisis intervention.—Each state, and sometimes locality, has specific regulations governing the handling of mentally ill individuals, including patients who exhibit self-destructive behavior.

16. b. state laws—Each state, and sometimes locality, has specific regulations governing the handling of mentally ill individuals, including patients who exhibit self-destructive behavior.

17. c. neurotransmitters.—Sometimes the cause of the disorder is an organic illness. Either an excess or, more commonly, a deficit of certain neurotransmitters results in some types of behavioral and psychiatric disorders.

18. d. migraine headaches.—One example is the use of antidepressants for treating migraine headaches.

19. a. pain.—Be alert for other possible causes of apparent emotional or psychiatric illnesses, especially in older patients. The most common "offenders" are medications and severe infections.

20. a. poor hygiene.—Some people with behavioral problems exhibit an abnormal lack of regard for their own personal hygiene.

21. d. Phobias—These fears can interfere with normal daily activities, affecting both personal and societal relationships.

22. b. when the patient exhibits a danger to others—The patient must be transported in any situation where the patient is a danger to himself or to others.

23. a. hypoxia—Anything that causes altered mental status should be considered as a possible cause of behavioral or psychiatric emergency.

24. b. delirium.—Delirium tremens is a violent delirium with tremors that is induced by excessive and prolonged use of alcohol.

25. d. Assuming the patient's actions were not an actual suicide attempt.—A common clinical myth is that people who engage in suicide gestures never really attempt suicide. This is a naïve and potentially deadly assumption.

26. d. suicide gesture—The person performs the act in a potentially reversible way, such as taking a small amount of pills.

27. c. to avoid accusations of sexual misconduct.—Sometimes emotionally disturbed patients (EDP) will accuse EMS personnel of sexual misconduct and this can help to reduce the risk of such an accusation.

28. a. Psychosis—The person truly believes his situation or condition is real. Often the psychotic person hears voices.

29. b. the "talk-down" technique.—This is done by gently and calmly talking to the person and reassuring him that everything is OK.

30. d. there are enough personnel to do the job.—Always follow local protocols on this procedure.

31. c. medication.—Be alert for other possible causes of apparent emotional or psychiatric illnesses, especially in older patients. The most common "offenders" are medications and severe infections.

32. d. mood—Mood disorders include depression, mania, and bipolar.

33. c. Addiction—A true addiction is a psychological and physical craving for the drug, as well as for the effect.

34. b. Intoxication—An abnormal state that is essentially a poisoning.

35. c. addiction—Addiction is a condition characterized by an overwhelming desire to continue taking a drug to which one has become "hooked."

36. b. worsens.—There is often an interrelationship between people with psychiatric disorders and substance abuse. In some cases, there is a direct cause–effect relationship. In other cases, the link is more anecdotal or based on stories of prior incidents.

37. d. posture.—For example, a paranoid individual may posture by keeping the face hidden and the extremities crossed close to the body.

38. c. confusion—Confusion results in bewilderment and the inability to act decisively.

39. c. affect—For example, a flat affect means a lack of any apparent verbal or body language expression of emotion.

40. d. engage in active listening—Other positive interview techniques include: engaging in active listening, being supportive and empathetic, limiting interruptions, allowing the patient to express anger and frustration verbally, forming an alliance with the patient, and avoiding continuous eye contact.

41. b. attempt to build a good rapport with the patient.— Attempt to do this by using positive therapeutic interviewing techniques that calm the patient and encourage him to cooperate with you.

42. c. keep talking to the patient—Continue to attempt to calm and reassure the patient and encourage him to cooperate with you.

43. c. Haldol and Versed.—Haloperidol (Haldol) and/or midazolam (Versed) either IM or IV are safe and effective chemical restraints for the violent and severely agitated patient.

44. b. women have better support systems.—Support systems (family, friends) are an integral part of a person's coping mechanism.

45. c. psychosomatic illness—The physical ailments are very real, despite the patient's emotional origin.

46. c. may develop violent behavior.—The aspects of domestic violence, pacing back and forth, and bragging about how tough she is are clues that a patient may develop violent behavior.

47. b. People with neurosis are not crazy.—Neurosis is a mental and emotional disorder that affects only part of the person's personality.

48. a. severely depressed.—Depression may present as another disease.

49. d. Phobias can interfere with daily living activities.—These fears are out of proportion to reality and compel the patient to avoid the feared object or situation.

50. a. They are used to encourage better patient responses.—These types of questions are used to allow the patient to express herself.

Chapter 30: Hematology

1. c. hematopoietic—The formation of blood or blood cells in the living body.

2. b. bone marrow.—The liver, spleen, and bone marrow make up the components of the hematopoietic system.

3. d. bone marrow.—The majority of blood cells are formed in the bone marrow.

4. c. 7.40—The average pH is slightly lower in venous than in arterial blood.

5. b. 70—In an adult man, this amount equals approximately five or six liters of blood. Women have slightly less, 65 cc per kg.

6. d. spleen.—The liver and the spleen produce red blood cells (RBCs) during fetal life. After birth, the majority of normal blood cell production occurs in the bone marrow in the long and flat bones.

7. b. stem cell.—All blood cells are derived from one common stem cell. This cell is capable of reproducing itself, but is also capable of differentiating into any of the marrow elements.

8. c. 120—After that, they are absorbed by tissues of the spleen.

9. a. bilirubin.—Cellular components are recycled and hemoglobin byproducts are excreted as bilirubin.

10. c. hematocrit.—Normal hematocrit (Hct) levels indicate a normal number of RBCs; a high Hct meant too many RBCs (polycythemia), and a low Hct level means too few (anemia).

11. d. anemia.—A high Hct meant too many RBCs (polycythemia), and a low Hct level means too few (anemia).

12. a. 36–46.—The normal range for men is slightly higher: 41–53.

13. c. 41–53.—The normal range for women is slightly lower: 36–46.

14. b. granulocytes.—Granulocytes are one of two types of white blood cells (WBCs).

15. b. monocytes.—Monocytes are one of two types of WBCs.

16. c. maintain host defenses against infection.— Leukocytes defend against infections, particularly bacterial infection.

17. c. kidneys and liver; bone marrow—Body feedback systems continuously monitor intravascular volume, as well as the numbers of circulating platelets and red and white blood cells. If more are needed, the kidneys and liver produce compounds that stimulate the bone marrow to manufacture additional cells.

18. a. humoral immunity.—Humoral immunity primarily involves antibodies that are produced by a specialized WBC, the B lymphocyte.

19. a. leukopenia.—This condition may result from congenital problems, acquired anemia, leukemia, viral infection, drug reaction, immunosuppression, destruction of WBCs in the peripheral blood, and pooling of WBCs.

20. b. 7–10—Platelets are formed from stem cells in the bone marrow and they are removed by the spleen.

21. c. anti-inflammatory drugs.—Many anti-inflammatory drugs and some herbals decrease the aggregation of platelets. Though this may have a beneficial effect (e.g., stoke and MI), these drugs may also result in a bleeding tendency.

22. c. Blood vessels dilate and develop increased permeability.—This response increases blood flow, producing the signs of heat and redness.

23. c. fibrin.—Intrinsic and extrinsic clotting systems are the chemical reactions that lead to the formation of fibrin. This substance completes the blood clot, which now consists of injured vascular epithelium, a platelet plug, and intertwined strands of clot formation.

24. b. red blood—Blood groups are classified into four types: type A, B, AB, and O.

25. b. acute hemolytic reaction—This type of reaction happens with blood type incompatibility. The severity of the reaction often depends on the amount of blood given. The transfusion must be stopped immediately.

26. b. stop the blood transfusion—An incompatibility reaction is very serious and accounts for over 50 percent of reported deaths related to transfusions.

27. d. O—Their blood may be given safely to people with any ABO blood type.

28. b. sickle cell crisis—All conditions may produce dyspnea. The severe abdominal pain is more specific to sickle cell crisis.

29. c. hemophilia.—A hereditary deficiency of clotting factors VIII resulting in excessive bleeding after minor wounds, insignificant trauma, and spontaneous bleeding into joints, abdomen, or central nervous system.

30. d. Leukemia—This type of cancer results in the rapid and uncontrolled proliferation of abnormal numbers and forms of leukocytes.

31. a. Fibrinolysis—Small injuries often lead to the activation of the clotting cascade. To prevent these small clots from developing into clinically significant thrombi, plasminogen is activated to form plasmin. Plasmin lyses the clots, returning things to a hemostatic baseline.

32. b. leukocytosis—A condition that results in too many WBCs.

33. c. eosinophils and basophils—Two types of granulocytes (WBCs) are important in allergic reactions.

34. b. hemoglobin.—The Hct and hemoglobin (Hb) are direct reflections of the number of RBCs. Each normal RBC contains the same amount of Hb. Thus, if we have a normal number of RBCs, the Hb concentration is normal.

35. b. Thrombocythemia—The platelets do not function properly and may form clots. The clots can form anywhere, but are mostly formed in the brain, hands, and feet.

Chapter 31: Gynecology

1. b. urethra—The urethra is part of the genitourinary tract.

2. a. ovaries—The ovaries produce sexual hormones and oocytes, the precursors to mature eggs.

3. c. Fertilization of the ovum usually occurs in one of the fallopian tubes.

4. a. fundus.—The main portion of the uterus is called the fundus.

5. c. endometriosis.—The relocated cells respond to the same hormonal stimuli as the normal cells. Symptoms include abdominal pain, pelvic pain, lower back pain, dysuria, irregular menses, and infertility.

6. a. the secretory phase.—This phase begins at the time of ovulation and lasts until the corpus luteum breaks down (about 12 days after ovulation).

7. d. Premenstrual dysphoric disorder—Formerly called premenstrual tension syndrome or PMS, the cause is not clear at this time.

8. d. aimed at relieving the symptoms.—The cause of premenstrual dysphoric disorder is not clear, so the treatment is aimed at relieving the symptoms. Analgesia, mild diuretics, and mood-lifting medications may be taken to relieve the symptoms.

9. a. estrogen—Estrogen also induces the development of female sexual characteristics.

10. b. progesterone.—Progesterone also helps to prevent rejection of the developing embryo or fetus.

11. d. PID—Pelvic inflammatory disease is an infection in the female reproductive and surrounding organs that can lead to complications such as sepsis and infertility.

12. d. chlamydia—Chlamydia infections remain the most common of all bacterial STDs occurring in both men and women.

13. c. urinary tract infection—UTIs may produce blood in the urine (hematuria).

14. b. bladder—The symptoms are urinary frequency and pain with urinations. The condition can be acute or chronic.

15. b. STDs—The other injuries are considered primary injuries from a sexual assault.

16. a. Place any items removed from the patient into separate bags.—Handle the clothing as little as possible, and bag each item separately. Avoid using plastic bags for blood-stained articles because they degrade the evidence with moisture.

17. b. providing emotional support.—The paramedic must treat the whole patient and respond to her physical and emotional needs.
18. a. one in three—It is also estimated that only 10–30% of these crimes are reported.
19. b. Menopause—In most women, menopause occurs in the late forties.
20. d. ruptured ovarian cyst—The other examples involve different body systems.
21. d. Mittelschmerz—The pain is self-limiting and benign. The complication that arises is making a differential diagnosis from other causes of abdominal pain.
22. b. Endomeritis—The infection can originate from an STD, trauma, use of an intrauterine device (IUD), or an abortion.
23. c. shock and death.—Uncontrolled bleeding can lead to hypovolemia, shock, and death.
24. d. too little or too much estrogen.—Other causes of DUB include infection, complications during pregnancy, tumors, or an ovary not releasing an egg during ovulation.
25. b. toilet paper—Other objects include crayons or marker caps. Tampons are a common object found in adolescents. Symptoms include vaginal bleeding and/or a foul discharge and smell.

Chapter 32: Non-Traumatic Musculoskeletal Disorders

1. c. uticaria.—General assessment findings and symptoms of non-traumatic musculoskeletal disorders include swelling, loss of movement, and circulatory changes.
2. b. osteomyelitis.—Your patient has a non-traumatic musculoskeletal disorder, which causes her chronic pain. This is most likely due to osteomyelitis.
3. c. carpal tunnel syndrome.—An overuse syndrome from constantly typing on a keyboard is called carpal tunnel syndrome.
4. a. cauda equina syndrome.—Each of the following (arthritis, gout, and rheumatoid) is a non-traumatic musculoskeletal disorder of the joints. Cauda equina syndrome is a disorder of the spine.
5. c. gangrene.—An example of a non-traumatic musculoskeletal disorder affecting soft tissue would be gangrene.
6. d. bursitis.—When a patient describes pain in his elbow after playing tennis for many hours, this could be due to bursitis.
7. b. gout.—An example of a non-traumatic musculoskeletal disorder that is related to the body's retention of uric acids in the blood, causing inflammation, is called gout.
8. d. kidneys.—The breakdown of muscle fibers from the disease rhabdomyolsis can cause serious damage to the patient's kidneys.
9. a. low-back pain.—The disorder that can be found in workers, such as paramedics, who lift improperly is low-back pain.
10. b. myalgia.—The symptom of muscle pain or aching is most common in myalgia.
11. c. arthritis.—The non-traumatic musculoskeletal disorder which effects the joints is arthritis.
12. b. flexor tenosynovitis.—The inflammation that can affect the tendons of the fingers is called flexor tenosynovitis.
13. d. overuse syndrome.—Peripheral nerve syndrome is an example of an overuse syndrome.
14. c. paronychia.—A skin infection occurring around the nails and cuticle is called paronychia.
15. b. gangrene—Of the following non-traumatic musculoskeletal disorders (gout, gangrene, bursitis, and osteoarthritis), gangrene is the one that involves tissue necrosis.

Chapter 33: Diseases of the Ears, Eyes, Nose, & Throat

1. b. sclera.—The white of the eye is a tough, fibrous coat that helps maintain shape of the eye. It is called the sclera.
2. c. pupil.—The circular adjustable opening within the iris through which light passes to the lens is called the pupil.
3. a. retina.—A delicate, 10-layered structure of nervous tissue that extends from the optic nerve is called the retina.
4. b. anterior chamber; aqueous humor.—The portion of the globe between the lens and the cornea is called the anterior chamber. It is filled with a clear watery fluid called aqueous humor.

5. c. secrete and drain tears from the eyes.—The purpose of the lacrimal system is to secrete and drain tears from the eyes.
6. d. conjunctivae.—The components of the lacrimal apparatus include the: lacrimal ducts, lacrimal sacs, and the lacrimal gland.
7. a. visual cortex of the brain.—The image on the retina is transmitted by the optic nerve to the visual cortex of the brain.
8. b. redness, lacerations, and discoloration.—When examining the eyes, check the globe for redness, lacerations, and discoloration.
9. c. DCAP-BTLS.—The exam for ocular function usually involves peripheral vision, visual acuity, and ocular motility.
10. c. diabetes.—The leading cause of adult blindness is diabetes.
11. b. anisocoria.—When the pupils are not equal in size, this condition is called anisocoria.
12. b. covering eyes with sterile moist pad and eye shield.—A 22-year-old female has sustained a burn to the eye from falling asleep in a tanning booth under UV light without the appropriate glasses on. Her eyes are dry and painful. The prehospital treatment should include covering eyes with sterile moist pad and eye shield.
13. c. tetracaine and Morgan® lens.—Irrigation of an eye which has been exposed to chemicals is best done with tetracaine and Morgan® lens.
14. a. conjunctivitis.—When the eye gets inflamed and looks pink, this is called conjunctivitis.
15. b. retinal detachment.—Serious injury to the eye from blunt trauma, due to a sport like boxing, can cause retinal detachment.

16. b. cochlea.—The inner ear consists of the semicircular canals and cochlea.
17. d. pinna.—Sound waves enter the ear through the pinna.
18. b. meniere's disease.—An inner ear disorder usually affecting middle-aged adults with symptoms of hearing loss, ear pressure, vertigo, and dizziness could be meniere's disease.
19. c. Eustachian tubes.—The pressure in your ears, when going up in an elevator in a high-rise building, is equalized by the eustachian tubes.
20. c. sinusitis.—Your patient is complaining of thick nasal discharge, facial pressure, headache, and fever. This is most likely sinusitis.
21. b. oculomotor nerve.—The oculomotor nerve is not a nerve involved in the nerve supply to the mouth and its structures.
22. d. thrush.—A yeast infection that causes white patches in the mouth or on the tongue is called thrush.
23. a. leukoplakia.—A smoker's disease that causes excess cell growth in the mouth, cheek, or gums and presents as white patches is called leukoplakia.
24. d. peritonsillar abscess.—A collection of infected material in the back of the throat caused by a bacterial infection which can be accompanied by facial swelling and chills is likely a peritonsillar abscess.
25. a. sleep apnea.—Causes of tempromandibular joint (TMJ) disorder include arthritis damage to the joint, injury to jaw, and muscle fatique from grinding or clenching teeth while sleeping.

Chapter 34: Shock & Resuscitation

1. c. three—Also referred to as decompensated shock, this stage of shock involves between 25% and 35% intravascular loss.
2. c. 25–35%—The patient will have the classic signs of hypovolemic shock.
3. b. two large bore IVs en route—Consider the need for IV fluid replacement en route to the hospital. If a patient is continuing to bleed, he can easily lose more blood in the time it takes to start the IV than the IV fluids will actually replace.
4. b. decompensated—When the body's compensatory mechanisms can no longer sustain the patient, decompensated shock will ensue (e.g., tachycardia, tachypnea, decreasing blood pressure, altered mental status, loss of distal pulses, and decreased urine output).
5. c. 70 cc—The stroke volume is the amount of blood ejected from the left ventricle with each contrac-

tion of the heart. This is usually approximately 70 cc of blood per beat, or approximately 4,900 cc per minute.
6. b. increasing the heart rate.—The heart rate can increase to improve the cardiac output (CO), or the systemic vascular resistance (SVR) can be increased through the constriction of the peripheral vessels.
7. b. increase in diastolic pressure—An early sign of hypovolemic shock is a narrowing pulse pressure. The systolic pressure drops slightly (due to volume loss) and the systolic pressure increases (representing vasoconstriction as a compensatory mechanism).
8. c. aerobic exercise on a regular basis—The body cannot increase the stroke volume on a moment's notice by a large amount. In order to increase the SV, you need to do aerobic exercise for more than

20 minutes, three or more times a week, for months. The effect of this type of exercise is the thickening of the left ventricle to increase the SV, making the muscle a more efficient pump.

9. b. vasoconstriction.—The alpha-1 effects of epinephrine cause vasoconstriction, an increase in peripheral vascular resistance, and an increase in afterload from arteriolar constriction.

10. c. positive dromotropic effects—The dromotropic response affects conductivity of the myocardium.

11. c. arginine vasopressin.—AVP, also known as antidiuretic hormone, is released from the anterior pituitary gland and increases free water absorption. It also decreases urine output and visceral vascular constriction.

12. d. angiotensin II.—It is also a positive inotrope (force of contraction) and chronotrope (rate of contraction).

13. b. hyperglycemic.—Insulin secretion is diminished by circulating epinephrine. Poor perfusion impairs the effect of insulin on peripheral tissue, leading to the failure of cells to take up glucose. This contributes to the hypoglycemic states seen following injury and volume loss.

14. c. myocardial blood supply increases.—In addition, there are capillary and cellular changes that ultimately lead to irreversible shock.

15. b. washout—The third of three phases the cells go through during decreased perfusion states. Here the post-capillary sphincter relaxes, causing hydrogen, potassium carbon dioxide, and thrombosed erythrocytes to wash out into the circulation. Metabolic acidosis results, and the CO drops even further.

16. b. vasomotor center failure.—This occurs in the stagnation (second) phase.

17. c. Irreversible—Even aggressive treatment at this stage does not result in a recovery. It is not possible in the out-of-hospital setting to differentiate decompensated shock from irreversible shock, so all patients should be managed aggressively.

18. a. chief complaint of chest pain—Cardiogenic shock is differentiated from hypovolemic shock by one or more of the following: complaint of dyspnea, chest pain, tachycardia, bradycardia, signs of CHF, and dysrhythmias.

19. d. flushed skin—Distributive shock is differentiated from hypovolemic shock by the presence of one or more of the following: warm, flushed skin, absence of tachycardia, and an MOI suggestive of vasodilation such as spinal cord injury, drug overdose, sepsis, or anaphylaxis.

20. b. presence of JVD—Obstructive shock can be differentiated from hypovolemic shock by the presence of distended neck veins and a narrowing pulse pressure, as seen with cardiac tamponade or tension pneumothorax.

21. a. isotonic—Normal saline or Ringer's lactate have the same tonicity (osmolarity) as plasma.

22. b. one-third—Consider the need for IV fluid replacement en route to the hospital. If a patient is continuing to bleed, she can easily lose more blood in the time it takes to start the IV than the IV fluids will actually replace.

23. a. interstitial space—Only about one-third of the infused fluid stays in the intravascular space, and it does not carry hemoglobin like a transfusion of whole blood does.

24. d. They do not carry hemoglobin.—Only about one-third of the infused fluid stays in the intravascular space, and it does not carry hemoglobin like a transfusion of whole blood does.

25. a. compensated—The compensated stage of shock involves 15–25% intravascular loss. The cardiac output is maintained by arteriolar constriction and a reflex tachycardia.

26. b. internal bleeding.—The potential for blood loss from femur fracture is approximately a liter, and intraabdominal bleeding can produce much more.

27. b. aortic arch—They sense a decreased flow and activate the vasomotor center, which, in turn, causes vasoconstriction of the peripheral vessels.

28. c. vasoconstriction of the peripheral vessels.—In addition, the sympathetic nervous system is stimulated.

29. c. adrenal glands.—The sympathetic nervous system sends the message from the brain down the spinal cord to the adrenal glands, which are located on top of the kidneys.

30. a. narrowing pulse pressure—The other events described are not signs that can be measured in the out-of-hospital setting.

31. a. endocrine responses.—These include the release of hormones: growth hormone, renin-angiotensin, glucagon, ACTH, and antidiuretic hormone.

32. b. 2–3—The fluid controversy is ongoing. Because only about one-third of the infused fluid stays in the intravascular space and does not carry hemoglobin, after two or three liters of a volume expander, the patient needs to receive fluid that carries hemoglobin (e.g., blood, blood products, or blood substitutes).

33. c. stabilization of pelvic fractures—Many EMS systems have relegated use of MAST/PASG to the stabilization of pelvic and femur fractures.

34. b. ACEP—The American College of Emergency Physicians still recommends that the MAST/PASG be available for immediate use in hospital EDs.

35. d. loss of vasomotor tone.—Distributive shock can occur with spinal injury, sepsis, and anaphylaxis.

36. c. Aldosterone—Secreted by the cells in the adrenal cortex, aldosterone protects the fluid volume.

37. a. arterioles in the kidney.—It is also a positive inotrope (force of contraction) and chronotrope (rate of contraction).

38. a. electrocution—A pre-morbid condition in an unhealthy patient would include congestive heart failure, renal failure, uncontrolled hypertension,

uncontrolled diabetes, obesity, electrolyte imbalance, drug toxicity, and stroke.

39. c. pulmonary embolus—Cardiac arrest in a healthy 35-year-old male patient is most likely to be caused by pulmonary embolus or ACS.

40. c. The heart is squeezed through direct compression between the sternum and the spinal column.—In respect to the physiology of blood flow during CPR, the heart pump theory states that the heart is squeezed through direct compression between sternum and spinal column.

41. c. high-quality chest compressions with a minimum of interruptions.—Of the steps in a resuscitation, high-quality chest compression with a minimum of interruptions has been proven to be the most effective technique.

42. c. epinephrine—Your 35-year-old male patient has been in cardiac arrest for about 10 minutes and CPR was started within the first few minutes of the arrest by a citizen. Your first consideration once venous access is acquired should be epinephrine.

43. a. defibrillating VF.—After the first 2 minutes of high-quality CPR, your concern in managing the patient who is in cardiac arrest should turn to defibrillating VF.

44. b. There is a return of spontaneous circulation.—You have been running a cardiac arrest on a 45-year-old female for the past 7 minutes when you notice that the ETCO$_2$ is beginning to improve. This is an indication of a return of spontaneous circulation, so you might want to reassess the pulse.

45. a. His electrolytes are abnormal.—His electrolytes are abnormal is least likely, but the other causes listed are considerations since there was significant trauma involved.

Chapter 35: Trauma Overview

1. c. transportation incidents.—From 2009 to 2010, the leading cause of work-related deaths was transportation incidents (39%).

2. a. MVCs, fire arms, and falls.—The top three causes of trauma deaths in all ages are: MVCs, fire arms, and falls

3. b. many MOIs have predictable patterns for specific injuries.—EMS providers are trained to consider the forces that were applied to the body and to look for specific injury patterns, even when the injuries are not visibly apparent.

4. d. Traumatic brain injury (TBI)—Recent estimates are that 1.7 million people annually sustain a TBI and 52,000 die.

5. b. anatomic structures that are involved.—The extent of damage caused by the energy absorbed by the body depends on the specific organs that have been affected.

6. a. convert the severity of an injury into a number.—Trauma scoring systems help clinicians speak a common language. More than 50 scoring systems have been published for the classification of trauma patients in the prehospital, emergency room, and intensive care settings.

7. a. MOI—Early recognition of the MOI and the possible injuries associated with those forces can help save the patient's life.

8. d. to help the paramedic decide whether to bring the patient to a trauma center.—Trauma scoring systems are also used for clinical decision making when the trauma patient has just arrived in the emergency department.

9. c. minimizing scene time when appropriate.—The golden hour is the first hour after the injury occurs. In serious trauma, the best chances of survival for the patient are a result of reaching the hospital's operating suite and having the bleeding controlled within that hour. EMS providers can do their part in helping achieve this goal (surgical intervention in <60 minutes) by limiting scene time to a "platinum ten" minutes. That's 10 minutes for assessment and management at the scene of a critical trauma patient.

10. d. White Paper.—Released in 1966, the White Paper depicted a very poor emergency care system and was credited as the "match that sparked" the future development of modern EMS systems.

11. c. data collection.—Trauma registries are reporting systems designed to collect trauma-related data in an effort to improve the quality and cost effectiveness of care and to aid in outcome research.

12. a. registry—Two software programs produced by the American College of Surgeons (ACS) are National Tracs® and the National Trauma Data Bank™.

13. c. Trauma centers must meet strict criteria to be designated a trauma center.—A trauma center is a hospital that has the capability of caring for the acutely injured patient. Trauma centers must meet strict criteria to use this designation. The criterion delineates the resources, personnel, equipment, and training necessary for an institution to provide quality trauma care.

14. c. traumatic cardiac arrest—These patients have extremely small chances of survival even with

brief periods of return of spontaneous circulation (ROSC). This is why they are transported to the nearest hospital.

15. a. access to a remote area—The other choices listed are contraindications or relative contraindications for air-medical transport.

16. a. traumatic cardiac arrest—These patients have little or no chance of survival from a possible reversal. This is why they are transported to the nearest hospital by ambulance.

17. d. Conservation of energy—This is one of the physical laws of energy. This is an important concept when you consider the MOI and the potential for injuries.

18. c. Newton's first law of motion.—One of the physical laws of energy. This is an important concept when you consider the MOI and the potential for injuries.

19. a. Kinetic energy—One of the physical laws of energy. This is an important concept when you consider the MOI and the potential for injuries.

20. c. Cavitation—Cavitation can be caused by both blunt and penetration trauma.

21. b. velocity—The value of speed (the velocity) is squared in the kinetic energy formula; the value of the mass is merely divided by two. The more speed involved, the greater the potential KE.

22. a. foot-pounds—Total kinetic energy is expressed in foot/pounds. Example: the impact of a person weighing (mass) 150 pounds moving at a speed (velocity) of 30 mph will strike with a force of 67,000 foot-pounds (total KE).

23. c. immediately after the injury is sustained—The golden hour is the first hour after the injury occurs.

24. a. The third collision occurs when the internal organs strike against the inside of the body.—The first collision is the car striking the concrete barrier; the second collision is the driver striking the steering wheel or dashboard. Any of the three collisions may result in severe damage.

25. d. Tumbling creates greater tissue damage.—The leading edge of the bullet does not enter the patient; rather, the bullet is tumbling through space and the entire side surface of the bullet can enter the body.

26. d. rapid acceleration and deceleration—The rear-end collision is where the rapid acceleration occurs (whiplash), and the stopping of the vehicle in the ditch is where the rapid deceleration should be suspected.

27. d. GSWs—Don't assume that a projectile, such as a bullet, always follows a straight path between the entrance and exit sites. Projectiles may ricochet inside the body, especially off bones, and travel many different pathways.

28. c. tertiary—In this phase, injuries can result from the patient becoming a flying object and striking other objects.

29. b. flying articles.—Injuries can be blunt from compression, or penetrating from lacerations.

30. a. high-power rifle—The more speed there is involved, the more energy there is to exchange with the body, and the higher the possibility for tissue damage.

31. d. 60-kg patient traveling at 60 mph—The more speed there is, the more energy there is. The value of speed (the velocity) is squared in the kinetic energy formula; the value of the mass is merely divided by two.

32. b. compression—In the primary phase of a blast, there is a pressure wave that causes major effects on the lungs and GI tract.

33. d. tertiary—In this phase, injuries can result from the patient becoming a flying object and striking other objects.

34. a. frontal—This is a common MOI. The rider is ejected up and forward with both legs striking the handle bars, resulting in bilateral femur factures.

35. b. rear-end—This is due to the whiplash effect of flexion and then extension. Head restraints, if properly positioned, can be helpful in reducing this type of injury.

36. c. smoke condition in the room in which the patient was found—With this common MOI, the paramedic should have a high index of suspicion that the patient has suffered smoke inhalation resulting in injury to the airways and difficulty breathing.

37. c. CO_2 inhalation—The inhalation of poisonous gases is very likely the cause of the patient's present state of unconsciousness.

38. d. the combination of forces involved—Getting a complete and accurate account of the incident is one of the best ways to suspect and look for injuries that may not be visibly apparent.

39. a. contusion, fracture, or rupture.—When a bullet is fired into the body, the energy forces from the bullet are transferred to the tissues. This causes momentary acceleration of tissue laterally away from the tract of the projectile, creating a cavity (cavitation).

40. d. type of empty shell casings—Shell casings may help providers understand the type of wound created (e.g., gunshot, buckshot, hand gun, or high-power rifle).

41. b. crush injuries—The initial impact with the leg, arm, shoulder, and hip against the car causes crush injuries. The fall and skid after the initial impact cause fractures and abrasions.

42. a. brain contusion—In the third collision, internal organs strike the body. This causes contusions, hematomas, and shearing of organs suspended by ligaments.

43. a. 10—The "platinum ten" minutes. In serious trauma, the best chances of survival for the patient are a

result of reaching the hospital's operating suite within the golden hour. EMS providers can help patients reach that goal by working within the first ten "platinum" minutes to get the patient off-scene and en route to the trauma center.

44. c. cavitation.—When a bullet is fired into the body, the energy forces from the bullet are transferred to the tissues. This causes momentary acceleration of tissue laterally away from the tract of the projectile, creating a cavity (cavitation).

45. b. lungs and GI tract—This type of MOI may cause injuries such as pneumothorax, ruptured organs, and an air embolism.

46. b. rupture of an organ or air embolism.—The lungs and the GI tract are the organs primarily affected.

47. d. being run over by the vehicle.—The other choices describe injuries that occur in the first and second phases of an auto–pedestrian collision.

48. c. 300—One of the key strategies for teaching motorcycle safety is educating the riders about wearing a helmet and protective gear when riding.

49. b. Airbags may produce minor facial and forearm abrasions.—These injuries are insignificant compared to the potential injuries that can result without the use of airbags.

50. a. They prevent hyperflexion of the upper torso.—The other choices are incorrect.

Chapter 36: Bleeding, Soft Tissue Trauma, and Burns

1. c. internal and external.—External bleeding is usually due to trauma, whereas internal bleeding can be from either trauma or a medical cause.

2. b. occult GI bleeding.—The most common site of nontraumatic bleeding is in the GI tract (e.g., peptic ulcer, diverticulosis, and esophageal varies).

3. b. artery.—Arterial bleeding is characterized as spurting or pulsing with each heartbeat.

4. a. crushing injury.—When treating a patient with a crush injury, one of the most important points is observing for the presence of ECG changes or dysrhythmias.

5. a. secondary infections.—Soft tissue injuries can be fatal, even without deep injuries.

6. b. physical forces—Activities such as contact sports and those involving high speed increase the risk of soft tissue trauma. MVCs, falls, assaults, and violence all contribute significantly to the risk of soft tissue injury.

7. c. superficial lesion—A lesion is an abnormal growth involving one or more layers of skin.

8. b. epidermis—The outer layer of skin.

9. a. dermis.—The layer of skin covered by the epidermis.

10. d. deep fascia—Binds together muscles and other internal structures.

11. a. tension lines.—There are two types of tension lines: static and dynamic. Static tension is the constant force due to the taut nature of skin. Underlying muscle contraction causes dynamic tension.

12. a. Hemostasis—In the first phase, there is reflex vasoconstriction for 10 minutes, and then clotting begins.

13. b. collagen synthesis.—One of the phases of normal wound healing.

14. a. Epithelialization—One of the phases of normal wound healing.

15. c. body region—Other factors that can affect wound healing include: static skin tension, dynamic skin tension, and pigmented and oily skin.

16. c. corticosteroids—Normal healing may be slowed if the patient is taking any of the following medications: corticosteroids, nonsteroidal anti-inflammatory drugs, penicillin, colchicines, anticoagulants, and antineoplastic agents.

17. c. acne—A number of medical conditions and diseases can affect normal wound healings.

18. c. human bites—Other wounds that have a high risk for infections include: bites from animals or humans, foreign bodies, wounds contaminated with organic matter, injected wounds, wounds with significant devitalized tissue, and crush wounds.

19. a. keloid scar.—These are more common in dark pigmented people and often occur on the ears, upper extremities, lower abdomen, and sternum.

20. b. cosmetically acceptable healing.—Plastic surgery is often requested for wounds to cosmetic regions such as the face, lip, and eyebrow.

21. a. degloving—Large, gaping wounds require closure (e.g., wounds over tension areas, degloving injuries, ring injuries, and skin tears).

22. b. hepatitis.—Hepatitis is easily transmitted by persons with no signs or symptoms of the disease. Health care providers are at risk of exposure when PPE is not used with every single patient.

23. a. contusion—With a contusion, the epidermis remains intact. Blood accumulates, causing pain and ecchymosis.

24. c. incision—These injuries are similar to lacerations except the wound ends are smooth and even. They

tend to heal better than lacerations due to the constriction of the vessels.

25. d. avulsion.—This type of injury can involve a small or large area of skin.

26. a. laceration.—The jagged wound is caused by forceful impact with a sharp object, and the ends usually bleed freely.

27. b. ring injury—The other injuries are all types of amputations.

28. c. secondary and tertiary—The secondary injuries are due to flying debris striking the patient, and the tertiary injuries are caused when the patient is thrown from the blast and strikes a hard object.

29. b. crush—The patient may develop "crush syndrome," also called traumatic rhabdomyolysis.

30. d. sodium bicarbonate to neutralize the buildup of acids.—When the cause of the crush injury is moved or lifted off, the patient may suddenly go into cardiac arrest due to the massive release of toxins from the ruptured muscles into the blood stream.

31. d. crush injury—Crush injuries occur as a result of compressive force sufficient to interfere with the normal metabolic function of the involved tissue. Prolonged compression can result from an improperly applied cast.

32. b. anaerobic metabolism—As a result of anaerobic metabolism, various compounds accumulate and cause local inflammation.

33. d. 6–8 hours—With compartment syndrome, a prolonged period of ischemia, greater than 6–8 hours leads to tissue hypoxia and anoxia, and ultimately cell death.

34. d. capillary hydrostatic—This causes ischemia in the affected muscle tissue.

35. a. palpation.—The "Ps" of compartment syndrome are the signs and symptoms a patient may experience: pain, paresthesia (the sensation of pins and needles), paresis (weakness), pressure, passive stretch pain, and pulselessness.

36. c. in a confined space.—The full effect of the blast is experienced within confined spaces. The patient also has an extremely high potential for inhalation injuries.

37. c. considering that both internal and external injuries are possible.—When you consider the MOI, remember the three phases of blasts and the injuries associated with each.

38. d. indirect pressure—The methods of hemorrhage control include: direct pressure, elevation, pressure dressing, pressure points, and tourniquet application.

39. b. promote localized clotting.—Once the bleeding has been stopped, normal wound healing begins with reflex vasoconstriction (hemostasis), and clotting begins.

40. d. The bandage should not occlude or impede arterial blood flow.—After applying a pressure bandage, check for a distal pulse. If there is no pulse, loosen the bandage enough for the return of the pulse.

41. c. pregnant trauma patient with an abdominal evisceration—A pressure dressing is indicated for hemorrhage control when direct pressure and elevation have not controlled the bleeding.

42. b. lose the limb to save the life.—Use of a tourniquet is considered a last resort of bleeding control. It is considered only after all other methods of bleeding control have failed.

43. a. the process to eliminate bacteria from the dressing material.—This type of dressing is used when infection is a concern.

44. a. passage of air—This type of dressing is useful for wounds involving the thorax and major vessels. It may prevent pneumothorax and air embolism.

45. d. non-adherent—This type of dressing is often used after wound closure.

46. b. adhesive—This type of dressing can also assist in controlling acute bleeding.

47. d. decreased risk of wound infection—The other choices are likely to occur with an improperly applied dressing.

48. b. Explain that a tetanus shot and sutures are necessary.—Transportation considerations for this type of wound include: the need for proper wound cleansing and dressing, the need for a tetanus booster, and the need for sutures due to the depth and location of the injury.

49. c. Do not allow the dressing to get wet.—A wet dressing will act as a wick and draw bacteria into the wound.

50. c. every 10 years—Currently, the recommendation for a booster is every 10 years.

51. a. covering the wound with a dry, sterile dressing.—Nonsterile dressings are used when something clean is acceptable and infection is not a concern.

52. b. be wrapped in sterile, moist gauze pad.—The amputated part should be wrapped in a sterile, moist gauze pad and placed in a plastic bag. Then, place the bag on ice. Be careful to ensure that the tissue does not freeze.

53. c. gangrene—Some experts recommend hyperbaric therapy to prevent gangrene and improve healing in crush injuries.

54. a. the observation of the presence of ECG changes or dysrhythmias.—Calcium chloride (1–3 cc IV in an adult) is indicated in this case. Of course, follow your local protocols.

55. b. subcutaneous layer—The other choices listed are the other layers of the skin (e.g., epidermis, dermis).

56. a. house—Each year, an estimated 1.25 million people are burned severely enough to seek treatment. Those who are at the highest risk are the elderly and children.

57. b. toddler and preschool—Smoke inhalation, scalds, contact, and electrical burns are especially likely to occur in children younger than 4 years old.

58. d. impairment of mobility or sensation.—Those who are at the highest risk for burns are the elderly (from impairment of mobility or sensation) and children (from child abuse).

59. c. turning down the thermostat on the hot water heater to 120°F.—Setting the thermostat to 100°F is the recommendation for preventing accidental burns.

60. a. decreased catecholamine release—An increase in catecholamine and dysrhythmias is a system complication of burn injuries.

61. c. full thickness—A full thickness burn involved all layers of the skin and may include charring of tissue.

62. b. deep fascia—This is a layer of connective tissue covering or binding body structures together.

63. b. second—Also referred to as a partial thickness burn.

64. c. eschar.—Eschar is the scab or immediate scar that forms on the skin following a burn injury.

65. a. body surface area burned.—The rule of nines is one method of estimating the amount of body surface area affected by a burn injury. There are two versions, one for adults and one for pediatrics.

66. b. requires transport to the nearest hospital.—Additional examples include: burns greater than 30% of BSA in adults, 15% of BSA in children, burns of the head or perineum, and burns associated with multiple trauma or serious medical problems.

67. b. the patient's gender—The other factors have a significant impact on the management and prognosis of the burn-injured patient.

68. c. the kidneys—Preexisting problems with the kidneys, lungs, or heart may make it difficult for the patient to handle the tremendous movement of body fluids that occurs with a burn injury.

69. d. 24%—The front and back of each lower leg is 6% (6 × 4). This equals 24% for both lower legs.

70. b. compensation—The phases of burn shock include the emergent, fluid shift, resolution, and hypermetabolic phases.

71. b. release of catecholamines—The patient will have tachycardia, tachypnea, mild hypertension, and anxiety.

72. c. fluid shift—During this phase, there is a massive shift of fluids from the intravascular to the extravascular space.

73. c. resolution—In this phase, the extravasation of fluid diminishes and equilibrium is reached between intravascular space and interstitial space.

74. a. carbon monoxide poisoning.—MOIs associated with inhalation injury include: toxic inhalations, smoke inhalation, carbon monoxide poisoning, thiocyanate intoxication, and thermal and chemical burns.

75. d. Eschar—The scar formation is thick and nonelastic. If large enough, it may impair circulation or respiration.

76. a. circulatory compromise—When this condition develops, the patient will require an escharotomy, a life- or limb-saving procedure in which physical cuts are made into the eschar formed on the skin with a scalpel.

77. b. fluid replacement amounts—This is a consideration in the management of the burn patient.

78. a. Maintain body heat.—Moving the patient to safety and stopping the burning process are the initial steps of care. Maintaining body heat, so the patient does not become hypothermic, is a priority over pain management.

79. b. determine fluid replacement—The formula is to administer four times the BSA, times the patient's weight in kilograms. The first half is given in the first 8 hours. For example, a 100-kg patient with 40% BSA full thick burns (4 × 40 × 100 = 16,000) should receive 8,000 cc in the first 8 hours.

80. c. crawling on the floor in a room with flames—The coolest area of a burning room is always the floor.

81. a. hoarseness—Other clues to look for include: singed nasal hairs, black soot in the sputum, stridor, and inspiratory wheezing.

82. c. hyperbaric oxygen—Though once reserved for only the very ill, some data suggest that treatment of patients with fairly low levels of carbon monoxide is also beneficial.

83. b. hot tar—Tar sticks to the skin, creating a longer exposure time. The temperature of hot tar ranges from 400°–500°F.

84. b. brushing it off and calling the poison control center for decon procedures.—Figure out what the chemical is before just washing it off. Some chemicals react with water and produce heat or develop a substance that is toxic to inhale.

85. a. continuous irrigation—Remove contacts and provide continuous irrigation. Take care with the runoff so as not to burn other areas of the body.

86. a. 1; 2—The burning effects of both of these substances can be minimized when the patient is instructed to avoid rubbing his eyes or face.

87. a. get the patient to blow his nose and spit out any residue.—The patient should also be instructed to avoid rubbing his eyes or face.

88. b. remove the lenses with a gloved hand or assist the patient in doing so.—The contact lens must be removed promptly to stop the burning process and allow for proper irrigation.

89. d. The path of electricity through the body may cause serious complications.—Always try to define the entry and exit points of the current because anything in the pathway is fair game for injury.

90. b. 1,000—The cause of death is usually attributed to the electrical effect on the heart, massive muscle destruction occurring from the current traveling through the body, or thermal burns from contact with the electrical source.

91. c. identify the source of the electricity prior to approaching the patient.—Personal safety first! Prior to approaching the patient, be sure you know what the source of the electricity injury was, and if it is still a live source.

92. b. less dangerous than AC.—The effects of AC on the body depend on the frequency. Low-frequency currents of 50–60 Hz, which are commonly used, are more dangerous than high-frequency currents, and are three to five times more dangerous than DC currents of the same voltage and amperage.

93. c. 60—Prolonged exposure causes more severe burns.

94. b. Escharotomy—A life-saving or limb-saving procedure in which the physician cuts into the eschar formed on the skin with a scalpel.

95. d. moist mucous membrane (mouth)—Body resistance is highest with dry, intact skin with thickly calloused areas (e.g., palm of the hand or sole of the foot).

96. a. anything in the path is "fair game" for injury.—The body is a great conductor of electricity. Assume that any tissue anywhere in the path of the current was damaged.

97. c. malocclusion—The other signs and symptoms are frequently associated with electrical injuries.

98. a. There is nothing you can do.—There is no treatment for preventing airway swelling with this MOI. The paramedic should assess the need for assisting ventilation and intubating, and provide what is necessary for the patient before the swelling becomes a complete airway obstruction. When the patient is conscious, sedation is often necessary. Call for the additional resources needed and follow local protocol.

99. a. lightning strike—Lightning rarely produces entrance and exit wounds. Typically, lightning flashes over the patient as opposed to achieving a direct hit.

100. c. The potential for internal injury is less than a thermal injury.—The potential for internal injury is often much greater. Thermal burns are typically associated with injury to the body's surface.

101. c. hands.—The hands, followed by the head, are the most common entry points. The most common exit point is the foot.

102. b. singed nasal hairs—This finding is more common with blast and inhalation injuries.

103. d. feet—The hands, followed by the head, are the most common entry points. The most common exit point is the foot.

104. a. ionization—Ionization can result from X-rays, gamma rays, and particle bombardment.

105. a. when the history is inconsistent with injuries—When a child's injuries or pattern of injuries do not appear to be consistent with the patient's, parent's, or caregiver's history of the MOI, the paramedic should consider the possibility of abuse.

Chapter 37: Chest Trauma

1. b. second—Head injuries are number one.

2. d. disruption of the bellows action.—The other conditions interrupt gas exchange rather than impair ventilations.

3. a. tearing of a great vessel.—Tearing occurs with rapid deceleration and penetrating MOIs.

4. b. tear—Tearing occurs with penetrating MOIs.

5. c. massive lung contusion to develop.—There is also a potential for respiratory burn injuries from the inhalation of superheated gases. Contusion or bruising reduces the area available to exchange oxygen and carbon dioxide (CO_2).

6. c. perforated lung tissue—The accumulation of air under the skin may also be caused by a tracheobronchial injury.

7. b. mesotendons—This is found in joints containing synovial fluid.

8. a. Sternocleidomastoid—A muscle used in breathing, as well as in flexion and extension of the head.

9. b. trapezius.—This muscle lies over the scapula.

10. d. mainstem bronchi.—It bifurcates (splits) into the right and left mainstem bronchi.

11. a. Parenchyma—The essential and distinctive tissue of a specific organ.

12. d. inferior vena cava.—The largest vein in the body returns blood to the right atrium of the heart.

13. a. aorta—The largest artery in the body.

14. b. trachea—The mediastinum contains the great vessels (e.g., aorta, vena cava, heart, esophagus, and trachea).

15. c. tension pneumothorax.—A tension pneumothorax develops in situations of penetrating trauma and blunt trauma. Morbidity is common; this injury should be considered an immediate life-threatening condition.

16. c. absence or presence of hyperresonance—Assessment findings in a patient with a tension pneumothorax include dyspnea, respiratory distress decreased or absent breath sounds, and hyperresonance. Signs of shock (a late sign), decreased

breath sounds, and hyperresonance to percussion on the same side of the chest means a tension pneumothorax until proven otherwise.

17. b. accessory muscles of breathing—These injuries can occur from deceleration, compression, or penetrating trauma.

18. b. carotid sinus—These constantly measure the CO_2 levels in the blood. Respiratory centers in the brain adjust the rate and depth of breathing to maintain normal CO_2 concentrations.

19. a. contusions on the lung tissue—Other mechanisms that can impair gas exchange as a result of chest trauma include collapsed alveoli (atelectasis) and blood accumulation, and disruption of the respiratory tract from a cut to the trachea or major respiratory anatomy.

20. b. Commodiocordis—Sudden cardiac arrest as a result of a blunt, non-penetrating blow to the chest with no injury to the ribs, sternum, or heart. The initial heart rhythm following the blow to the chest is ventricular fibrillation.

21. a. splenic rupture.—The spleen lies beneath the lower ribs and is highly susceptible to laceration and rupture from blunt trauma. Because it is highly vascular, it can produce life-threatening hemorrhage.

22. a. expand all the air sacs.—This will help prevent atelectasis and pneumonia from developing.

23. b. four to nine—The most common locations of rib fractures are in the axillary line and around the sternum.

24. c. severe trauma—These ribs are protected by the clavicle. The force required to fracture these ribs is significant.

25. c. 20–40—Mortality is increased with advanced age, seven or more ribs fractured, three or more associated injuries, shock, or a head injury.

26. d. The arterial blood flow is impaired, resulting in a ventilation–perfusion mismatch.—This type of injury impairs venous return.

27. a. pulmonary contusion—These contusion causes a decrease in the lung compliance and hemorrhage in the intra-alveolar capillaries and alveolus, making it even more difficult to ventilate and exchange gases at the cellular level.

28. d. deceleration compression—This occurs when the chest strikes the steering wheel or dashboard. This is a very serious injury that involves a 25–45% mortality rate.

29. c. because of the associated injuries.—If the thorax receives enough force to fracture the sternum, then we must assume that the same force was transmitted to the heart, great vessels, lungs, and diaphragm.

30. b. shoulder or arm on the affected side.—An abnormal accumulation of air in the apexes of the chest can cause pain in the shoulder or arm on the affected side.

31. c. hypoventilation.—Ventilation–perfusion mismatch occurs as a result of shunting, hypoventilation, hypoxia, and the development of a large, functional dead space.

32. b. respiratory effort is ineffective.—If the size of the hole is greater than the glottic opening, little to no air comes in through the glottis.

33. d. a serious reduction in cardiac output caused by deformation of the vena cava reducing preload.—The mediastinum shifts to the contralateral side, and this leads to right-to-left intrapulmonary shunting and hypoxia.

34. b. hyporesonance and mediastinal shift to the ipsilateral side—These findings should be detected on the affected side.

35. d. 50—Hemothorax can occur from penetrating or blunt trauma to the lung, chest wall vessels, the intercostal vessels, or the myocardium itself.

36. a. 2,000–3,000—A large volume of blood can bleed into the pleural space and chest cavity.

37. c. parenchyma.—The pulmonary parenchyma is a low-pressure vascular system. When a massive hemothorax is present, consider another cause for the bleeding (e.g., great vessel or heart).

38. b. respiratory distress.—The major problem associated with a developing hemothorax is the progression of shock and respiratory compromise.

39. b. positive pressure ventilation.—Airway and ventilatory management are first and foremost. Positive pressure ventilation may be helpful to re-expand the injured lung, which in turn may help reduce the bleeding.

40. c. the high incidence of other associated injuries.—The mortality is between 14–20%.

41. d. cyanosis to the face and neck—The other findings are typical with pulmonary contusion.

42. d. abdominal—Patients with pulmonary contusions also tend to have other severe thoracic and abdominal injuries. Always assume multiple potential injuries are present.

43. a. prevent the kinking of the great vessels.—It attaches the great vessels at the base of the heart.

44. b. ventricular diastolic filling—The accumulation of fluid in the pericardial sac impairs diastolic filling of the heart, with a subsequent decrease in cardiac output.

45. c. JVD and narrow pulse pressure.—Other signs and symptoms may include: respiratory distress and cyanosis of the head, neck, and upper extremities, pulsusparadoxus, ECG changes, and Beck's triad.

46. b. myocardial contusion—If the thorax receives enough force to fracture the sternum, then we must assume that the same force was transmitted to the heart, great vessels, lungs, and diaphragm. The fractured ribs are more local over the heart. Myocardial and pulmonary contusions are very likely.

47. a. sinus tachycardia without obvious hypovolemia.—Other ECG changes to be alert for as a clue to this problem include: persistent tachycardia, ST segment elevation, T wave inversion, right bundle branch block (RBBB), atrial flutter or fibrillation, and PVCs or PACs.

48. d. pain management and considering antidysrhythmics.—Treatment of the patient with suspected myocardial contusion involves airway and ventilation control. Administer high-concentration oxygen and evaluate the need for intubation. Administer fluids, manage pain, and consider medications to control cardiac arrhythmias.

49. c. CHF or pulmonary edema—The history of a recent trauma and a new onset of CHF or pulmonary edema are clues to a possible myocardial rupture.

50. b. falls.—This is a very critical injury, where 85–95% of the patients die instantaneously.

51. d. 85–95—Aortic dissections are present in 15% of all blunt trauma deaths.

52. b. The patient described the pain as a "tearing" sensation.—The most common sign is pain with a sudden and intense onset. The patient may complain of a "ripping" or "tearing" sensation.

53. c. Trendelenburg position—This position may make the respiratory distress worse. Gravity will push the abdominal contents and diaphragm further up into the chest cavity, impeding expansion of the lungs.

54. a. cardiac event.—Other signs and symptoms may include: chest pain, fever, hoarseness, dysphagia, respiratory distress, shock, subcutaneous emphysema, and ECG changes.

55. c. chest—The chest contains the lungs and heart. Traumatic asphyxia causes direct pressure on these organs, crushing them and creating a backflow of blood into the jugular veins (increased venous pressure).

56. a. IV fluids for hypotension.—Airway and ventilatory management are primary, as with any patient. After the compression is released, typically the patient will experience hypotension, which should be managed with IV fluids.

57. c. both blunt and penetrating chest trauma.—This type of injury occurs in less than 3% of chest injuries, but has a mortality rate of greater than 30%.

58. d. tachy-brady dysrhythmias—The tear from this injury can occur anywhere along the tracheobronchial tree. There is a rapid movement of air into the pleural space, often making the tension pneumothorax refractory to needle decompression.

59. c. penetrating trauma.—Penetrating trauma from a bullet or a knife can cause an esophageal injury.

60. a. diaphragmatic injury.—When the MOI causes a high-pressure compression to the abdomen, the result can be a diaphragmatic rupture with extravasation of abdominal contents into the chest.

Chapter 38: Nervous System and Head, Facial, Neck, and Spine Trauma

1. c. airway compromise.—Consider the ABCs. With this type of injury, there is a high risk of potential for complications of the patient's airway.

2. d. gunshot wounds (GSW).—The other choices are not examples of penetrating MOIs; they are blunt trauma.

3. d. cervical spine injury—The paramedic must take C-spine precautions with any patient who has an MOI with a blunt force above the shoulders.

4. d. there is an associated injury to the major blood vessels.—Throat injuries may be fatal, usually due to associated injury to the airway or the main blood vessels (e.g., carotid and jugular). Vocal cord injury may lead to hoarseness or respiratory compromise.

5. d. hyphema—A collection of blood in the front of the eye.

6. c. blowout fracture.—A blowout fracture occurs because blunt trauma is applied to the eye socket.

7. a. punch—More severe injuries to the mouth are rare and often involve penetrating trauma.

8. a. complicated airway.—LeFort fractures are based on X-ray or CT scan findings. These injuries involve the mouth, nose, eyes, and cheeks.

9. c. X-ray or CT scan findings.—Some experts now contend that the differentiation is artificial and not helpful.

10. d. cranial nerves 1–5.—The vagus nerve (tenth) is the only cranial nerve that extends out of the skull into the thorax.

11. c. external—The key assessment point is to note if CSF is draining from the ear.

12. b. eardrum.—The key assessment point is to determine if there is acute gross hearing loss.

13. d. cones.—Conical-shaped photoreceptive cells in the retina are called the cones.

14. d. cornea—The cornea can be easily injured from exposure to chemicals and other substances, or from blunt force trauma.

15. b. Eyelids—Also called palpebra.

16. b. rods—Rod-shaped photoreceptive cells in the retina.

17. a. hypoglossal—The pair of twelfth cranial nerves, which are the motor nerves that supply the muscles of the tongue and hyoid.

18. a. hyoid.—The only unarticulated bone in the body.

19. b. malocclusion.—Determine if the malocclusion is normal for the patient or new as a result of traumatic injury.

20. c. movement from conjugate gaze of the uninjured eye.—Conjugate gaze refers to the use of both eyes to look steadily in one direction.

21. c. million—Most head injuries are minor. Major head injury is the most common cause of death from trauma in trauma centers. Statistics show that over 50% of all trauma deaths involve a head injury.

22. b. males; 15–24—Also at high risk are infants, school-age children, and the elderly.

23. a. MVC.—Other common MOIs for head injury include: sports, falls, and penetrating trauma from GSWs.

24. d. galea—It is comprised of the hair and subcutaneous tissue, which contains the major scalp veins that, when injured, can bleed profusely.

25. c. be strong yet light in weight.—The head also has sinuses (hollow cavities) that help to lighten the weight.

26. b. cerebrum—This area of the brain contains the cortex controls that are responsible for voluntary skeletal movement and the level of awareness component of consciousness.

27. c. occipital—This area of the brain is the origin of the optic nerves.

28. c. III; X—The third cranial nerve controls pupil size. The tenth cranial nerve is the vagus, which innervates the sinoatrial (SA) and atrioventricular (AV) nodes, as well as the stomach and GI tract. Stimulation of this nerve causes bradycardia.

29. d. reticular activating system—The RAS is responsible for the level of arousal and must be intact for cortical function to maintain wakefulness.

30. a. venous blood vessels that reabsorb CSF.—The arachnoid member is the middle layer of the meninges and loosely covers the central nervous center.

31. c. 20—The brain also requires many nutrients, (e.g., glucose and thiamine), but does not have the ability to store nutrients.

32. c. autoregulation—Perfusion of the brain can be affected by conditions that interfere with cerebral perfusion pressure (CPP), such as edema, bleeding, or hypotension.

33. a. coup—Coup injuries develop directly below the point of impact.

34. b. concussion—A concussion results in a transient episode of neuronal dysfunction with a rapid return to normal neurological activity. The injuries

are most commonly the result of blunt trauma to the head.

35. b. focal—Focal injuries are specific, grossly observable brain lesions (e.g., cerebral contusion, intracranial hemorrhage, and epidural hematoma).

36. d. Diffuse axonal injury.—It is often a mild or classic concussion, but it can be moderate or severe.

37. b. concussion—The injuries are most commonly the result of blunt trauma to the head. The patient is often initially confused and disoriented and may not remember the event.

38. c. Battle's sign—This is a finding (bruising behind the ear) associated with a basilar skull fracture.

39. a. linear—Leaking of SCF may not occur for 24 hours. If there are no other associated injuries, there is typically no danger.

40. a. Acute subdural—This type of hemorrhage results from the rupture of bridging veins between the cortex and dura and may be acute, chronic, or delayed.

41. b. tachycardia.—Bradycardia would be a more typical finding due to pressure on the vagus nerve.

42. a. 4–6—This response is a late and ominous finding associated with brain herniation.

43. d. elevated blood pressure—The usual response within the brain is elevated BP due to the loss of cerebral autoregulation. This is the only way that the body can continue perfusion to the injured tissue.

44. d. cerebral cortex and upper brain stem—The effects of an expanding hematoma on the cerebral cortex and upper brain stem may include Cushing's reflex and reactive pupils, and Cheyne–Stokes respirations may be present. Initially, the patient will have a purposeful response to pain. As the mental status deteriorates, this sensation is lost and the patient withdraws from pain. Flexion or decorticate posturing will occur in response to a painful stimuli.

45. a. Vegetative functions are temporarily impaired because of the pressure.—At this late point in brain herniation, the patient's injury is not considered survivable.

46. b. 8–12.—A severe head injury is less than 8.

47. c. subarachnoid—The arachnoid membrane is composed of venous blood vessels that reabsorb CSF.

48. a. pads of the fingers—When the depression is visually obvious, there is no reason to palpate the site. When performing a focused exam of the skull for a possible injury, use the pads of the fingertips, which are dexterous and sensitive enough to assess a potential skull depression without causing further injury.

49. c. tachycardia and tachypnea—Bradycardia and abnormal respirations are associated with enlarging intracranial hematomas.

50. a. frontal lobe—Trauma to this area of the brain may result in personality changes, placid reactions, or seizures.

51. b. aggressive hyperventilation.—It is now believed that hyperventilation produces a marked reduction in cerebral blood flow. Decreased cerebral blood flow may lead to or exacerbate ischemia, enhancing rather than reducing injury. It also decreases coronary perfusion pressure in cardiac arrest.

52. a. another organ or injuries besides the brain.— Typically, bleeding from the head is not significant enough to produce hypotension.

53. d. paralysis prior to intubation—Pharmacological-induced paralysis keeps the patient from becoming anxious and combative, both of which can worsen head injury.

54. b. only when hypoglycemia is confirmed.— Exogenous glucose can increase brain swelling and should only be administered when hypoglycemia can be confirmed.

55. b. assure adequate tidal volume.—Ensure a patent airway, adequate ventilation, and oxygenation.

56. a. systolic; 70—Ensure adequate circulation, but do not administer too much fluid. Manage hypotension with fluid boluses, not to exceed a systolic of 90–100 mmHg in the adult male patient.

57. c. nasal intubation—Ensure an adequate airway, but avoid nasal intubation because it may increase the ICP.

58. a. the history of the MOI—Getting a good story of the MOI may be the only way to recognize the presence of brain injury.

59. c. 5—Eye response = 1, verbal response = 1, motor response = 3, for a total of 5.

60. a. linear—This is the most common type of skull fracture and can only be determined by X-ray. If there are no associated injuries, the fracture may be missed. Getting a good story of the MOI may be the only way to recognize the presence of brain injury.

61. b. men, 16–30—This occurs primarily due to sports, as well as inexperienced and immature drivers.

62. c. 25—This includes bystanders pulling patients out of cars and swimming pools without proper spinal immobilization.

63. d. all of the above.—Nerves and blood vessels are also interconnected with the spine. Injury to any of these components may result in neck or back pain.

64. b. posterior longitudinal.—The four key ligaments that support the spine are the anterior and posterior longitudinal ligaments, and the cruciform and accessory atlantoaxial ligaments.

65. c. cruciform.—Cruciate means shaped like a cross. This very complete ligament supports the atlas vertebra.

66. c. axis.—The atlas is the first cervical vertebra and the axis is the second.

67. d. transverse.—The atlantoaxial ligament attaches the axis and atlas, as well as the transverse ligament that serves to hold the odontoid process close to the anterior arch.

68. a. dens—A fracture of the odontoid process results in death in most cases.

69. b. thoracic.—The spine is thickest in this area and has the additional protection of the ribs.

70. c. thirty-one—Also called peripheral nerves, they exit the spinal cord between each of the vertebra.

71. a. coccyx—The coccyx joins with the sacrum from above and is the terminus of the spine.

72. b. transverse process.—These processes can fracture and break off as a result of blunt force trauma.

73. b. spinous process.—These processes can fracture and break off as a result of blunt force trauma.

74. d. nucleus pulposus.—Trauma, degenerative disk disease, and improper lifting may cause herniation (a tear in the capsule enclosing the nucleus pulposus) of the intervertebral disk.

75. c. L-2—The spinal cord ends at the level of second lumbar vertebra.

76. b. It is manufactured in the ventricles of the brain.— CSF protects and supports the brain and spinal cord. CSF is completely replaced several times a day.

77. a. white matter.—The white matter is located in the anatomical spinal tracts, which are longitudinal bundles of myelinated nerve tracts. Myelin is a soft, white, fatty substance that forms a thick sheath around certain nerves. The gray matter is located in the core of the cord.

78. b. ascending nerve tracts.—There are two groups of ascending nerve tracts: spinothalmic tracts and the fascicular gracilis and corneatus tracts.

79. c. descending nerve tracts.—The descending nerve tracts carry motor impulses from the brain to the body. There are three groups: corticospinal, reticulospinal, and rubrospinal tracts.

80. a. a group of nerve fibers with a similar function— The funiculi function like a coaxial cable. They conduct sensory impulses from the skin, muscle tendons, and joints to the brain for interpretation as sensations of touch, pressure, and body movement.

81. c. conduct impulses of pain and temperature to the brain.—The lateral and anterior spinothalmic tracts are located in the lateral and anterior funiculi, and the impulses cross over at the spinal cord.

82. b. dermatome.—Dermatomes can be mapped out by the level of the spinal nerve. They are a useful tool to determine the specific level of spinal cord injury (SCI).

83. d. T-4—The motor and sensory dermatomes at the nipple line are located at the fourth thoracic vertebra.

84. a. C-3—The nerve roots C-3, C-4, and C-5 have a relationship to the motor function of the diaphragm.

85. b. resistance to movement.—Two exceptions for not moving a patient into a normal anatomical position

for immobilization are extreme pain or resistance from the bones in gently moving the neck.

86. d. Have the patient sign a refusal for the collar and immobilize her without it.—Any competent adult patient has the right to refuse any or all care offered.

87. b. The patient experienced hyperflexion.—The classic "lipstick" sign results from hyperflexion of the head as it is forced down to the chest with rapid acceleration.

88. b. thoracic—Paraplegia can occur with transection of the lumbar level, as well. When a patient has a complete spinal cord transection, all cord-mediated functions below the transection are permanently lost.

89. c. The spinal cord may be injured without accompanying bone or soft tissue injury.—The other statements are inaccurate.

90. d. it should not be used at all—If the decision is made to immobilize a patient in the field, the patient should get both a collar and spine board.

91. b. full spinal immobilization with the parent providing support—The patient has more than one indication for providing full spinal immobilization (e.g., fall from twice his height and loss of consciousness).

92. c. mental status—A patient who is alert, calm, cooperative, sober and oriented, and has had no loss of consciousness is considered reliable and able to refuse any or all care.

93. c. fully immobilize the spine.—New neck pain or tenderness after any MOI is an indication for the application of full spinal immobilization.

94. b. Tender areas may not hurt unless palpated.—Always palpate over the spinous processes before concluding that a patient has no neck pain. Some providers simply ask the patient and never perform a physical exam.

95. b. paresthesia in the left leg after, not before, immobilization—A change in the patient's condition that is more severe is significant. Recognizing the change is good assessment; correcting the problem is good care.

96. a. vertical compression of the spine—Also referred to as axial loading, usually to the top of the head from a sudden deceleration (e.g., a brick falling onto someone's head). It may cause a compression fracture without an SCI or a crushed vertebral body with an SCI.

97. d. distraction of the neck—This type of force may cause a stretching of the spinal cord and supporting ligaments (e.g., hanging that did not break the odontoid).

98. a. rotational neck injury—T-bone collisions are associated with excessive rotation of the neck beyond the normal range of motion. A rupture of the supporting ligaments may also occur.

99. a. concussion.—The spinal cord can be injured in a number of ways. A cord concussion is a temporary disruption of cord-mediated functions.

100. b. spinal shock.—Spinal shock refers to a temporary loss of all types of spinal cord functions distal to the injury. The patient will be flaccid and paralyzed distal to the injury site. It is important to manage the patient carefully to avoid a secondary injury.

101. d. Brown–Sequard syndrome—This syndrome is caused by a penetrating injury that produces a partial transection of the spinal cord. It is referred to as a hemisection of the cord and involves only one side of the cord.

102. c. variable segment instability.—The degeneration of a disc may cause the vertebrae to come in closer contact with one another.

103. c. 60–90—The usual cause is a lumbar nerve root problem. This syndrome affects men and women equally up to the age of 60, when it increases in women.

104. b. The head moves around inside the helmet.—The helmet is not the right size when the head moves around and should be removed in order to properly immobilize the cervical spine.

105. b. spondylolysis—A structural defect of the spine involving the lamina or vertebral arch. It usually occurs between the superior and inferior articulating facets.

106. a. palliative care—The goal is to make the patient comfortable by decreasing any pain or discomfort from movement.

107. c. metastasis—Tumors are often accidentally discovered with an X-ray following a traumatic event.

108. b. 10; 15—This is a major reason for placing a patient with a suspected SCI on a backboard. This neutral position allows the most space for the cord, helping to reduce excess pressure and cord hypoxia.

109. c. They totally eliminate neck movement.—Cervical collars alone do not totally eliminate neck movement. They are used together with an immobilization device to prevent neck movement.

110. b. airway management—When the airway cannot be adequately managed with the helmet in place, it must be removed promptly without causing further injury.

111. a. compensating shock—Rapid extrication should only be used with the critical patient or when hazardous conditions will further harm the patient or rescuers.

112. c. Passenger involved in a high-speed MVC complaining of a headache after the collision.—The MOI is one of the most significant factors in the assessment and treatment of any trauma patient.

113. c. when it is necessary for the patient to be supine—In most cases, a toddler can be immobilized in a child seat. If it becomes necessary for the child to

be placed in the supine position, the child should be rapidly extricated out of the car seat onto a backboard.

114. b. position is the most comfortable for the patient.—This position is uncomfortable for most patients. Many patients complain of increased pain after being immobilized.

115. a. The goal is to prevent further injury.—Preventing secondary injury following the primary injury is paramount. The first step is to recognize the actual or potential primary injury and manage it appropriately.

116. d. lumbar and cervical—These areas of the spine are most susceptible to injury.

117. a. Palpate over each of the spinal processes.—Each process is palpated for deformity, step-offs, and free-moving bones.

118. b. foot dorsiflexion.—The patient is asked to pull up and push down against the resistance of the examiner's hands.

119. a. directions of force.—These forces include: acceleration, deceleration, flexion, hyperflexion, extension, hyperextension, vertical compression, distraction, and deformation.

120. b. neurogenic shock—A temporary loss of the autonomic function of the cord at the level of injury that controls the cardiovascular function.

Chapter 39: Abdominal and Genitourinary Trauma

1. a. second—Major hemorrhage can occur rapidly and go unrecognized. This is why abdominal trauma is a major cause of trauma death and the second leading cause of preventable trauma death.

2. b. 1.5—The adult abdominal cavity can hide a significant blood loss easily before showing any signs of distention.

3. d. associated chest injuries.—Based on the MOI, certain syndromes are common. People with abdominal injuries often have a chest injury, as well.

4. c. MOI—When the MOI is penetrating, the obvious wound is the clue to potential injury to underlying organs. When the MOI is blunt, the potential for injury is often underappreciated or not recognized at all.

5. c. rapid deceleration—MVCs often produce the rapid deceleration that can cause these types of injuries.

6. b. jejunum—The jejunum has larger, thicker walls, and is more vascular than other sections of the small intestine.

7. c. ileum—This section lies between the jejunum and the large intestine.

8. b. hernia repair—Surgical repair of a hernia.

9. a. liver—The liver is very vascular, and the blood loss from an injury can be fatal.

10. a. Visceral—The visceral peritoneum receives input from both sides of the spinal cord. This causes pain to present as diffuse rather than localized.

11. a. somatic—Somatic pain is caused by direct irritation of the parietal peritoneum. As such, it is more localized. Visceral pain is more diffuse.

12. d. liver and gallbladder—These organs are located in the upper-left quadrant of the abdomen.

13. b. intraperitoneal bleeding and/or irritation.—The location of pain often does not correspond to the actual source. However, there are referral patterns and pain associated with many conditions.

14. a. Cullen's sign.—This sign may be identified 12–24 hours after the initial injury.

15. c. testicular torsion—This condition is usually unilateral. Frequently, the patient complains of a sudden onset of extreme pain in his testicle, occurring during or after physical exertion.

16. c. Move the patient into his position of comfort, then administer analgesia and an antiemetic.—Management is primarily palliative to decrease any pain or discomfort and ease the nausea.

17. c. Manage his pain and transport gently.—Testicular torsion is an acute urological emergency that threatens the male's future reproductive capability. Manage the patient's pain and nausea while transporting to the hospital.

18. a. prompt surgery.—Even with prompt treatment, some studies report a semen analysis to be abnormal after unilateral torsion.

19. a. perforations and hemorrhage.—Perforations are common in both males and females. They are caused by foreign objects inserted into the vagina or rectum. Signs and symptoms include acute abdominal pain, tachycardia, tachypnea, fever, and a rigid abdomen.

20. b. contamination from fecal matter—All of the signs and symptoms described above are due to contamination from fecal matter.

21. a. Keep the patient in a position of comfort.—Monitor the patient for signs of shock, and treat for shock if present.

22. d. nausea and vomiting.—Treat nausea with an antiemetic.

23. c. intra-abdominal bleed.—Isolated head injury rarely causes hypotension. Intra-abdominal bleeding must be suspected when signs of shock are present but no other apparent cause for bleeding can be immediately discovered.

24. c. IV fluid replacement.—This should be done en route to the hospital.
25. d. peritonitis.—This can result at a later point, as a result of the infection from perforation.
26. c. 35%—Maternal circulation increases by nearly 50% by full term. She can lose a significant amount of blood before signs and symptoms begin to appear.
27. a. uterine inversion.—A condition where the uterus turns inside out after delivery.
28. b. shoulder—This is an established referral pattern of pain associated with diaphragmatic irritation.
29. c. pancreas—The other organs are located in the abdominal cavity.
30. d. Ileus—A bowel obstruction that is painful and impairs peristalsis.
31. b. evisceration—The patient has a slash of the abdomen allowing some abdominal contents to slip or protrude out. This is called an abdominal evisceration.

32. c. treat for shock—From a management perspective, the highest priority for the treatment of the patient would be to treat for shock since he does not need ventilator assistance at this point.
33. d. apply an occlusive dressing to the wound—The treatment of the actual wound found in the patient should be an occlusive dressing to minimize infection and keep the air out.
34. c. high priority as he is having difficulty compensating—On reassessment, the patient has rapid and shallow respirations; a weak, fast, and thready pulse; and his systolic BP is starting to drop. He is bleeding significantly, so as a high priority and moving from compensated to decompensated shock, get him moving right away.
35. d. OR of the trauma center.—Definitive care for the patient will need to be provided in the OR of the trauma center.

Chapter 40: Orthopedic Trauma

1. b. become more porous.—This causes the bones to become brittle.
2. a. bony thorax.—The thorax protects the vital organs in the chest (e.g., heart, lungs, aorta, and vena cava).
3. d. clavicle and scapula.—This structure supports the upper extremity.
4. a. tendons—The tendon allows for power of movement across the joints.
5. b. fibrous, cartilaginous, and synovial.—These are the structural classifications of joints.
6. d. producing red blood cells.—Bones also store salts (e.g., calcium) and metabolic materials.
7. a. parts of a long bone.—The ends, shaft, and covering of long bones.
8. a. Metaphysis—The area of the bone that transitions between the epiphysis and the diaphysis.
9. c. the olecranon—The process on the ulna that articulates with the humerus and forms the elbow.
10. d. ulna shaft—The radius is the bone on the thumb side of the lower arm.
11. a. acromioclavicular joint.—The joint connecting the acromion and the clavicle.
12. b. pelvis—If the fracture is complicated, such as one that severs the femoral artery, the patient can easily bleed to death.
13. d. femur—The femur is the bone of the upper leg.
14. b. condyle—The distal ends of the femur and humerus have condyles.
15. a. anterior; medial malleolus—The shinbone.
16. c. suspect significant amount of energy caused the injury.—Because children are continuously growing, most body structures have not matured. Incomplete calcification of bones makes them

softer and less likely to fracture than adult bones. Therefore, when a deformity of a bone is apparent, you must suspect that a significant amount of energy was involved in the injury and that there may also be accompanying internal injury as well.
17. d. posterior; lateral—The smaller of the two lower leg bones.
18. c. axial—The three muscle types are cardiac, skeletal, and smooth.
19. a. Smooth—Smooth muscle can relax or contract to alter the inner lumen diameter of vessels.
20. b. cartilage.—A cartilaginous joint is one in which there is cartilage connecting the bones.
21. c. Ligaments—A sprain is an injury to the ligaments around a joint.
22. b. Smooth muscle—Found in the lower airways, blood vessels, and intestines. It is under the control of the autonomic nervous system.
23. c. padded by cartilage.—Ligaments hold the joints together.
24. a. automaticity.—Only cardiac muscle has this capability.
25. b. Skeletal muscle—Smooth muscle includes the major muscle mass of the body and allows for mobility.
26. c. elbow and knee.—The hip and shoulder are ball and sockets joints, and the digits are pivot joints.
27. a. symphysis—The articulation of bones may be formed of cartilage.
28. b. gomphoses.—An example of gomphoses is teeth in the jawbone.
29. c. Syndesmoses—Bone ends that are connected by ligaments.
30. d. synovial—Examples of synovial joints include: hinge, pivot, saddle, and ball-and-socket joints.

31. c. greenstick—The fracture appears similar to how a live green tree splits.

32. d. synovial—The knee, hip, fingers, and shoulder are examples of synovial joints.

33. b. transverse—These types of fractures are obvious and gross, and may be open or closed.

34. a. 500—A complicated fracture involving a laceration to an artery can produce life-threatening hemorrhage.

35. a. subluxation.—A subluxation usually produces a great amount of damage and instability.

36. b. dislocation.—When the bone is moved from its normal position within a joint, it becomes dislocated.

37. b. Achilles rupture — The Achilles tendon is the largest tendon in the body. It connects the calf muscle to the heal bone. It can be ruptured by a sudden force on the foot or ankle. The patient may feel a pop or snapping sensation followed by immediate pain and weakness in the calf.

38. b. tibia; posterior—Dislocation of the knee and elbow is serious because they have a high probability of blood vessel and nerve damage.

39. c. brachial artery and blood supply to the arm.—Dislocation of the knee and elbow is serious because they have a high probability of blood vessel and nerve damage.

40. d. patellar tendon dislocation—The patellar tendon is actually a ligament, which connects the patella and the tibial tubercle. A patellar tendon dislocation, also called jumper's knee due to the MOI by which it can occur. On physical exam, active knee extension is impossible and flexion is limited because of pain.

41. b. bursitis and gouty arthritis.—Tendonitis is another common cause.

42. d. relieve the muscle spasms that can worsen the injury.—Controlling the spasm of the strong muscles surrounding the femur helps to minimize overriding by the broken bone ends.

43. d. transportation is long or delayed.—Delayed or prolonged transport may require a different approach. Follow your local protocol.

44. a. a knee dislocation involves the tibia popping out of the knee joint.—A patella dislocation is the movement of the kneecap from its normal position.

45. a. pelvic—Many EMS systems have relegated use of MAST/PASG to the stabilization of the pelvic or bilateral femur fractures.

46. b. Loosen the sling, then swathe and reassess.—If this does not work, consider repositioning the extremity and reassessing.

47. b. tissue hypoxia and anoxia.—A prolonged period of ischemia, greater than 6–8 hours, leads to tissue hypoxia and anoxia, and ultimately cell death.

48. d. forearm.—Commonly occurs from falls, skating, snowboarding, and skiing. Wrist guards significantly reduce the risk of Colles' fractures.

49. c. allowing the bone to protrude through the skin.—Open fractures become complicated because of the significant risk of infection.

50. c. fracture of the radius or ulna—Compartment syndrome can occur as a result of fractures with significant bleeding, in any extremity, a badly bruised muscle, and crush injuries.

Chapter 41: Environmental Trauma

1. d. atmospheric pressure.—The other choices are predisposing risk factors.

2. c. small children and geriatrics—People at the extremes of age are at greater risk for environmental emergencies. Older patients lose their ability to internally regulate their temperature, and small children have large body surface area and a very limited ability to compensate for acute major changes in temperature.

3. c. cancer—Anyone who has a serious underlying medical condition, especially if he is undernourished, is more susceptible to environmental influences.

4. b. diabetes—Many diabetics have a decreased sensation in the extremities.

5. a. tricyclic antidepressants—Many common medications have anticholinergic side effects. The result is an impaired ability to sweat and dissipate heat.

6. b. diving—Diving illness and high-altitude illness are examples of pressurization illnesses.

7. c. hypothalamus—The hypothalamus senses when the skin is too hot or cold and sets in motion a series of responses designed to warm or cool the body, all without conscious effort.

8. c. underactive thyroids—Underactive thyroids (hypothyroidism) can slow the metabolism down; therefore, the body is producing less heat and the person feels cold even in warm environments when others around them do not.

9. c. metabolic—This includes the breakdown of glucose, proteins, and fats to energy.

10. a. Thermoregulation—As the body temperature increases, changes occur in each organ system. If an individual gradually exposes himself to a hot environment, the body acclimates or becomes used to the heat.

11. a. convection—Heat is gained or dissipated from the body by four mechanisms: radiation, conduction, convection, and evaporation.

12. b. conduction.—The transmission of heat from warmer to cooler objects in direct contact.

13. d. evaporation—High humidity seriously impairs heat dissipation because evaporation occurs slowly.

14. a. dehydration.—The patient loses significant fluid and electrolytes, especially sodium. The result is increased concentrations of sodium (sometimes potassium) in the serum, with resultant symptoms.

15. b. diaphoresis and flushing.—Increased skin temperature and flushing may be present.

16. b. disrupt sodium concentrations.—People who are acclimatized to warm temperatures are less likely to suffer heat illness. Proper acclimatization requires at least a week of gradually increasing heat exposure.

17. a. urban—Cold stress among the elderly, intoxication, or debilitation can cause fatal hypothermia (urban hypothermia).

18. b. exhaustion—A more severe loss of fluid and salt than occurs in heat cramps. Some patients simply develop dehydration without further signs or symptoms of heat exhaustion.

19. a. treat for dehydration.—There is a high incidence of heat exhaustion in young children, individuals on water pills, and the debilitated (who are unable to maintain an adequate oral water intake), or those having prolonged bouts of diarrhea.

20. c. hypothermia—This finding is common in people who are relatively immobile, such as in a nursing facility.

21. c. antihistamines—The anticholinergic side effects impair the ability to sweat and dissipate heat.

22. a. take diuretics.—There is a high incidence of heat exhaustion in young children, individuals on water pills, and the debilitated (who are unable to maintain an adequate oral water intake), or those having prolonged bouts of diarrhea. Some patients simply develop dehydration without further signs or symptoms of heat exhaustion.

23. a. pyrogens—Fever usually results from an infection, though other illnesses (e.g., hyperthyroidism) may also increase the body temperature.

24. b. heat stroke—When the body's temperature continues to rise with a failing thermoregulatory system multi-organ damage and hemorrhage occur and can be fatal.

25. a. wool—A natural fiber wool is an excellent clothing material for cold and wet conditions.

26. d. anesthetic medications—Without prompt treatment to correct the problem, this condition can quickly become life threatening.

27. d. AMI—There are many common predisposing factors for hypothermia, including: extreme ages (young/old), medications, accidents, limited mobility, chronic disease, and low income. Acute MI is not a common predisposing factor.

28. b. signs and symptoms.—The severity of hypothermia is determined by the CBT and the presence of signs and symptoms. There is no reliable correlation between signs or symptoms and a specific CBT. Always obtain a reliable CBT reading.

29. b. it is impossible to tell how much current passed through vital organs.—There are too many variables to know exactly how much current passes through vital organs, even if the shock was witnessed.

30. b. subacute—Comes on over minutes to hours. The prognosis may be better than the acute onset form, unless the patient is not rescued or treated for a long period of time.

31. d. urban—This occurs to individuals who may be inside but lack appropriate thermoregulation.

32. a. stroke.—Endocrine disorders (hypothyroidism, malnutrition, and hypoglycemia) may cause hypothermia as well.

33. b. ventricular fibrillation—It may occur as the CBT drops, but it is more common in the rewarming phase.

34. a. Cold may affect the potency of first-line cardiac drugs.—Avoid lidocaine and procainamide in hypothermia because they paradoxically lower the VF threshold, increasing resistance to defibrillation. Follow your local protocols.

35. b. V-fib and asystole.—The risks of V-fib are related both to the depth and duration of hypothermia. Severe hypothermia mimics clinical death. It may be impossible to distinguish a patient who is still alive, but profoundly hypothermic, from the victim of a cardiac arrest.

36. d. the patient is handled roughly during care and transport.—There is no increased risk of inducing V-fib from orotracheal or nasotracheal intubation as long as the patient is adequately preoxygenated.

37. b. hypothermic—Many immersion victims are hypothermic.

38. d. stop ongoing heat loss.—Remove the patient from the cold environment.

39. c. ice crystals—These crystals damage the blood vessels and other tissues.

40. a. deep frostbite skin has a white, waxy appearance.—Generally there is also a complete loss of sensation that does not recover within a short period.

41. b. lack of oxygen.—The patient may say that the affected area feels "like a stump." This feeling is due to a lack of oxygen in the affected area.

42. a. the use of alcohol and mind-altering drugs.—Studies have shown that anywhere from 35–75% of drowning victims have elevated blood-alcohol levels.

43. a. they may appear normal and unaffected.—Secondary drowning may occur within a few minutes or up to 4 days later, and present in the form of pulmonary edema or aspiration pneumonia after a successful recovery from the initial incident.

44. b. hypoxia.—The mechanisms of lung damage from seawater and freshwater submersion are very different, but the endpoints are the same: decreased pulmonary compliance results in pulmonary edema and hypoxia.

45. a. metabolic acidosis.—No matter the type of water involved, the endpoints in submersion are metabolic acidosis, pulmonary edema, and aspiration injuries. Cerebral hypoxia often precipitates neurogenic pulmonary edema, worsening an already bad situation.

46. b. secondary.—Secondary drowning is the recurrence of respiratory distress after a successful recovery from the initial incident. It can occur within a few minutes or up to 4 days later.

47. d. nitrogen—The nitrogen bubbles form in the blood stream and can cause serious problems including embolism, brain injury, paralysis, blindness, and death.

48. b. time to the first spontaneous gasp following removal from the water.—The shorter this period, the better the neurological prognosis.

49. c. Secondary—The patient develops pulmonary edema or aspiration pneumonia after a successful recovery from the initial incident.

50. c. self-contained underwater breathing apparatus.—SCUBA.

51. c. Dalton's law—Room air, for example, is a mixture of nitrogen and oxygen. The total pressure in a diving tank equals the sum of each individual partial pressure.

52. a. Boyle's—In other words, as the pressure increases, the gas volume decreases.

53. a. decrease; expand.—This relates to Boyle's law of gases.

54. c. pneumothorax—Failure to exhale upon ascent from a dive causes the lungs to expand and pop.

55. b. nitrogen bubbles—Also called "the bends." This releases previously absorbed excess nitrogen from the tissues into the bloodstream in the form of bubbles.

56. a. bends.—Pain in the legs or joints is present in 90% of the cases. The most commonly involved joint is the shoulder, though multiple joints may be involved in serious cases. Recurrent pains are common.

57. b. Henry's—Henry's law states that, at a constant temperature, the solubility of any gas in a liquid is directly proportional to the pressure of the liquid. The deeper one dives, the greater the pressure and threat the soluble gas that becomes dissolved in the blood and tissue.

58. b. Asthma—Mucous plugs can trap air that cannot be exhaled properly during ascent.

59. a. air embolism—This is the most serious diving-related emergency. Because divers most commonly ascend in a vertical position, bubbles of air in the bloodstream often travel to the brain.

60. c. Consider decompression therapy.—Hyperbaric O_2 is beneficial for both air embolism and decompression sickness.

61. d. ruptured eardrum from barotrauma—This is a pressure-related injury that occurs when the air in the middle ear can't escape through the Eustachian tube and ruptures the eardrum.

62. d. air embolism—Even late recompression of decompression sickness problems can be accomplished with relief of symptoms and morbidity.

63. a. lack of recognition of symptoms.—Often there is wishful thinking that symptoms will just go away.

64. b. decompression sickness—The most common and often life-threatening injury associated with scuba diving is decompression illness, which is either decompression sickness or arterial gas embolism.

65. b. descent—Gas-associated problems (hypoxia due to equipment failure or carbon monoxide poisoning) commonly occur at this point also.

66. d. high-altitude pulmonary edema (HAPE)—HAPE occurs when increased pulmonary artery pressures develop from hypoxia. This leads to the release of various vasoactive substances that increase alveolar permeability. Fluids leak into the alveoli, and pulmonary edema occurs.

67. b. hypoxia.—The most common altitude syndromes are acute mountain sickness (AMS), high-altitude pulmonary edema (HAPE), and high-altitude cerebral edema (HACE).

68. a. skydiving—High-altitude illness occurs as a result of decreased atmospheric pressure that causes hypoxia. Typical skydiving does not allow enough time in the conditions that would cause these syndromes.

69. a. AMS—This condition occurs after rapid ascent by an unacclimatized person to altitudes in excess of 8,000 feet.

70. a. administer high-flow oxygen.—The most important treatments are rapid descent and oxygen.

71. a. helium—Liquid helium is the coldest known fluid and is used as a coolant in cryogenics. Skin contact can cause dry skin, rash, contact dermatitis, and frostbite.

72. a. eyes.—Ultraviolet radiation can easily damage the cornea causing pain, changes in vision, or loss of vision. Sources include the sun, sun lamps, halogen lamps, welder's arc, photographer's flood lamps, light from transilluminators, and UV germicidal lamps just to name a few.

73. c. ears and sinuses—Squeeze syndromes are caused by excess pressure involving the ears and sinuses.

74. c. His glucose stores are depleted.—As the energy stores (liver and muscle glycogen) are exhausted, shivering will cease and the CBT will drop.

75. a. impaired thinking—Nitrogen narcosis, often referred to as "rapture of the depths," is the development of an apathetic, slight euphoric mental state due to the

narcotic effect of dissolved nitrogen. This effect is analogous to excessive ethanol levels.

76. c. 55—High humidity seriously impairs heat dissipation because evaporation occurs slowly.

77. b. drink warm fluids.—Warm fluids will help warm the patient and restore energy.

78. c. providing high-quality CPR—Continue CPR and stabilize the spine due to the MOI.

79. a. gastric distention—The stomach may contain water from the drowning and aggressive ventilations, and overfill as a result. Consider abdominal decompression.

80. a. decompress the stomach.—The stomach may contain water from the drowning and aggressive ventilations, and overfill as a result. Consider abdominal decompression.

Chapter 42: Special Consideration in Trauma and Multisystem Trauma

1. a. kinematics of trauma.—Looking at a trauma scene and attempting to determine what injuries might have resulted is examining the kinematics of trauma.

2. c. weight—The weight of an item/patient and its speed contribute to the kinetic energy at a trauma call.

3. b. velocity.—Another term for the speed the projectile was traveling that needs to be taken into consideration when determining the potential injury is the velocity.

4. d. fragmentation.—In the instance of penetrating trauma, when a projectile causes bones to break and cause secondary injuries, this is referred to as fragmentation.

5. b. cavitation.—The momentary acceleration of tissue away from the tract of the projectile is known as cavitation.

6. a. low—When a patient has a penetrating injury that was caused by a stabbing with a steak knife, this was most likely low-energy (<200 feet per second) trauma.

7. c. high-energy trauma.—When a patient sustains penetrating trauma from a military (rifle) weapon, it is most likely high-energy trauma.

8. b. roll-over—The greatest potential for occupant ejection, if unrestrained, occurs in a roll-over collision.

9. b. side impact—The side impact collision often presents with patient injuries such as fractured humerus, rib injuries, and hip injuries.

10. c. rotational—An impact where the vehicle spins around the point of impact and the injuries of the unrestrained occupant are unpredictable is called a rotational impact.

11. c. chest.—Your patient was the driver of a frontal collision and was not restrained. Most likely if the windshield is cracked, he may have sustained injuries to his head, neck, and chest.

12. a. the need to bandage all the soft tissue injuries.—When a patient sustains multisystem trauma from an automobile crash, the paramedic should consider: spinal immobilization, the appropriate transportation destination, and the mechanism of injury and kinematics. Bandaging all the soft tissue injuries is not a high priority.

13. b. A team of surgeons is needed to treat the multisystem trauma patient.—It is important to consider transporting the multisystem trauma patient to the trauma center because a team of surgeons is needed to treat the multisystem trauma patient.

14. c. blast—Aside from a motor vehicle crash, a good example of a mechanism that has significant potential to produce multisystem trauma would be a blast injury.

15. a. total body surface area.—Each of the following is a consideration in the extent of the injuries with an explosion or blast injury: the blast wave damage, the blast winds damage, the heat generated, and ground shock.

Chapter 43: Obstetrics

1. b. embryo.—During the embryonic period, all the major organ systems begin to develop.

2. d. returning oxygenated blood from the placenta to the fetus.—The two arteries return deoxygenated blood from the fetus to the placenta.

3. a. zygote.—After fertilization, the zygote begins cell division and forms a hollow ball called a blastocyst as it moves into the uterine cavity, where it implants on the uterine wall.

4. a. pregnancy—Amenorrhea, or the suppression of menstruation, is normal during pregnancy and abnormal in other circumstances.

5. b. abruptio placenta.—Abruptio is characterized by severe constant pain with or without bleeding and occurs after 20 weeks' gestation.

6. b. Treat for shock and begin transport.—The premature separation causes blood loss that is not always apparent because it may be trapped behind

the placenta. If the separation is complete, most often the fetus will die.

7. b. destroy fetal cells.—After the termination of any pregnancy, either by birth or abortion, the mother is given an injection of immune globulin to suppress her immune response.

8. c. pulmonary embolism—This condition occurs frequently and has a high mortality rate. It results from a blood clot in the pelvic circulation. This can occur during pregnancy, labor, or postpartum.

9. d. rapid transport for a life-threatening condition.— Appropriate treatment includes high-concentration oxygen and vascular access with gentle but rapid transport to an appropriate facility.

10. a. hypertension—Pregnancy-associated hypertension (140/90 mm Hg) is an indication of possible toxemia. Preexisting hypertension requires close monitoring.

11. d. growing tissue may destroy maternal structures.— Ectopic means "out of place". In ectopic pregnancy, the fertilized egg attaches somewhere outside of the uterus and as it grows it will eventually burst the organ that contains it, causing severe life-threatening bleeding for the mother.

12. a. spine—Rubbing the patient's lower back during labor can help to ease the discomfort.

13. c. oxytocin—Stretch receptors in the uterine walls sense the increased stretch produced by the movement of the uterus, and this triggers the pituitary gland to secrete the hormone oxytocin.

14. b. Labor is 2 weeks early, but the mother is mentally competent and refuses.—Any adult patient who is alert and competent has the right to refuse any or all care offered.

15. d. holding one hand on the baby's head while the mother is pushing.—This may help to reduce tearing of the perineum.

16. b. inspect for a nuchal cord.—Nuchal cord is common and must be recognized and corrected quickly to prevent strangulation and hypoxia.

17. a. laterally.—The baby's head will turn to the left or right, then the shoulders will appear.

18. a. reflex and color.—Each sign is rated 0, 1, or 2, depending on the findings at 1 and 5 minutes after birth.

19. c. the baby will be easier to manage and assess.— Typically there is no hurry to cut the cord, unless the baby or mother is in distress. If the cord is not cut

immediately, the infant should be kept at a level lower than the placenta to prevent placental transfusion.

20. b. at a lower level than the placenta—This is a gravity thing. If the baby is raised above the level of the placenta, the baby's blood will drain out.

21. c. umbilical vein cannulation—Umbilical vein cannulation is preferred in neonatal resuscitation because the vein is so easy to identify and cannulate. The skill does take practice, and a special umbilical catheter is used.

22. c. the right side of the board elevated slightly.—This position helps to keeps the fetus off the mother's vena cava in an effort to allow adequate blood return to the heart.

23. a. aggressive fluid replacement.—Appropriate management of this patient includes aggressive management of the ABCs and rapid transport to a trauma center.

24. d. in the clinical setting and not in the field.— Assessing the fetal heart rate is the standard of care in the clinical setting to determine if the fetus is in any distress.

25. d. shunting of blood from the fetus.—The mother's body will begin to decrease circulation to non-vital organs (skin and GI) when it goes into shock. In a state of shock, the mother's body treats the fetus as a foreign object and shunts blood from the placenta to its own heart, brain, and lungs.

26. b. Prepare for imminent delivery.—A multiparous woman will know when she is about to deliver. Listen to her, and prepare to assist with the delivery. This can be done in the ambulance, and transport may be started.

27. c. Observe the birth canal for crowning.—Crowning is a clear indication that birth is about to happen.

28. b. Treat for shock and begin transport.—Significant blood loss can occur with postpartum hemorrhage, and this must be managed aggressively. If possible, bring the placenta to the hospital for inspection. An incomplete placenta could be the cause of the bleeding, and inspection can help rule out a cause.

29. b. cover the protruding tissue with moist, sterile dressings.—This is a true emergency that requires aggressive treatment and rapid transport.

30. c. Allow the cord to deliver and support the body.—The head may require extra attention in passing through the vaginal opening. Support the body to prevent tearing of the neck muscles and blood vessels.

Chapter 44: Neonatal Care and Pediatrics

1. a. umbilical vein—The umbilical vein, which leads from the placenta to the fetus is different from other veins in that it carries oxygenated blood rather than deoxygenated blood to the right atrium of the heart.

2. c. ductus venosus—In utero, the ductus venosus empties into the inferior vena cava.

3. a. foramen ovale—The opening in the septal wall between the right and left atria in the fetus.

4. a. persistent fetal circulation—Hypoxia or acidosis can trigger the pulmonary vascular bed to constrict and reopen the ductus arteriosus, creating fetal circulation as in utero. The danger here is that the majority of the circulation is then shunted from the right heart to the left heart, bypassing the lungs.

5. c. stimulating the newborn to breathe.—In addition, the baby must be kept warm and assisted with oxygenation and ventilation as required.

6. d. apnea of infancy.—This condition usually resolves itself, but does need to be monitored until such time.

7. a. caffeine—Additional treatments include positioning the child on its back to sleep, and continuous positive airway pressure (CPAP).

8. b. three—The extra genetic material disrupts their physical and cognitive development.

9. d. flat facial profile with a small nose and depressed nasal bridge—The tongue is very large, the eyes have an upward slant and a small fold on the inner corners, and the ears are small with an abnormal shape (dysplastic ears).

10. d. an excessive space between the large and second toe.—Other distinguishing features include: a single deep crease across the palm of the hand, overall weak body muscle tone, and excessive ability to extend the joints.

11. b. exposed spinal structures.—There are three common types of spina bifida: occulta, meningocele, and myelomeningocele.

12. b. no prenatal care—Inadequate or no prenatal care is an avoidable factor that can affect childbirth.

13. b. prolonged labor—Other factors include: preterm labor, prolapsed cord, abnormal limb or fetal presentation, meconium staining or aspiration syndrome, and a mother's use of narcotics just before delivery.

14. a. Birth defects—Approximately 1 in 33 infants born annually in the United States are born with birth defects. Birth defects are the leading cause of infant death with 1 in 5.

15. b. Multiple fetuses—This is a significant antepartum factor that classifies a newborn as high risk.

16. a. dry and stimulate—After completing the initial steps and the infant does not respond, more aggressive interventions will be necessary and will include ventilation, chest compression, and medications.

17. b. infant feeding problems—Prenatal drug use increases the risk of miscarriage, premature labor, fetal stroke, death, abruptio placenta, low birth weight, birth defects, feeding problems, sleep disorders, SIDS, and the slowed development of motor skills.

18. d. respiratory effort, pulse rate, and skin color.—The primary assessment is the same as with any other patient: airway, breathing, and circulation.

19. c. appearance, pulse, grimace, activity, and reflex.—APGAR is assessed and given a score of 0, 1, or 2 at 1 and 5 minutes after birth.

20. d. metabolic—Specific tests vary from state to state.

21. b. poor growth and mental retardation.—This is an example of a condition that may be screened for at birth.

22. a. low birth weight, small head, and small eye openings—Fetal alcohol syndrome (FAS) results from maternal alcohol consumption. Even the consumption of very small amounts of alcohol during pregnancy can have serious effects on a developing fetus.

23. d. central nervous system problems.—Even the consumption of very small amounts of alcohol during pregnancy can have serious effects on a developing fetus. Children with FAS can have problems with learning, memory, attention span, communication, vision, or hearing.

24. c. decreased mental status of the newborn—Maternal narcotic use within 4 hours of delivery can depress the fetus and is associated with respiratory depression at birth.

25. c. Administer oxygen, assist ventilations, and administer Narcan®.—Treatment is similar to adult narcotic overdose.

26. b. always have their own placenta.—This is an accurate statement.

27. b. fractured clavicle—This occurs when the shoulders are too large to fit through the birth canal.

28. b. Assist with ventilations by bag mask.—The next step in resuscitation is to assist with ventilations by bag mask. If this fails to stimulate the child to breathe and increase the heart rate, compressions are started.

29. d. Start CPR.—If assisted ventilations fail to stimulate the child to breathe and increase the heart rate, compressions are started.

30. a. keeping the baby warm and continuing oxygen delivery.—Follow local protocols and medical direction for additional interventions.

31. c. fluid imbalance—Airway and fluid imbalance problems are the most common potentially life-threatening disorders that affect neonates.

32. b. surfactant—Surfactant is not present in adequate quantities until after 34 weeks' gestation.

33. c. umbilical—An opening or weakened muscles around the bellybutton permit a bulge when the infant cries, coughs, or strains.

34. a. hypoglycemia.—Additional causes include alcohol or drug withdrawal and, less commonly, genetic or metabolic disorders.

35. b. immature thermoregulatory system.—An infection from a virus or bacteria is the most common cause of fever in neonates. Due to the immature thermoregulatory system, any fever is serious and requires evaluation.

36. d. before, during, and after.—This is a fact.

37. c. bilirubin.—This condition usually disappears within 5–7 days after birth. The most common treatment is exposing the infant to ultraviolet lights to help break down the extra bilirubin so the baby's liver can process it.

38. c. 2–3 days—Jaundice occurs when a baby's immature liver cannot dispose of excess bilirubin.

39. a. drug withdrawal.—Complications can result from the aspiration of vomitus, electrolyte imbalance, or dehydration due to the loss of fluids.

40. d. electrolyte imbalance.—A congenital abnormality of the pyloric valve (pyloric stenosis) leads to vomiting within a few days after birth.

41. b. all stools are loose.—A general guideline is to consider more than six stools a day to be excessive.

42. b. hernias.—Intestinal obstruction and congenital abnormalities are other causes of abdominal distention in the neonate.

43. b. to watch the baby's airway.—Full stomachs and vomiting go hand in hand with babies.

44. c. toddler—Generally speaking, toddlers do not like to be touched by strangers or separated from their parents. They do not like their clothing removed, they frighten easily, and they often overreact. They do not want to be "suffocated" by an oxygen mask.

45. c. preschool—Children in this age group may believe that their illness is a punishment for being bad. They fear pain, blood, and permanent injury.

45. d. adolescent—They want to be treated as adults. They may feel they are indestructible, but may also have fears of permanent injury and disfigurement.

47. b. 6—A stuffy nose or mucus in the nose can be a complete, serious airway obstruction.

48. a. head injury.—In a healthy infant, the fontanels are normally soft and flat. They may sink when dehydrated or in shock, and bulge when crying or when there is increased pressure in the head (ICP).

49. b. Abdominal or "belly breathing" is normal in this age group.—The infant's respiratory muscles are not well developed, and they use their abdominal muscles to help them breathe. The infant becomes fatigued easily, and, in cases of severe respiratory distress, as the child attempts to compensate, sternal retractions occur.

50. a. They do not have the ability to shiver to create body heat.—Infants have immature and underdeveloped thermoregulatory systems, making it difficult for them to maintain their body temperature.

51. d. Trauma—The leading cause of trauma death in pediatrics is MVCs.

52. a. respiratory depression—Many of the ingested products cause life-threatening symptoms in the respiratory, CNS, and circulatory systems.

53. b. Injuries to the head, face, and neck occur with more frequency in children than in adults.—Due to the relatively larger size of the child's head, face,

and neck, these areas are injured more frequently than in adults.

54. a. during the winter months.—Other risk factors that have been identified include: male, premature, and low-birth weight infants are at high risk; infants with respiratory infection are at high risk; and maternal smoking, placing the infant on the stomach, and a family history of SIDS are also high risks.

55. b. viral infections.—Cold or flu are the most common triggers. Other common triggers include: exposure to smoke, irritants, or strong odors; exercise; allergies; respiratory infections; and stress or emotions.

56. a. headache and muscle ache.—Stomachache and lack of energy are also common physical complaints.

57. a. emotional—Child abuse and neglect occur when a child is injured or allowed to be injured by someone who was entrusted with their care.

58. b. the location and color of each bruise.—Be objective and report exactly what you see.

59. b. signs of malnourishment—The others are signs of physical abuse.

60. a. severe head trauma.—Because infants have weak neck muscles and heads that are proportionately larger than their bodies, small rips and tears occur in the brain. This can result in a subdural hematoma from the bleeding, swelling of the brain (edema), and/or retinal hemorrhages.

61. b. under 1 year old when trauma is inflicted.—Other predisposing risk factors include: male child (60%), young parents, families below the poverty level, and a baseline with a preexisting medical or physical disability.

62. a. the same—The risk factors vary in each age group.

63. c. meningitis—To date, there is no vaccination for meningitis.

64. a. rash and feces.—The disease is spread by direct contact with rashes and fecal matter. Frequent hand washing helps to prevent the spread of this disease.

65. c. saliva or blood.—This disease is spread by direct contact with blood and saliva.

66. c. meningococcemia meningitis—This type of bacterial meningitis requires special isolation procedures, because it is highly contagious.

67. a. Febrile seizures have no lasting neurological effects.—These seizures are associated with a rapid rise in body temperatures. The post-ictal period is usually brief, but the child remains tired from the event.

68. d. Asthma—Asthma can occur at any age but is prominent in the 3-to 12-year-old age group.

69. b. presenting with Reye's syndrome.—This disease process affects multiple body systems and is characterized by severe edema of the brain, increased ICP, hypoglycemia, and liver dysfunction. The cause is unknown, but it is usually associated with

a previous viral infection. There is also an association between the administration of aspirin for fever, particularly with flu and chicken pox.

70. b. IV fluids and seizure precautions.—Out-of-hospital treatment is supportive of the ABCs, with IV fluids and seizure precautions.

71. c. inflammation, excess mucus production, and bronchoconstriction—To date, it is still unknown what causes asthma. However, there are various triggers that are well known.

72. c. Bronchiolitis—Bronchiolitis is produced by a viral infection. Symptoms are often indistinguishable from asthma.

73. d. asthma attack—Air trapping and difficulty exhaling are major characteristics of asthma.

74. c. nebulized Ventolin.—Keep the child calm and provide continuous nebulized bronchodilators (e.g., albuterol, ipratropium, epinephrine, or levalbuterol).

75. d. Pneumonia—Ask about a recent history of upper respiratory infection.

76. d. As airways enlarge, some children outgrow the condition.—There is a tendency for some children to outgrow the condition.

77. c. decreased level of consciousness.—When the child can no longer compensate and becomes physically exhausted, ventilatory failure and respiratory arrest quickly follow.

78. a. prolonged infection.—Sepsis, metabolic disorders, or brain disorders affecting thermoregulatory centers can be the cause of hypothermia in pediatrics.

79. c. hyperglycemic.—High blood sugar, excess thirst (polydipsia), and urination (polyuria) are the signs of new onset diabetes mellitus.

80. d. while the fetus is developing in utero.—These defects occur while the child is developing and are present at birth.

81. a. disrupt normal blood flow.—There are more than thirty-five different types of heart defects.

82. a. stenosis.—Many conditions can be corrected surgically due to significant advances in surgery.

83. d. asystole.—Irregular rhythms, murmurs, and bundle-branch blocks are generally not as common in children as adults.

84. c. hypoxia—Hypoxia leads to acidosis and suppression of the SA node, causing bradycardia. Correction of the hypoxia with oxygen usually corrects the bradycardia.

85. b. conjunctivitis.—Also called pink eye.

86. d. dehydration.—A common childhood condition caused by one or a combination of the following: fever, nausea, vomiting, diarrhea, burns, loss of appetite, and poor feeding.

87. d. gentle cooling measures—Febrile seizures, in most cases, do not require aggressive or invasive treatment modalities. Gentle cooling and fever reducers (acetaminophen) work in most cases. If seizures persist, Valium is indicated.

88. c. epiglottitis.—A relatively rare, potentially life-threatening infection that causes a severely inflamed and swollen epiglottis. Infection can occur at any age, but 3–6 years of age is the most common.

89. b. Visualize the airway for an obstruction.—Allow the child to take the most comfortable, but safe, position. Keep the child calm, and avoid alarming the child by looking in the airway, slamming ambulance doors, using excessive speed, or using the siren.

90. a. Consider the use of blow-by oxygen.—It is paramount to keep the child calm and avoid agitating him, as this can worsen the condition. The swollen epiglottis has the potential to completely obstruct the airway.

91. a. immediate but calm transport.—The safest means of transport is to use the child's own car seat. The child is familiar with its own seat and tends to stay calm there. Keep a parent next to the child, within the patient's eyesight.

92. b. the patient's mental status.—Respiratory depression and depressed mental status are the concerns with methadone overdose.

93. c. 0.1 mg/kg naloxone.—If respiratory depression needs to be reversed, administer naloxone slowly to bring the patient to a more alert status. Be prepared to manage an agitated and possible physical patient!

94. b. head, chest, and lower extremities—By the MOI, head injury is probably the reason for unconsciousness. The size of the patient places the child at risk for specific injury patterns that involve the head, chest, and lower extremities.

95. b. Waddel's triad.—The child is tall enough that the bumper strikes the femurs (1); the child is thrown up onto the hood, striking the chest (2); and the child is thrown to the ground, where he strikes his head (3); creating a predictable triad of injuries.

96. d. a shunt that drains into the abdomen.—Hydrocephalus is treated with surgical placement of a shunt or ETV. It is not a cure and rarely does treatment last a lifetime without complications.

97. d. malfunction of the shunt.—Signs and symptoms vary from person to person and can include headache, nausea, vomiting, sleepiness, personality changes, coma, and death.

98. d. Respiratory syncytial virus—Respiratory syncytial virus (RSV) is a viral disease of the lungs and the leading cause of lower respiratory tract infections in infants and young children.

99. c. digestive system.—CF affects the cells of the sweat glands in the skin, lungs, liver, pancreas, reproductive, and digestive systems. Children with CF have problems gaining weight.

100. a. thick mucus traps bacteria.—CF causes the body to produce mucus that is thick and sticky. The two organs most affected are the lungs and pancreas causing digestive problems. The thick mucus in the lungs traps bacteria causing infections.

Chapter 45: Geriatrics

1. d. Gerontology—The comprehensive study of aging and the problems associated with aging.
2. b. loss of elastic fiber.—The loss of sebaceous glands and vascularity in the skin affects thermoregulation.
3. b. decreased muscle and bone mass.—Consistent weight-bearing exercise can slow this process.
4. c. the chest wall becomes stiff and rigid, increasing the risk for fractures.— Other age-related changes affecting the respiratory system include: decreased gag reflex, which increases the risk of aspiration; diminished lung capacity with the loss of elasticity; and decreased cilia, which increases the risk of infectious pulmonary disease.
5. b. catecholamine—Cardiac output decreases with age, and coronary artery disease predominates in the elderly.
6. d. increased depression—The other choices are sociological rather than psychological.
7. a. decrease in thyroid function.—These changes bring about a long list of symptoms: fatigue, weakness, cold intolerance, muscle and joint aches, hypertension, and many more.
8. b. the drop in sexual hormone levels.—The ovaries begin to produce less of the three sex hormones: estrogen, androgen, and progesterone.
9. c. menopausal syndrome.—Some of the symptoms include: fatigue, depression, headaches, irritability, nervousness, insomnia, stress, incontinence, decreased sexual drive, and vaginal dryness.
10. b. five—Most of the baby boomer generation will be age 65 or older by this year.
11. d. Rheumatoid arthritis—Also called RA, it is an inflammatory disease that affects joints in the body, causing pain, deformity, and destruction of the joint.
12. c. quadruple—Depressive symptoms are an important indicator of the general well-being and mental health of older Americans.
13. a. heart disease—Risk factors for heart disease include obesity, hypertension, diabetes, smoking, elevated cholesterol, poor diet, and lack of exercise.
14. d. brain and vessels tear on the sharp, bony edges inside the skull.—The brain atrophies (shrinks) with age. The subdural space enlarges, and veins become stretched. When the patient experiences rapid acceleration or deceleration forces, the brain and vessels tear on the sharp, bony edges inside the skull.
15. b. Younger adults tend to die from ACS rather than heart failure.—Heart failure is more common in those over 65. The underlying cause of heart failure may be from an acute MI, dysrhythmia, aneurysm, anemia, fever, or hypertension.
16. a. diminished pain perception.—A decreased catecholamine response affects the ability to increase the heart rate in response to stress and exercise.

This may mask the typical pain a younger person might experience. Certain medications (beta-blockers) have the same effect.

17. c. hypertension—One of the main problems associated with hypertension is that it is often asymptomatic until severe complications (e.g., stroke) occur.
18. d. pulmonary embolism—The history suggests pulmonary embolism: a patient that presents with difficulty breathing that progressively worsens, pleuritic chest pain, anxiety, leg pain, and typically no cough or fever. Often the patient is overweight with a history of heart failure, recent surgery or immobilization, and estrogen use.
19. a. IV access only.—The patient has a cardiac history with respiratory distress. She also has a history that suggests the possibility of a pulmonary embolus. Contact medical control for early notification and any other orders.
20. d. neurologic—Behavioral emergencies include: anxiety, paranoia, hostility, wandering, and uncooperativeness; psychiatric—depression; and metabolic—dehydration, infection, and drug toxicity.
21. b. injuries from falling.—Emergencies in Parkinson's patients usually result from falls, dementia, and dysphagia.
22. b. Alzheimer's—A major, leading cause of death in the elderly. It can run its course in just a few years or last as long as 20 years; the average is 9 years.
23. c. Depressive symptoms—Higher rates of depressive symptoms are associated with higher rates of physical illness, functional disability, and higher health care resource usage.
24. a. hypothermia.—Symptoms associated with hypothyroidism include: fatigue, weakness, cold intolerance, muscle and joint aches, hypertension, and many more.
25. c. Dementia—Some causes of dementia include: drugs, chemicals, toxins, metabolic disorders, infections, stroke, tumors, trauma, emotional problems, vision or hearing deficits, and nutritional deficits.
26. c. hemorrhoids and colorectal cancer.—Other common causes include: peptic ulcer, diverticular disease, and angiodysplasia.
27. a. bowel obstruction—Signs and symptoms of a bowel obstruction are acute onset of pain, cramps, vomiting, distention, and constipation.
28. b. stable with a bowel obstruction—The patient states that she is in a lot of pain. The acute onset of pain with cramps suggests a bowel obstruction. Her vital signs are stable.
29. d. hydrocodone—Pain medications (e.g., codeine) often cause constipation.
30. b. Paget's disease—For bone diseases, Paget's is second only to osteoporosis in frequency.

31. c. ibuprofen—This is one of the most common non-steroidal anti-inflammatories (NSAIDs). The most serious side effect of NSAIDs is GI bleeding.

32. d. drug toxicity.—Geriatric patients have a higher risk of an adverse reaction. If a patient is taking a medication, assume that it could be contributing to just about any health problem.

33. d. senior retirement facilities—The other choices are types of nursing homes, to which federal regulations apply.

34. a. intermediate care facility—This is one type of nursing facility.

35. b. shingles—The same virus that causes chickenpox causes herpes zoster. Pain along the site of future eruptions typically precedes the rash by 2–30 days. The rash follows the past of one or more dermatomes in a unilateral pattern.

36. b. the tasks of daily living.—Affective disorders, such as forgetfulness, distractibility, or difficulty following directions, interfere with the tasks of daily living. Injuries commonly occur with driving, falling, wandering, and cooking.

37. a. digitalis—With aging, there is a decrease in circulation as well as renal and liver functions, which in turn causes a decrease in the metabolic rate and results in more drugs in the system. The increased amount of drugs in the system can reach lethal levels, commonly referred to as drug toxicity. Some of the most common drugs that produce drug toxicity are digitalis, lidocaine, and various beta-blockers.

38. c. Pressure sores—The greatest incidence occurs in those of 65 years of age. Prevention is the best medicine.

39. c. severe infection.—Because of a decrease in the function of the thermoregulatory system and the body's impaired ability to maintain homeostasis, even a modest elevation or subnormal temperature is an indication for concern. This is especially true when it is associated with confusion, loss of appetite, or other behavioral changes. Consider that hypothermia in the elderly is due to a severe infection (e.g., pneumonia, urinary tract infections, and sepsis) until proven otherwise.

40. d. family members.—Abusers can be anyone that an older person comes in contact with.

41. d. and once infected the victim will develop chickenpox.—Herpes zoster or shingles can be spread from an affected person to babies, children, immunosupressed persons, and adults who have not had chickenpox. Instead of developing shingles, these people develop chickenpox. Later in life the virus reemerges as shingles.

42. b. obtaining infectious pulmonary diseases.—The cilia in the airway act as a filter. When the filter and cough reflex become less effective, the risk of developing a respiratory illness increases. A diminished gag reflex increases the risk of aspiration.

43. a. cause any additional injury.—The older patient can be very fragile. Bones can be easily fractured during a move.

44. c. urinary tract infection—The very warm skin combined with the altered mental status indicate a possible infection. UTIs are common in elderly women, especially when they are inactive or have limited mobility. Additional causes of acute infection include: UTI, pneumonia, sepsis, viral infections, meningitis, encephalitis, malaria, and cerebral abscess.

45. b. vertebral fractures.—Hip fractures in older people increase their mortality significantly during the following year. This is true even if the patient is in good health prior to suffering the fracture.

46. a. developing dementia—Dementia is not a normal part of aging. In fact, only 30% of patients over 85 years of age show a significant progressive decline in cognitive function.

47. c. hypoglycemia—Hypoxia and hypoglycemia must be ruled out first in any patient with altered mental status, not just the elderly.

48. a. embolism—Problems that arise with VADs are due to infection, clotting, dislodgement, extravasations, hemorrhage, embolism, or an infusion given too rapidly.

49. d. ventilatory support as needed and rapid transport.—Making sure the patient is getting adequate oxygenation and ventilation is the primary goal in managing an embolism.

50. b. Diabetes—Complications of diabetes lead to many other diseases.

Chapter 46: Patients with Special Challenges

1. c. sensorineural—One of two types of hearing impairments. The nervous system is unable to perceive or transmit sound impulses due to damage to nerve or brain tissue.

2. d. unless you are making direct eye contact.—Many people with borderline hearing impairment are unaware that they have a problem. If a patient frequently asks you to repeat what you said, suspect a hearing impairment.

3. b. Speaking slowly with exaggerated lip movement.—Many deaf and hearing-impaired people are able to read lips. Speak slowly, but do not exaggerate your

lip movements. Lip readers are trained to read normal lip movement, not exaggerated ones.

4. c. strokes and CNS infections.—The two most common etiologies of visual impairment are injury and disease.

5. a. acute head injury—Sometimes acute head injury may cause transient blindness.

6. a. fluency—Stuttering may also be associated with psychiatric or developmental disorders.

7. a. aphasia.—Common causes include: stroke, head injury, brain tumor, delayed development, hearing loss, lack of stimulation, or emotional disturbance.

8. b. dysarthria.—An articulation disorder; patients often have slurred, indistinct, slow, or nasal-sounding speech. .

9. d. voice production—Though the neuromuscular pathways are intact, voice production disorders result from factors that impair the proper functioning of the vocal cords.

10. a. hearing loss with an acute onset—An acute loss is often associated with an emergent event (e.g., trauma or stroke).

11. a. a low metabolic rate.—Other etiologies include excess insulin production and the use of steroids.

12. c. psychoses—The person with psychoses truly believes his situation or condition is real.

13. b. talk—In a drug-induced psychosis, hallucinogens or stimulant agents cause the patient to lose touch with reality. Often, the patient develops hyperactive and sometimes dangerous behavior.

14. b. the brain.—Developmental disabilities result in an inability to learn at the usual rate.

15. b. occur in the victim's home.—Most cases of elder abuse occur in the victim's home by family, other household members, or paid caregivers.

16. d. deficiency of neurotransmitters.—Psychosis is when the patient has no concept of reality. This condition may also be induced by drugs.

17. a. maladaptive behavior.—This means that a person is unable to properly adapt to various challenging circumstances for a variety of different reasons.

18. a. Decreased range of motion may limit the physical exam.—More time than usual may be necessary to complete a physical exam and to move the patient.

19. a. transdermal medication patches.—Be alert for these, as they are not always obvious. Too much pain medication can cause altered mental status, respiratory depression, and other problems necessitating the call for EMS.

20. c. understands everything you say and do.—Cerebral palsy is a nonprogressive disorder of movement and posture. Most patients are highly intelligent.

21. b. is prone to mood disorders.—This is a common problem associated with multiple sclerosis patients.

22. a. many common medications may worsen an exacerbation.—Always contact medical control prior to administering any drugs other than oxygen.

23. a. catheters—If present, catheters may need attention. Problems with shunts may also be the purpose of an EMS call, but care of these problems is managed in the hospital.

24. a. 6–12 months—The phrase "terminally ill" is subject to widespread interpretation. For EMS providers, it usually means the patient has a condition that, regardless of any current available treatment, will result in death within the next 6–12 months.

25. a. DNAR status.—The most important consideration for the paramedic is a clear understanding of the patient's "end of life" decisions. Follow your local protocol for "no code," "living will," and other related determinations. Whenever possible, follow the patient's wishes.

26. c. try to convince him that his health should be the first priority.—Competent patients do have the right to refuse any or all care offered. When a patient has a financial concern, knowledge about your local resources may make the difference.

27. b. Acknowledge that the competent patient has a right to refuse care.—Competent patients do have the right to refuse any or all care offered.

28. b. There are signs of neglect.—Signs of neglect by a caregiver include: being left dirty or unbathed, unsafe living conditions, malnutrition, dehydration, unsuitable clothing, unsanitary living conditions, or untreated physical problems.

29. b. high-pitched—This is why you should avoid shouting and use low-pitched sounds directly in the ear canal.

30. b. multiple sclerosis—Many disease processes cause both temporary and permanent vision loss.

31. c. Pad the contractures and use extra care during the move.—Gentle handling may take extra time, but it is necessary. Make the patient as comfortable as possible and never force an extremity, as it may cause an injury.

32. a. respiratory support—This may include oxygenation, assisted ventilation, CPAP, or suctioning.

33. b. pointing to an area of the body before touching it.—A calm and professional manner goes far. Facial expressions are universal.

34. d. culture-based preferences may conflict with a paramedic's learned medical practice.—Be aware of cultural differences, but not to the point of limiting your thinking about the other person.

35. c. Notify the nurse you gave report to.—Mandatory reporting requirements for EMS providers vary from state to state, but usually EMS providers have a requirement to make a report or personally nofity a mandated reporter (e.g., physician or nurse) in the receiving facility.

36. d. appropriately sized diagnostic devices.—One example is the need for an extra-large blood pressure cuff.

37. b. has concurrent multiple health problems.—With little or no access to preventive care, homeless people often suffer from several ailments simultaneously. The problems are often complex and interrelated.

38. a. describe everything she is going to do before actually doing it.—Don't hesitate to ask patients about the best way you can help them navigate.

39. b. hospice programs—Hospices also provide services for the patient's family.

40. a. may not exhibit the normal pain response.—Some patients with autism do not have normal sensations and may not feel cold, heat, or pain in a typical manner and may fail to recognize pain in spite of significant pathology being present.

41. b. obstructed tubing—Problems arise with airway devices when they are improperly placed or become obstructed, and when oxygen tubing becomes blocked or the oxygen runs out.

42. a. involving the alert and oriented patient in any decisions regarding movement and transport.—Chances are good that the patient has gone through the move before. The patient often knows more about his own particular needs than you do.

43. a. psychotic person—When psychosis is drug induced (e.g., hallucinogens or stimulants), it is common for the patient to develop hyperactive and sometimes dangerous behavior.

44. c. 20–30%—There are numerous underlying and often related causes.

45. d. economic—Hospice programs and services provide significant support for the dying person and the family members as the death experience come to a culmination.

46. c. BiPAP—Both BiPAP and CPAP may be administered by nasal cannula or face mask without endotracheal intubation.

47. a. apnea monitor.—These devices are used at home to monitor babies who have infantile apnea and with adults who have sleep apnea.

48. b. drooping eyelids and difficulty swallowing.—Patients may have vision problems, difficulty speaking, chewing, or swallowing.

49. b. supportive care and transport.—Other accommodations will vary depending on the presentation.

50. c. There has been a recent change in the patient's behavior.—There is no typical appearance or presentation for previously head-injured patients. Ask about the patient's baseline mental status and behavior, and if there have been any recent changes. This is of concern and most likely the reason EMS has been called.

51. b. UTI and urinary retention.—These devices may be short or long term.

52. c. leaking catheter—The other choices may be discovered during an assessment but are not problems associated with failure of the device.

53. b. choose the place to die and time of death.—The patient also has the right to: know the truth, confidentially and privacy, consent to treatment, and determine the disposition of his body.

54. b. five—When a person first learns he is dying, he typically experiences shock and disbelief. Then acceptance comes after moments or months, and the person enters the second state, "anger." Bargaining is followed by depression. Finally, acceptance is achieved in the final stage of detachment.

55. b. anger.—Many dying patients experience anger as well as the other stages: shock, bargaining, depression, and acceptance.

56. b. ostomy.—Ostomys are common in the home care setting.

57. a. VAD—VADs and medication ports are common in home care settings. They are used to administer medication, maintain long-term vascular access, and provide nutritional support.

58. c. systemic infection—The signs and symptoms suggest a systemic infection.

59. a. they often know more about the patient's special needs than anyone else.—Do not hesitate to ask for their expertise, if needed.

60. a. Wait for hospice to arrive and then leave.—Sometimes the family gets nervous and calls EMS. Hospice serves an important role, and EMS providers should cooperate fully with the family and hospice representatives to comply with the patient's wishes.

Chapter 47: Principles of Safety: Operating an Ambulance and Air Medical

1. b. State—Minimum standards for ambulance operations specify the worst they could let things get and still be allowed to operate.

2. d. ambulance design and manufacturing requirements.—These specifications are an attempt to influence safety standards, as well as standardize the look of ambulances.

3. d. as a risk-management tool.—Completing the ambulance equipment and supply checklist helps make the work environment safer for the EMS provider.

4. c. stop to assess damage, render aid, and exchange information.—An ambulance is not exempted from leaving the scene of an accident, even when a patient is on board.

5. a. routinely checking expiration dates.—Many expiration dates fall at the beginning or end of the month.

6. c. after the transport of any patient with a potentially communicable disease.—OSHA is charged with setting and enforcing standards for worker safety.

7. b. cleaning requirements.—This plan must also state how personnel should clean up a blood spill in the ambulance.

8. b. ambulance deployment.—Deployment is often based on the location of existing facilities to station the ambulance, location of hospitals, geographic considerations, and the anticipated call volume in each area of the community.

9. d. Reserve capacity—Some services ask off-duty personnel to carry pagers or sign up for backup coverage.

10. b. system status management.—This is one method of deployment that has become popular in recent years.

11. a. its resources.—The standards of reliability of a response agency take into consideration the percentage of the time that high-priority calls are responded to within an agreed-upon system response time.

12. b. low-level disinfection.—This product is designed for low-level disinfection.

13. a. sterilization.—Sterilization kills all forms of microbial life on medical instruments.

14. c. due regard.—Due regard is a responsibility that the operator of an emergency vehicle takes on when operating an emergency vehicle.

15. b. higher—Nowhere in the motor vehicle laws does it say any other driver is responsible for the safety of all other motorists.

16. c. the posted parking regulations.—Some allow exemptions from posted speed limits, the posted direction of travel, and the requirement to stop and wait at a red light.

17. c. 50–100—Do not rely solely on the lights and siren to alert the other motorists. Be sure to leave plenty of room around your vehicle and get a face-to-face commitment from other drivers that they understand where your vehicle is going.

18. c. head injury with AMS—The patient with a head injury and AMS gets the air medical transport. Cardiac arrest victims are not flown, and the toddler and 10-year-old patient are stable and can go by ground transport.

19. a. increase its visibility.—Alternating headlamps should only be used on nighttime calls if they are installed in a secondary lamp.

20. a. 50 feet in front of—Park at least 50 feet in front of the wreckage if your ambulance is the first emergency vehicle on the scene, so your warning lights can warn approaching motorist before flares can be set up.

21. d. Maryland—The Maryland state police medevac program continues to set the gold standards, which other programs try to emulate.

22. b. identify the location and size of the ambulance.—The vehicle must be clearly visible from 360° to all other motorists.

23. c. open rear doors—Always assume that oncoming traffic does not see you, and that, even if they do, they often won't pull over or slow down.

24. a. remote regions, such as parts of Alaska.—In addition, these aircraft are often used to bring critical patients who sustain serious medical emergencies or injuries while traveling from faraway places back to a hospital closer to their home.

25. b. limited treatment area in the aircraft.—Depending on the specific aircraft used, the cabin size can place limitations on the crew members, equipment carried, and configuration of the stretcher in the aircraft.

26. c. 100 + 100—All EMS providers should be capable of selecting a landing zone (LZ) and describing the terrain, major landmarks, estimated distance to the nearest town, and other pertinent information to the pilot of the helicopter on a designated frequency.

27. a. Convert IV bags over to pressure infuser bags.—Problems arise during ascent and descent when pressures change with altitude.

28. d. strengthen the safety of the aviation transport environment.—CAAMS also serves to promote the highest quality of patient care.

29. a. cabin size.—Depending on the specific aircraft used, the cabin size can place limitations on the crew members, equipment carried, and configuration of the stretcher in the aircraft.

30. d. vital for the safety and health of you, your crew, and the patient.—The steps you take to prepare your ambulance for going into service will help to ensure the safety and health of you, your crew, and the patient.

Chapter 48: Incident Management, Multiple Casualty Incidents

1. b. multiple casualty incident—Sometimes the term *MCI* is used for a mass casualty incident. This is misleading because it gives providers the impression that the MCI plan should be saved for the "big one."

2. a. specific location of the incident.—The report should also include the extent of the incident and the approximate number of patients.

3. d. closed—An example of a closed incident is an overturned bus where there is limited access to the passengers inside.

4. b. equipment and facilities.—ICS also consists of procedures for controlling personnel and communications.

5. c. the requirement for management and operations no longer exists.—Though originally developed for the fire service, ICS has been adapted to serve all emergency response disciplines.

6. b. Planning—Planning is also responsible for the collection, evaluation, dissemination, and use of information about the development of the incident and the status of the resources.

7. b. span of control—It can be very easy to lose track of your workers at an incident if they are not assigned to small units.

8. d. developing the incident action plan.—The IC is also responsible for assessing incident priorities and determining the strategic goals.

9. a. making it easy to identify the command officers.—These can be easily donned over the uniform and outer coat.

10. c. triage—It is not a good idea to take a physician or nurse who is not familiar with the workings of your EMS system and put her in a sector officer position.

11. b. they do not take any training to use.—Triage tags can be very useful tools. The hardest part is getting the crews to pull them out and start using them.

12. d. commanders can critique without the fear of offending anyone.—There is something to be learned from each incident so we can do a better job the next time. In a nonthreatening manner, the commanders of each emergency service should schedule a critique to discuss the incident.

13. d. the function they serve.—During an MCI is not the time to begin figuring out another agency's "code system."

14. c. to work cooperatively with other emergency commanders—Responsibilities also include managing the EMS response, designating the EMS division or sector officers, and establishing a command post and remaining there.

15. a. open—An open incident is one where the patients are accessible and the EMS providers will have safe access to the patients.

16. c. logistics—The size of the incident will help determine when and how much logistics are required.

17. d. unified command.—A unified command structure is the more common and key component of an ICS.

18. b. unified command post.—This means that all involved agencies contribute to the command process by determining the overall goals and objectives, joint planning for tactical activities, and maximizing the use of all assigned resources at the incident.

19. d. simple triage and rapid transport.—The START process permits a few rescuers to triage large numbers of patients very rapidly.

20. a. the most serious patients are treated and transported first.—In situations where there are many serious patients and limited ambulances, the very critical patients who have a small chance of survival are given the lowest priority.

21. a. to never let the driver, keys, or stretcher get separated from their ambulance.—This mistake has resulted in unnecessary fatalities and delays in patient care.

22. a. create a safe perimeter.—Paramedics are trained to the HAZMAT awareness level, which means they have the knowledge to recognize a hazardous scene, call for more help, establish a safe perimeter, and not enter unless they have a higher level of training and the proper equipment.

23. c. operations, planning, logistics, and finance.—The four major components utilized during the management of a large MCI are operations, planning, logistics, and finance.

24. d. 28-year-old female with a swollen and deformed ankle and abrasions on both hands—This patient has minor injuries and none that affect the ABCs.

25. a. 8-year-old female having difficulty breathing from an asthma attack—This patient is having a breathing problem, which makes her a high priority in need of immediate care.

Chapter 49: Vehicle Extrication

1. c. awareness—Awareness-level training implies enough knowledge to comprehend the hazards and realize that additional expertise is needed to effect the rescue.

2. c. the patient's medical condition—Because there is no rescue if there is no patient, all rescues should be driven by patient need. Just as in patient care, the first concern is rescuer safety.

3. b. when it is or is not safe to gain access.—One of the major benefits of rescue awareness training is to avoid a provider attempting a rescue for which he is not trained.

4. a. helmets and eye protection—Personal safety must be the paramount issue in any rescue situation. For most rescues, the minimum PPE should include eye protection, a helmet, and the appropriate gloves.

5. b. They do not withstand severe impact.—The best rescue helmets have a four-point, nonelastic suspension system, in contrast to the two-point system found in construction hard hats.

6. a. ANSI.—The eye protection should include both goggles, vented to prevent fogging, and industrial safety glasses held by an elastic band. These should be ANSI (American National Standards Institute) approved.

7. d. industrial safety glasses.—The face shield on most fire helmets is inadequate protection for your eyes.

8. c. leather work gloves.—In addition to disposable rubber or latex gloves for standard precautions purposes, leather work gloves, such as those used for gardening, are usually best for protection against cuts and punctures.

9. a. provide limited flash protection.—These materials provide limited flash protection and should be strongly considered as part of the EMS provider's personal protection.

10. b. aluminized rescue blankets—A variety of protective blankets should be available to shield patients from debris, fire, or weather. Aluminum rescue blankets protect from fire, heat, or glass dust.

11. c. backboards—Short and long backboards and other commonly found equipment can be used as shields to protect patients.

12. c. surgical mask—Surgical masks or commercial dust masks are adequate for most occasions. These should be routinely supplied to all EMS units.

13. c. SOPs.—Standard operating procedures should include sections on all types of anticipated rescue and specify the required safety equipment, particular actions required or prohibited, and any rescue-specific modifications in assignments. SOPs should include a statement requiring a safety officer and describing his relationship to command.

14. d. arrival and size-up, hazard control, and gaining access to the patient.—The last four phases are medical treatment, disentanglement, patient packaging, and transportation.

15. d. safety officer.—The safety officer should be someone with the knowledge and authority to intervene in unsafe situations.

16. b. provide immense psychological support.—This is especially true in situations where the patient is entrapped and disentanglement will take a significant amount of time.

17. b. Improvement of personnel safety and operational success.—Preplan also generates ideas on the efficient use of existing personnel and equipment, and anticipates the need for additional equipment, rescuers, or expertise.

18. a. conduct a scene size-up.—The first arriving crew must immediately establish medical command and conduct a scene size-up to determine the number of patients and appoint a triage officer and other personnel as necessary.

19. c. creating a safe perimeter.—The EMS provider's approach should be limited to creating a safe perimeter, attempting to identify the substance involved from a safe position, and keeping bystanders and EMS personnel away from the hot zone.

20. c. Wearing the appropriate PPE—Additional precautions include making sure all EMS personnel are clearly visible and always alert to traffic.

21. c. an on-scene SAR specialist.—If possible, ask dispatch to send an on-scene specialist (search and rescue team member) to meet the crew. Search dogs, electronic detection devices, or an experienced search manager may be required to find the patients.

22. a. after gaining access—After gaining access, medical personnel can begin to make patient contact. No EMS provider should enter an area to provide patient care unless she is protected from hazards with PPE and has the technical skills to reach, manage, and remove patients safely.

23. c. protected from hazards with PPE.—All EMS personnel must have on the PPE appropriate for the specific type of rescue.

24. c. disentanglement.—Disentanglement literally means removing the wreckage from the victim, not the other way around.

25. c. disentanglement—The methods used to disentangle the patient must each be analyzed for their risk versus benefit to the patient's medical needs and the estimated time they take to perform.

26. b. means of egress.—Some patient packaging can be more complex than others, considering the specialized rescue techniques required to get them out of the situation they were found in.

27. d. traffic—The greatest concern is the traffic itself. Studies have shown that drivers who are drugged, intoxicated, or tired actually drive right into the emergency lights.

28. a. the risk of fire or explosion.—There may be a natural gas or high-pressure tank at risk of fire or explosion. Electrical vehicles have storage cells that may be very dangerous.

29. b. not be directly exposed to traffic.—Ambulance lights to warn traffic are often obstructed when the doors are open for loading.

30. b. turn on only a minimum of warning lights.—When too many lights are used, it is very confusing and blinding to the oncoming traffic.

31. a. direct the flow of traffic away from emergency workers.—As soon as the first unit arrives on the scene, flares or cones should be placed to direct traffic away from the collision.

32. a. The potential for a fire hazard is increased.—Under each vehicle is a catalytic converter (which has a temperature around 1,200°F), which is a good source of ignition for a fire.

33. b. If loaded, they may release when unexpected.—The bumpers on many vehicles have pistons in them and are designed to withstand a slow-speed collision to limit the damage to the front or rear of the vehicle. Sometimes these bumpers become loaded in the crushed position and do not immediately bounce back out.

34. d. it can inflate when not expected.—Airbags that have not deployed during a collision, have been known to deploy in the middle of extrication.

35. b. stabilize the vehicle.—Remember to turn off the ignition and set the vehicle in park. If trained to do so, temporarily stabilize the vehicle with ropes, chocks, or a come-a-long until the vehicle rescue team has arrived at the scene.

36. c. Stabilize the vehicle with cribbing.—Setting cribbing and chocking the wheels are simple measures the paramedic can take to stabilize a vehicle.

37. b. firewall.—The firewall can collapse on a patient's legs when involved in a high-speed, head-on collision. Sometimes the patient's feet may go through the firewall.

38. c. Nader pin.—The Nader pin must be disengaged to make it possible to pry the door open unless hydraulic jaws are used.

39. b. safety—The safety glass that is used in the windshield is designed to crack when struck with an object such as a flying stone. When shattered or broken, safety glass stays intact.

40. a. tempered; sharp—Tempered glass is used in the side and rear windows of a vehicle, and is designed to withstand blows with a blunt object without breaking.

41. d. Nader pin—The Nader pin must be disengaged to make it possible to pry the door open unless hydraulic jaws are used.

42. d. try to open all four doors first.—Always try to open a door that may be unlocked prior to breaking any glass.

43. c. gain access through the window farthest away from the patient.—This reduces the risk of furthering injury to those inside.

44. b. inner circle.—The inner circle is where the rescue takes place. The outer circle is where equipment staging and additional personnel should wait until they are assigned a duty.

45. b. low angle.—The types of hazardous terrain are divided into low angle, high angle, or flat with obstructions.

46. b. Stokes®—The Stokes® stretcher is the standard for rough terrain evacuation. It provides a rigid frame for patient protection and is easy to carry with an adequate number of personnel.

47. a. wire and tubular metal.—The wire-mesh Stokes® baskets are the strongest of the types and provide better air and water flow through the basket.

48. c. six—There should be a minimum of six personnel on the Stokes®, and extra teams of six should be rotated in situations where there is a long way to carry the basket.

49. a. haul on the lines as instructed.—Any rescue requiring hauling needs plenty of helpers to assist with the hauling.

50. b. reposition dislocations.—Additional skills the paramedic may utilize on patients who require an extensive evacuation time include: long-term hydration management, cleansing and care of wounds, removal of impaled objects, pain management, hypothermia management, and management of crush injuries and compartment syndromes.

Chapter 50: Hazardous Material Awareness

1. b. 473—Competencies for EMS Personnel Responding to Hazardous Materials Incidents established two levels of EMS hazmat responders above the awareness level and was the first NFPA standard to specifically address EMS workers.

2. c. 704—The other choices relate to other NFPA standards.

3. b. First responder operations—At this level, a trained person can also carry out basic decontamination procedures.

4. d. the level of training the paramedic has and the local hazmat plan.—Paramedics are trained to the hazmat awareness at the minimum. This level of training means they have the knowledge to recognize a hazardous scene, call for more help, and not enter unless they have advanced training and proper equipment. The level of response and participation is predetermined in many communities.

5. b. five—First responder awareness, First responder operations, hazardous material technician, hazardous material specialist, and on-scene incident commander.

6. a. *North American Emergency Response Guidebook*—A well-known and used reference for identifying hazardous materials found in transport.

7. d. nonflammable.—Gases are classified as: poison A, flammable gas, nonflammable gas, and corrosive gas.

8. c. MSDS—material safety data sheets—a list of detailed information about a substance to be used when exposure occurs with that product. Employers are required to keep these on the work site.

9. a. gross—Gross decon is a rapid removal of the material by removing clothing, shoes, and jewelry and then using water to flush away as much of the substance as possible. When the patient is able, they should be instructed to do this themselves to reduce the chance of contaminating others.
10. a. Poison actions—The factors that affect poison actions are: dose, route of exposure, synergistic effects, and toxicity.
11. b. chemical—Training requirements are a significant factor that limits field decontamination.
12. a. two—Patient condition can limit the decontamination process. The more stable a patient is, the more thorough the decon that can be completed.
13. d. eight—Patient condition can limit the decontamination process. The more stable a patient is, the more thorough the decon that can be completed.
14. b. topical—Other common decon solutions are tincture of green soap, isopropyl alcohol, and vegetable oil.
15. d. milk—Milk may be used to transport a tooth that has been accidentally displaced.
16. d. reactivity.—The placards are colored and indicate specific hazards. Red = fire hazard; blue = health hazard; and yellow = reactivity hazard.
17. b. zones—These safety zones are designated as hot, warm, and cold.
18. d. Instruct the patient to remove contaminated shoes and clothing.—At this level of training, the paramedic can keep unnecessary people away from the hazard and provide first aid by having victims move into fresh air.
19. a. Dose response—Understanding this helps to determine the level of decontamination required.
20. d. critical patient condition.—The more stable a patient is, the more thorough the decon that can be completed.
21. d. threshold limit value-ceiling.—Exposure to higher concentrations must not occur.
22. c. Permissible exposure limit—The PEL is primarily intended as an exposure guide rather than as an absolute exposure limit.
23. b. get everyone out of the residence.—The responders and the victims of a possible exposure should be removed immediately. The longer the exposure, the more serious their condition may become.
24. d. Code of Federal Regulations (CFR)—EMS agencies must follow CFR 1910.1200 (the Right to Know Law) and CFR 1910.120 (Emergency Response to Hazardous Substance Releases).
25. d. Chemical Manufacturers Association—The telephone number is 1-800-424-9300.
26. d. stage equipment in the cold zone of the operation.—The cold zone is the area of the operation furthest from the exposure point. It is the safe area for personnel and their equipment.
27. d. The product may ignite other combustible materials.—Product flammability warnings include the following information: may cause fire or explosion, may ignite other combustible materials and may be ignited by heat, sparks, or flames.
28. c. take the patient through their own decon procedures—An emergency department with the resources will have the patient proceed through a designated procedure within its own facility for additional decon.
29. c. incident management system (IMS)—Each community needs to have an IMS that has been practiced and is understood by all of the providers within the agencies that could respond to an event in and around the community.
30. b. avoid any exposure to yourself and your crew.—Safety first for yourself and crew. At the hazmat awareness level, the paramedic is trained to recognize a hazardous scene, call for more help when needed, and not enter unless he has advanced training and the proper equipment.

Chapter 51: Terrorism and Disasters

1. c. Terrorism—Terrorism has become extremely heightened in recent years.
2. b. nerve agents, blister agents, and blood agents.—Chemical agents are classified into six categories: nerve agents, blister agents, blood agents, chokingagents, irritating agents, and incapacitating agents.
3. b. with information obtained from dispatch.—Attempt to use all available resources, such as law enforcement, prior to arrival at the scene, as well as on scene.
4. b. retreat right away.—When you are concerned for your safety, don't ever hesitate to run away.
5. c. a nerve agent.—Nerve agents usually over stimulate the release of chemical neurotransmitters, causing muscles and certain glands of the body to overreact.
6. c. out of sight of the scene.—Do not become an additional distraction for law enforcement.
7. a. Stand to the side of the door before ringing or knocking.—A simple form of concealment that could safe your life.
8. d. attempt to identify signs of specific agent exposure.—This action will assist with the safety and protection of responders while they provide treatment and decontamination.

9. a. exact location.—If you are struck by a vehicle, you may not be able to give the exact location.

10. b. driver would normally expect the police to approach on the driver's side.—Avoid actions that make you look like a threat (law enforcement).

11. c. have a portable radio in hand.—This way you can call for help. Many radios have an emergency button that can be activated with one finger.

12. b. reporting to command and then to an assigned sector (group).—The role of the paramedic in this type of incident is similar to that in other incidents. Upon arrival at the scene, report to command and then to any area designated by command.

13. a. nausea and vomiting.—Later effects include; continued nausea, vomiting, diarrhea, loss of appetite, weakness, internal bleeding, fever, destruction of bone marrow, seizures, and possible coma.

14. a. injuries from an explosion.—Meth labs contain highly flammable chemicals that can explode easily.

15. d. decrease the amount of time spent near the source—Some basic ways to reduce exposure to radiation include: increasing the distance from the source, decreasing the amount of time spent near the source, and using a shield as a barrier between yourself/patients and the source.

16. c. booby traps to be set—The occupants of the labs are often armed and otherwise violent people.

17. c. potential for street violence.—Many of the gangs are heavily involved in drug trafficking and use underage children (minors) to conduct most of the violence.

18. c. colors—EMS providers must be careful to show respect to the colors or face deadly repercussions.

19. d. leave immediately and call law enforcement.—It is suggested that the incident command system be initiated and hazmat asked to respond, as well as the fire department.

20. b. the DEA—The local or state police may notify the Drug Enforcement Administration (DEA), which has responsibility for and expertise in this particular area.

21. d. hours to days.—Victims of exposure to biological agents have delayed onset of symptoms. Some early effects may be seen within 4–6 hours; other effects may take days or weeks.

22. c. the potential for a secondary device.—Secondary devices are bombs placed at the scene that are designed to have a delayed explosion after the primary explosion. The paramedic must be alert to the potential for a secondary device.

23. c. Protect the victim by getting between the victim and the abuser.—One of the most potentially dangerous situations to be in is the "middle" of a domestic disturbance. Always have a backup plan, radio in hand, and another unit at your side.

24. c. avoidance is always preferable to confrontation.—Be aware of the proper tactical response to avoid danger and know how to deal appropriately with danger in situations where it cannot be avoided.

25. b. make sure the EMD does not send any further EMS units directly into the scene.—Don't let your co-workers walk into a situation you are retreating from.

26. a. Concealment is positioning the paramedic or crew behind an object that hides them from the view of others.—Concealment offers no ballistic protection should the perpetrator begin firing a weapon at you.

27. d. Throw the equipment to slow or trip the aggressor.—Try to wedge the stretcher in the doorway to block the aggressor.

28. b. that too much protection can create additional hazards.—Using unnecessary levels of PPE may cause additional hazards for the responders such as heat, stress, dehydration, and limited visibility and mobility.

29. c. tactical EMS.—Tactical EMS is provided in a violent or tactically "hot" zone. This requires a working relationship with the law enforcement team, as well as special training.

30. a. CONTOMS—CONTOMS stands for Counter Narcotic and Terrorism Operational Medical Support program.

31. b. cutting along the seam of the clothing.—Protect the evidence by avoiding ripping or cutting through a knife or bullet hole.

32. a. a paper bag.—The moisture in plastic bags can break down the evidence. Better yet, have the law enforcement officer assist you so it is handled in the manner that she prefers.

33. b. nerve agent — Care for nerve agent exposure includes airway management, the use of an antidote kit containing atropine and pralidoxime and packaged as Mark 1 Kit, and Valium (diazepam).

34. c. destroying or "smudging" the perpetrator's prints.—Touch as little as possible.

35. c. keeping a safe stance with feet apart, ready to react.—This, together with keeping your hands out of the pockets and not hanging onto equipment, can help you to keep your balance and be ready to run.

36. c. there is a possibility of carbon monoxide poisoning in all the victims of this fire.—Victims who have been in a confined space where smoke and fire were present are at risk for carbon monoxide inhalation and should be evaluated for it.

37. d. wind direction—Wind directions can change the dynamics of a HAZMAT incident very rapidly. Wind direction is routinely monitored during outside HAZMAT incidents for this reason.

38. d. search and rescue specialists—If possible, SAR specialists should be requested to the scene. These teams have specialized training and resources such as search dogs and electronic detection devices.

39. a. becoming involved in preplanning and training.—Preplanning and training are the best way to prepare for disaster operations.

40. a. work best when plain English only is used.—"Keep it simple and clear with plain English" is the concept used in such emergencies.

Chapter 52: Basic and Advanced Cardiac Life Support Review

1. c. basic life support.—Together with advanced cardiac life support (ACLS), it is part of the emergency cardiac care provided to patients experiencing symptoms of a heart attack. BLS is used interchangeably with the old phrase basic cardiac life support (BCLS) when discussing cardiac care. BLS is often used to refer to the technique of cardiopulmonary resuscitation (CPR) when managing a cardiac arrest.

2. a. emphasizing that all rescuers should push hard and fast.—The better and faster the compressions, the more blood flow they will produce.

3. b. acute coronary syndrome.—An acute coronary syndrome (ACS) is a catch-all term devised to emphasize that many times it is impossible to tell the difference between unstable angina and infarction.

4. a. 2—Studies have shown that the effectiveness of chest compressions deteriorate rapidly as the rescuer tires. The new recommendation is for the rescuers to switch, without interruption, every 2 minutes.

5. a. one second per breath.—When the adult patient has a pulse, but is not breathing, rescue breaths should be given over 1 second every 5–6 seconds.

6. a. 30:2 for all rescuers.—This change emphasizes the importance of maximizing chest compressions without interruptions for all rescuers.

7. c. based on scientific evidence.—This evidence was reviewed and scientific consensus obtained from the international resuscitation community.

8. b. IIa.—An example of a class IIa treatment is that each rescue breath be given over 1 second.

9. c. IIb.—An example of a class IIb treatment is for the health care provider to use the jaw-thrust without head extension in the patient with a suspected cervical spine injury.

10. d. Indeterminate.—Often these are ideas at a preliminary research stage, promising but in need of more research at a higher level. Thus, the AHA and resuscitation experts cannot make a recommendation for or against at this time.

11. a. all rescuers deliver one shock followed by immediate CPR for 2 minutes.—The new recommendation is for single shocks, followed by immediate CPR and rhythm checks assessed every 2 minutes.

12. b. IIb—EMS providers should be prepared to temporarily act as family advocates until additional help arrives for grief support (chaplain, family minister, or other family members) and management of the body (medical examiner, coroner, and police).

13. b. IIa—Another example of a class IIa treatment is chest compressions delivered at a rate of 100 per minute.

14. c. every 3–5 seconds.—When the infant or child patient has a pulse, but is not breathing, rescue breaths should be given over 1 second every 3–5 seconds.

15. c. take less than 10 seconds.—Interruptions in chest compression should occur as infrequently as possible and take no more than 10 seconds.

16. d. allows the heart to fill with blood.—If the chest does not recoil, the heart will not receive adequate venous return and the subsequent compression will not produce adequate cardiac output.

17. a. it impedes blood return to the heart.—Overinflation of the lungs increases intrathoracic pressure, and this prevents adequate filling of the heart with blood.

18. b. DNAR order.—It is the responsibility of the health care provider to search for and honor a DNAR that is deemed valid.

19. c. consensus standards.—They are based on the ILCOR consensus and the science of resuscitation.

20. d. 360 J.—This is a change from the 2000 Guidelines. The recommended dose for initial and subsequent shocks using monophasic waveform is 360 J.

21. d. 360 J.—The recommended dose for initial and subsequent shocks using monophasic waveform is 360 J.

22. c. a low body temperature—In some instances hypothermia can mimic clinical death. The saying goes, "They are not dead until they are warm and dead."

23. b. 2 minutes of CPR—In the out-of-hospital setting, all rescuers should provide five cycles or approximately 2 minutes of CPR prior to using the AED.

24. b. defibrillation—Early defibrillation is the single acute intervention that really makes a difference in saving lives from sudden cardiac arrest.

25. d. 1—Since 2003, the use of AEDs is recommended for children 1year and older in sudden cardiac arrest.

26. c. removing barriers to implementing PAD—Limited funds are better spent on removing the barriers to training the lay public in CPR and public access defibrillation (PAD). Clearly, all the medications do not help save as many patients as getting the defibrillator operator there faster.

27. c. patients 1 year old to the onset of puberty.—The change applies to victims of cardiac arrest from about 1 year old to the onset of puberty or adolescence, as defined by the presence of secondary sex characteristics.

28. a. a child with previous ACS—The major exception to the phone-fast rule is those children under 8 years old who are known to be at risk for ventricular fibrillation (VF) or ventricular tachycardia (VT), who have a history of cardiac dysrhythmias, or those with congenital heart disease who experience sudden witnessed collapse.

29. c. poisoning or drug overdose—These patients tend to be hypoxic and have the best chance of survival when CPR is provided in the first few minutes of sudden cardiac arrest.

30. d. all of the above.—The technique of providing ventilations with a bag mask requires routine practice and is a fundamental skill that should be mastered by all health care providers.

31. b. about 18 inches above the head of the patient—The ventilator should be positioned approximately 18 inches above the head of the patient; hyperextend the airway and use the weight of the left arm, which is sealing the mask, to hold the airway in the hyperextended position. The other hand can be used to squeeze the bag against itself.

32. b. The jaw thrust can be used for one-rescuer bag mask technique on a trauma patient.—It is not possible to do a jaw thrust, jutting both sides of the jar anterior, with only one hand.

33. d. chest should rise visibly.—With supplemental oxygen attached to the bag mask, smaller tidal volumes (400–600 ml) are acceptable. The rescuer should still be able to see the chest rise and maintain the patient's oxygen saturation at greater than 90%.

34. a. two rescue breaths—After the two rescue breaths are given, the rescuer should immediately begin chest compressions in cycles of 30:2.

35. d. they were frequently wrong in their assessment—This step was taking too long to perform and was too often performed incorrectly. The goal now is to deliver chest compressions rapidly and without delays.

36. a. 150 J.—An initial dose of 150–200 J is recommended when using a biphasic truncated exponential waveform, and 120 J for a rectilinear biphasic waveform.

37. b. reposition the neck and reattempt to ventilate.—Blind finger sweeps should not be used on any patient.

38. a. 2 J/kg.—Subsequent doses should be 4 J/kg.

39. b. chest compressions may be helpful.—Chest compressions generated at least as high or higher intrathoracic pressures than abdominal thrusts. Therefore, the chest compressions used in CPR are helpful in dislodging an FBAO in the unresponsive patient.

40. d. in the center of the chest between the nipples—This position has not changed in the new Guidelines.

41. d. at least 100—This rate changed in the Guidelines 2010.

42. b. 15:2.—For infants less than 1year old, the compression to ventilation ratio is 5:1.

43. b. the heel of one or two hands to compress the lower half of the sternum.—The placement of the hand or hands should be at about the nipple line.

44. a. two-thumb-encircling-hands chest technique.—The Guidelines still recommends this as the primary method for compressions for the neonate.

45. b. the LMA and Combitube® are better than bag mask.—Evidence shows that under certain clinical conditions, both the LMA and Combitube® are clinically equivalent to the ET tube.

46. d. the agency's medical director—Prior to making this decision, many factors must be considered by the medical director using the quality improvement process.

47. b. evidence-based—The Guidelines were developed using an evidence-based rigorous review of the published scientific evidence and studies on resuscitation.

48. a. 1: 6–8—Once an advanced airway has been inserted, the rescuer delivers one ventilation every 6–8 seconds, and the compressor continues without interruption.

49. a. bag mask—The bag mask provides effective ventilations when used by properly trained providers who practice the skill.

50. a. an IV or IO.—Medications administered through an IV or IO provide a more predictable delivery and pharmacologic effect.

51. c. resume CPR for five cycles, and then reanalyze the rhythm and check pulse.—Pulse and rhythm are not checked after the shock; rather, they are checked after five cycles of CPR, or about 2 minutes.

52. b. capnography—Capnography provides $EtCO_2$ readings in two forms; one is a number and the other is a wave form or graph.

53. d. This device requires extensive training to use.—This device is easy to use and does not require extensive training. The device is inserted blindly and does not require a mask seal to ventilate.

54. d. during CPR, as soon as possible after rhythm checks.—The emphasis is to minimize interruption of compressions. Therefore, medications should be administered during CPR, as soon as possible after rhythm checks.

55. b. Vasopressin—A single dose may be given to replace either the first or second dose of epinephrine in VF/pulseless VT, asystole, or PEA arrest.

56. d. all of the above.—There are possible benefits of induced hypothermia for 12–24 hours for patients who have an ROSC, but who remain comatose after a reversal of a cardiac arrest.

57. a. is very difficult to accurately dose to the patient's weight.—The use of high-dose epinephrine is not recommended (class III) for all of the other reasons listed.

58. b. Amiodarone—Amiodarone is preferred (class IIb), but lidocaine may be used when amiodarone is not available.

59. a. routine suctioning is no longer recommended.—The recommendation is to avoid routine suctioning of meconium staining.

60. c. the patient takes warfarin—Contraindications for fibrinolysis include: bleeding or clotting problems on blood thinners, pregnancy, history of serious systemic disease, recent surgery or trauma, and BP greater than 180 systolic or 110 diastolic.

61. d. Magnesium sulfate—This drug is recommended for use in cardiac arrest when the rhythm is torsades de points or when you suspect the patient has hypomagnesemia.

62. c. Vasopressin—This drug may be used as an alternative vasopressor to epinephrine in adult cardiac arrest with shock-refractory VF. It may also be useful in cardiac arrest with asystole and PEA rhythms.

63. d. All of the actions listed above are appropriate and should be done.—If possible, one crew member or the EMS supervisor should talk with the family and explain what treatment is being provided, what the most likely outcome is, and answer questions, clarify information, and comfort the family.

64. a. acute coronary syndromes.—An acute coronary syndrome (ACS) is a catch-all term devised to emphasize that many times it is impossible to tell the difference between unstable angina and infarction.

65. c. primary angioplasty and intra-aortic balloon placement.—Patients with large anterior infarctions, systolic BP <100 mmHg, heart rates over 100, or rales greater than one-third of the lung fields should also be considered for transfer to these specialty facilities.

66. c. 3 hours of the onset of stroke symptoms.—These patients should be triaged with the same urgency as acute ST segment elevation MI (STEMI).

67. a. systemic alkalosis.—The treatment of choice is the induction of a systemic alkalosis with a pH of 7.50 to 7.55.

68. a. ventricular dysrhythmias.—Cocaine has both alpha and beta stimulatory effects.

69. d. beta-blocking agents as a second-line therapy when the first-line treatment fails.—Beta-blockers are relatively contraindicated, and propranolol should definitely not be used for cocaine intoxication.

70. a. aspirin—All patients with signs and symptoms of ACS, including non-Q wave MI, should receive aspirin and beta-blockers in the absence of contraindications.

Appendix B:
Tips for Preparing for
a Practical Skills Examination

Paramedic courses are designed to cover specific objectives, as outlined in the DOT National Standard Curriculum and 2009 National Emergency Medical Services Education Standards. The latest version of the Paramedic Instructional Guidelines often will take around 1,800 hours of lecture, lab, clinical, and internship to accomplish.

During a paramedic course, many educators teach the core curriculum and provide enrichment material as time, resources, and experience permit. Near the end of a paramedic program, which may have taken a year or two to complete, it is typical for the educator to change his or her style of teaching and prep for the exam. That is to say, instructors will provide examples of the material to be tested on state and national exams, and give tips on how to take the written exams. He or she may hold one or more practice skills sessions and a mock practical exam to help the students prepare. Limited time and resources often do not allow for as much practice time for skills as some students would like. In preparing for the practical skills exam, we have included some tips to help you get ready.

If you haven't done so already, obtain a copy of the skills testing sheets to be used for *your* practical skills exam and carefully read the instructions well before the day of the practical skills exam. Note that each exam skills sheet has items that are identified as critical pass or fail items. These items are usually bolded for easy identification. These items include taking or verbalizing BSI (standard precautions) or scene safety, as well as other critical tasks. National Registry skills sheets will also list "critical criteria" at the bottom of each skills sheet. This is a list of items that were not performed and should have been. When an evaluator checks one of these items, the candidate will fail the station.

Often the course instructor will hand out a set of the skills testing sheets to be used for the state and/or registry exam during or near the end of the course, and you will be given an opportunity to practice the skills in lab using the testing sheets. We strongly recommend that you take every opportunity provided during the

course to do this. In addition, find one or more students or experienced paramedics to practice skills with. Study groups are usually a helpful strategy. While you demonstrate the skill, have another person use the testing sheet to evaluate your performance. Be tough on each other in a friendly way! Pay close attention to the critical failure items and then focus on obtaining every available point.

Prior to the day of the practical skills exam, make certain you are familiar with the location of the exam. Arrive 15 minutes early on the day of the exam. Bring a copy of the skills sheets with you to review while you are waiting. On the testing day, be patient and prepare to be at the testing site for most of the day. As you already are aware, practical skills testing typically takes a lot of time. In addition to bringing the skills sheets to review, bring a book, a drink, lunch, good humor, and plenty of patience.

On the day of the practical exam, if you have the option of choosing the order of the testing stations, there are two theories we recommend. The first one is this: if you are a little nervous and you want to build your confidence, start with a short skill station like one of the EMT skills. This is a skill you have successfully completed in the past. From there, continue to build your confidence by selecting the stations that you feel you can complete without difficulty.

The second theory we recommend is selecting the most difficult stations and completing those first. For most people, the dynamic cardiology and assessment stations seem the most difficult because they have the most steps and take the longest to complete. Once these stations are complete, you can breathe a little easier while completing the remaining stations.

If you do not have the option of choosing the order of skills to be tested, do not worry; at this point, you have prepared and are ready for each skills station. During the exam, the evaluators are instructed not to advise you if you have passed or failed a skills station until you have finished testing at all of the stations, so don't expect them to. If you fail a station early in the testing, you may become distracted and fail another.

Once in the station, you will be read a set of instructions and given the opportunity to ask questions for clarification and to check the equipment provided. I recommend that you do this, especially if you are the first candidate of the day coming into a station. The evaluator has been instructed to make sure that the equipment is functioning properly and that there are no distractions for the candidates. They are not there to trip you up, but occasionally a blood pressure cuff is broken and is not detected prior to starting the exam.

In the patient assessment station, we recommend that you ask if the injuries or significant signs that you are supposed to detect are going to be visible with moulage or by another method. This is a common area where problems can occur. Verbalize the steps and tasks you complete as if you are talking to a new partner. After a long day of testing, evaluators become fatigued just like you. If an evaluator happens to have his or her head turned while you are performing a critical step, he or she will hear you verbalizing it.

If you should have to repeat a station, know the retest policy and do not overreact. You have spent a lot of time training and should persevere rather than throwing in the towel over one bad day! Remember, we humans do make mistakes occasionally. The key is how you learn from your mistakes, correct them, and move forward.

Lastly, get some sleep before the examination. Try to get a good night's rest two nights before the exam, in addition to the night before. Many people are very nervous about test taking and do not sleep well the night before, no matter what. Getting good sleep two nights before does help.

Best of luck, and be prepared!

—Bob and Kirsten

Appendix C:
National Registry Practical Examination Sheets

National Registry of Emergency Medical Technicians
Advanced Level Psychomotor Examination

ALTERNATIVE AIRWAY DEVICE (SUPRAGLOTTIC AIRWAY)

Candidate: _____ Examiner: _____
Date: _____ Signature: _____
Device: _____

NOTE: If candidate elects to initially ventilate with BVM attached to reservoir and oxygen, full credit must be awarded for steps denoted by "**" so long as first ventilation is delivered within 30 seconds.

Actual Time Started: _____

	Possible Points	Points Awarded
Takes or verbalizes body substance isolation precautions	1	
Opens the airway manually	1	
Elevates tongue, inserts simple adjunct [oropharyngeal or nasopharyngeal airway]	1	
NOTE: Examiner now informs candidate no gag reflex is present and patient accepts adjunct		
**Ventilates patient immediately with bag-valve-mask device unattached to oxygen	1	
**Ventilates patient with room air	1	
NOTE: Examiner now informs candidate that ventilation is being performed without difficulty and that pulse oximetry indicates the patient's blood oxygen saturation is 85%		
Attaches oxygen reservoir to bag-valve-mask device and connects to high-flow oxygen regulator [12–15 L/minute]	1	
Ventilates patient at a rate of 10–12/minute with appropriate volumes	1	
NOTE: After 30 seconds, examiner auscultates and reports breath sounds are present and equal bilaterally and medical direction has ordered insertion of a supraglottic airway. The examiner must now take over ventilation.		
Directs assistant to pre-oxygenate patient	1	
Checks/prepares supraglottic airway device	1	
Lubricates distal tip of the device [may be verbalized]	1	
NOTE: Examiner to remove OPA and move out of the way when candidate is prepared to insert device.		
Positions head properly	1	
Performs a tongue-jaw lift	1	
Inserts device to proper depth	1	
Secures device in patient [inflates cuffs with proper volumes and immediately removes syringe or secures strap]	1	
Ventilates patient and confirms proper ventilation [correct lumen and proper insertion depth] by auscultation bilaterally over lungs and over epigastrium	1	
Adjusts ventilation as necessary [ventilates through additional lumen or slightly withdraws tube until ventilation is optimized]	1	
Verifies proper tube placement by secondary confirmation such as capnography, capnometry, EDD or colorimetric device	1	
NOTE: The examiner must now ask the candidate, "How would you know if you are delivering appropriate volumes with each ventilation?"		
Secures device or confirms that the device remains properly secured	1	
Ventilates patient at proper rate and volume while observing capnography/capnometry and pulse oximeter	1	

Actual Time Ended: _____ **TOTAL** 19

Critical Criteria
____ Failure to initiate ventilations within 30 seconds after taking body substance isolation precautions or interrupts ventilations for greater than 30 seconds at any time
____ Failure to take or verbalize body substance isolation precautions
____ Failure to voice and ultimately provide high oxygen concentration [at least 85%]
____ Failure to ventilate the patient at a rate of 10–12/minute
____ Failure to provide adequate volumes per breath [maximum 2 errors/minute permissible]
____ Failure to pre-oxygenate patient prior to insertion of the supraglottic airway device
____ Failure to insert the supraglottic airway device at a proper depth or location within 3 attempts
____ Failure to inflate cuffs properly and immediately remove the syringe
____ Failure to secure the strap (if present) prior to cuff inflation
____ Failure to confirm that patient is being ventilated properly (correct lumen and proper insertion depth) by auscultation bilaterally over lungs and over epigastrium
____ Insertion or use of any adjunct in a manner dangerous to the patient
____ Failure to manage the patient as a competent EMT
____ Exhibits unacceptable affect with patient or other personnel
____ Uses or orders a dangerous or inappropriate intervention

You must factually document your rationale for checking any of the above critical items on the reverse side of this form.

(Reprinted with permission of the National Registry of Emergency Medical Technicians.)

National Registry of Emergency Medical Technicians
Advanced Level Practical Examination

BLEEDING CONTROL/SHOCK MANAGEMENT

Candidate: _____   Examiner: _____

Date: _____   Signature: _____

TimeStart: _____

	Possible Points	Points Awarded
Takes or verbalizes body substance isolation precautions	1	
Applies direct pressure to the wound	1	
NOTE: The examiner must now inform the candidate that the wound continues to bleed.		
Applies tourniquet	1	
NOTE: The examiner must now inform the candidate that the patient is exhibiting signs and symptoms of hypoperfusion.		
Properly positions the patient	1	
Administers high-concentration oxygen	1	
Initiates steps to prevent heat loss from the patient	1	
Indicates the need for immediate transportation	1	
Time End:_____ TOTAL	7	

CRITICAL CRITERIA

_____ Did not take or verbalize body substance isolation precautions
_____ Did not apply high concentration of oxygen
_____ Did not control hemorrhage using correct procedures in a timely manner
_____ Did not indicate the need for immediate transportation

You must factually document your rationale for checking any of the above critical items on the reverse side of this form.

(Reprinted with permission of the National Registry of Emergency Medical Technicians.)

National Registry of Emergency Medical Technicians
Advanced Emergency Medical Technician Psychomotor Examination

CARDIAC ARREST MANAGEMENT/AED

Candidate: _____ Examiner: _____

Date: _____ Signature: _____

Actual Time Started: _____

	Possible Points	Points Awarded
Takes or verbalizes appropriate body substance isolation precautions	1	
Determines the scene/situation is safe	1	
Attempts to question any bystanders about arrest events	1	
Checks patient responsiveness	1	
Assesses patient for signs of breathing [observes the patient and determines the absence of breathing or abnormal breathing (gasping or agonal respirations)]	1	
Checks carotid pulse [no more than 10 seconds]	1	
Immediately begins chest compressions [adequate depth and rate; allows the chest to recoil completely]	1	
Requests additional EMS response	1	

Performs 2 minutes of high-quality, 1-rescuer adult CPR
    Adequate depth and rate (1 point)
    Correct compression-to-ventilation ratio (1 point)
    Allows the chest to recoil completely (1 point)
    Adequate volumes for each breath (1 point)
    Minimal interruptions of less than 10 seconds throughout (1 point)
	5	

NOTE: After 2 minutes (5 cycles), patient is assessed and second rescuer resumes compressions while candidate operates AED.		
Turns-on power to AED	1	
Follows prompts and correctly attaches AED to patient	1	
Stops CPR and ensures all individuals are clear of the patient during rhythm analysis	1	
Ensures that all individuals are clear of the patient and delivers shock from AED	1	
Immediately directs rescuer to resume chest compressions	1	

Actual Time Ended: _____   **TOTAL**   18

Critical Criteria

____ Failure to take or verbalize appropriate body substance isolation precautions
____ Failure to immediately begin chest compressions as soon as pulselessness is confirmed
____ Failure to deliver shock in a timely manner
____ Interrupts CPR for more than 10 seconds at any point
____ Failure to demonstrate acceptable high-quality, 1-rescuer adult CPR
____ Failure to operate the AED properly
____ Failure to correctly attach the AED to the patient
____ Failure to assure that all individuals are clear of patient during rhythm analysis and before delivering shock(s) [verbalizes "All clear" and observes]
____ Failure to immediately resume compressions after shock delivered
____ Failure to manage the patient as a competent EMT
____ Exhibits unacceptable affect with patient or other personnel
____ Uses or orders a dangerous or inappropriate intervention

You must factually document your rationale for checking any of the above critical items on the reverse side of this form.

(Reprinted with permission of the National Registry of Emergency Medical Technicians.)

DYNAMIC CARDIOLOGY

Candidate:_____   Examiner:_____

Date:_____   Signature:_____

SET #_____

Level of Testing: ☐ NREMT-Intermediate/99   ☐ NR-Paramedic

Actual Time Started:_____

	Possible Points	Points Awarded
Takes or verbalizes infection control precautions	1	
Checks patient responsiveness	1	
Checks ABCs [responsive patient] – or – checks breathing and pulse [unresponsive patient]	1	
Initiates CPR if appropriate [verbally]	1	
Attaches ECG monitor in a timely fashion [patches, pads, or paddles]	1	
Correctly interprets initial rhythm	1	
Appropriately manages initial rhythm	2	
Notes change in rhythm	1	
Checks patient condition to include pulse and, if appropriate, BP	1	
Correctly interprets second rhythm	1	
Appropriately manages second rhythm	2	
Notes change in rhythm	1	
Checks patient condition to include pulse and, if appropriate, BP	1	
Correctly interprets third rhythm	1	
Appropriately manages third rhythm	2	
Notes change in rhythm	1	
Checks patient condition to include pulse and, if appropriate, BP	1	
Correctly interprets fourth rhythm	1	
Appropriately manages fourth rhythm	2	
Orders high percentages of supplemental oxygen at proper times	1	
Actual Time Ended: _____ TOTAL	24	

CRITICAL CRITERIA

_____ Failure to deliver first shock in a timely manner
_____ Failure to verify rhythm before delivering each shock
_____ Failure to ensure the safety of self and others [verbalizes "All clear" and observes]
_____ Inability to deliver DC shock [does not use machine properly]
_____ Failure to demonstrate acceptable shock sequence
_____ Failure to order initiation or resumption of CPR when appropriate
_____ Failure to order correct management of airway [ET when appropriate]
_____ Failure to order administration of appropriate oxygen at proper time
_____ Failure to diagnose or treat 2 or more rhythms correctly
_____ Orders administration of an inappropriate drug or lethal dosage
_____ Failure to correctly diagnose or adequately treat v-fib, v-tach, or asystole
_____ Failure to manage the patient as a competent EMT
_____ Exhibits unacceptable affect with patient or other personnel
_____ Uses or orders a dangerous or inappropriate intervention

You must factually document your rationale for checking any of the above critical items on the reverse side of this form.

(Reprinted with permission of the National Registry of Emergency Medical Technicians.)

National Registry of Emergency Medical Technicians
Advanced Level Psychomotor Examination
INTRAVENOUS THERAPY

Candidate: _____   Examiner: _____

Date: _____   Signature: _____

Level of Testing: ☐ NREMT-Intermediate/85   ☐ NRAEMT   ☐ NREMT-Intermediate/99   ☐ NREMT-Paramedic

Actual Time Started: _____

	Possible Points	Points Awarded

Checks selected IV fluid for:
  -Proper fluid (1 point)
  -Clarity (1 point)
  -Expiration date (1 point)
	3	

Selects appropriate catheter	1	
Selects proper administration set	1	
Connects IV tubing to the IV bag	1	
Prepares administration set [fills drip chamber and flushes tubing]	1	
Cuts or tears tape [at any time before venipuncture]	1	
Takes or verbalizes body substance isolation precautions [prior to venipuncture]	1	
Applies tourniquet	1	
Palpates suitable vein	1	
Cleanses site appropriately	1	

Performs venipuncture
  -Inserts stylette (1 point)
  -Notes or verbalizes flashback (1 point)
  -Occludes vein proximal to catheter (1 point)
  -Removes stylette (1 point)
  -Connects IV tubing to catheter (1 point)
	5	

Disposes/verbalizes proper disposal of needle in proper container	1	
Releases tourniquet	1	
Runs IV for a brief period to assure patent line	1	
Secures catheter [tapes securely or verbalizes]	1	
Adjusts flow rate as appropriate	1	
Actual Time Ended: _____ **TOTAL**	22	

NOTE: Check here ☐ if candidate did not establish a patent IV within 3 attempts in 6 minutes. Do **not** evaluate the candidate in IV Bolus Medications.

Critical Criteria

____ Failure to establish a patent and properly adjusted IV within 6-minute time limit
____ Failure to take or verbalize appropriate body substance isolation precautions prior to performing venipuncture
____ Contaminates equipment or site without appropriately correcting the situation
____ Performs any improper technique resulting in the potential for uncontrolled hemorrhage, catheter shear, or air embolism
____ Failure to successfully establish IV within 3 attempts during 6-minute time limit
____ Failure to dispose/verbalize disposal of blood-contaminated sharps immediately in proper container at the point of use
____ Failure to manage the patient as a competent EMT
____ Exhibits unacceptable affect with patient or other personnel
____ Uses or orders a dangerous or inappropriate intervention

You must factually document your rationale for checking any of the above critical items on the reverse side of this form.

INTRAVENOUS BOLUS MEDICATIONS

Actual Time Started: _____

	Possible Points	Points Awarded
Asks patient for known allergies	1	
Selects correct medication	1	
Assures correct concentration of medication	1	
Assembles prefilled syringe correctly and dispels air	1	
Continues to take or verbalize body substance isolation precautions	1	
Identifies and cleanses injection site closest to the patient [Y-port or hub]	1	
Reaffirms medication	1	
Stops IV flow	1	
Administers correct dose at proper push rate	1	
Disposes/verbalizes proper disposal of syringe and needle in proper container	1	
Turns IV on and adjusts drip rate to TKO/KVO	1	
Verbalizes need to observe patient for desired effect and adverse side effects	1	
Actual Time Ended: _____ **TOTAL**	12	

Critical Criteria

____ Failure to continue to take or verbalize appropriate body substance isolation precautions
____ Failure to begin administration of medication within 3-minute time limit
____ Contaminates equipment or site without appropriately correcting the situation
____ Failure to adequately dispel air resulting in potential for air embolism
____ Injects improper medication or dosage [wrong medication, incorrect amount, or pushes at inappropriate rate]
____ Failure to turn-on IV after injecting medication
____ Recaps needle or failure to dispose/verbalize disposal of syringe and other material in proper container
____ Failure to manage the patient as a competent EMT
____ Exhibits unacceptable affect with patient or other personnel
____ Uses or orders a dangerous or inappropriate intervention

You must factually document your rationale for checking any of the above critical items on the reverse side of this form.

p309/05-11

(Reprinted with permission of the National Registry of Emergency Medical Technicians.)

JOINT IMMOBILIZATION

Candidate: _____ Examiner: _____

Date: _____ Signature: _____

Actual Time Started: _____	Possible Points	Points Awarded
Takes or verbalizes appropriate body substance isolation precautions	1	
Directs application of manual stabilization of the injury	1	
Assesses distal motor, sensory, and circulatory functions in the injured extremity	1	
NOTE: The examiner acknowledges, "Motor, sensory, and circulatory functions are present and normal."		
Selects the proper splinting material	1	
Immobilizes the site of the injury	1	
Immobilizes the bone above the injury site	1	
Immobilizes the bone below the injury site	1	
Secures the entire injured extremity	1	
Reassesses distal motor, sensory, and circulatory functions in the injured extremity	1	
NOTE: The examiner acknowledges, "Motor, sensory, and circulatory functions are present and normal."		
Actual Time Ended: _____ TOTAL	9	

Critical Criteria

___ Did not immediately stabilize the extremity manually
___ Grossly moves the injured extremity
___ Did not immobilize the bone above and below the injury site
___ Did not reassess distal motor, sensory, and circulatory functions in the injured extremity before and after splinting
___ Failure to manage the patient as a competent EMT
___ Exhibits unacceptable affect with patient or other personnel
___ Uses or orders a dangerous or inappropriate intervention

You must factually document your rationale for checking any of the above critical items on the reverse side of this form.

(Reprinted with permission of the National Registry of Emergency Medical Technicians.)

National Registry of Emergency Medical Technicians
Advanced Level Psychomotor Examination

LONG BONE IMMOBILIZATION

Candidate: _____   Examiner: _____

Date: _____   Signature: _____

Actual Time Started: _____

	Possible Points	Points Awarded
Takes or verbalizes appropriate body substance isolation precautions	1	
Directs application of manual stabilization of the injury	1	
Assesses distal motor, sensory, and circulatory functions in the injured extremity	1	
NOTE: The examiner acknowledges, "Motor, sensory, and circulatory functions are present and normal."		
Measures the splint	1	
Applies the splint	1	
Immobilizes the joint above the injury site	1	
Immobilizes the joint below the injury site	1	
Secures the entire injured extremity	1	
Immobilizes the hand/foot in the position of function	1	
Reassesses distal motor, sensory, and circulatory functions in the injured extremity	1	
NOTE: The examiner acknowledges, "Motor, sensory, and circulatory functions are present and normal."		

Actual Time Ended: _____   **TOTAL**   10

Critical Criteria

___ Did not immediately stabilize the extremity manually
___ Grossly moves the injured extremity
___ Did not immobilize the joint above and the joint below the injury site
___ Did not immobilize the hand or foot in a position of function
___ Did not reassess distal motor, sensory, and circulatory functions in the injured extremity before and after splinting
___ Failure to manage the patient as a competent EMT
___ Exhibits unacceptable affect with patient or other personnel
___ Uses or orders a dangerous or inappropriate intervention

You must factually document your rationale for checking any of the above critical items on the reverse side of this form.

(Reprinted with permission of the National Registry of Emergency Medical Technicians.)

National Registry of Emergency Medical Technicians
Advanced Level Psychomotor Examination
ORAL STATION

Candidate: _____ Examiner: _____

Date: _____ Signature: _____

Scenario: _____

Actual Time Started: _____

	Possible Points	Points Awarded
Scene Management		
Thoroughly assessed and took deliberate actions to control the scene	3	
Assessed the scene, identified potential hazards, did not put anyone in danger	2	
Incompletely assessed or managed the scene	1	
Did not assess or manage the scene	0	
Patient Assessment		
Completed an organized assessment and integrated findings to expand further assessment	3	
Completed primary survey and secondary assessment	2	
Performed an incomplete or disorganized assessment	1	
Did not complete a primary survey	0	
Patient Management		
Managed all aspects of the patient's condition and anticipated further needs	3	
Appropriately managed the patient's presenting condition	2	
Performed an incomplete or disorganized management	1	
Did not manage life-threatening conditions	0	
Interpersonal relations		
Established rapport and interacted in an organized, therapeutic manner	3	
Interacted and responded appropriately with patient, crew, and bystanders	2	
Used inappropriate communication techniques	1	
Demonstrated intolerance for patient, bystanders, and crew	0	
Integration (verbal report, field impression, and transport decision)		
Stated correct field impression and pathophysiological basis, provided succinct and accurate verbal report including social/psychological concerns, and considered alternate transport destinations	3	
Stated correct field impression, provided succinct and accurate verbal report, and appropriately stated transport decision	2	
Stated correct field impression, provided inappropriate verbal report or transport decision	1	
Stated incorrect field impression or did not provide verbal report	0	

Actual Time Ended: _____ **TOTAL** **15**

Critical Criteria
_____ Failure to appropriately address any of the scenario's "Mandatory Actions"
_____ Failure to manage the patient as a competent EMT
_____ Exhibits unacceptable affect with patient or other personnel
_____ Uses or orders a dangerous or inappropriate intervention
You must factually document your rationale for checking any of the above critical items on the reverse side of this form.

p308/10-11

(Reprinted with permission of the National Registry of Emergency Medical Technicians.)

National Registry of Emergency Medical Technicians
Advanced Level Psychomotor Examination

PATIENT ASSESSMENT - MEDICAL

Candidate: _____   Examiner: _____

Date: _____   Signature: _____

Scenario: _____

Actual Time Started: _____

	Possible Points	Points Awarded
Takes or verbalizes body substance isolation precautions	1	
SCENE SIZE-UP		
Determines the scene/situation is safe	1	
Determines the mechanism of injury/nature of illness	1	
Determines the number of patients	1	
Requests additional help if necessary	1	
Considers stabilization of spine	1	
PRIMARY SURVEY		
Verbalizes general impression of the patient	1	
Determines responsiveness/level of consciousness	1	
Determines chief complaint/apparent life-threats	1	

Assesses airway and breathing
    -Assessment (1 point)
    -Assures adequate ventilation (1 point)
        -Initiates appropriate oxygen therapy (1 point)
	3	

Assesses circulation
    -Assesses/controls major bleeding (1 point)   -Assesses skin [either skin color, temperature, or condition] (1 point)
    -Assesses pulse (1 point)
	3	

Identifies priority patients/makes transport decision	1	
HISTORY TAKING AND SECONDARY ASSESSMENT		

History of present illness
    -Onset (1 point)   -Severity (1 point)
    -Provocation (1 point)   -Time (1 point)
    -Quality (1 point)   -Clarifying questions of associated signs and symptoms as related to OPQRST (2 points)
    -Radiation (1 point)
	8	

Past medical history
    -Allergies (1 point)   -Past pertinent history (1 point)   -Events leading to present illness (1 point)
    -Medications (1 point)   -Last oral intake (1 point)
	5	

Performs secondary assessment [assess affected body part/system or, if indicated, completes rapid assessment]
    -Cardiovascular   -Neurological   -Integumentary   -Reproductive
    -Pulmonary   -Musculoskeletal   -GI/GU   -Psychological/Social
	5	

Vital signs
    -Pulse (1 point)   -Respiratory rate and quality (1 point each)
    -Blood pressure (1 point)   -AVPU (1 point)
	5	

Diagnostics [must include application of ECG monitor for dyspnea and chest pain]	2	
States field impression of patient	1	
Verbalizes treatment plan for patient and calls for appropriate intervention(s)	1	
Transport decision re-evaluated	1	
REASSESSMENT		
Repeats primary survey	1	
Repeats vital signs	1	
Evaluates response to treatments	1	
Repeats secondary assessment regarding patient complaint or injuries	1	
Actual Time Ended: _____		
CRITICAL CRITERIA **TOTAL**	48	

_____ Failure to initiate or call for transport of the patient within 15-minute time limit
_____ Failure to take or verbalize body substance isolation precautions
_____ Failure to determine scene safety before approaching patient
_____ Failure to voice and ultimately provide appropriate oxygen therapy
_____ Failure to assess/provide adequate ventilation
_____ Failure to find or appropriately manage problems associated with airway, breathing, hemorrhage or shock [hypoperfusion]
_____ Failure to differentiate patient's need for immediate transportation versus continued assessment and treatment at the scene
_____ Does other detailed history or physical examination before assessing and treating threats to airway, breathing, and circulation
_____ Failure to determine the patient's primary problem
_____ Orders a dangerous or inappropriate intervention
_____ Failure to provide for spinal protection when indicated

You must factually document your rationale for checking any of the above critical items on the reverse side of this form.

(Reprinted with permission of the National Registry of Emergency Medical Technicians.)

National Registry of Emergency Medical Technicians
Advanced Level Psychomotor Examination

PATIENT ASSESSMENT - TRAUMA

Candidate: _____ Examiner: _____

Date: _____ Signature: _____

Scenario # _____

Actual Time Started: _____   NOTE: Areas denoted by "**" may be integrated within sequence of primary survey

	Possible Points	Points Awarded
Takes or verbalizes body substance isolation precautions	1	
SCENE SIZE-UP		
Determines the scene/situation is safe	1	
Determines the mechanism of injury/nature of illness	1	
Determines the number of patients	1	
Requests additional help if necessary	1	
Considers stabilization of spine	1	
PRIMARY SURVEY/RESUSCITATION		
Verbalizes general impression of the patient	1	
Determines responsiveness/level of consciousness	1	
Determines chief complaint/apparent life-threats	1	
Airway -Opens and assesses airway (1 point) -Inserts adjunct as indicated (1 point)	2	
Breathing -Assess breathing (1 point) -Assures adequate ventilation (1 point) -Initiates appropriate oxygen therapy (1 point) -Manages any injury which may compromise breathing/ventilation (1 point)	4	
Circulation -Checks pulse (1point) -Assess skin [either skin color, temperature, or condition] (1 point) -Assesses for and controls major bleeding if present (1 point) -Initiates shock management (1 point)	4	
Identifies priority patients/makes transport decision based upon calculated GCS	1	
HISTORY TAKING		
Obtains, or directs assistant to obtain, baseline vital signs	1	
Attempts to obtain sample history	1	
SECONDARY ASSESSMENT		
Head -Inspects mouth**, nose**, and assesses facial area (1 point) -Inspects and palpates scalp and ears (1 point) -Assesses eyes for PERRL** (1 point)	3	
Neck** -Checks position of trachea (1 point) -Checks jugular veins (1 point) -Palpates cervical spine (1 point)	3	
Chest** -Inspects chest (1 point) -Palpates chest (1 point) -Auscultates chest (1 point)	3	
Abdomen/pelvis** -Inspects and palpates abdomen (1 point) -Assesses pelvis (1 point) -Verbalizes assessment of genitalia/perineum as needed (1 point)	3	
Lower extremities** -Inspects, palpates, and assesses motor, sensory, and distal circulatory functions (1 point/leg)	2	
Upper extremities -Inspects, palpates, and assesses motor, sensory, and distal circulatory functions (1 point/arm)	2	
Posterior thorax, lumbar, and buttocks** -Inspects and palpates posterior thorax (1 point) -Inspects and palpates lumbar and buttocks area (1 point)	2	
Manages secondary injuries and wounds appropriately	1	
Reassesses patient	1	
TOTAL	42	

Actual Time Ended: _____

CRITICAL CRITERIA

_____ Failure to initiate or call for transport of the patient within 10-minute time limit
_____ Failure to take or verbalize body substance isolation precautions
_____ Failure to determine scene safety
_____ Failure to assess for and provide spinal protection when indicated
_____ Failure to voice and ultimately provide high concentration of oxygen
_____ Failure to assess/provide adequate ventilation
_____ Failure to find or appropriately manage problems associated with airway, breathing, hemorrhage or shock [hypoperfusion]
_____ Failure to differentiate patient's need for immediate transportation versus continued assessment/treatment at the scene
_____ Does other detailed history or physical exam before assessing/treating threats to airway, breathing, and circulation
_____ Failure to manage the patient as a competent EMT
_____ Exhibits unacceptable affect with patient or other personnel
_____ Uses or orders a dangerous or inappropriate intervention

You must factually document your rationale for checking any of the above critical items on the reverse side of this form.

(Reprinted with permission of the National Registry of Emergency Medical Technicians.)

PEDIATRIC INTRAOSSEOUS INFUSION

Candidate: _____ Examiner: _____

Date: _____ Signature: _____

Actual Time Started: _____	Possible Points	Points Awarded
Checks selected IV fluid for: -Proper fluid (1 point) -Clarity (1 point) -Expiration date (1 point)	3	
Selects appropriate equipment to include: -IO needle (1 point) -Syringe (1 point) -Saline (1 point) -Extension set or 3-way stopcock (1 point)	4	
Selects proper administration set	1	
Connects administration set to bag	1	
Prepares administration set [fills drip chamber and flushes tubing]	1	
Prepares syringe and extension tubing or 3-way stopcock	1	
Cuts or tears tape [at any time before IO puncture]	1	
Takes or verbalizes appropriate body substance isolation precautions [prior to IO puncture]	1	
Identifies proper anatomical site for IO puncture	1	
Cleanses site appropriately	1	
Performs IO puncture: -Stabilizes tibia without placing hand under puncture site and "cupping" leg (1 point) -Inserts needle at proper angle (1 point) -Advances needle with twisting motion until "pop" is felt or notices sudden lack of resistance (1 point) -Removes stylette (1 point)	4	
Disposes/verbalizes proper disposal of needle in proper container	1	
Attaches syringe and extension set to IO needle and aspirates; or attaches 3-way stopcock between administration set and IO needle and aspirates; or attaches extension set to IO needle [aspiration is not required for any of these as many IO sticks are "dry" sticks]	1	
Slowly injects saline to assure proper placement of needle	1	
Adjusts flow rate/bolus as appropriate	1	
Secures needle and supports with bulky dressing [tapes securely or verbalizes]	1	
Actual Time Ended: _____ **TOTAL**	24	

Critical Criteria

____ Failure to establish a patent and properly adjusted IO line within 6-minute time limit
____ Failure to take or verbalize appropriate body substance isolation precautions prior to performing IO puncture
____ Contaminates equipment or site without appropriately correcting the situation
____ Performs any improper technique resulting in the potential for air embolism
____ Failure to assure correct needle placement [must aspirate or watch closely for early signs of infiltration]
____ Failure to successfully establish IO infusion within 2 attempts during 6-minute time limit
____ Performs IO puncture in an unacceptable manner [improper site, incorrect needle angle, holds leg in palm and performs IO puncture directly above hand, etc.]
____ Failure to properly dispose/verbalize disposal of blood-contaminated sharps immediately in proper container at the point of use
____ Failure to manage the patient as a competent EMT
____ Exhibits unacceptable affect with patient or other personnel
____ Uses or orders a dangerous or inappropriate intervention

You must factually document your rationale for checking any of the above critical items on the reverse side of this form.

(Reprinted with permission of the National Registry of Emergency Medical Technicians.)

National Registry of Emergency Medical Technicians
Advanced Emergency Medical Technician Psychomotor Examination

PEDIATRIC RESPIRATORY COMPROMISE

Candidate: _____   Examiner: _____
Date: _____   Signature: _____

Actual Time Started: _____

	Possible Points	Points Awarded
Takes or verbalizes body substance isolation precautions	1	
Verbalizes general impression of patient from a distance before approaching or touching the patient	1	
Determines level of consciousness	1	
Assesses the airway [looks for secretions and signs of foreign body airway obstruction; listens for audible noises and voice sounds]	1	
Assesses breathing [checks rate, rhythm, chest excursion, audible noises]	1	
Attaches pulse oximeter and evaluates SpO$_2$ reading	1	
NOTE: Examiner now informs candidate, "Pulse oximeter shows a saturation of 82%."		
Selects proper delivery device and attaches to oxygen	1	
Administers oxygen at proper flow rate [blow-by oxygen, non-rebreather mask]	1	
Checks pulse	1	
Evaluates perfusion [skin color, temperature, condition; capillary refill]	1	
Obtains baseline vital signs	1	
NOTE: Examiner now advises candidate that patient begins to develop decreasing SpO$_2$, decreasing pulse rate, see-saw respirations, head bobbing, drowsiness, etc.		
Places patient supine and pads appropriately to maintain a sniffing position	1	
Manually opens airway	1	
Considers airway adjunct insertion based upon patient presentation [oropharyngeal or nasopharyngeal airway]	1	
NOTE: Examiner now informs candidate no gag reflex is present and patient accepts airway adjunct. The patient's respiratory rate is now 20/minute.		
Inserts airway adjunct properly and positions head and neck for ventilation	1	
Selects appropriate BVM and attaches reservoir to oxygen flowing at 12–15 L/minute	1	
Assures tight mask seal to face	1	
Assists ventilations at a rate of 20/minute and with sufficient volume to cause visible chest rise	1	
Ventilates at proper rate and volume while observing changes in capnometry/capnography, pulse oximeter, pulse rate, level of responsiveness	1	
NOTE: The examiner must now ask the candidate, "How would you know if you are ventilating the patient properly?"		
Calls for immediate transport of patient	1	

Actual Time Ended: _____   **TOTAL**   20

Critical Criteria

___ Failure to initiate ventilations within 30 seconds after taking body substance isolation precautions or interrupts ventilations for greater than 30 seconds at any time
___ Failure to take or verbalize body substance isolation precautions
___ Failure to voice and ultimately provide high oxygen concentration [at least 85%]
___ Failure to ventilate the patient at a rate of 20/minute
___ Failure to provide adequate volumes per breath [maximum 2 errors/minute permissible]
___ Failure to recognize and treat respiratory failure in a timely manner
___ Insertion or use of any airway adjunct in a manner dangerous to the patient
___ Failure to manage the patient as a competent EMT
___ Exhibits unacceptable affect with patient or other personnel
___ Uses or orders a dangerous or inappropriate intervention

You must factually document your rationale for checking any of the above critical items on the reverse side of this form.

© 2011 National Registry of Emergency Medical Technicians, Inc., Columbus, OH
All materials subject to this copyright may be photocopied for the non-commercial purpose of educational or scientific advancement.   p314/10-11

(Reprinted with permission of the National Registry of Emergency Medical Technicians.)

National Registry Practical Examination Sheets   **427**

National Registry of Emergency Medical Technicians
Advanced Level Psychomotor Examination

PEDIATRIC (<2 yrs.) VENTILATORY MANAGEMENT

Candidate: _____ Examiner: _____

Date: _____ Signature: _____

NOTE   If candidate elects to ventilate initially with BVM attached to reservoir and oxygen, full credit must be awarded for steps denoted by "**" so long as first ventilation is delivered within 30 seconds.

Actual Time Started: _____

	Possible Points	Points Awarded
Takes or verbalizes body substance isolation precautions	1	
Opens the airway manually	1	
Elevates tongue, inserts simple adjunct [oropharyngeal or nasopharyngeal airway]	1	
NOTE: Examiner now informs candidate no gag reflex is present and patient accepts adjunct		
**Ventilates patient immediately with bag-valve-mask device unattached to oxygen	1	
**Ventilates patient with room air	1	
NOTE: Examiner now informs candidate that ventilation is being performed without difficulty and that pulse oximetry indicates the patient's blood oxygen saturation is 85%		
Attaches oxygen reservoir to bag-valve-mask device and connects to oxygen regulator [12–15 L/minute]	1	
Ventilates patient at a rate of 12–15/minute and assures visible chest rise	1	
NOTE: After 30 seconds, examiner auscultates and reports breath sounds are present, equal bilaterally and medical direction has ordered intubation. The examiner must now take over ventilation.		
Directs assistant to pre-oxygenate patient	1	
Identifies/selects proper equipment for intubation	1	
Checks laryngoscope to assure operational with bulb tight	1	
NOTE: Examiner to remove OPA and move out of the way when candidate is prepared to intubate		
Places patient in neutral or sniffing position	1	
Inserts blade while displacing tongue	1	
Elevates mandible with laryngoscope	1	
Introduces ET tube and advances to proper depth	1	
Directs ventilation of patient	1	
Confirms proper placement by auscultation bilaterally over each lung and over epigastrium	1	
NOTE: Examiner to ask, "If you had proper placement, what should you expect to hear?"		
Secures ET tube [may be verbalized]	1	

Actual Time Ended: _____   **TOTAL**   17

CRITICAL CRITERIA

_____ Failure to initiate ventilations within 30 seconds after applying gloves or interrupts ventilations for greater than 30 seconds at any time
_____ Failure to take or verbalize body substance isolation precautions
_____ Failure to pad under the torso to allow neutral head position or sniffing position
_____ Failure to voice and ultimately provide high oxygen concentrations [at least 85%]
_____ Failure to ventilate patient at a rate of 12–15/minute
_____ Failure to provide adequate volumes per breath [maximum 2 errors/minute permissible]
_____ Failure to pre-oxygenate patient prior to intubation
_____ Failure to successfully intubate within 3 attempts
_____ Uses gums as a fulcrum
_____ Failure to assure proper tube placement by auscultation bilaterally **and** over the epigastrium
_____ Inserts any adjunct in a manner dangerous to the patient
_____ Attempts to use any equipment not appropriate for the pediatric patient
_____ Failure to manage the patient as a competent EMT
_____ Exhibits unacceptable affect with patient or other personnel
_____ Uses or orders a dangerous or inappropriate intervention

You must factually document your rationale for checking any of the above critical items on the reverse side of this form.

(Reprinted with permission of the National Registry of Emergency Medical Technicians.)

National Registry of Emergency Medical Technicians
Advanced Level Psychomotor Examination

SPINAL IMMOBILIZATION (SEATED PATIENT)

Candidate: _____ Examiner: _____

Date: _____ Signature: _____

Actual Time Start: _____	Possible Points	Points Awarded
Takes or verbalizes body substance isolation precautions	1	
Directs assistant to place/maintain head in the neutral, inline position	1	
Directs assistant to maintain manual immobilization of the head	1	
Reassesses motor, sensory, and circulatory functions in each extremity	1	
Applies appropriately sized extrication collar	1	
Positions the immobilization device behind the patient	1	
Secures the device to the patient's torso	1	
Evaluates torso fixation and adjusts as necessary	1	
Evaluates and pads behind the patient's head as necessary	1	
Secures the patient's head to the device	1	
Verbalizes moving the patient to a long backboard	1	
Reassesses motor, sensory, and circulatory function in each extremity	1	

Actual Time End: _____   **TOTAL**   12

CRITICAL CRITERIA

_____ Did not immediately direct or take manual immobilization of the head
_____ Did not properly apply appropriately sized cervical collar before ordering release of manual immobilization
_____ Released or ordered release of manual immobilization before it was maintained mechanically
_____ Manipulated or moved patient excessively causing potential spinal compromise
_____ Head immobilized to the device before device sufficiently secured to torso
_____ Device moves excessively up, down, left, or right on the patient's torso
_____ Head immobilization allows for excessive movement
_____ Torso fixation inhibits chest rise, resulting in respiratory compromise
_____ Upon completion of immobilization, head is not in a neutral, inline position
_____ Did not reassess motor, sensory, and circulatory functions in each extremity after voicing immobilization to the long backboard
_____ Failure to manage the patient as a competent EMT
_____ Exhibits unacceptable affect with patient or other personnel
_____ Uses or orders a dangerous or inappropriate intervention

You must factually document your rationale for checking any of the above critical items on the reverse side of this form.

(Reprinted with permission of the National Registry of Emergency Medical Technicians.)

Candidate: _____   Examiner: _____

Date: _____   Signature: _____

Actual Time Started: _____

	Possible Points	Points Awarded
Takes or verbalizes body substance isolation precautions	1	
Directs assistant to place/maintain head in the neutral, inline position	1	
Directs assistant to maintain manual immobilization of the head	1	
Reassesses motor, sensory, and circulatory function in each extremity	1	
Applies appropriately sized extrication collar	1	
Positions the immobilization device appropriately	1	
Directs movement of the patient onto the device without compromising the integrity of the spine	1	
Applies padding to voids between the torso and the device as necessary	1	
Immobilizes the patient's torso to the device	1	
Evaluates and pads behind the patient's head as necessary	1	
Immobilizes the patient's head to the device	1	
Secures the patient's legs to the device	1	
Secures the patient's arms to the device	1	
Reassesses motor, sensory, and circulatory function in each extremity	1	

Actual Time Ended: _____   **TOTAL**   14

CRITICAL CRITERIA

_____ Did not immediately direct or take manual immobilization of the head
_____ Did not properly apply appropriately sized cervical collar before ordering release of manual immobilization
_____ Released or ordered release of manual immobilization before it was maintained mechanically
_____ Manipulated or moved patient excessively causing potential spinal compromise
_____ Head immobilized to the device **before** device sufficiently secured to torso
_____ Patient moves excessively up, down, left, or right on the device
_____ Head immobilization allows for excessive movement
_____ Upon completion of immobilization, head is not in a neutral, inline position
_____ Did not reassess motor, sensory, and circulatory functions in each extremity after immobilizing patient
          to the device
_____ Failure to manage the patient as a competent EMT
_____ Exhibits unacceptable affect with patient or other personnel
_____ Uses or orders a dangerous or inappropriate intervention

You must factually document your rationale for checking any of the above critical items on the reverse side of this form.

(Reprinted with permission of the National Registry of Emergency Medical Technicians.)

National Registry of Emergency
Advanced Level Psychomotor Examination

STATIC CARDIOLOGY

Candidate: _____ Examiner: _____

Date: _____ Signature: _____

SET # _____

Level of Testing: ☐ NREMT-Intermediate/99   ☐ NREMT-Paramedic

Note: No points for treatment may be awarded if the diagnosis is incorrect.
Only document incorrect responses in spaces provided.

Actual Time Started: _____

	Possible Points	Points Awarded
STRIP #1		
Diagnosis:	1	
Treatment:	2	
STRIP #2		
Diagnosis:	1	
Treatment:	2	
STRIP #3		
Diagnosis:	1	
Treatment:	2	
STRIP #4		
Diagnosis:	1	
Treatment:	2	
Actual Time Ended: _____ **TOTAL**	12	

p307/07-11

(Reprinted with permission of the National Registry of Emergency Medical Technicians.)

National Registry of Emergency Medical Technicians
Advanced Level Psychomotor Examination

VENTILATORY MANAGEMENT - ADULT

Candidate: _____   Examiner: _____

Date: _____   Signature: _____

NOTE: If candidate elects to ventilate initially with BVM attached to reservoir and oxygen, full credit must be awarded for steps denoted by "**" so long as first ventilation is delivered within 30 seconds.

Actual Time Started: _____

	Possible Points	Points Awarded
Takes or verbalizes body substance isolation precautions	1	
Opens the airway manually	1	
Elevates tongue, inserts simple adjunct [oropharyngeal or nasopharyngeal airway]	1	
NOTE: Examiner now informs candidate no gag reflex is present and patient accepts adjunct		
**Ventilates patient immediately with bag-valve-mask device unattached to oxygen	1	
**Ventilates patient with room air	1	
NOTE: Examiner now informs candidate that ventilation is being performed without difficulty and that pulse oximetry indicates the patient's blood oxygen saturation is 85%		
Attaches oxygen reservoir to bag-valve-mask device and connects to oxygen regulator [12–15 L/minute]	1	
Ventilates patient at a rate of 10–12/minute with appropriate volumes	1	
NOTE: After 30 seconds, examiner auscultates and reports breath sounds are present, equal bilaterally and medical direction has ordered intubation. The examiner must now take over ventilation.		
Directs assistant to pre-oxygenate patient	1	
Identifies/selects proper equipment for intubation	1	
Checks equipment for: -Cuff leaks (1 point) -Laryngoscope operational with bulb tight (1 point)	2	
NOTE: Examiner to remove OPA and move out of the way when candidate is prepared to intubate		
Positions head properly	1	
Inserts blade while displacing tongue	1	
Elevates mandible with laryngoscope	1	
Introduces ET tube and advances to proper depth	1	
Inflates cuff to proper pressure and disconnects syringe	1	
Directs ventilation of patient	1	
Confirms proper placement by auscultation bilaterally over each lung and over epigastrium	1	
NOTE: Examiner to ask, "If you had proper placement, what should you expect to hear?"		
Secures ET tube [may be verbalized]	1	
NOTE: Examiner now asks candidate, "Please demonstrate one additional method of verifying proper tube placement in this patient."		
Identifies/selects proper equipment	1	
Verbalizes findings and interpretations [checks end-tidal CO_2, colorimetric device, EDD recoil, etc.]	1	
NOTE: Examiner now states, "You see secretions in the tube and hear gurgling sounds with the patient's exhalation."		
Identifies/selects a flexible suction catheter	1	
Pre-oxygenates patient	1	
Marks maximum insertion length with thumb and forefinger	1	
Inserts catheter into the ET tube leaving catheter port open	1	
At proper insertion depth, covers catheter port and applies suction while withdrawing catheter	1	
Ventilates/directs ventilation of patient as catheter is flushed with sterile water	1	

Actual Time Ended: _____   **TOTAL**   **27**

CRITICAL CRITERIA

_____ Failure to initiate ventilations within 30 seconds after applying gloves or interrupts ventilations for greater than 30 seconds at any time
_____ Failure to take or verbalize body substance isolation precautions
_____ Failure to voice and ultimately provide high oxygen concentrations [at least 85%]
_____ Failure to ventilate patient at a rate of 10–12/minute
_____ Failure to provide adequate volumes per breath [maximum 2 errors/minute permissible]
_____ Failure to pre-oxygenate patient prior to intubation and suctioning
_____ Failure to successfully intubate within 3 attempts
_____ Failure to disconnect syringe **immediately** after inflating cuff of ET tube
_____ Uses teeth as a fulcrum
_____ Failure to assure proper tube placement by auscultation bilaterally **and** over the epigastrium
_____ If used, stylette extends beyond end of ET tube
_____ Inserts any adjunct in a manner dangerous to the patient
_____ Suctions patient excessively
_____ Does not suction the patient
_____ Failure to manage the patient as a competent EMT
_____ Exhibits unacceptable affect with patient or other personnel
_____ Uses or orders a dangerous or inappropriate intervention

You must factually document your rationale for checking any of the above critical items on the reverse side of this form.

(Reprinted with permission of the National Registry of Emergency Medical Technicians.)

Note to all students/readers: *These sheets were current at the time this book was printed. They do change and it is always prudent to check the National Registry or your State EMS website for the most recent version!*

Appendix D: Glossary

AAA (abdominal aortic aneurysm) Damage to the wall of the aorta, which causes a thinning of the wall and a large bubble that becomes a pulsatile mass in the patient's abdomen. If the AAA should leak or burst, it can be rapidly fatal.

abandonment Leaving a patient who requires medical care without turning him over to the proper medical care provider.

ABCD survey The survey that is taught in the ACLS course, which includes assessing and managing the airway, breathing, circulation, and defibrillation as needed.

abrasion Damage to the outermost layer of skin due to shearing forces.

abruption placenta The premature separation of the placenta.

absence seizure A type of seizure in which the patient stares off into space or seems to be daydreaming; common in children; once called petit mal.

accommodation The ability of the lenses of the eyes to adjust in order to focus on objects at different distances.

ACD-CPR Active compression–decompression CPR technique.

ACLS (advanced cardiac life support) Training required of medical professionals in the resuscitation of acute cardiac events and ECG dysrhythmias that may be life threatening.

ACS See *acute coronary syndromes*.

acuity Clarity or sharpness of vision.

acute coronary syndrome (ACS) A broad category of cardiovascular disorders associated with coronary atherosclerosis that may develop a spectrum of clinical syndromes representing varying degrees of coronary artery occlusion. These syndromes include unstable angina, non-Q wave MI, Q wave MI, and sudden cardiac death.

acute life-threatening event See *ALTE*.

acute mountain sickness See *AMS*.

acute myocardial infarction See *AMI*.

acute pulmonary edema (APE) A rapid onset of fluid in the alveoli and interstitial tissue of the lungs.

AD (affective disorders) Disorders that affect the patient's temperament.

adrenal gland disease A disease that affects the adrenal gland, such as Cushing's syndrome or adrenal insufficiency.

adrenal insufficiency The inadequate production of adrenal hormones (primarily cortisol and aldosterone).

advanced cardiac life support See *ACLS*.

advanced directive A document or order prepared at the request of the patient, an authorized family member or legal representative, or the physician to ensure that certain treatment choices are followed at a time when the patient is unable to speak for himself.

advanced life support See *ALS*.

adventitious Abnormal.

advocate Someone who looks out for the needs of others who are not in a position to look out for themselves for various reasons, such as ignorance, incapacity, underage, or misfortune; also, to look out for another.

AED (automated external defibrillator) A device designed to be applied by electrode pads to the chest of a pulseless patient, which will rapidly analyze if the ECG is a shockable rhythm and, if so, guide the user with voice prompts through clearing the patient and then administering a shock to the heart.

AEIOUTIPS The mnemonic used to remember the many possible reasons a person may experience an altered mental state: alcohol, epilepsy, infection, overdose, uremia, trauma, insulin, psychosis, stroke.

affect The emotional mindset prompting an expressed emotion or behavior.

agonal respirations Dying breaths; irregular and progressively slowing breaths. Often called gasps.

air embolism A potentially life-threatening condition in which a bubble of air has collected in the patient's vessels. This can be caused by a scuba incident, a slashed neck vein, or accidental injection of air into a vein.

allergy A reaction from the body after an exposure to a foreign substance.

ALS (advanced life support) The care provided to patients with acute emergencies that involve invasive therapies such as medication administration and inserting an advanced airway device.

ALTE (acute life-threatening event) In the newly born, an event involving a combination of apnea, choking, gagging, and change in color and muscle tone, which is not a sleep disorder.

altered mental status The mental status of a patient whose level of consciousness is anything other than alert (oriented to person, place, and day).

altitude illness Sickness brought on in high altitudes where there is decreased atmospheric pressure. This condition is usually a result of flying in an unpressurized airplane or mountain climbing without first acclimatizing.

Alzheimer's disease A disorder that affects approximately four million Americans, involving cortical atrophy and a loss of neurons in the frontal and temporal lobes of the brain.

American Sign Language (ASL) A communication technique in which the hands and arms are used to sign words or phrases for individuals who are deaf or hard of hearing.

Americans with Disabilities Act (ADA) Federal legislation that regulates the rights of individuals with disabilities to ensure that these individuals have access to equipment and information that can improve their ability to function and interact.

AMI (acute myocardial infarction) The death of cardiac muscle tissue, usually due to a blockage of the blood flow through one of the coronary arteries.

amnesia Forgetting; usually the loss of short-term memory immediately after striking one's head.

amputation Complete loss of a limb or other body part.

AMS (acute mountain sickness) A combination of intracerebral edema and acute pulmonary edema, which is experienced by climbing very tall mountains without first acclimatizing.

anaphylaxis The most severe type of reaction to an allergen, involving cardiovascular collapse.

anemia of pregnancy An increase in the total blood volume that occurs during pregnancy without a proportionate increase in hemoglobin, creating a dilution effect.

angioedema Cutaneous swelling that most often affects the face, neck, head, and upper airways.

anisocoria Unequal pupils; normal in a small percentage of the population or may indicate a central nervous system disease.

antepartum factors Those medical history factors that may seriously affect pregnancy and labor. Some are controllable (e.g., drug use and smoking) while others are not (e.g., diabetes, placenta previa , or abruptio placentae).

anterior cord syndrome A partial transaction caused by bone fragments or pressure on spinal arteries. It involves loss of motor function and the sensation of pain, temperature, and heavy touch.

antibody A protein substance formed by the body in response to antigens that have entered the body.

antigen A foreign substance that, when introduced to the body, causes the production of antibodies.

antisocial behavior A period that some adolescents go through in which they have an identity crisis or act out against society and its rules. This typically peaks around the eighth or ninth grade.

aortic dissection A splitting of the wall of the aorta, usually due to systemic hypertension and a weakness in the wall. This can lead to a tearing or leaking of the vessel, which can be rapidly life threatening.

APCO Association of Public-Safety Communications Officials.

APE (acute pulmonary edema) Fluid that has rapidly gathered in the alveoli and interstitial tissue of the lungs from a backup of the blood in the left side of the heart. Primarily found in cardiac patients, but can also be found in patients with altitude sickness and narcotic overdose.

APGAR scoring system A well-accepted assessment scoring system for newborns that assigns a rating of 0, 1, or 2 to each of the following signs: color, pulse, reflex, muscle tone, and respirations. The APGAR score is measured at 1 minute and 5 minutes after birth.

aphasia A defect or loss of the ability to either say or comprehend words. The person may have difficulty reading, writing, speaking, or understanding the speech of others.

apical pulse The kick of the left ventricle, which can be felt at the point of maximal impulse on the lower-left chest wall.

apnea A cessation of breathing.

apnea monitor A device that is designed to alert the family members or health care providers that a patient has stopped breathing. These devices are often used with premature infants and patients with sleep disorders.

apothecary system The system used prior to the metric system, involving units of measure such as minims, fluidrams, fluidounces, pints, and gallons.

arterial gas (air) embolism The most serious diving-related emergency, caused by failing to exhale on ascent with a resultant expansion of air in the lungs, causing alveoli to rupture and allow air to escape.

arterial tourniquet A band of cloth or bandage that is tied so tightly that it occludes the blood flow to an extremity. This is a form of bleeding control considered a last resort where the choice would be to potentially sacrifice the limb to save the life.

ascending nerve tracts Nerve tracts that carry impulses from body parts and sensory information to the brain.

ascites An abnormal accumulation of fluid in the peritoneal cavity.

aspirate To inhale vomitus, blood, or other secretions into the lungs.

assault and battery Striking out at someone or verbally accosting them with the intent to cause harm. In some states, these crimes are illegal against emergency service providers and carry higher penalties.

asthma A form of reversible obstructive lung disease; a multifactorial hypersensitivity reaction causing constriction of the bronchioles and difficulty breathing.

asystole The lack of a cardiac rhythm; cardiac standstill or flatline.

ataxia An abnormal gait that appears wobbly and unsteady, as when one is intoxicated or heavily medicated.

atelectasis Collapse of lung tissue.

atherosclerosis The plaque that forms on the inside of the arteries, also referred to as hardening of the arteries. Cholesterol, fat, and other blood components build up in the walls of the arteries. As the condition progresses, the arteries to the heart may narrow, reducing the flow of oxygen-rich blood and nutrients to the heart.

atrial fibrillation An ECG dysrhythmia common in the elderly, which originates in the atria and is irregular; involving a fibrillating atria.

atrophy A decrease in cell size leading to a decrease in the size of the tissue and organ.

ATV (automatic transport ventilator) A positive pressure ventilation device that automatically cycles based on the setting of the volume and the rate per minute.

aura A sensation (e.g., color, lights) experienced just before a seizure.

auscultation To listen with a stethoscope, as in breath sounds, blood pressure, and heart sounds.

autoimmunity When a person's T cells or antibodies attack them, causing tissue damage or organ dysfunction.

automated external defibrillator See *AED*.

automatic transport ventilator See *ATV*.

automaticity The unique ability of the heart muscle tissue to generate impulses.

AVPU An abbreviation for the mini-neuro exam used by the EMS provider during the initial assessment of a patient: alert, verbally responsive, painful response, unresponsive.

avulsion Loose or torn tissue.

awareness-level training As specified in the OSHA regulation CFR 1910.120, the level of training for first responders to hazardous materials incidents where the responders may come in contact with an incident but will be in the cold zone and have no responsibility for patient decontamination.

BAAM® (Beck Airway Airflow Monitor) A small device that fits onto the end of the tracheal tube and is designed to make a noise (like a kazoo) when the patient breathes or when the provider who is attempting to place a tracheal tube through the nasal route locates the glottic opening.

Babinski's reflex An abnormal response of dorsiflexion of the big toe and fanning of all the toes when the outer surface of the sole is firmly stroked from the heel to the toe; indicates a disturbance in the motor response in the central nervous system.

bag mask ventilation Formerly called the BVM, or bag-valve-mask, the Guidelines 2005 have standardized this terminology as the bag mask device or bag mask ventilation.

bag-valve-mask (BVM) See *bag mask ventilation*.

barrel chest The shape of the chest in a COPD patient who has chronically retained air in his lungs for an extended period of time.

baseline vital signs The first set of a patient's vital signs measured.

biological clock The term used to describe the time when a woman is approaching the end of her child-bearing years.

Biot's respirations An irregular but cyclic pattern of increased and decreased rate and depth of breathing, with periods of apnea.

black stool Dark, black, or tarry stool may indicate upper GI bleeding or the ingestion of iron or bismuth preparation, such as antacids.

blast injuries The injuries that occur as the result of an explosion, which are often compounded by occurring within a confined space, causing further injury from the pressure.

blood glucose A measurement of the sugar found in the patient's venous or capillary blood on a test strip or a glucometer.

blood pressure The pressure (systolic) within the arteries when the left ventricle pumps blood into the systemic system, and the pressure (diastolic) in the system during the relaxation of the left ventricle.

BLS (basic life support) 1. CPR; 2. The care provided by emergency medical responders and EMT, which does not involve invasive interventions.

body language The expression of thoughts or emotions by means of posture or gestures.

body recovery A rescue effort in which it has been determined that the injuries to the patient are mortal wounds or the patient is obviously deceased. All safety must be taken, and this is not a rush that would ever put rescuers in jeopardy.

body surface area (BSA) The amount of skin surface on the body; used to measure the area burned on a person's body.

bone marrow The substance within the shaft of the long bones where red blood cells develop.

bones The strong, fibrous framework of the body. They protect vital organs and provide a structure for muscles to allow movement, as well as for red blood cells to develop.

bowel sounds The sounds of the bowel digesting food, which can be heard by listening with a stethoscope. This is rarely done in the out-of-hospital setting.

bradypnea Slow breathing.

brain abscess A serious condition that can develop within the brain, with signs and symptoms of fever, headache, and possibly sinusitis. The patient may also have a seizure, depending on the location where the abscess develops.

brain herniation A life-threatening injury to the brain, which causes a hematoma and swelling to push brain tissue through the tentorium.

brain stem Helps to connect the hemispheres of the brain. The parts of the brain stem include the midbrain, pons, and medulla oblongata.

Braxton Hicks contractions Irregular and inconsistent contractions; also called false labor.

breath sounds Upon auscultation with a stethoscope, the sound of the air flowing through the patient's lower airways. Depending on the specific location, the sounds can differ slightly.

bronchiolitis A viral infection of the bronchioles that causes swelling of the lower airways.

Brown-Sequard syndrome A syndrome caused by a penetrating injury that produces a partial transection of the spinal cord. It is referred to as a hemisection of the cord and involves only one side of the cord.

bruit A swishing turbulent sound heard over the arteries that indicates blockage of blood flow.

BS (blood sugar) A measurement of the sugar in the patient's bloodstream, as determined by a glucometer or chemical strip from a drop of blood.

BSI (body substance isolation) The level of precautions designed to protect the provider from body substances (e.g., blood, urine, vomit, saliva, etc.). This is used when the rescuer is not able to determine what a liquid substance might be, to which he could potentially be exposed.

CAD (computer-aided dispatch) system A dispatch system where the computer has digitalized locations in the response area and is able to make recommendations to the dispatcher based on available units and their specific locations.

CAD Coronary artery disease.

cancer Includes a large number of malignant neoplasms. The prognosis depends on the extent of its spread when found, metastases, and the effectiveness of treatment.

capillary refill time The amount of time it takes for the capillaries in the fingertips to fill with blood after being temporarily squeezed. Normal capillary refill time is less than 2 seconds.

capnography A measurement of the level of carbon dioxide exhaled by the patient.

capnometer A device that has a digital readout of end-tidal carbon dioxide.

cardiac enzyme testing When cardiac muscle dies, enzymes are released in the blood stream. The measurement of CK-MB (creatine kinase; M, muscle; B, brain) over a 12- to 24-hour period.

cardiac muscle The heart muscle that has the unique ability to generate and conduct electrical impulses.

cardiac tamponade An accumulation of fluids or a loss of blood into the pericardial sac.

cardiac valves The valves between the chambers, and at the entry and exit of the heart. Designed to prevent backflow of blood into the chamber or vessel from which it came.

cardiogenic shock Hypotension due to a massive ACS or the cumulative effect of multiple MIs, leaving a critical mass of ineffective pumping muscle.

cardiomegaly An increase in heart size, for any number of reasons.

cardiomyopathies Incurable diseases of the heart that ultimately lead to congestive heart failure, ACS, or death.

cardiopulmonary resuscitation (CPR) The technique of providing a combination of high-quality chest compressions and artificial ventilations on a pulseless patient. A simplified technique known as "hands-only" CPR does not include the ventilations and is taught primarily to the general public.

carotid artery disease (CAD) Deterioration in the carotid artery as a result of blockage or breakdown in the vessel that can result in inadequate blood flow and blood supply to the organs of the body.

carpopedal spasms Spasmodic contractions of the hands, wrists, feet, and ankles associated with alkalosis and hypocapnia.

cartilaginous joints Joints in which there is cartilage connecting the bones.

catecholamines Various substances that function as hormones, or neurotransmitters, or both (e.g., epinephrine or norepinephrine).

CE (continuing education) Updates, reviews, and new training on relevant topics for the health care provider. Some providers renew their licenses or certifications based on a specific number of CE hours and topics.

cellular adaption When cells are exposed to adverse conditions, they go through a process of adaption. In some situations, they change permanently; in others, they change their structure and function only temporarily.

cellular environment The distribution of cells throughout the body; the change in cell distribution with aging and disease.

cellular immunity Also known as cell-mediated immunity, the portion of our immune system that primarily involves cells.

cellular injury May result from various causes, such as hypoxia (the most common cause), chemical injury, infectious injury, immunological injury, and inflammatory injury.

central cord syndrome Partial transaction usually occurs with a hyperextension of the cervical region. The patient may have weakness or paresthesia in the upper extremities but normal strength in the lower extremities.

central nervous system (CNS) The brain and spinal cord.

cerebellum The portion of the brain responsible for balance, coordination, and equilibrium.

cerebrospinal fluid (CSF) A clear body fluid, manufactured in the ventricles of the brain, that bathes the brain and spinal cord.

cerebrovascular accident (CVA) A stroke in which there is an interruption of blood flow to an area of the brain, caused by an embolus, hemorrhage, or thrombus.

cerebrum The portion of the brain responsible for thought and higher cognition.

chemical injury Injury and ultimately destruction of cells by chemicals. Chemical carcinogens, cancer-causing agents, can be found everywhere in our environment.

chemical restraint The use of a sedative medication to calm a violent patient.

chemoreceptors Receptors found in the aortic arch and carotid sinus, which analyze the chemistry of the blood and report the findings to the brain.

CHEMTREC A resource that emergency responders to a chemical spill can call for consultation and advice. This hotline, which is open 24 hours a day, 365 days a year, was developed by chemical manufacturers.

Cheyne–Stokes respirations A rhythmic pattern of gradually increased and decreased rates and depths of breathing, with periods of apnea.

CHF (congestive heart failure) Heart failure in which the heart is unable to maintain an adequate flow of blood through the body. Excess fluid collects in the dependent parts of the body, such as the ankles or sacral area, if the patient is bedridden.

chief complaint (CC) The reason EMS was called; best told in the patient's own words.

cholesterol An odorless, white, waxy, powdery substance, needed by the body in small quantities; found in foods.

cholinergic receptor Activated by the involvement of the neurotransmitter acetylcholine.

chronic bronchitis An inflammation of the bronchial tubes causing a productive cough that lasts at least 3 months and reoccurs for 2 or more years.

chronic obstructive pulmonary disease (COPD) A form of obstructive lung disease (e.g., emphysema, chronic bronchitis, asbestosis, or black lung) that is progressive and irreversible.

Cincinnati prehospital stroke scale A prehospital stroke assessment tool.

circadian rhythms Regular changes in mental and physical characteristics that occur in the course of a day (circadian is Latin for "around the day").

CISM (critical incident stress management) A technique for defusing and debriefing stress in emergency responders as a result of major incidents such as the death of a coworker, pediatric catastrophes, or MCIs.

clarification A communication technique in which the EMS provider asks the patient for more information to determine whether his interpretation is accurate.

clean accident An incident that involves an explosion or spill, which does not involve hidden hazards (such as radioactive particles) that could easily spread to those exposed.

cleft lip A birth defect; a cosmetic problem that appears as a separation in the lip.

cleft palate A birth defect; a split in the palate that creates an opening between the mouth and the nose. The opening may be unilateral, complete, or incomplete.

closed fracture A broken bone that has not, as yet, punctured the skin.

closed question A type of question that requires only a "yes" or "no" response or a one- or two-word response; also known as a direct question.

clot–busters Drugs designed to rapidly thin the blood; typically called fibrinolytics or thrombolytics.

CNS (central nervous system) The brain and spinal cord.

CO (cardiac output) The stroke volume times the heart rate.

Combitube® A dual lumen airway that is considered one of the few acceptable advanced airway devices used by out-of-hospital personnel.

communication process The process by which a sender encodes a message to be decoded by an intended receiver, who in turn provides feedback.

compartment syndrome The edema and ischemia caused to the soft tissue by pressure or heavy weight on top of it. The tissue pressure rises above the capillary hydrostatic pressure, resulting in ischemia to the muscle.

compensated shock The early phase of the shock syndrome, in which the patient is able to sustain her systolic BP and adequately perfuse the brain.

comprehensive examination and health assessment An examination of the body as a whole.

compression–ventilation (CV) ratio The number of chest compressions administered to the patient during CPR compared to the number of rescue breaths. For adults, children, and infants, during single-rescuer CPR, this ratio is 30:2.

concealment Positioning oneself behind an object that hides one from the view of others. This offers no ballistic protection.

concussion An injury that shakes up the brain but usually does not involve long-term injury to the brain itself.

conductivity The ability of tissues, such as heart muscle tissue, to allow electrical current to flow through.

confidentiality Keeping the private information that was shared with you about a patient private.

confined-space rescue Access and removal of a patient from a space that is often a low-oxygen environment. A confined space is not designed for people to be in it, and the rescue requires specialty equipment and training.

congenital bleb A birth defect causing a weak spot on the surface of the lung that can burst, causing a pneumo-thorax.

congenital heart defects Problems with the heart that a patient is born with (e.g., valves not operating properly, holes in the wall of the chambers).

conjugate gaze The normal position of the eyes.

connective tissue Stellate or spindle-shaped cells with interlacing processes that support and bind together other tissues of the body.

consensual light reflex Constriction of both pupils when a light is shone into one eye; a normal response.

consent Permission from an adult to treat a patient.

contained incident A hazmat or MCI that is an isolated area, where all the patients are in one place and not spread out. An example would be an incident on a ferry boat, where all the patients are currently on the boat.

contamination That which is soiled, stained, or containing a potentially hazardous material that could be a danger to the patient and others.

CONTOMS program Counter Narcotic and Terrorism Operational Medical Support program.

contracoup An injury to the brain that develops on the opposite side of the point of impact.

contusion A closed, soft-tissue injury in which cells are damaged and blood vessels are torn.

converge To move closer together; normal movement of the eyes as an object comes closer to the face.

COPD (chronic obstructive pulmonary disease) A lung disease, such as emphysema, chronic bronchitis, asbestosis, or black lung, which involves progressive deteriorating of the lung tissue.

coronary heart disease (CHD) Caused by the narrowing of coronary arteries. In time, the inadequate supply of oxygen-rich blood and nutrients damages the heart muscle and can lead to chest pain and heart attack, and possible death.

coup An injury to the brain that develops directly beneath the point of impact.

coup-contra coup A type of head injury that results when the head is struck on one side, and the force of the impact causes injury to the side that was struck as well as to the opposite side.

cover To hide behind something that conceals a person as well as provides protection from bullets (e.g., a brick wall as opposed to a curtain).

CPR (cardiopulmonary resuscitation) The technique of providing a combination of high-quality chest compressions and artificial ventilations on a pulseless patient.

CQI (continuous quality improvement) A process designed to review and attempt to improve the work or product provided to your customers.

crackles A sound similar to that made by the crumpling up of a candy wrapper, usually heard on expiration; also called rales.

cranial nerves The twelve pairs of nerves that come directly out of the brain, which innervate mostly the head, face, and shoulders, and control sensory and motor functions.

crepitation The sound or sensation of broken bone ends grating on each other.

crisis An internal experience that can create reactions such as severe anxiety, panic, paranoia, or some other brief psychotic event.

croup A viral respiratory infection often caused by other types of infection, such as an ear infection, that results in swelling of the vocal cords, trachea, and upper airway tissues and, thereby, a partial obstruction of the airway.

crushing injury A closed, soft-tissue injury resulting in organ rupture and severe fractures from a crushing force.

CSF (cerebrospinal fluid) Fluid manufactured in the brain's ventricles that circulates around the outer coverings of the brain and spinal cord.

Cullen's sign Ecchymosis in the periumbilical region (around the belly button), indicating internal bleeding.

CUPS A system used in EMS to prioritize patients by severity of presenting problem: critical, unstable, potentially unstable, and stable.

Cushing's triad Three assessment findings that, when displayed together, indicate increasing intracranial pressure (ICP): rising blood pressure, decreasing pulse rate, and changes in the respiratory pattern.

cystitis An inflammation of the urinary bladder.

DAI (diffuse axonal injury) The effect of acceleration or deceleration on the brain. Often a mild or classic concussion, though it can be moderate or severe.

DAN® The Diver's Alert Network; a resource for injured divers and those who provide emergency care for them.

DCAP-BTLS A mnemonic for assessment points in the examination of soft tissue: deformities, contusions, abrasions, penetrations or punctures, burns, tenderness, lacerations, and swelling.

DCI (decompression illness) A sickness occurring during or after ascent, secondary to a rapid release of nitrogen bubbles. Also called the bends.

DEA (Drug Enforcement Agency) Part of the Homeland Security Agency; responsible for enforcing the drug laws.

decerebrate A form of neurological posturing characterized by the patient's stiffly extending both the arms and legs and retracting the head.

decode To interpret a message.

decompensated shock The late phase of shock, when the body is no longer able to maintain the systolic blood pressure and adequately perfuse the brain.

decon To remove a hazardous material from a patient who has been exposed by washing and rinsing him with the appropriate agent in the warm zone of a hazmat.

decorticate A form of neurological posturing characterized by the patient's flexing the upper extremities to the torso, or core of the body, while extending the lower extremities.

degenerative disc disease A common disk problem in patients over 50 years of age. It is a narrowing of the disk that results in variable segments of instability.

degloving Type of open, soft-tissue injury in which the epidermis is removed.

delegation of authority The granting of medical privileges by a physician, either online (direct) or off-line (indirect), to an EMS provider to perform skills or procedures within the EMS provider's scope of practice.

delusion A false personal belief or idea that is portrayed as true.

demand valve A ventilator with a valve that opens to allow self-administered oxygen when the patient creates a negative pressure against the valve or "demands" oxygen by inhaling through the mask. This device is not used for resuscitation of a nonbreathing patient unless it has a positive pressure feature with a triggering device for the health care provider to use to ventilate the patient.

dementia A condition of decaying mentality that is characterized by marked decline from the individual's former intellectual level and often by emotional apathy.

depression 1. A depression downward and inward; 2. a psychiatric disorder marked by sadness, inactivity, and difficulty with thinking and concentration.

dermatomes The areas on the surface of the body that are innervated by afferent fibers from one spinal root.

descending nerve tracts The tracts that carry motor impulses from the brain to the body. The three groups include the corticospinal, reticulospinal, and rubrospinal tracts.

detailed physical examination (DPE) A component of the patient assessment, to be conducted on trauma patients who have significant MOI; this should be done only while en route to the hospital.

developmentally disabled Term used to describe an individual with impaired or insufficient development of the brain, resulting in an inability to learn at the usual rate.

diabetic ketoacidosis (DKA) During hypoglycemia, the inability of patients with diabetes to metabolize fat.

diagnosis The identification of a specific disease or condition; usually made after the medical team has evaluated the entire situation; the determination, by a physician, of the medical problem that a patient is experiencing.

dialysis A general term for a method, involving a semipermeable membrane, used to separate smaller particles from larger ones in a liquid mixture.

diarrhea Abnormally frequent intestinal evacuations with liquid stool.

diastolic The residual blood pressure in the arterial system as the left ventricle relaxes.

diffuse axonal injury (DAI) Injury to brain tissues that results from rapid acceleration or deceleration on the brain.

diffusion The process where particles of liquids, gases, or solids intermingle as a result of their spontaneous movement caused by thermal agitation; in dissolved substances, the movement from regions of higher to lower concentrations.

digital intubation A blind form of intubation that involves using the fingers.

diplopia Double vision.

dirty accident An incident involving a bomb or chemical spillage that is laced with radioactive particles that are extremely hazardous.

disentanglement To carefully remove the parts of a vehicle that a patient is wrapped around or pinned underneath in order to release the patient.

disinfection To free from infection and destroy harmful microorganisms.

dislocation Displacement of one or more of the bones at a joint.

distress Pain or suffering affecting the body.

diverge To move apart; normal movement of the eyes as they focus on a distant object.

diving emergencies Any one of a number of injuries or illnesses that can occur during underwater diving (e.g., the bends, nitrogen narcosis, overpressurization injuries).

dizziness The sensation of unsteadiness and the sensation of movement within the head.

DKA See *diabetic ketoacidosis*.

DNAR (do not attempt resuscitation) order An order in a patient's chart that was prepared after consultation with the patient or her legal proxy and physician, based on the wishes of the patient that a resuscitation not be attempted should she go into cardiac arrest.

DNR (do not resuscitate) order The current terminology is DNAR.

domestic violence Physical, sexual, or emotional violence, within an adult partner relationship.

Doppler ultrasound A device used for physical examination that monitors the Doppler effect. The Doppler effect is a change in frequency during which waves (sound or light) from a given source reach an observer, while the source and the observer are in rapid motion with respect to each other, so that the frequency increases or decreases according to the speed at which the distance is decreasing or increasing.

DOT-KKK-1822 The Federal Ambulance Specifications.

Down syndrome Moderate to severe mental retardation caused by trisomy of the human chromosome 21, in which a person often has slanting eyes, a broad, short skull, and broad hands with short fingers.

DPE (detailed physical examination) The head-to-toe examination that is done on the trauma patient with significant MOI en route to the hospital.

DPL (diagnostic peritoneal lavage) A procedure that is done on patients with abdominal trauma and suspected internal organ injury to see if there is bleeding into the abdomen.

drowning To suffocate in water or some other liquid.

due regard A legal term found in most state's motor vehicle laws describing the level of responsibility of an operator of an emergency vehicle (i.e., with *due regard* for the safety of all other motorists).

duty to act A legal term that describes the level of responsibility of an EMT or paramedic when on duty and receiving a call.

dysarthria An abnormal articulation of speech due to disturbances in muscle control.

dysphagia Difficulty swallowing.

dysphasia Abnormal speech due to lack of coordination and failure to arrange words in the proper order.

dysphonia Discomfort when speaking due to laryngeal disease.

dysplasia Abnormal growth or development of cells.

dyspnea Difficulty breathing.

dysrhythmias An irregular electrocardiogram.

dysuria Difficulty urinating.

eclampsia An attack of convulsions due to toxemia of pregnancy.

ECF (extracellular fluid) The fluid outside the cells.

ECG (electrocardiogram) The tracing made by an electrocardiograph of the electrical potential occurring within the heart.

edema An abnormal collection of serous fluid in a connective or serous tissue.

EGTA (esophageal-gastric tube airway) An advanced airway device that is a class III device and may be harmful to use in the field.

Einthoven's triangle Dr. William Einthoven, the inventor of the ECG machine, described the placement of the first three standardized leads (lead I, II, and III) as a triangle over the body and around the heart.

electro-mechanical disassociation (EMD) A lack of an association between the electrical activity and the mechanical activity of the heart, resulting in a cardiac standstill or lack of perfusion. The terminology was changed to pulseless electrical activity, or PEA.

emancipated minor A child under the age of 18 who has legally declared himself free of his parents. In most states, this also includes a pregnant female or one who is the mother of a child.

EMD Emergency medical dispatcher.

emergency doctrine The type of consent given for emergency intervention for a patient who is physically or mentally unable to provide expressed consent; also called implied consent. This type of consent remains in effect for as long as the patient requires lifesaving treatments.

Emergency Medical Services Systems Act The law enacted by each state to allow for a designated lead agency (e.g., health, emergency management, DOT, etc.) to supervise and coordinate the development of the EMS system.

emotional disorder Also called a "mental disorder," any disturbance of emotional balance manifested by maladaptive behavior and impaired functioning (e.g., depression).

empathy A sensitivity to and an understanding of another person's feelings.

emphysema A chronic lung disease that results from a destruction of the walls of the alveoli.

EMS-C (Emergency Medical Services for Children) Act Passed in 1983, this act (PL-98-555) was designed to improve the care of children.

EMS Command The overall leader of the EMS response at the scene of an MCI.

EMT One of the four national levels of EMS provider (EMR, EMT, advanced EMT, paramedic) that has training curriculum developed by the U.S. Department of Transportation. The EMT-Basic is the program designed as the minimum training level required to work or volunteer on an ambulance; skills involved in the training revolve around that role.

encode To determine what terms to use to convey a message.

endocrinology The study of the endocrine glands.

endometriosis The presence and growth of functioning endometrial tissue in places other than the uterus, which often results in severe pain and infertility.

Endotrol® tube A specialized endotracheal tube that has a small ring with a connection to the tip of the tube. This is particularly helpful, when doing a blind nasal intubation, in directing the tip of the tube into the glottic opening.

end-tidal carbon dioxide (EtCO$_2$) The concentration of carbon dioxide (CO$_2$) in the exhaled gas at the end of the exhalation.

enhanced 911 A system of alerting emergency services by the public in communities where the 911 uniform access number is in place. In the enhanced version, the software places the caller's location (based on the phone he or she is calling from) on the dispatcher's CRT screen.

enteral drug administration Administering medicine that is swallowed and then passes through the stomach and intestines.

environmental emergencies A group of illnesses that relate to extreme conditions of the weather or activities that occur outdoors (e.g., drowning, submersion, heat-related illness, hypothermia and frostbite, diving accidents, etc.).

EOA (esophageal obturator airway) A class III airway device that may be considered harmful to use in the field.

epidemiology A study of the causes and trends of injury or illness and disease.

epidural hematoma An injury to the brain that involves an arterial tear resulting in increased intracranial pressure.

epiglottitis A rare, life-threatening infection causing severe inflammation and swelling of the epiglottis.

epilepsy A disease that involves convulsions that can be controlled by taking anticonvulsants.

Epi-pen® Designed for patients who are highly allergic; the pen is a self-injector of epinephrine for anaphylaxis.

epistaxis A nose bleed.

error of commission or omission Negligent acts, for which a provider could be sued, that involve going beyond the scope of practice (commission) and not providing treatment at the level of the standard of care by eliminating vital steps (omission).

escharotomy A surgical incision into necrotic tissue of a burn to expand the tissue and decrease ischemia from a circumferential burn.

esophageal intubation detector (EDD) device An airway tool with either a bulb syringe or a rigid syringe that is used to determine whether an endotracheal tube is in the trachea or esophagus.

esophageal tracheal combitube (ETC; see Combitube®) The esophageal tracheal combitube is referred to as the Combitube® throughout the Guidelines 2005 publication.

ethics The study of hard decisions that are not defined by laws but are considered the right thing to do, involving values and morals.

etiology The cause of a disease or condition.

ET tube A clear plastic tube that is designed to be passed through the vocal cords and glottic opening to assist with ventilations directly into the patient's lungs.

eupnea Normal breathing.

eustress The normal stress of life that is necessary to function.

EVOC (emergency vehicle operator course) A training program that involves both a didactic and lab (hands-on) component, developed by the U.S. DOT and designed to improve the driving skills of the operator of an emergency vehicle. Three versions of the course focus on a specific audience and type of vehicle (e.g., police, firefighters, EMS workers).

exacerbation An increase in the seriousness of a disease or disorder.

extracorporal CPR The technique of cardiac compressions that is employed when a patient arrests during open chest surgery.

extraocular muscles (EOMs) Muscles that produce movement of the eyes.

extravasate Escape of fluid, such as blood from a vessel into the surrounding tissues.

extubation The removal of a tube, such as the ET tube, from the trachea or when incorrectly inserted from the esophagus.

facilitation The method in which EMS providers speak and use posture and actions to encourage the patient to say more.

false imprisonment To take someone someplace and keep him or her there against his or her will, without consent (e.g., kidnapping).

FAS (fetal alcohol syndrome) A group of birth defects, including mental retardation, deficient growth, and defects of the skull, face, and brain, that tends to occur in the infants of women who consume a large amount of alcohol during pregnancy.

FAST Abbreviation used in stroke assessment to remind the provider of facial droop, abnormal speech, smile, and time, which are components of the Cincinnati prehospital stroke scale.

fat One of the essential nutrients that supplies calories to the body. Fat provides nine calories per gram, more than twice the number provided by carbohydrates or protein. Small amounts of fat are necessary for normal body function.

FCC (Federal Communications Commission) The federal agency responsible for allocating and supervising the radio airwaves and frequencies.

febrile seizures The convulsions in an infant, which are a result of the rapid rise in temperature from a fever.

feedback A receiver's response to a message.

festination An abnormal gait that appears uneven and hurried, as seen in Parkinson's patients.

fetal alcohol syndrome See *FAS*.

fetal distress A fetus may be stressed while in the uterus due to a number of reasons (e.g., post-term gestation over 42 weeks, maternal supine hypotensive syndrome, eclampsia, umbilical cord obstruction or prolapse, placental insufficiency, hypoxia, drug effects, or bacterial sepsis).

fetal heart rate (FHR) The heart rate of a fetus.

fetal heart tones (FHTs) The heartbeats of a fetus.

fibrinolysis The body's natural and normal way of preventing excess blood clot formation.

fibrous joints Joints that are connected by fibrous tissue, such as the immovable sutures that are located in the skull.

Fick principle Oxygen transport principle that states that adequate cellular perfusion requires four components to be present and working: an adequate oxygen supply, oxygen exchange in the lungs, the circulation of oxygen to the cells, and an adequate number of red blood cells.

field impression A working diagnosis to determine the cause of a patient's condition.

"fight or flight" response The hormonal response to stress that can affect the EMS provider's decision-making ability both positively and negatively.

first-party caller An emergency call to the EMS dispatcher or 911 operator that comes directly from the patient.

First responder awareness level Level at which an EMS provider is trained to recognize a hazardous materials incident, back off, and call for help.

First responder operations level Level at which an EMS provider is trained to perform risk assessment, to select and don appropriate personal protective equipment, and to contain the scene and carry out basic decontamination procedures.

flail segment A section of the rib cage that has two or more ribs broken in two or more places, creating a paradoxical movement of the broken section as the patient breathes; also called a flail chest.

flow-restricted, oxygen-powered ventilation device (FROPVD) Used for mechanical positive pressure ventilation of a patient in the out-of-hospital setting. The Guidelines 2005 refer to these devices as manually triggered, oxygen-powered, flow-limiting resuscitators.

FLSA (Fair Labor Standards Act) The FLSA is the federal law that regulates minimum wages and overtime in the workplace.

flu Influenza, or the flu, is a specific type of viral infection that may affect both the upper (e.g., dry, hacking cough with diffuse muscle aches) and lower respiratory tracts (e.g., pneumonia).

fluid wave test A special procedure that is performed on the abdomen to test for ascites.

focal head injury Injury to the brain tissues resulting in lesions.

focused history and physical examination (FH&PE) A component of patient assessment that varies depending on whether the patient has a medical or trauma complaint. If trauma, the MOI is determined, vital signs are taken, and a history of presenting illness is determined on the basis of OPQRST. Has been updated to be called the secondary assessment.

FOIA (Freedom of Information Act) A law that allows the general public to obtain copies of government documents.

food poisoning Gastroenteritis or a more severe infection caused by pathogens in spoiled or improperly prepared food.

foreign body airway obstruction (FBAO) The blockage of the upper airways due to the inhalation of objects such as a large bolus of meat, a coin, or a balloon. These are classified as mild or severe.

fractures Broken bones.

frontal lobotomy A surgical procedure designed to disconnect the frontal cerebral lobe, which houses inhibition and extreme emotional reactions, from the rest of the brain. This is a last resort in the psychiatric patient prone to fits of anger.

FROPVD See *flow-restricted, oxygen-powered ventilation device.*

frostbite A local cold injury ranging from superficial to partial thickness to full thickness. At risk are the very old and very young, as well as those who are outdoors in very cold and windy temperatures with hands or face exposed.

fundus The top of the uterus.

gallstones Also referred to as cholelithiasis, these are caused by the precipitation of substances contained in bile such as cholesterol and bilirubin.

GAS (general adaptation syndrome) GAS is a long-term physiological response pattern to adaption. The response is mediated by cortisol release from the adrenal cortex.

gastric distention The bloating of the stomach with air and food, which leaves the patient prone to regurgitation.

gastric ulcers Ulcerations of the stomach caused by the bacterium *Helicobacter pylori* (*H. pylori*).

gastroenteritis A general term that includes many types of infections and irritations of the digestive tract.

gastroenterology The study of the digestive system and its workings.

GCS (Glasgow coma scale) A numerical score to quantify the severity of an altered mental status resulting from head injury, utilizing the sum of the following three variables: best eye opening response (4 to 1), best verbal response (5 to 1), and best motor response (6 to 1). Scores can range from 3 to 15.

general impression The EMS provider's first impression of the patient to determine the priority of care, taking into consideration the environment and the patient's chief complaint.

generalized seizure A type of seizure that involves the entire brain and is classified as complete motor seizure, absence seizure, or atonic seizure; once called grand mal.

geriatrics The study of the elderly.

gerontology The study of the problems of all aspects of aging.

GI bleed Hemorrhaging from an ulceration of the stomach or other GI tract structures.

glaucoma A disease in which elevated pressure in the eye, due to an obstruction of the outflow of aqueous humor, damages the optic nerve and causes visual defects.

Global Med-Net A medical information service with a toll-free phone number that EMS providers can call to obtain a patient's complete medical profile using the patient's member identification number.

glucose meter A handheld glucose meter, which is a relatively accurate method to determine the range of a person's glucose.

golden hour The optimum limit of 1 hour between time of injury and surgery at the hospital.

Good Samaritan law A state law designed to provide legal protection and limited immunity from civil suits for individuals who stop at the scene of an accident to render first aid.

governmental immunity A specific state law designed to provide legal protection and limited immunity for local government employees.

gravida The total number of pregnancies a woman has had.

gray matter The gray fibers of the CNS including the cerebral cortex, basal ganglia, and parts of the brain and spinal cord.

Grey-Turner's sign Ecchymosis in the flanks and periumbilical areas that is a late sign of internal bleeding.

grieving A process in response to the death or dying of a loved one, which includes the stages of shock, denial, anger, bargaining, depression, and acceptance.

grunting A sound that results from breathing out against a partially obstructed epiglottis.

guarding A particular position of comfort to protect a body part from pain.

Guidelines 2010 The American Heart Association's latest issue of the resuscitation and emergency cardiovascular care treatments, which are based upon the latest science as well as the consensus of the International Liaison Committee on Resuscitation (ILCOR) councils.

gynecology The study of problems associated with the female reproductive system and its structures.

HACE (high-altitude cerebral edema) Swelling of the brain caused by failing to properly acclimate to high altitudes.

HAPE (high-altitude pulmonary edema) Swelling and fluid collected in the lungs caused by failing to properly acclimate to high altitudes.

hazardous material (hazmat) Any substance that can cause injury or death to an individual who has been exposed to the substance.

HDL cholesterol High-density lipoprotein, which helps carry the "bad cholesterol" away from the walls of the arteries and returns it to the bloodstream, thus preventing buildup of cholesterol in the artery walls.

headache Pain in the head that may be caused by one of a number of conditions such as: cerebral aneurysm, glaucoma, meningitis, migraine, stress, subarachnoid, temporal arteritis, temporomandibular joint syndrome, trauma, and trigeminal neuralgia.

health care power of attorney A durable power of attorney or health care proxy allows a person to designate an agent to act in cases where the person is unable to make decisions for him- or herself.

health care professional (HCP) One who confirms to the standards of a health care profession to provide quality patient care.

health care proxy The person who has the legal authority to make medical decisions for a patient should he or she become incapacitated.

heart sounds The sounds of the valves closing, heard through a stethoscope, during the pumping phases of the heart.

heat illness Medical condition sustained from exposure to extremely hot weather conditions or environmental conditions, such as heat exhaustion or heat stroke.

HEENT An acronym for head, eyes, ears, nose, and throat.

HELP position The heat-escape lessening position, which involves floating with the head out of the water and the body in a fetal tuck.

hematocrit The number of red blood cells (RBCs) in the peripheral blood.

hematology The study of the blood and its medical conditions.

hematoma A collection of blood beneath the skin.

hematopoietic system The system that produces blood cells.

hemoglobin and hematocrit (H&H) Hemoglobin is the part of the red blood cell that contains iron and carries oxygen to the lungs and tissues. Hematocrit is the percentage of the whole volume of blood contributed by cells.

hemophilia Hereditary deficiency of clotting factors IVVV (hemophilia A) or IX (hemophilia B).

hemoptysis Coughing up blood from the respiratory tract.

hemothorax Blood in the chest cavity.

hepatitis An inflammation of the liver causing an acute or chronic potentially life-threatening condition.

hepatojugular reflux Observing the jugular veins while simultaneously performing a deep palpation on the upper-right quadrant of the abdomen for 30–60 seconds.

herniated intervertebral disk Damage to the disk that can allow leakage of the fluid in the disk. This is a very painful injury or condition that can easily be aggravated by simply bending the wrong way.

HHNC (hyperosmolar hyperglycemia nonketotic coma) Results from a relative insulin deficiency that leads to marked hyperglycemia and the absence of ketones and acidosis.

high-frequency chest compressions An experimental type of CPR involving over 120 chest compressions per minute.

history of the present illness (HPI) Specific patient information about the current illness or condition.

HIV (human immunodeficiency virus) The virus that has been found to be the cause of acquired immunodeficiency syndrome (AIDS).

homeostasis The effort and mechanisms of the body to keep its environment "normal."

hospice The psychological, physical, spiritual, and pain management support for a terminally ill patient and his or her family.

HPV Human papillomavirus.

HTN Hypertension.

humane restraints Wide leather or cloth restraints that are used to tie a patient in the supine or seated position onto a stretcher. It is not appropriate to use one pair of handcuffs to restrain a patient with a medical or psychiatric problem in front of or behind his/her back. It is reasonable to use two pairs of handcuffs to restrain the patient in the supine position to a long backboard.

humoral immunity Also known as antibody-mediated immunity, primarily involves antibodies that are produced by a specialized WBC, the B lymphocyte.

Huntington's disease A rare hereditary disorder involving chronic progressive chorea, psychological changes, and dementia.

hypercapnia An abnormally high concentration of carbon dioxide in the blood.

hypercarbia Carbon dioxide retention.

hydrocephalus An increase in the amount of CSF due to either a blockage or decreased reabsorption.

hydrophobia Another name for rabies, a viral infection of the central nervous system.

hyperbaric chamber therapy A chamber used to treat conditions brought on by scuba accidents and carbon monoxide poisoning. Under pressure, it is possible to help the oxygen attach to the hemoglobin receptor sites on the red blood cells.

hyperglycemia An elevated blood sugar level often found in diabetics or patients who have problems with their pancreas or insulin production.

hypernatremia A high sodium level.

hyperplasia An increase in the number of cells due to hormonal stimulation. The excess growth often causes tumors that may be malignant or benign.

hypersensitivity Any bodily response to any substance to which a patient is abnormally sensitive.

hypertensive emergency A life-threatening, sudden, and severe increase in BP that can lead to serious, irreversible end-organ damage within hours if left untreated.

hypertrophy An increase in the size of the cell leading to an increase in tissue and organ size.

hyperventilation A respiratory rate greater than that required for normal body function.

hyphema Bleeding into the anterior chamber of the eye.

hypocapnia An abnormally low concentration of carbon dioxide in the blood.

hypoglycemia A low blood sugar level, often found in patients with a history of diabetes after a period of exercising or not eating.

hyponatremia A low sodium level.

hypothermia A generalized low body temperature and the associated condition it causes.

hypothyroidism Also called myxedema, a clinical syndrome due to a deficiency of thyroid hormone.

hypoventilation Irregular and shallow breathing.

hypovolemic shock Poor peripheral perfusion due to a loss of blood volume.

hypoxemia A lack of oxygen in the blood (e.g., carbon monoxide taking up all the oxygen receptor sites on the hemoglobin).

hypoxia Inadequate oxygenation of the blood cells.

IAC-CPR Interposed abdominal compressions CPR technique.

iatrogenic disorder A medical condition that is caused by the care provided by a health care provider.

IBS (irritable bowel syndrome) A condition characterized by recurrent abdominal pain, usually crampy in nature, and diarrhea, often alternating with periods of constipation.

ICF (intracellular fluid) The fluid within the cells. Water moves between the ICF and the extracellular fluid by osmosis.

ICS (incident command system) See *IMS*.

ictal phase The period during a seizure attack.

ILCOR (International Liaison Committee on Resuscitation) The group of resuscitation councils and experts that develops the Consensus on Science, on which the American Heart Association's Guidelines are based.

illusions Misperceptions of actual existing stimuli by any sense.

immune system The body's complex system that acts to fight off foreign substances and disease-causing agents.

immunizations Injections of medications designed to prevent infectious diseases (e.g., tetanus, diphtheria, hepatitis B).

immunologic injury When cellular membranes are injured by direct contact with the cellular and chemical components of the immune or inflammatory process, such as phagocytes, histamine, antibodies, and lymphokines.

impaled object An object that has pierced and become fixed in the skin and tissues.

IMS (incident management system) The system used to coordinate the efforts at a disaster or major incident. It involves command and the four key functional areas of finance, logistics, operations, and planning, as well as a module design for escalation and de-escalation as the incident warrants; previously called incident command system, or ICS.

incident command system (ICS) See *IMS*.

incident report The appropriate documentation, aside from the PCR, that EMS agencies prepare in unusual instances or for reportable cases (e.g., infectious disease exposure, work injury or fatality, multiple casualty incident).

incision A clean break in the skin, usually made by a knife.

index of suspicion Injury patterns associated with specific mechanisms of injury from which the EMS provider can anticipate the potential for shock or other problems.

infants According to the American Heart Association, a child is considered an infant from the release of the initial hospitalization to 1 year of age.

infectious and communicable diseases Conditions that can be transmitted from person to person. A communicable disease can be transmitted directly or indirectly from one person to another. An infectious disease is an illness caused by an invasion of the body by an organism such as a virus, bacteria, or fungus.

inflammatory injury Inflammation is a protective response that can occur without bacterial invasion. This occurs when cellular membranes are injured by direct contact with the cellular and chemical components of the inflammatory process.

initial assessment (IA) The second component of patient assessment; an orderly and sequential examination with correction of life-threats and determination of the patient's priority. This is now called the primary assessment.

injury Blunt or penetrating trauma that has damaged a body part.

inspection The first step in the examination of a patient, which involves looking at the body part and comparing it to the other side (e.g., right leg to left leg).

interstitial fluid The fluid that is found between the cells of the body.

intracranial hemorrhage Bleeding into the head, usually developing a collection of blood that is named in relation to the meninges (e.g., subdural, epidural).

involuntary commitment Each state law may differ on this, but a patient can be committed to a mental health facility for an evaluation, against his or her will, on the order of a county mental health physician.

IPPB (intermittent positive-pressure breathing) Indicated when a conscious or unconscious adult patient needs a high volume of high-concentration oxygen. It is not indicated with noncompliant patients who are breathing but fight the device.

IQ (intelligence quotient) One of the standardized tests commonly used to identify mental retardation. When the IQ exam is administered, a tested IQ of 70 is considered the upper line for those needing special care and training.

irreversible shock The phase of shock when the patient has attempted to compensate but his mechanisms have been overwhelmed, and the damage occurring at the cellular level is irreversible.

ischemia Tissue that is starved of oxygen but the damage is not yet permanent.

isoimmunity Formation of antibodies or T cells directed against antigens on another person's cells.

isotonic fluid volume The fluid in the extracellular compartment that can shift into the cells or vascular space. An isotonic fluid excess represents an increase in both sodium and water in the ECF compartment. This is commonly caused by kidney, heart, or liver failure.

ITD (impedance threshold device) A valve that is designed to improve coronary perfusion and is easily employed during CPR.

jaundice Caused by an excess of bilirubin, this is a yellowish pigment to the skin. This condition is common with liver disease and in premature infants during their initial hospitalization.

JVD (jugular vein distention) The external, noninvasive measurement of CVP. With the patient placed in the semi-Fowler's position, distension indicates increased CVP.

KE (kinetic energy) Energy that is absorbed by the body in a car crash or a penetrating or blunt injury. It is calculated by multiplying half the mass by the velocity squared.

Kehr's sign Abdominal pain that radiates to the left shoulder, which may be an indication of intraperitoneal bleeding.

keloid scar formation The excessive accumulation of scar tissue that extends beyond the original wound border is called a keloid scar.

kinesthetic Refers to the sense of body position.

Kussmaul's respirations Air hunger.

labor The pain and contractions of the uterus while the cervix dilates to allow expulsion of the fetus. It is divided into three stages.

laceration A break in the skin; can be deep or superficial and usually has uneven edges.

lactose intolerance A very common GI abnormality affecting almost half the world's population. Patients get bloating, pain, and diarrhea, sometimes violent, within minutes to hours after eating the sugar lactose that is found in milk and cheese.

laryngeal spasm A closure of the vocal cords and surrounding muscles. It may be caused by the trauma of an overly aggressive intubation attempt.

laryngectomy A surgical removal of the larynx, often due to cancer of the throat.

latex A natural sap from the rubber tree used to make natural rubber products.

LDB-CPR CPR compressions that employ a load-distributing band or vest CPR device.

LDL cholesterol The "bad cholesterol" or low-density lipoprotein that carries the largest amount of cholesterol in the blood and is responsible for depositing cholesterol in the artery walls. An elevated LDL cholesterol level is associated with risk of heart disease.

LeFort classifications Named after French surgeon Leon LeFort, a classification of facial fractures.

leukocytes Includes the two white blood cell types: granulocytes and monocytes.

leukotriene blockers Produced during asthma attacks; anti-inflammatory drugs that either block the leukotriene receptor or the substance that synthesizes leukotrienes.

Levine's sign Presentation of a sick-looking patient who places a clenched fist over the sternum to describe chest pain.

libel An act in which a person's character or reputation is injured by the false or malicious written words of another person.

life expectancy The amount of time remaining before a person is expected to die.

life span The total duration of one's life from birth to death.

lightning injuries An electrical burn injury from a strike, or from being very close to a strike, of a lightning bolt.

limbic system Located in the diencephalon, the limbic system is comprised of several brain structures that are involved with emotions.

lipids Fatty substances that are present in blood and body tissues and include cholesterol and triglycerides.

lipoproteins Protein-coated packages that carry fat and cholesterol through the body. Lipoproteins are classified by their density.

living will An advanced directive that states the type of lifesaving medical treatment a patient wants or does not want to be employed in case of terminal illness.

LMA (laryngeal mask airway) An advanced airway device that is used on unconscious or non-breathing patients to improve ventilation. Its use is recommended for patients with an empty stomach, as aspiration is a concern if the patient regurgitates.

loaded bumper A shock-absorbing bumper on a motor vehicle that has been compressed and can release suddenly without warning.

LOC (level of consciousness) The patient's mental status, usually described using the acronym AVPU.

Los Angeles prehospital stroke screen (LAPSS) An out-of-hospital ministroke assessment tool.

Lyme disease An infection that is transmitted by ticks. Flu-like symptoms and muscle joint aches follow, with or without a rash. The infection can lead to AMS, paralysis, paresthesia, stiff neck, sensitivity to light, dysrhythmias, and chest pain.

LZ (landing zone) The location where a helicopter can safely land. It needs to be flat, wide, or obstruction free, and approximately $100' \times 100'$.

malpractice Dereliction of professional duty.

manic-depressive disorder A major mental disorder characterized by fits of mania and periods of depression.

manual spinal motion restriction (MSMR) Phrase that is now used in the Guidelines 2005, instead of the terminology "spinal immobilization," as it is more accurate.

Marfan's syndrome Inherited disease of the connective tissue characterized by elongated long bones and ocular and circulatory defects.

MAST/PASG Military antishock trousers/pneumatic antishock garment.

McBurney's point A landmark on the abdomen associated with the late pain of appendicitis; an imaginary triangle on the anterior quadrant, from the navel out to the right superior iliac spine.

MCI (multiple casualty incident) An incident involving many patients.

MD (muscular dystrophy) Any of a group of hereditary diseases characterized by progressive muscular wasting.

mechanical piston device A device used for CPR, such as the life vest or the Thumper®.

meconium The greenish, tar-like substance that an infant may be covered with at birth. It is thought to be the result of fetal distress.

medical command At a major incident, the leader of the EMS personnel who should be working with the incident commander in the command post.

medical direction Either online or off-line input or physician direction of EMS providers in their care of patients.

MedicAlert® Foundation An organization that maintains a 24-hour emergency response center with a toll-free phone number that EMS providers can call to obtain information on patients who wear medical identification necklaces or bracelets with an identifiable symbol.

medical monitoring At a hazmat incident or fire rehab sector, the monitoring of the firefighter's vital signs or the hazmat team prior to suiting up and after removing the suits. This is conducted in the cold zone.

Medical Practice Act The state law that specifies exactly what a health care provider is allowed to do in his or her work environment.

melena Blood in stool.

meninges The three layers that cover the brain and spinal cord.

meningitis An inflammation of the meninges that can be caused by a bacteria or virus. Bacterial meningitis is highly communicable and may be fatal if not aggressively treated in the hospital setting.

menopause The period of natural cessation of menstruation occurring between the ages of 45 and 50.

menstrual cycle The entire cycle of physiological changes from the beginning of one cycle to the beginning of the next.

mental retardation Subaverage intellectual ability that is equal to or below an IQ of 70 and is present from birth.

mental status (MS) Determination of whether a patient is alert and oriented.

message The points being conveyed by a sender to a receiver.

metabolic acidosis A shift in the body's pH caused by the metabolic processes, producing a pH under 7.35.

metabolic alkalosis A shift in the body's pH caused by the metabolic processes, producing a pH over 7.45.

metaplasia The transformation of one tissue into another (e.g., cartilage into bone); the abnormal replacement of cells by another type of cell.

MI (myocardial infarction) A heart attack where cardiac cells are deprived of oxygen for a long enough time that they begin to die.

middle meningeal artery The artery in the temporal skull that is usually the cause of an epidural hematoma, due to a blow to the temporal skull.

minimum data set The data elements defined by the federal government to be placed on all standardized prehospital care reports in the United States.

minute volume The amount of gas inspired in a minute.

mitral valve prolapse Also referred to as a floppy mitral valve, which has been associated with Marfan's syndrome, osteogenesis imperfecta, and other connective tissue disorders.

mittelschmerz Abdominal pain in the middle of the menstrual period usually associated with ovulation.

MODS (multiple organ dysfunction syndrome) A new diagnosis (since 1975) that involves the progressive failure of two or more organ systems after severe illness or injury.

MOI (mechanism of injury) The forces that cause an injury, which can be predictive of the extent of the injury patterns (e.g., type of collision, speed and type of penetrating projectile, distance of fall).

monocyte A large leukocyte with finely granulated chromatin dispersed throughout the nucleus.

monounsaturated fat Slightly unsaturated fat that is found in greatest amounts in foods from plants, including olive and canola oil. When substituted for saturated fat, monounsaturated fat helps to reduce blood cholesterol.

morbidity The extent of injury in groups of patients caused by trauma or medical conditions.

Morgan lenses® A special contact lens that is designed to allow flushing of the eye that has been exposed to chemicals or a burn injury.

mortality The death rate of patients caused by injuries or medical conditions.

MS (mental status) The state of a patient's level of consciousness as described using AVPU.

MS (multiple sclerosis) A demyelinating disease marked by patches of hardened tissue in the brain or spinal cord. It is associated with paralysis and muscular jerking or tremors.

MS-ABC The plan for the initial assessment of a patient involving an assessment of the mental status, airway, breathing, and circulation.

multiparous Term used to describe a woman who has given birth.

musculoskeletal trauma An injury to the bones or muscles such as a sprain, strain, dislocation, or a fracture.

myelin A soft, white, fatty sheath around the protoplasmic core of the myelinated nerve.

myxedema Severe hypothyroidism characterized by a firm, inelastic edema, dry skin and hair, and loss of mental and physical vigor.

NAERG (*North American Emergency Response Guidebook*) The book that should be carried in every emergency vehicle to identify the most commonly found hazardous materials in transport on the highways.

NALS (neonatal advanced life support) A training program focused on the initial hospitalization of an infant.

narrow complex SVT A category of rapid ECG rhythms presumably originating from the atria.

nasal cannula A basic oxygen-administration device used on patients who will not tolerate a mask or who require only small percentages of oxygen.

nasal flaring Widening of the nostrils during breathing.

nasal pharyngeal airway (NPA) A basic airway adjunct designed to be lubricated with a water-soluble gel and then inserted into the nares.

nasotracheal intubation An advanced procedure that involves a blind insertion of a tube down the nares, listening for air movement, while attempting to insert the distal end into the glottic opening.

nature of the illness (NOI) The condition or chief complaint of the patient.

nausea The sensation that a patient describes of feeling like he or she could vomit.

near drowning A patient who was submersed under water for a long enough period of time to need emergency medical care and possibly rescue breathing or CPR.

needle cricothyrotomy The last-resort technique in a patient with a complete airway obstruction or in whom tracheal intubation is otherwise impossible.

needle stick injuries A potentially serious exposure if the needle or sharps has been contaminated with a patient's blood. Work practices should be engineered to minimize these injuries by placing the sharps immediately into a container as part of the procedure.

neglect A form of abuse where necessary care is not provided.

negligence Providing care improperly or eliminating essential steps. To prove negligence, the plaintiff must show that the provider had a duty to act, breached his or her duty, an injury occurred, and the breach of duty caused the injury.

neonatal sepsis Severe, overwhelming infection in a neonate (birth to 1 month).

neoplasm A new growth of tissue serving no physiological function.

neurogenic shock A form of shock, often called fainting or syncope, due to disorders of the nervous system with an absence of sympathetic response. Three assessment findings that, when displayed together, indicate neurogenic shock are decreasing blood pressure, decreasing pulse rate, and decreasing respiratory rate.

neurological posturing Positioning of the patient as a reflex in response to pain. Examples include decorticate and decerebrate posturing, or the fetal position.

neurology The study of the nervous system and its components and function in sickness and health.

neurons The basic unit of the nervous system.

NHTSA (National Highway Traffic Safety Administration) A division of the U.S. Department of Transportation where the EMS initiatives are coordinated at the federal level.

nitrogen narcosis (rapture of the deep) A state of euphoria or exhilaration occurring when nitrogen enters the blood stream at approximately seven times the atmospheric pressure during a diving incident.

non-rebreather mask A basic oxygen-therapy appliance used by all levels of out-of-hospital and in-hospital providers to administer high concentrations of oxygen to the breathing patient.

North American Emergency Response Guidebook See NAERG.

nosocomial disorder A medical condition that originates in the hospital setting.

NPA (nasal pharyngeal airway) A basic airway adjunct designed to be lubricated with a water-soluble gel and then inserted into the nares.

NPO (nothing by mouth) A hospital order for patients who are going to surgery or have a medical condition that does not allow them to take in any food or drink.

NREMT (National Registry of EMTs) The organization that provides a standardized examination and practical skills examination for the first responders, EMT-basics, EMT-intermediates, and paramedics of many states.

NSTEMI An acute myocardial infarction that does not show ST-segment elevation on the ECG.

nulliparous Term used to describe a woman who has never given birth.

nutrition The act or process of being nourished with food and drink that are required to survive.

nystagmus A fine motor twitching of the eyeball, normal during extreme lateral gaze but not in any other position.

obesity A condition characterized by excessive body fat.

objective information Data representing the clinical signs that can be observed and measured by the examiner, such as the pulse, respiratory rate, and blood pressure.

obstetrics The branch of medical science that deals with birth, pregnancy, and its complications.

obstructive airway disease A medical condition that causes constriction, spasms, or thick secretions and inflammation of the airways.

occlusive dressing A covering to apply to a puncture wound that will not allow air to pass through the hole. Many services use Vaseline gauze for this purpose.

ongoing assessment (OA) The assessment of the patient that is normally conducted en route to the hospital involving serial vital signs, reassessment, and checking on interventions. This is now referred to as reassessment.

OPA (oropharyngeal airway) A basic airway adjunct used on patients with no gag reflex to help keep the tongue away from the back of the throat.

opacification The forming of cataract cloudiness, impairing vision.

open-ended question A type of question that requires a narrative form of response.

open fracture A break in a bone that has punctured the skin with the bone ends.

open pneumothorax Air in the chest due to a penetrating wound, allowing air to enter the chest cavity.

OPQRRST An elaboration of the chief complaint, including: onset; provocation; quality; region, radiation, relief, recurrence; severity; time.

ophthalmoscope A tool used by health care personnel to perform a detailed examination of the eye.

organ donors Patients who have agreed to donate their organs should they die in a fatal accident or from a fatal medical condition, so others may benefit from them.

orthopnea The abnormal condition in which a patient must sit or stand to breathe comfortably.

orthostatic changes An increase in heart rate and a decrease in blood pressure when a patient rises from a supine or sitting position.

orthostatic hypotension A drop in the patient's blood pressure when he or she stands up; usually due to internal bleeding.

OSHA (Occupational Safety and Health Administration) A program of the U.S. Department of Labor that is designed to protect the employee from the employer and assure that the workplace is a safe environment.

osmosis Movement of a solvent across a semipermeable membrane into a solution of higher-solute concentration to equalize the concentrations of solute on the two sides of the membrane.

osteoporosis A condition, primarily affecting older women, that causes decreased bone mass and density, resulting in bones that break more easily.

otorrhea A discharge from the ear.

otoscope A tool used by health personnel to perform a detailed examination of the ear.

out-of-hospital care The term that has replaced prehospital care in the Guidelines 2005. This seems to be the direction of most of the national organizations in respect to care provided outside of the hospital.

overdose An excessive and dangerous, potentially lethal, dose of a drug.

oxyhemoglobin saturation curve A sigmoid-shaped curve that represents the percentage saturation of hemoglobin by oxygen on the vertical axis and the partial pressure of oxygen (PO_2) in arterial blood on the horizontal axis.

pacemaker An implanted device that is designed to provide an electrical impulse to pace the heart when the normal conduction cells are not functioning properly.

pacemaker cells The cells in the heart that generate the electrical impulses. Typically assembled in nodes (e.g., SA node, AV node).

palliative care Treatment that reduces the violence of a disease without actually curing the disease.

PAR (primary area of responsibility) The territory in which a roving ambulance is assigned to stay within when not assigned to an actual call.

paradoxical motion Seen when a free-floating section of the rib cage moves in the opposite direction of the rest of the rib cage during respirations.

paralytic ileus A twisted and paralyzed bowel.

paraplegia The inability to move the legs after an injury or illness involving the spine.

parenteral drug administration The introduction of a medication to the body outside of the GI tract (e.g., IV medications).

parity The total number of births a woman has had.

Parkinson's disease A chronic, progressive nervous disease involving tremors and muscular weakness.

paroxysmal nocturnal dyspnea (PND) A form of transient pulmonary edema that wakes the patient during the night with severe shortness of breath; associated with heart failure.

partial seizure A type of seizure that occurs only in a particular area of the brain, so the patient remains conscious and the effects are apparent only in a specific area of the body.

pathogenesis The origination or development of a disease.

pathologic fracture A break in a bone weakened by disease.

pathology The study of disease and its effect on the anatomy and physiology of the organism.

pathophysiology The study of the irregular or abnormal functioning of the body or its organ systems.

patient advocacy A key part of the EMS provider's role in lobbying for the most appropriate care for his or her patient in a busy health care facility.

patient assessment The methodical process by which a patient's condition is evaluated.

PCC (poison control center) A resource of information on poisons and their management.

PCI Percutaneous coronary intervention, such as coronary catheterization for the diagnosis and management of ACS.

PE (pulmonary edema) The collection of fluid in the lungs usually due to heart failure or pump failure, although it is occasionally found in narcotic overdoses and high-altitude sickness.

PEA (pulseless electrical activity) An ECG found on a patient in cardiac arrest that shows some electrical activity but not enough to cause sufficient pumping to move the blood. Previously called electromechanical dissociation, or EMD.

peak flow A measurement of how rapidly a patient can exhale.

pediatrics The study of the care of healthy and sick children.

penetration A break in the skin due to an object's being forced into and tearing the skin and internal organs.

pepper spray Used by the police as an irritant to the eyes to disperse a potentially violent crowd without doing any long-term, serious medical damage to the victims.

percussion A step in the examination of the patient that involves tapping the body to listen for dull or hollow sounds.

perfusion Blood flow to the tissues of the body.

peritonitis Inflammation of the peritoneum.

PERRLA An acronym for documenting normal findings related to the eyes: pupils equally round, reactive to light and accommodation.

personal protective equipment (PPE) Items that can be worn to protect the EMS provider from harm from bodily fluids or hazardous substances, such as disposable gloves, eye shields or goggles, masks, and gowns.

pertinent negatives Symptoms the patient does not have that may be relevant to the case (e.g., a patient struck his head but did not lose consciousness).

PFDs (personal flotation devices) A life preserver that should be worn whenever rescue personnel are near or around water.

pH The scale of a chemical's acidity or alkalinity (acid or base), where the body's normal pH is defined as between 7.35 and 7.45.

pharmacodynamics The division of pharmacology dealing with reactions between drugs and organisms.

pharmacokinetics The study of bodily absorption, distribution, metabolism, and excretion of drugs.

pharmacology The study of drugs, their functions, and their medical applications to treatment.

phlebitis The inflammation of a vein.

phobia An exaggerated and often incapacitating fear.

PID (pelvic inflammatory disease) An infectious disease in the female reproductive and surrounding organs that can lead to complications including sepsis and infertility.

piloerection A reflexive response to cold; also known as goose pimples.

placenta previa Abnormal attachment of the placenta near the opening of the birth canal, which can cause the placenta to precede the delivery of the infant.

plague An acute febrile, infectious, and highly fatal disease caused by a gram positive bacteria.

plantar reflex A reflex that is assessed on both conscious and unconscious patients with suspected spinal cord injury. With the end of a capped pen, a light stroke is drawn up the lateral side of the sole of the foot and across the ball of the foot, like an upside-down letter J. The normal response is plantar flexion of the toes and foot.

plasma A combination of 91% water and 9% proteins found in the blood.

platelets Particles in the blood responsible for forming the initial blood clot.

platinum ten minutes The optimum limit of 10 minutes at the scene with a critical trauma patient; used in both Montana's and New York State's critical trauma care courses.

pleural friction rub A grating sound in the chest caused by inflamed pleural surfaces.

pleurisy Inflammation of the lining of the lungs.

pleuritic pain Pain caused by any condition that causes inflammation in the lung or heart that extends to the pleural surfaces of the lung.

PMH (past medical history) Relevant recent surgeries, illnesses, trauma, periods of immobilization or hospitalizations, changes in mental status or physical ability, and changes in medication or daily routine/activity.

PMS (premenstrual syndrome) Varying symptoms manifested by some women prior to menstruation that may include emotional instability, irritability, insomnia, fatigue, anxiety, or depression. Previously referred to as premenstrual tension syndrome, this is now called premenstrual dysphoric disorder.

PMS (pulses, motor function, and sensory function) When evaluating the distal circulation and nervous system function, especially before and after applying a splint, the PMS should be evaluated.

PND (paroxysmal nocturnal dyspnea) The shortness of breath that occurs during the night, often waking the patient up.

pneumonia An inflammation of the lungs commonly caused by bacteria, a virus, or other pathogens.

pneumothorax A collection of air or gas in the pleural space of the chest, causing one or both lungs to collapse.

PNS (peripheral nervous system) The twelve pairs of cranial nerves and 31 pairs of peripheral nerves existing between each vertebrae of the spinal column.

point of maximal impulse (PMI) The point on the chest where the impulse of the left ventricle is felt most strongly.

poisoning Connotes exposure to a substance that is generally only harmful and has no usual beneficial effects.

polypharmacy (polymedication) The administering or taking of many medications concurrently, often for the same condition.

polyunsaturated fat Highly unsaturated fat that is found in food products derived from plants, including sunflower, corn, and soybean oils. Like monounsaturated fat, this is a healthier alternative to saturated fat.

positive findings Information obtained in the focused history and physical examination that is clearly relevant to the chief complaint.

post-ictal The third phase of a seizure, during which the patient is extremely exhausted and confused while slowly regaining consciousness.

preeclampsia A disorder of the last trimester marked by edema, hypertension, and proteinuria. Formerly called toxemia of pregnancy.

preexcitation syndrome See *WPW (Wolf-Parkingson-White) syndrome*.

prehospital care The term "out-of-hospital setting" has replaced "prehospital care."

prehospital care report (PCR) A report that should be completed on every call; an accurate and thorough documentation of the assessment findings and field management of the patient.

pre-ictal phase The period before a seizure attack.

prejudice Preconceived notions, judging patients by stereotypes, and intolerance to cultural diversity.

preload The degree of stretch in a cardiac contraction.

premature infant An infant born prior to full term (i.e., before 36 weeks).

presbycusis Normal hearing loss that occurs with aging.

pressure dressing A sterile gauze applied to a soft-tissue injury designed to provide continuous bleeding control to assist in the clot formation.

preterm labor True labor that occurs before 38 weeks' gestation.

Prinzmetal's angina An atypical form of angina caused by the vasospasm of otherwise normal coronary arteries.

profession A "calling" requiring specialized and specific academic preparation.

prognosis Prediction of the outcome of the problem.

pronator drift A test used to assess focal weakness. The patient is asked to extend both arms out in front of him, with palms up, while both eyes are closed. If one arm "drifts" lower or the palm turns down, this is considered a deficit.

proprioception The perceptions concerning movements and position of the body.

protected airway Rather than saying "secure the airway" or "protect the airway," the phrase "insert or pass an advanced airway" is used, because terminology like "secure" or "protect" may give a false sense of security to the provider.

protective custody When police take someone into custody for the purpose of protecting that person from him- or herself, or others, or to have the person evaluated.

protocol The treatment guidelines that are agreed upon for a typical patient presentation. These are a form of indirect or off-line medical control.

PSVT See *reentry SVT*.

psychosis A serious mental disorder characterized by a loss of contact with reality.

PTACD–CPR CPR employing a device to provide phased thoracic-abdominal compression–decompression.

PTL (pharyngotracheal lumen airway) A dual lumen airway that is blindly inserted into the patient when other forms of advanced airways are not available. These are no longer commonly used by out-of-hospital providers.

pulmonary circulation The circuit of blood flow between the heart and the lungs.

pulmonary contusion A common serious injury from blunt thoracic trauma.

pulmonary edema The filling of the lungs with fluid in the interstitial space, the alveoli, or both.

pulmonary embolism (PE) A serious condition caused by a foreign body (e.g., a clot) that lodges in the pulmonary capillary bed.

pulse deficit A result of the irregular filling of the ventricles; present when there is a slower distal pulse compared to the core pulse (apical).

pulse oximetry A technique used to measure the percentage of hemoglobin saturated with oxygen.

pulseless ventricular tachycardia (VT) An ECG generating in the ventricles, which is generally over 180 beats per minute and is not able to produce effective cardiac pumping. It is considered a shockable rhythm.

pulsus differens A condition in which the pulses on either side of the body are unequal.

pulsus paradoxus (also called **paradoxical pulse**) A pulse that diminishes during the inspiration phase of breathing.

puncture A break in the skin as a result of an object's being forced into the skin.

pursed-lip breathing Exhaling past partially closed lips to build up air pressure in the lungs.

quadriplegia The inability of a patient to move his or her four extremities due to an injury or medical condition affecting the cervical spine.

quality assurance (QA) A program that looks closely at the medical care given to assure that the highest quality is provided and to make improvements to the care on an ongoing basis.

quality improvement (QI) A program that looks closely at the medical care provided in order to strive to improve the quality of care so excellence can be achieved on a regular basis.

rabies (also see **hydrophobia**) A viral infection transmitted through saliva of an infected animal. It is fatal in humans if not aggressively treated.

radiating pain Pain or discomfort that spreads from the source to another area (e.g., ischemic chest pain radiating down the left arm).

radiation exposure Injuries and medical ailments caused by excessive exposure to ionizing radiation. The extent of the injury is a function of the duration of exposure and the types of particles to which a person is exposed (e.g., alpha, beta, or gamma).

rales See *crackles*.

range of motion (ROM) The area and span of motion of the joints.

rapid extrication The procedure for removing a patient found in the seated position from a vehicle using only a long backboard, a rigid cervical collar, and three to four trained EMS providers. This is only done if the patient is unstable, as in all other cases the vest-type device (i.e., KED) should be utilized.

rapid physical examination (RPE) A systematic, quick examination of the major body sections (head, neck, chest, abdomen, pelvis, back, buttocks, and extremities) for injuries, conducted on the medical patient who is not responsive (e.g., hypoglycemia, hypothermia, or postictal state).

rapid takedown technique The procedure for carefully moving a patient who has a suspected spine injury from the standing position to the supine position on a long backboard. This procedure requires a rigid cervical collar, a long backboard, and three trained EMS providers.

rapid trauma assessment (RTE) A quick head-to-toe assessment conducted on a trauma patient with significant mechanism of injury involving the major body sections (head, neck, chest, abdomen, pelvis, back, buttocks, and extremities).

rapid trauma examination (RTE) A systematic, quick examination of the major body sections (head, neck, chest, abdomen, pelvis, back, buttocks, and extremities) for injuries.

rapture of the deep See *nitrogen narcosis*.

reciprocity The ability of one's certification or license to be utilized between one state and another. This is a function of the use of a standardized training curriculum (e.g., DOT) and the specific rules of each state.

reentry SVT Previously called PSVT, a tachycardic rhythm caused by a reentry circuit originating from above the ventricles, as depicted on the ECG.

referred pain Pain that originates in one area of the body that is also sensed in another area.

reflection A communication technique in which the EMS provider repeats the patient's words to encourage further discussion.

reflex arc An involuntary or immediate response to a stimulus.

refractory period Not responding or yielding to treatment.

regurgitation Backward flow, as in the return of stomach contents into the esophagus.

respiration The chemical and physical processes in which an organism acquires oxygen and eliminates carbon dioxide.

respiratory acidosis A condition in which the body's pH falls below 3.35, primarily as a result of not breathing enough.

respiratory alkalosis A condition in which the body's pH rises above 3.45, primarily from breathing too much.

respiratory distress The sensation of dyspnea or the signs of difficulty breathing (e.g., tripod position, intercostal separations, grunting, cyanosis, etc.).

restraints Supplies or devices used to tie a patient for the purpose of protecting the patient or others from violence. When dealing with injured or medical patients, humane restraints (e.g., wide bands of cloth, sheets, leather restraints) are used instead of handcuffs.

retraction A pulling in of skin in the suprasternal, subclavicular, and intercostal areas during inhalation.

revised trauma score (RTS) A numerical grading system used for triage and to predict patient outcomes, developed by Howard Champion, MD; see also trauma score.

Reye's syndrome An acute, frequently fatal childhood syndrome marked by encephalopathy, hepatitis, and fatty accumulations in the viscera; thought to be caused by excess administration of salicylates to children.

Rh A factor in the blood, derived from the rhesus monkey, that is inherited.

rhabdomyolysis An acute, potentially fatal disorder involving disintegration of skeletal muscles and urine excretion of the muscle pigment myoglobin.

rheumatic heart disease A manifestation of rheumatic fever consisting of inflammatory changes and damaged heart valves.

rhonchi Rattling noises in the upper airways caused by mucus or other secretions; singular rhonchus.

right-sided heart failure A potential backup of fluid into the systemic system that is also referred to as cor pulmonale.

RMA (refusal of medical assistance) The term used when a patient does not want to give consent to a specific treatment (e.g., an IV or cervical collar) or transport to a hospital.

ROSC (return of spontaneous circulation) The phrase used when a cardiac arrest patient's pulses return.

rotavirus A virus that causes acute gastroenteritis in children.

RSI (rapid sequence induction) The use of medications to paralyze and cause amnesia when it is medically necessary to rapidly intubate a patient.

rubberneckers Individuals who pose a traffic hazard when passing the scene of an accident so they can get a look at the damage and rescue taking place.

rule out Process by which a diagnosis is made in the cardiac care unit in order to determine a definitive diagnosis.

S1 A normal heart sound; the first sound heard, which is produced by the atrioventricular valves.

S2 A normal heart sound; the second sound heard, which is produced by the semilunar valves.

safety A key concern at any EMS or rescue operation to assure that procedures are done in the least potentially harmful manner possible. Some agencies appoint a safety officer at major incidents.

SAMPLE history An acronym for the information needed to assess and manage an incident or complaint: signs and symptoms, allergies, medications, pertinent past medical history, last oral intake, events leading up to this incident.

saturated fat Usually solid at room temperature. This is commonly found in animal products, such as meat, poultry, egg yolks, and dairy products. It is also found in a few vegetable products, such as coconuts and cocoa. Saturated fat raises blood cholesterol more than anything else in the diet.

scalp The skin and hair on the outside of the cranium; provides a protective layer against minor blunt trauma to the head.

scaphoid abdomen A sinking, or concave, shape to the abdomen.

scene choreography An important element of the management of the health care providers who are administering care to a patient.

scene size-up The first component of patient assessment, which involves determining whether the location, or environment, is safe for the responders and the patient.

SCI (spinal cord injury) A laceration, bruise, cut, or compression injury to the spinal cord that can have devastating implications for the patient.

SCIWORA (spinal cord injury without radiographic abnormalities) A potential problem in children, where the vertebrae can slip out of place and then return on their own to the appropriate positioning, leaving a damaged or severed cord behind.

scope of practice As usually defined in state laws, the extent to which health care providers can practice within their specific state.

SCUBA (self-contained underwater breathing apparatus) The tank and regulator that allows an underwater diver to breathe for extended periods of time without returning to the surface.

second-party caller A call for emergency services made by the bystander or family member and not the patient.

seizure An attack or sudden onset of disease. A convulsion or epileptic attack classified into different types (e.g., absence, clonic, focal motor, generalized tonic-clonic, or partial focal seizure).

semantics The study of the meanings in language.

serial vital signs All measurements after, or comparisons against, the baseline measurements.

sexual abuse Abuse of a sexual nature.

shaken baby syndrome Bleeding into the skull of an infant from damage to the bridging veins on the outside of the brain, due to picking up the child and shaking him or her continuously.

sharp A device, such as a needle, that could puncture the skin and may transmit pathogens.

shipping papers The documentation of potentially hazardous materials on a ship, train, truck, or plane.

shock 1. The body's response to low perfusion states, which involves an initial compensation phase followed by decompensation, and then an irreversible or terminal phase, if not properly managed early on; 2. an electrical injury; 3. treatment of a "shockable" ECG in a pulseless patient.

SIDS (sudden infant death syndrome) The sudden death of an otherwise healthy infant.

sign A finding that can be measured accurately by hand or with a measuring device such as a blood pressure cuff.

silent myocardial infarction (MI) An ACS with atypical signs and symptoms; common among elderly and diabetic patients.

simple pneumothorax An injury or medical condition that causes air to enter the chest cavity. The simple pneumothorax is a respiratory problem; because it does not continue to suck air into the chest, it does not proceed to move the mediastinum or turn into a tension pneumothorax.

sinus arrhythmia A cardiac rhythm, typical in children and healthy adults, characterized by a regular rate that increases and decreases rhythmically with breathing.

skeletal muscle The voluntary (striated) muscle that moves the long bones.

skin CTC (color, temperature, and condition) Assessment that the EMS provider can do to determine circulatory status.

skin lesions Breaks or injuries to the skin, such as papule, scale, crust, patch, plaque, wheal, cyst, bulla, pustule, fissure, ulcer, vesicle, and macule.

skin turgor An indication of the patient's state of hydration.

skull The outer cover of bone that encases the brain; consisting of the bones of the face and the cranium.

skull fracture Isolated linear, nondepressed fractures with an intact scalp that are common and do not require treatment. However, life-threatening intracranial hemorrhage may result if the fracture causes disruption of the middle meningeal artery or a major dural sinus.

small-volume nebulizer Another form of administering oxygen combined with medicine (e.g., Albuterol).

smooth muscle Found in the lower airways; vessels and intestines can relax or contract to alter the inner lumen of the vessels.

sniffing position A position of the head and neck used to help visualize the vocal cord during intubation.

soft spots The fontanelles are the membrane-covered spaces between the incomplete ossified cranial bones of an infant.

soft tissue trauma Injuries to the skin, which are open or closed.

somatic pain Pain caused by irritation of pain fibers in the parietal peritoneum; tends to be localized to the area of pathology.

SOPs (standard operating procedures) The policy that an agency uses to define the steps they would like personnel to take when confronted with a particular situation or operating a specific device (e.g., SOP on wearing seat belts).

span of control In the incident command system, it is recognized that emergency managers can effectively lead and communicate with approximately five to seven people each. Keeping this in mind: the incident commander at a school bus rollover should not attempt to talk to all fifty emergency personnel at the scene; rather, he or she should communicate with the staging officer, the triage officer, the transport officer, the treatment officer, and the other service leaders (police and FD) at the command post.

spastic hemiparesis An abnormal gait with unilateral weakness and foot dragging.

spina bifida A birth defect where the infant is born with exposed spinal structures.

spinal immobilization See *manual spinal motion restriction.*

sprain An injury to the ligaments around a joint; marked by pain, swelling, and the dislocation of the skin over the joint.

staging Effectively parking resources (e.g., emergency vehicles) within a few minutes of the incident rather than cluttering up the actual incident site. This way, they can be moved in as they are needed, and traffic flow may be maintained.

START An acronym for simple triage and rapid treatment; a system used to triage patients in a multiple-casualty incident.

status asthmaticus A severe, prolonged asthma attack that does not respond to standard medications.

status epilepticus Two or more seizures occurring without full recovery of consciousness between attacks, or continuous seizure activity for 10 minutes or more.

STDs (sexually transmitted diseases) Common examples: AIDS, bacterial vaginosis, chancroid, chlamydial infections, cytomegalovirus infections, genital herpes, genital warts, gonorrhea, granuloma inguinale, hepatitis, leukemia, lymphoma, myelopathy, lymphogranuloma venereum, molluscum contagiosum, pubic lice, scabies, syphilis, trichomoniasis, and vaginal yeast infections.

STEMI An acute myocardial infarction that shows ST-segment elevation on the ECG.

steppage gait An abnormal gait in which the person appears to be walking up steps when on an even surface.

sterilization To disinfect equipment in a manner that kills all germs.

stethoscope A device that is used to listen to the patient's heart or lung sounds.

stings Punctures made by an insect.

Stokes–Adams syndrome Syncope or convulsions caused by complete heart block and a pulse rate of forty or less.

stress A factor that induces bodily or mental tension.

striae Atrophic lines or streaks from a rapid or prolonged stretching of the skin.

stridor A high-pitched sound associated with upper airway obstruction.

stroke The result of any process that causes disruption of blood flow to a particular part of the brain.

stroke volume The normal amount of blood ejected from the left ventricle with each contraction of the heart (approximately 70 cc in the adult).

subcutaneous emphysema Air bubbles under the skin resulting from a pneumothorax; sometimes exhibits as crackling like Rice Krispies® or the sensation of plastic packing bubbles.

subdural hematoma An injury to the brain resulting in bleeding from the rupture of bridging vessels between the cortex and dura mater.

subjective information Data obtained from the patient and commonly referred to as the symptoms; this cannot be measured by the EMS provider.

subluxation Partial dislocation of a joint that usually has a great amount of damage and instability.

substance abuse Abuse of drugs, including alcohol and tobacco.

substance dependence A psychological craving for, or a psychological reliance on, a chemical agent resulting from abuse or addiction.

suctioning The use of an aspirator or suction device to remove fluid or small solid particles from a patient's airway.

suicide An attempt to take one's life.

supine hypotension A drop in blood pressure that occurs during the third trimester of pregnancy, when the mother is supine, because the weight of the fetus lies on the inferior vena cava.

supplemental See *supplementary*.

supplementary Increasing the percentage of inspired oxygen. The previous term used was "supplemental," though the correct term, "supplementary," is now used throughout the Guidelines 2005.

sympathy An expression of sorrow for another's loss, grief, or misfortune; implies having feelings and emotions similar to or shared with another person.

symphysis pubis The area of the anterior pelvis where the two pubic bones grow together.

symptom A subjective finding that the patient tells the EMS provider.

symptomatic bradycardia A heart rate below 60 in an adult patient, in which the patient has an altered mental status, difficulty breathing, hypotension, or chest pain. This may include an AV block on the ECG.

syncope Fainting.

synovial joints A joint filled with fluid that lubricates the articulated surfaces.

system status management A method of deploying ambulances that involves assigning them to very specific locations and reassigning their locations as the call volume changes throughout the day.

systolic The peak blood pressure in the arterial system as the left ventricle contracts.

tachypnea Rapid, shallow breathing.

tactile fremitus A vibration of the chest wall during breathing that can be felt by the examiner, often associated with inflammation, infection, or congestion.

tactile intubation Involves placing the first two digits into the mouth to push the tongue down.

TB (tuberculosis) An infection of the lungs that presents as a severe cough, a hemoptysis, chest pain, fever and night sweats, chills, weakness, loss of appetite, and weight loss.

tear gas The chemical used by police to gain control of an angry crowd. Causes a burning sensation that usually lasts for about an hour.

technical terminology Language or professional jargon that has meaning only for the medical community or professional group.

temperature The measurement of the degree of hot or cold in the body. The core temperature is the most accurate, and is approximately 98.6°F.

tension pneumothorax A life-threatening condition resulting from air or gas trapped in the pleural space of the chest and causing collapse of one or both lungs, movement of the mediastinum, and a dramatic decrease in cardiac output.

tenting Characteristic of skin that has poor turgor or a connective tissue disease; the skin remains in a tent position when pinched and does not return to normal.

terminal illness Usually means that the patient has a condition that, regardless of any currently available treatment, will result in her death in the next six to twelve months.

testicular torsion Occurs when a testicle twists on its pedicle, leading to acute ischemia.

tetanus A ubiquitous bacteria that pops up in many places at the same time and is potentially fatal. Prophylaxis is recommended every 10 years.

thalidomide A sedative that was banned in the 1960s because it caused severe birth defects.

thermal regulation The process by which the body controls its heat loss and gain.

third collision When the internal organs strike against the inside of the body in a motor vehicle crash.

thoracic trauma Injury, either blunt or penetrating, that occurs to the chest cavity or chest wall.

thyroid disease Entropy and the over- or underproduction of hormones produced by the thyroid gland leading to hypothyroidism, hyperthyroidism, a goiter, or thyroid cancer.

thyrotoxicosis A general term for the overactivity of the thyroid gland, or hyperthyroidism.

TIA (transient ischemic attack) A ministroke; a temporary occlusion of an artery to the brain caused by a blood clot.

tiered response A response to an EMS incident that involves multiple units of different training levels arriving at different times.

tilt test A test used to assess heart rate and blood pressure for orthostatic changes when a patient rises up from a lying position.

toddler A child between the ages of 2 and 4 years.

tolerance The capacity to assimilate a drug continuously in large doses.

tonicity 1. The normal condition of tension during the slight continuous contraction of skeletal muscles; 2. the effective osmotic pressure.

tonsils A small mass of lymphoid tissue, especially the palatine tonsil.

total cholesterol The total of the HDL cholesterol, LDL cholesterol, and VLDL cholesterol.

toxicology The study of the harmful effects of chemicals on the body.

transfer of command The passing of the command function to a more superior or experienced leader in such a way as to minimize the interruption in the flow of the incident; occurs at a major incident, where the incident command system has been implemented.

transient ischemic attack (TIA) A temporary interruption of blood flow to an area of the brain; may be a precursor to a major cerebrovascular accident.

trauma center A hospital that has the capability of caring for the acutely injured patient.

trauma registry A computer database with relevant data elements for research on the trauma care provided by regional trauma centers.

trauma score An assessment tool that assigns a numerical value to represent the extent of injury on the basis of respiratory rate and chest expansion, capillary refill, and blood pressure ranges; also known as the revised trauma score.

traumatic asphyxia Sudden compression to the chest that causes the blood to rush backward into the systemic circulation. These patients often appear blue above the chest.

traumatic brain injury (TBI) A blunt or penetrating injury to the brain.

Trendelenburg position The shock position where the patient is lying down with his legs raised approximately 18 inches above the rest of the body.

trending Changes over time observed by the comparison of multiple sets of vital signs and/or assessments to establish a diagnostic picture of the patient's status.

triage A French word that means "to sort."

triglycerides Fat-like substances that are carried through the bloodstream to the tissues. Much of the body's fat is stored in the form of triglycerides for later use as energy.

trimester One of the 3-month segments of pregnancy.

tripod position A sitting position often assumed by patients who are having difficulty breathing; leaning forward, with elbows outward and hands on knees.

trismus Difficulty in opening the mouth due to tonic spasm of the muscles of mastication.

true labor Persistent, regular contractions.

turnout gear Protective personal gear used for fire rescue (e.g., boots, pants, helmet, coat, gloves).

tunnel vision The making of judgments or determinations on the basis of history and past experiences with an individual or an event.

tympany A drum-like sound.

unified command The command of a major incident that involves the police, fire, and EMS leadership working together to resolve the situation.

universal precautions Taking the appropriate precautions as a standard procedure when handling all patients, in order to protect the rescuer from body substances. The current term used is *standard precautions*.

unsaturated fat Usually liquid at refrigerator temperature. This is primarily found in vegetable products and includes either monounsaturated or polyunsaturated fats.

up triaging A concept used in medicine that means that if a patient's presenting problem could be either more or less serious, the patient should be managed as having the more serious of the two possibilities until the patient's condition has been absolutely determined.

URI Upper respiratory infection.

urology The study of the urinary system and excretion of fluids from the body.

urticaria The hives that develop as a sign of a severe allergic reaction.

U.S. Pharmacopoeia The book that lists all official drug names.

UTI Urinary tract infection.

VADs Vascular access devices.

ventilation The physiological process where air in the lungs is exchanged with atmospheric air.

vertigo A vestibular disorder that includes motion sickness, in which the patient expressed a false sensation of motion.

Vial of Life® A rolled piece of paper with pertinent medical information about the patient that is kept in a plastic tube similar to a prescription drug container. Patients are often told to keep this in their refrigerator for ease of EMS providers locating them.

virulence How strong a virus is; the degree of disease-producing capability of a microorganism.

visceral pain Pain caused by the stretching of nerve fibers surrounding either solid or hollow organs in the abdomen; this type of pain is often poorly localized and diffuse.

vital signs Pulse, blood pressure, and respirations, often considered the starting point for assessment and a gauge of a person's health status.

VLDL cholesterol Very-low-density lipoprotein that carries cholesterol and triglycerides for later use as energy.

vomiting The active process of expelling the contents of the stomach.

Waddell's triad An injury pattern seen in children that involves the legs, chest, and head.

wheezing A continuous whistling sound caused by narrowing of the lower airways, usually heard at the end of exhalation.

withdrawal 1. The act of removing or discontinuing; 2. a pathologic detachment or retreat from emotional involvement with people or the environment.

WPW (Wolff–Parkinson–White) syndrome Congenital heart condition with an anomalous AV excitation that is marked by irregular heartbeat and distorted patterns of ECG (e.g., shortened P-R and prolonged QRS); also called preexcitation syndrome.

THE COMPLETE

STRESS

MANAGEMENT

WORKBOOK

THE COMPLETE
STRESS
MANAGEMENT
WORKBOOK

YOUR PERSONAL
STEP-BY-STEP PROGRAM FOR HANDLING
THE STRESS IN YOUR LIFE

DR. THOMAS WHITEMAN, DR. SAM VERGHESE, AND RANDY PETERSEN

ZondervanPublishingHouse
Grand Rapids, Michigan
A Division of HarperCollinsPublishers

The Complete Stress Management Workbook
Copyright © 1996 by Thomas A. Whiteman, Samuel Verghese, and Randy Petersen

Requests for information should be addressed to:

ZondervanPublishingHouse
Grand Rapids, Michigan 49530

ISBN: 0-310-20115-2

Edited by Robin Schmitt and Sandra Vander Zicht
Interior design by Sherri L. Hoffman
Interior art by Adam Bloom

Printed in the United States of America

96 97 98 99 00 01 02 /❖ DH/ 10 9 8 7 6 5 4 3 2 1

To the memory of Barbara Sandel Wirth,
who taught us much about managing stress
with enthusiasm and joy

Introduction

If you want to learn about stress, talk to a metallurgist.

With metal, there is *stress* and there is *strain*. When metal is feeling stress, it is experiencing great pressure. Strain is when the metal begins to move, to buckle under that pressure. Metallurgists also talk about a *yield point*. Up to that point, there may be great pressure on a piece of metal, even to the point of slight bending—but it's temporary bending; the metal retains its shape. Beyond the yield point, however, the metal is changed. It is bent or cracked.

You're under stress. Because you've picked up this book, we assume that you're feeling considerable stress. You've decided you need help in handling it, and you've come to the right place.

The Complete Stress Management Workbook will not take all your stress away. That would be impossible. But we'll urge you toward specific techniques, attitudes, and habits that will help to *manage* your stress. If you apply them, these principles will turn your strain back into manageable stress and keep you well on the safe side of your personal yield point.

This is not the sort of book you read at bedtime and yawn and say, "That's nice." This is a book you *do*. There are surveys and suggestions and diets and exercises and journal entries and self-evaluations within each chapter. The more you put into this book, the more you'll get out of it. We suggest that you write "stress management" into your weekly (if not daily) schedule for the next six months or so. Set aside the time to read *and do* this book.

We are Christians and we assume you are, too. There's a major spiritual component of stress—anxiety. And there's a spiritual aspect of stress management—trust. You'll find these themes interwoven throughout this workbook. But that's not the whole story. God has made us as complex spiritual-physical-intellectual-emotional beings. Stress affects every area of our being and is affected by every area. For that reason, we can't just throw Bible verses at you and say, "Trust God more." You *should* trust God more, but you know that. Here are ways to *practice* that trust in your day-to-day activities.

Stress is not a sin. Jesus himself faced so much stress in the Garden of Gethsemane that "his sweat was like drops of blood falling to the ground" (Luke 22:44). Mark records that Jesus was "deeply distressed and troubled" and told his disciples, "My soul is overwhelmed with sorrow to the point of death." He fervently begged God to remove the burden he had to face (Mark 14:33–36).

Chances are, you will never face that level of stress, but you probably do become "deeply distressed and troubled" when you encounter difficult situations. Stress is something that comes upon us. The question is, What do we do with it? That's when we can make sinful choices—worry, pursue unhealthy "escapes" such as alcohol or drugs, or lash out in anger. Or we can make righteous choices, managing our stress in healthy, God-honoring ways.

So don't feel guilty for having stress in your life. Instead, be diligent about making good choices in dealing with that stress. This book is designed to help you make those choices.

Three of us have written this book. Thomas Whiteman, a psychologist, has focused on those chapters involving changes in attitude and relationship. Samuel Verghese, a specialist in the medical aspects of stress, including nutrition, exercise, and brain activity, has prepared the chapters on those specific topics and has offered valuable input for the other chapters. Writer Randy Petersen has put it all together.

We believe that personal examples are crucial to any book like this, so we have freely used material from our own lives and experiences. To protect the privacy of some of our clients and friends, we have changed their names and some details as we've told their stories, but the essence of each anecdote is true.

May God richly bless you, granting you peace and joy as you read and work through this book. May he grant you peace.

Thomas Whiteman
Samuel Verghese
Randy Petersen

1

What Is Stress?

Stressed out! You've been there, haven't you? You know what it's like to have a million things to do in the next week, or fifty things to do in the next hour, or thirteen in the next minute. You know all about deadlines stampeding toward you like buffalo, or fires that must be put out immediately to save your company or your home, or children who are even now at your elbow demanding attention *right now* or else they will be emotionally scarred for life.

You know what that's like.

There are some people who can afford to spend a lot of time meditating on the Twenty-third Psalm when they feel pressure. This book is not for those people. It's for you, someone whose only journey through "green pastures" is when you have to cut the grass. And as for "still waters," your schedule has been downright turbulent since you turned twelve.

You've grown used to this supersonic lifestyle. You hate it but you love it, too. It's hard to take a day off. Your vacations tend to be working vacations. Either you bring along your laptop or you take command of your troops—er, your family—and order them, "Have fun *NOW!* Or else we're all going home!"

You're an LP record (remember those?) played at 45rpm. You fast-forward through the video of your life. Your date book is so full, you

11

could use it for wallpaper. You're the life of the party or the rising star or the hardworking executive or the supermom, but sometimes you just get really tired. And one of these days, you'll crash.

Stress is a part of life. It can be, in fact, a *good* part of life, though you may not feel that way right now.

This book is an early-warning system. It will help you change your life. You can be healthier and happier and get more done in less time. Like so many things in life, stress management is a matter of making good decisions. And the first good decision is to do this book. Don't just *read* it, *do* it.

We suggest that you slot into your date book a half hour a week to go through this book. That should take you a chapter at a time through the insights and exercises we offer. It will be worth it.

ELIMINATING STRESS

Every so often you'll hear a person talk about trying to "eliminate" stress from his or her life. Suddenly the person doesn't return phone calls, drops out of committees and clubs, or starts working at home. While those may be very good things to do, such people will not—*cannot*—succeed in eliminating stress from their lives. It's a logical impossibility. If you eliminate all stress from your life, you don't have a life—you're dead.

Stress is a part of life. It can be, in fact, a *good* part of life, though you may not feel that way right now.

Say you're driving down the road and a car suddenly veers in front of yours. You have to respond quickly—and you do, slamming on the brakes to avoid a collision.

What happens in those few moments? In a word, your body is *energized* to do what it has to do, using God-given instincts to respond to danger. Your heart beats faster, pumping adrenaline through your system, which gives you a temporary ability to see more clearly, think more sharply, and act with more strength and speed.

The car that cuts you off is a *stress producer,* creating a temporary stressful situation for you. You react with a *stress response* as your body gears up to avoid danger.

There's actually a complex chemical procedure that happens in a moment like that. When you sense a sudden threat, one part of the brain (the hypothalamus) sends a hormone (CRF) that stirs the anterior pituitary gland to send another hormone (ACTH) to wake up *another* part of the brain (the adrenal cortex), which produces another hormone (cortisol aldosterone). This hormone essentially provides battle fuel. It increases blood sugar, breaking down the proteins and fats in your system, pumps up your blood pressure, and diverts resources from your immune system in order to meet the immediate challenge.

The autonomic nervous system is activated (which is why you often act instinctively in such situations, without planning your actions). Ultimately, adrenaline and other stimulants flood the bloodstream, increasing your body's metabolism. You are ready for fight or flight, whichever you choose. On the highway, of course, you just need to slam on the brakes and hold on tight.

But what happens *after* this near accident? It takes a while for your body to return to normal. The adrenaline is still surging through your system after the momentary danger has passed. Your heart is still racing. You have a death grip on the steering wheel. Your mind replays the moment again and again. Though the stress producer is long gone, you are still in your stress response.

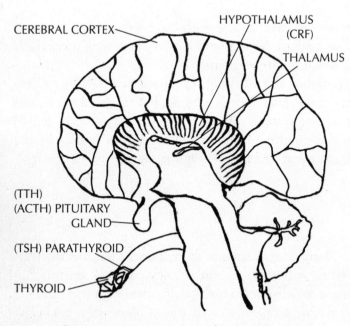

CEREBRAL CORTEX

HYPOTHALAMUS (CRF)

THALAMUS

(TTH) (ACTH) PITUITARY GLAND

(TSH) PARATHYROID

THYROID

The Brain, Hormones, and Stress Reaction

It may take a half hour for your heart rate to get back to normal. It may take all day. And when you do recover, how do you feel? Tired. When you get home from that harrowing drive, you just want to lie down for a while. Or you get to work and you just can't get anything done. But after you've had some time to rest up again, you're fine. That's a normal stress cycle. There's nothing unhealthy about it.

The problem occurs when there are too many stress producers in your life. Your body never has a chance to get through the cycle. You get home after that drive and your child has cut himself and needs stitches, or you get to the office and learn that the Albuquerque plant has run out of semiconductors and you're losing a million bucks a minute. It's as if cars were cutting you off on a regular basis. Your body gears up to meet the challenge and never comes down. Your stressful response becomes a nonstop way of life. Your heart rate stays high, your blood pressure stays up, your body is energized for too long a period of time. It has no chance to rest.

After a while we fool ourselves into thinking that this high level of stress response is *normal*. When the crises fade, we should be able to come back down and recover from the temporary stress response—*but we've forgotten how to relax*. So we create new crises. We worry too much. We hurry too much. We create impossible expectations. We drink coffee and we smoke cigarettes to keep our bodies on red alert.

While the human stress response is a good thing, stress problems occur when we have too much of this good thing.

Orthopedic doctors will diagnose "stress fractures" when a bone cracks because too much weight is put on it. This often happens to athletes who jump or run or hit with great force, repeatedly, day after day weakening the bone that bears the main weight of those motions. Finally the bone cracks.

Construction engineers have to deal with "stress cracks" in concrete foundations, roads, or bridges. It's a matter of too much weight regularly put upon a surface, which finally weakens.

Our bodies are designed to withstand occasional stress. We can handle the car that veers in our lane once in a while, but repeated stress puts too much pressure on our systems. When our bodies are *always* geared up for confrontation, something eventually has to give. It may be the heart, the stomach, the mind, the nerves—but some sort of "stress fracture" will occur.

MANAGING STRESS

What's the answer? Many people attempt to **reduce** the number of stress producers in their lives, with mixed results. They cut back on their involvements. They may even turn down high-paying (and high-pressure) job opportunities. These are the people who walk out of rooms saying, "I can't deal with this right now."

Reducing the number of stressful situations in which you find yourself is part of a good strategy for dealing with stress, but only part. There will always be stressful situations. And there will be rooms you can't walk out of. While it may be wise to stay out of superstress jobs, every job has its share of stress. Stress avoidance is good when you can do it, but it's not the complete answer.

Others try to *ignore* stressful situations by taking drugs to dull their senses. It seemed as if every movie made in the fifties and sixties had a character saying, "It's been a rough day. I need a drink." In the seventies and eighties it became, "Where's my Valium?" (Now, of course, it's Prozac.) The clear lesson is this: You can cope with stress by trying to forget about your troubles, using alcohol or medication to do so. But this solution is also unsatisfactory. When you wake up, you'll still have your problems—along with a nasty hangover. Drugs and alcohol often cause far more problems, creating situations that are even more stressful.

The main component of effective stress management is this: equipping your mind and body to deal with the stresses that come your way.

What you need to do is to *manage* your stress. While this may involve reducing your involvement in stressful situations or ignoring a few minor stresses, the main component of effective stress management is this: equipping your mind and body to deal with the stresses that come your way.

Mind *and* body. Stress is not just in your head, though the way you think about the stressors in your life is very important. You also need to train your body to be ready for stress and to return to normal after a stressful experience. That's what makes this book a "complete" guide. We'll deal with spiritual, cognitive, and physical issues.

STRESS PRODUCERS AND OUR RESPONSES

So what is stress?

It's hard to pin down. We might talk about the "stress experience" that begins with some event (a stress producer) and includes our normal responses to that event (momentary energizing of our systems). The stress experience becomes unhealthy when the response is prolonged or out of proportion.

Staying with our traffic analogy, if you are still focusing on that near accident two days later, and if your heart is still racing from that experience, there's something wrong—your stress response is going on for too long. Or if you get angry at every stoplight that turns red for you, seething and cursing as you wait for green, then your response is out of proportion—there's something wrong.

We'll discuss our stress management strategies later, but for now it will help to distinguish between the stress *producers* and our stress *responses*. We can attack the stress experience from both sides, but more effectively from the response side.

Maybe you have said, "I have too much stress in my life." What did you mean by that? You probably meant that there are too many stress producers in your life—and that may be true. You can take steps to remove yourself from some stressful situations. But you can also begin to change the way you respond to those stress producers.

Some people hate to speak in public. Anne is like that. If you asked her to stand up and say a few words in church, it would be a major stress experience for her (we've seen it happen). The very thought of addressing a crowd gets her palms sweating, her heart galloping. But when she's chatting with a few friends, she's quite talkative. She has no problem sitting in a restaurant with four or five pals and talking freely, but something changes when she has to address twenty or thirty people in a more formal setting.

What's the difference? Is there something inherently stressful about public speaking? Apparently not. Other people handle public speaking easily, with no stress, enjoying the crowds. And Anne herself can talk in front of people—just not a crowd of people.

The difference is in the response. Anne gets stressed out at the thought of speaking in public because she focuses on all the things that can go wrong. She concentrates on her own perceived ineptitude and the possibility of embarrassment. She *makes* public speaking stressful by responding to it as a threat.

Others see no threat in the crowd. Focusing on the message that has to be delivered, they don't even think of their own ineptitude (though in some cases they probably should).

So even this common stress producer—public speaking—is a stress producer only because people respond to it that way. Anne is not really being "stressed out" by the experience; she is stressing *herself* out in response to the experience.

We're not saying that all stress producers are imaginary; there are plenty of events that pack their own real wallop. The death of a loved one, being fired from a job, a move, a deadline, a traffic accident—all these carry a certain weight that we need to bear *temporarily*.

But stress is not simply something that happens to us. It's also how we react to those things that happen. Some of our responses are instinctive, autonomic, but other responses—especially those that last over a period of time—are matters of choice. In most cases, we can choose to be stressed or not to be stressed.

And that is stress management.

YOUR TURN

1. List below the names of nine adults you know fairly well. These people may be in your family, in your neighborhood, at work, or at church. (Leave the short spaces blank for now.)

   _____   _____

   _____   _____

   _____   _____

   _____   _____

   _____   _____

   _____   _____

   _____   _____

   _____   _____

   _____   _____

2. Now think about the stress producers in these people's lives (as far as you know). Would you say they have a *high* level of stress producers in their lives, a *low* level, or something in between? (Don't judge whether they *act* "stressed out" but whether their lives are filled with things that cause most people stress—tough job, many commitments, family troubles, frequent crises or losses, etc.)

In the small space to the right of each name above, put one of the following symbols:

H—for high level of stress producers

MH—for medium high level

M—for medium

ML—for medium low

L—for low

3. Now rewrite that list below in order of the level of stress producers, from high to low, *and put yourself in the list at the appropriate point.* Who has the most stress producers in his or her life? (Put all these H's at the top of your new list.) Who has the least? (Put all the L's at the bottom.) And where do you think you fall? (For now leave the short space at the right, "Response," blank.)

Producers	Names	Response
_____	_____	_____
_____	_____	_____
_____	_____	_____
_____	_____	_____
_____	_____	_____
_____	_____	_____
_____	_____	_____
_____	_____	_____
_____	_____	_____
_____	_____	_____

4. Now, on the right above, grade each person on the basis of *how stressed they seem to be.* Use the same H to L scale and consider their behavior (and your own). Do they seem to deal with the pressures of life calmly, or are they often anxious, fretting, complaining, etc.?

The point is that people don't always react as you would expect them to. Some people have many stressors but exhibit little stress, while others have relatively pressure-free lives but still respond stressfully to little things that occur. Remember: stress does not just happen to you; it also involves how you respond to what happens.

5. What are the three most stressful things that have happened to you in the last year? List these (in a few words) in the spaces at left.

   _____ _____

   _____ _____

   _____ _____

6. How did you handle these stresses? In the spaces at right above, using a simple A to F letter grade (as in school), give yourself a rating for how you dealt with these challenges.

7. What are the three most stressful things that have happened to you in the last *week*? List these in the spaces at left.

   _____ _____

   _____ _____

   _____ _____

8. What did you do in response to these things? Did you vent anger, worry, blame yourself, get drunk, run away—what? In a word or two for each, describe your response in the space at right above.

9. What effect does stress have on you? Consider the five statements below and indicate how true they are of you. Use a 1 to 5 scale, 1 being "most true of you."

   _____ I tend to worry a lot.

   _____ I have physical problems related to stress.

   _____ Stress hurts my job performance.

   _____ When stressed, I get very angry at people around me.

   _____ Stress is hurting my family relationships.

2

How Stressed Are You?

Have you ever been out driving on a turnpike or freeway and suddenly noticed you were going a lot faster than you intended? You started out with the intention of driving the speed limit (or thereabouts), but the traffic around you was going faster, so you naturally sped up to keep pace. Suddenly you realized you were going seventy or eighty. If you were having a really bad day, the cop behind you realized this as well.

How does this happen?

There's a sort of theory of relativity at work here. You don't realize how fast you're traveling because everyone else is going that fast. You're just keeping pace.

Life is like that sometimes. Your schedule gets fuller and fuller. Your days are crammed with activities and concerns. Your life is going eighty miles an hour, but you don't realize it at first, *because everyone else is going that fast, too.*

Your boss demands fourteen-hour days, and you have to go along with that, because everyone else does. The neighbors enroll their children in nine different clubs and sports, so that seems normal to you. (You certainly don't want to deprive your kids of the full experience of childhood.) Your church asks you to serve on three different committees, and that's only reasonable, since everyone else is similarly overcommitted.

It used to be that when you were asked, "How are you?" your answer was "Fine." Now it's "Busy."

People are living and working under overwhelming stress, and they don't even realize it, because they feel they should be able to handle those pressures. The years of pressure erode their physical and mental health, but they ignore the warning signs. In their efforts to keep up with the "traffic" around them, they deny that there's a problem.

Your life is going eighty miles an hour, but you don't realize it at first, because everyone else is going that fast, too.

Imagine that you're driving that highway in a 1972 Pinto. The car starts to rattle at about forty miles an hour, but you can't be bothered by that. At sixty, a warning light appears on the dashboard. You're pushing the engine too hard, but cars are still passing you, so you keep your foot on the accelerator. At eighty miles an hour, the car is internally hemorrhaging, but hey, you're making great time.

Until the car just stops.

It helps to take inventory every so often, to look for warning signs, to check out your stress level. The very fact that you're reading this book is a good sign. You recognize that stress is a problem you need to manage. The next step is to determine *how big* a problem.

It's time to take inventory. The personal stress inventory on the following pages will help us get started.

PERSONAL STRESS INVENTORY

Statements are presented in groups of three, with a point value for each statement. Read all three statements and decide which one matches your situation the best. Then write that point value in the space.

1.

____ My family causes me many difficulties and offers little support. 1

____ My family causes me a substantial amount of difficulty but also offers some support. 5

____ My family causes me little difficulty and offers great support. 10

2.

____ I don't allow family problems to interfere with my work. 10

____ I minimize family problems interfering with my work. 5

____ Family problems interfere with my work. 1

3.

____ I don't take work problems home. 10

____ I take some work problems home. 5

____ Recently I have been taking most work problems home. 1

4.

____ I often have trouble sleeping, because I think about problems of the day. 1

____ I sometimes have trouble sleeping, because I think about problems of the day. 5

____ My daily problems hardly ever affect my sleep. 10

5.

____ I am almost always on time for work and other events. 10

____ I am late for work and other events a fair amount of time. 5

____ I am often late for work and other events. 1

6.

___ I love the work I do each day. 10

___ I usually have a good attitude about the work I have to do each day. 5

___ I hate the work I do each day. 1

7.

___ I like myself. 10

___ I usually accept myself. 5

___ I don't like myself. 1

8.

___ I am assertive. 10

___ I try to be assertive. 5

___ I am increasingly passive. 1

9.

___ People know they can call on me for anything. 1

___ People too often ask me for help, but I find it hard to say no. 5

___ Occasionally people ask me for help, and sometimes I have to say no. 10

10.

___ In most situations, I look at the positive side. 10

___ I try to focus on the positive things around me. 5

___ I tend to focus on the negative things in my life. 1

11.

___ I always strive for perfection. 1

___ I frequently strive for perfection. 5

___ I am realistic in the goals I set for myself. 10

12.

　　____ I am a good communicator. 10

　　____ I try to communicate well. 5

　　____ I find it difficult to communicate. 1

13.

　　____ I always have too much to do. 1

　　____ I often have too much to do. 5

　　____ Occasionally I have too much to do, but then I try to cut back. 10

14F. (For female respondents)

　　____ As a woman, I feel I need to outperform men. 1

　　____ As a woman, I feel some responsibility to represent my gender well at work and in society. 5

　　____ I accept my unique abilities and try to use them well. 10

14M. (For male respondents)

　　____ As a man, I feel a major responsibility to solve all my family's problems. 1

　　____ As a man, I feel I have a special responsibility to provide for my family. 5

　　____ I accept my unique abilities and try to use them well. 10

15M. (For married respondents)

　　____ I feel a lot of pressure from my spouse. 1

　　____ I feel some pressure from my spouse. 5

　　____ I feel minimal pressure and considerable support from my spouse. 10

15S. (For single respondents)

　　____ I am enjoying my singleness thoroughly. 10

_____ I occasionally feel hassled by the dating scene (or fears that I will never marry). 5

_____ I often worry that I will never find a spouse. 1

15D. (For recently divorced respondents)

_____ My divorce has left me with many worries, doubts, fears, and grudges. 1

_____ I'm getting better, but I still feel tremendously harried because of my divorce. 5

_____ I believe I have come through the pain of divorce all right and I'm stronger now. 10

16.

_____ I feel very appreciated for all that I do. 10

_____ I sometimes feel appreciated for things I do. 5

_____ People hardly notice anything I do. 1

17.

_____ I am good at delegating responsibilities to others. 10

_____ I sometimes delegate responsibilities to others. 5

_____ I seldom delegate responsibilities to others. 1

18.

_____ I always try to please the people around me. 1

_____ I often try to please the people around me. 5

_____ I care what people think, but I know I can't please everyone. 10

19.

_____ I accept changes pretty easily. 10

_____ Change is difficult, but I try to accept it. 5

_____ I find change extremely difficult to accept. 1

20.

_____ I try to make sure everyone knows what's going on with everyone else. 1

_____ I attempt to communicate the important news of people's lives with others who need to know. 5

_____ I try to avoid gossip. 10

21.

_____ I meet deadlines pretty easily. 10

_____ I meet deadlines, even if I have to work all night. 5

_____ I am always missing deadlines. 1

22.

_____ I talk easily about my feelings. 10

_____ It is sometimes hard to talk about my feelings, but I try. 5

_____ I very seldom tell anyone how I'm feeling. 1

23.

_____ I get along well with the people I work with. 10

_____ I usually get along with my coworkers. 5

_____ I often have trouble with my coworkers. 1

24.

_____ I get along well with my neighbors. 10

_____ I usually get along with my neighbors. 5

_____ I often have trouble with my neighbors. 1

25.

_____ I get along well with the people at church. 10

_____ I usually get along with the people at church. 5

_____ I often have trouble with the people at church. 1

26.

_____ I find my daily work challenging. 10

_____ I find my daily work semichallenging. 5

_____ My daily work is increasingly underchallenging. 1

27.

_____ I am often sick. 1

_____ I get sick from time to time. 5

_____ I seldom get sick. 10

28.

_____ I usually take some medication to get through the day. 1

_____ I occasionally take medication to get through the day. 5

_____ I hardly ever take medication to get through the day. 10

29.

_____ I get a headache nearly every day. 1

_____ I often get headaches. 5

_____ I seldom get headaches. 10

30.

_____ My hands often feel cold. 1

_____ My hands occasionally feel cold. 5

_____ My hands hardly ever feel cold. 10

31.

_____ I increasingly notice my heart pounding. 1

_____ I sometimes notice my heart pounding. 5

_____ I hardly ever notice my heart pounding. 10

32.

_____ I concentrate well on what I have to do. 10

_____ I can keep my mind on one thing fairly well. 5

_____ I find it hard to concentrate on one thing. 1

33.

_____ I am normally calm and relaxed. 10

_____ I am nervous and tense once in a while. 5

_____ I am nervous and tense every day. 1

34.

_____ I don't drink any more than one or two cups of coffee a day. 10

_____ I like three or four cups of coffee each day. 5

_____ Each day, I need more than five cups of coffee. 1

35.

_____ I don't consume any alcoholic beverages. 10

_____ I consume a couple of drinks at work. 5

_____ I can't function without consuming at least two drinks a day. 1

36.

_____ I limit sweets, salts, cholesterol, saturated fats, and low-fiber foods. 10

_____ I try to limit these foods when possible. 5

_____ I am increasingly careless about what I eat. 1

37.

_____ I don't smoke. 10

_____ I smoke sometimes. 5

_____ I smoke every day. 1

38.

_____ I take a few brief time-outs each day. 10

_____ I take time out to relax once in a while. 5

_____ I hardly ever take time to relax. 1

39.

_____ I am presently close to my ideal weight. 10

_____ I am presently 5–8 lbs. over my ideal weight. 5

_____ I am at least 15 lbs. over my ideal weight. 1

40.

_____ I am careful to get some kind of exercise three or more times a week. 10

_____ I do some kind of exercise if I feel like it. 5

_____ I don't do any kind of special exercise. 1

41.

_____ I am a high achiever. 10

_____ I am an average achiever. 5

_____ I am achieving less and less. 1

42.

_____ I have a good, nourishing relationship with God. 10

_____ I have an acceptable but not exciting relationship with God. 5

_____ I increasingly find it hard to believe that there's a God who cares for me. 1

43.

_____ I have a good friend to lean on. 10

_____ I can find a good friend to lean on. 5

_____ I can't think of a good friend to lean on. 1

44.

___ I am not a procrastinator. 10

___ I am occasionally a procrastinator. 5

___ I am increasingly becoming a procrastinator. 1

___ I'll tell you tomorrow. 0

45.

___ I am good at putting things in their places. 10

___ I try to put things in their places. 5

___ I increasingly misplace things. 1

46.

___ I am good at anticipating and preparing for difficult circumstances that may arise. 10

___ I try to prepare for difficult circumstances. 5

___ I am increasingly surprised by difficult circumstances. 1

47.

___ I am increasingly irritable. 1

___ I am irritable sometimes. 5

___ I am hardly ever irritable at work. 10

48.

___ I am satisfied with my job. 10

___ Sometimes I think about finding another job. 5

___ I often think about finding another job. 1

49.

___ I find love and joy at my church. 10

___ I occasionally find love and joy at my church. 5

___ It is frustrating, even draining, to go to church these days. 1

50.

_____ I am satisfied with my home. 10

_____ Sometimes I get dissatisfied and want to move. 5

_____ I often think about moving to another home. 1

51.

_____ There is room for advancement at my job. 10

_____ There may be room for advancement at my work; I'm not sure. 5

_____ I am in a dead-end place of employment. 1

52.

_____ I frequently get angry at people around me. 1

_____ I occasionally get angry at people around me. 5

_____ I rarely get angry at people around me. 10

53.

_____ I have a good sense of humor. 10

_____ I try to have a good sense of humor. 5

_____ It's difficult for me to have a sense of humor. 1

54.

_____ When wronged, I forgive fairly easily. 10

_____ When wronged, I forgive, but reluctantly. 5

_____ When wronged, I find it nearly impossible to forgive. 1

55.

_____ I often regret things I have done in the past. 1

_____ Occasionally, regrettable things from the past come to mind when I don't want to think about them. 5

_____ I have let go of my negative past. 10

56.

____ I fear that God will not approve of me unless I do a lot of work for him. 1

____ I feel a strong compulsion to work tirelessly for the Lord and the church. 5

____ I feel loved and accepted by God, whatever I accomplish. 10

57.

____ I often get angry at other drivers on the road. 1

____ I occasionally get angry at other drivers. 5

____ I seldom get angry at other drivers. 10

58.

____ My last vacation was a time of much-needed rest. 10

____ My last vacation was somewhat restful but also a lot of work. 5

____ Vacation? What's a vacation? 1

59.

____ I am aware of most of the things that cause me stress. 10

____ I am aware of some of the things that cause me stress. 5

____ I have no clue about the things that cause me stress. 1

60.

____ I am taking definite steps to better my life. 10

____ I am thinking about taking definite steps to better my life. 5

____ I have too many problems and don't know where to start bettering my life. 1

WHAT YOUR SCORE MEANS

Now that you have completed the personal stress inventory, take a deep breath, smile, and add up all the values you wrote down.

Total score: _____

Now consult the scale below to find out what your score means.

Job Stress Scale

450–600. You are in excellent shape, stresswise. You can smile. This range indicates a low, healthy level of stress symptoms. Keep up the good work. You are flexible and generally satisfied with your home, family, and job.

350–449. You are doing fine. This range represents moderate levels of stress symptoms. You may attempt to reach a still lower level of stress manifestations in certain areas of your life. You are positive and mostly satisfied at home and work.

300–349. You are a little above the moderate stress range. You are a candidate for a few stress symptoms unless you take steps to improve. You may be frustrated and bored with your home or work situation, but you can make things better quickly.

250–299. You are experiencing certain stress symptoms that may become a threat to your body, mind, work, and relationships in the long run. You may be negative and show a lack of cooperation with others at work or home. You're not in the danger zone yet, but you should make serious attempts to manage your stress levels.

180–249. You are experiencing a great deal of stress. This score represents a high probability for stress-related illnesses. You are fatigued and experiencing dissatisfaction at home or work.

100–179. You are definitely experiencing slow burnout. You may be encountering chronic, high-level stress symptoms with increasing frequency. It is very likely that you will experience some stress-related disease in the future. You also seem to have difficulty interacting with others. Take immediate action.

60–99. You are burning out rapidly. You have low self-esteem. This range is a clear indication of dangerous and excessive levels of stress. At this level, people experience numerous stress symptoms, family problems, increased absenteeism from work, and possibly some illnesses. Seek immediate help.

3

What Is Stress Management?

Today's world pulsates with work and worries. There is always too much to do—and so much that can go wrong. Stress can be induced by a variety of things: pollutants in the air and water; carcinogens in our food; noisy, crowded living conditions; rush-hour traffic; stress-filled working environments; the daily news of urban decay, tragic accidents, violence, and terrorism; not to mention the anxiety due to our own unmet needs.

The pressure builds with each new day. What can we do about it?

Stress is a fact of life. Stressful situations will occur. But too many people respond to stress by doing things that actually make it worse. They deny it, repress their worries, make themselves even busier, or indulge in addictive-compulsive behavior.

If this describes you, then you need to find successful coping strategies. By tracing the roots of your worries and by redirecting your destructive impulses into positive action, you can begin to rise above your daily pressures. But how is this done?

Humans are complex physical, chemical, psychological, and meta-physical units, not just scrap heaps of spare parts. Therefore we need to consider the brain, mind, body, and spirit together. Stress attacks all of these areas, so stress management must involve a multifaceted approach.

PRESSURE AND PAINKILLERS

Carl, age forty-seven, a tall, athletic man, was plagued by insomnia, headaches, pains, and fatigue—the symptoms had lasted for about two years. It was difficult for him to fall asleep at night, and even more difficult to get out of bed in the morning. Frequently he became irritable and lost control of his emotions. Such physical and psychological trouble affected his work as vice president of a major company. It also spoiled his social and family relationships.

Fatigue, insomnia, and incapacitating headaches, accompanied by momentary memory loss from time to time, made Carl's life miserable. He went to parties but couldn't enjoy them. He went on vacation with his family but missed the fun. After sitting down in the office of Samuel Verghese (one of this book's authors), Carl said, "It seems doctors can't agree on what causes my problems. I can't figure out what is wrong with me."

His reaction to this condition ranged from denial to anxiety to hopelessness. Like many of those who suffer from stress-related symptoms, Carl had gone from doctor to doctor, searching for an explanation for his problems. After many tests and drug treatments, Carl's physician had concluded that the problems were not physical but psychological. So Carl went to a psychiatrist for a period of time, with only short-term relief. The psychiatrist advised him to try relaxation, biofeedback, meditation, nutritional modification, or stress management.

That's when he came to Samuel. In Carl's first two visits, they talked about his family atmosphere, working environment, friends, recreational activities, nutritional issues, allergies, and other daily habits. They were looking for clues to the events that triggered or reinforced his symptoms and disorders.

- Carl woke up early each morning and drove an hour to his job.
- There was a great deal of pressure in this job.
- Carl was also experiencing midlife crisis.
- As far as he knew, there was no one else in his family who had similar problems, so this was a lonely struggle for him.

- The physical symptoms of Carl's stress caused him pain and concern, thus intensifying the stress that caused them.

Carl disclosed that he had tried many painkillers, such as Percodan, Inderal, and Demerol, on and off for two years, with little success. His psychiatrist also gave him antidepressants and muscle-relaxant drugs, such as paxil, to keep his aches and anxieties under control. But these medications made Carl's mind tired and dull, and upset his stomach. This roller-coaster ride of doctors and medications had just added to his stress, and yet no one had helped him fully cure the insomnia, chronic pain, and fatigue that were interfering with his everyday activities.

> **We need to consider the brain, mind, body, and spirit together. Stress attacks all of these areas, so stress management must involve a multifaceted approach.**

THE SYMPTOMS

Together, Samuel and Carl soon began to zero in on Carl's symptoms. His headaches were not migraines, which tend to appear suddenly, causing throbbing, rhythmic pain, usually on one side of the head. His severe headaches were normally the result of tension built up over the course of a day. Sometimes, however, he would wake up with them.

Carl's insomnia was also stress related, though it was exacerbated by a lack of calcium, magnesium, and other nutrients. He suffered from cardiac arrhythmia (irregular heartbeat) and high blood pressure (an average of 190 over 99). In addition, he was having sexual difficulties and digestive troubles.

At Carl's urging, Samuel arranged several tests. Carl was willing to pay any fee to discover explanations for his disorders. The tests included blood, urine, stool, saliva, sweat, yeast, hormones, nutrition, and psychochemicals. (In most cases, there is no need for such extensive tests. Carl's case was complex, and he was eager to be thoroughly tested.)

In the meantime Carl took acidophilus (dried yogurt) for his digestive troubles. Since Carl had taken heavy doses of antibiotics, antidepressants, and headache medications, the good bacteria in his stomach was very low. Therefore he required the additional acidophilus to colonize the intestinal tract for more efficient and complete digestion.

When his digestion improved, Carl took various nutrients to enhance the energy-producing mechanism in the tissues that helps the body to handle stress: vitamin C to increase resistance to infection; B complex for his nerves; chromium complex and Vanadium sulfate to regulate the highs and lows of blood sugar to reduce fatigue; coenzyme Q_{10} (coQ_{10}), Vitamin E, selenium, L-Taurine, and L-carnitine to strengthen his heart muscles, improve circulation, and help stabilize the cardiac arrythmias, and boost the immune system. Since he was not allergic to any food group, he was urged to eat a wider range of foods. Finally, he was given a natural sleeping pill containing catnip, valarian root, hops, passionflower, chamomile, skullcap, GABA and 1 mg. of melatonin. Due to Carl's low level of energy, Samuel had wondered about his thyroid function. When the test results arrived, he did have certain biochemical imbalance.

Carl did not have diabetes but had borderline hypoglycemia and hypothyroidism. The allergy test showed no major reactions to the food he ate or the air he breathed. His high-density lipoprotein (HDL) count was lower than normal, and his low-density lipoprotein (LDL) count was high. When blood contains too much LDL, it can accumulate inside the artery walls.

Samuel recommended that he install a good water purifier at home to provide filtered water. Carl started a low-sugar, low-fat, complex-carbohydrate nutritional plan combined with kelp to meet the physical and mental demands placed on him. He was encouraged to a take a few days off from work to relax and enjoy physical exercise. All of these were carried out under the supervision of a group of specialists.

CARL'S SELF-IMAGE AND SELF-ESTEEM

In one of their sessions together, Samuel and Carl decided to look at Carl's self-image. Self-image, of course, refers to the pictures of ourselves we have in our minds. Self-esteem varies slightly from self-image, referring to the assessment of our value, potential, abilities, limitations, emotional and physical resources, and worthiness. While self-image is a description of ourselves, self-esteem involves self-evaluation and assessment. These are closely related and overlap quite a bit, and they both are constantly changing, since they are regularly influenced by our changing life experiences. Depending upon its content (faulty, realistic, or in between these perspectives), our total self-concept can either help or hinder every facet of our lives.

What was the connection between Carl's stress-related problems and his self-image? Carl's self-image in certain areas did not match reality. For a period of time, he refused to accept the fact that he needed professional help. He felt that he was self-sufficient and qualified to diagnose himself. He rejected the feedback from his caring wife, family members, and friends. (In this, Carl represents many men who ignore the sincere concerns of their wives or friends.)

> **Self-image can be a lens through which a person views everything else.**

Carl's self-esteem was lopsided in a number of other areas as well. While he was overconfident in some matters, he lacked confidence where he was truly talented. He did not fully appreciate himself and his accomplishments.

Self-image can be a lens through which a person views everything else. Carl's inaccurate view of himself was causing him additional stress. At work, he would set impossible goals and then hate himself for failing to reach them. Carl would see nearly every issue at home or in the office as a referendum on his own value. That made every situation a personal crisis, adding to his stress.

THE COMPLETE APPROACH

Carl gives us a great example of the multifaceted nature of stress. In addition to his increasing physical problems, he had problems with self-image and relationships. It would be easy to blame his stress level on his demanding job or his midlife crisis, but there were many other factors as well. Some of these seem to be *results* of stress, and others are *causes,* but sometimes it's hard to distinguish. A sort of downward spiral can occur as stress symptoms cause greater stress, which causes worse symptoms, and so on.

As we try to untangle the situation, we have to approach it from all angles, easing the stress where we can and getting down to the root causes.

You have already learned the difference between *stress producers* and *stress responses*. Now here's another distinction: stress producers involve both *stress events* and *stress situations*, and these are affected by *stress catalysts*.

Stress Events

A stress event is a momentary crisis. Your child is injured, friends show up unannounced for dinner, you're in a traffic accident. It may be serious or silly, but your blood pressure goes up all the same. The moment calls for quick thinking and decisive action, and your body gears up for that. This is perfectly healthy.

The event happens and it's over with. It may last a minute or a day or even a week, but there is an end to it. Life gets back to normal.

The healthy cycle of response to a stress event involves the instinctive response, the recovery, and a return to equilibrium.

We have already discussed the *instinctive response,* the series of chemical messages in the brain that send hormones racing through the bloodstream, energizing the body. You have little control over this—it happens when you sense danger. But you have some control over (a) how often you sense danger, and (b) what you do with all that energy.

Some people are just plain timid. They imagine danger all around them. Consider two men walking down a dark street. One knows the area—it's his neighborhood. The other is a stranger. When a car backfires a block away, the stranger jumps, his heart doing the mambo. The other guy just laughs, "That must be Tony's old crate."

Same street. Same sound. But one imagines danger and the other doesn't.

Many a Christian will mask his or her true emotions out of a desire to be a "victorious believer" who does not succumb to the trials of life.

Some people view life as a dark street, and they jump at the slightest provocation. Your response to the danger may be instinctive, but you may be able to change the trigger on that instinctive response.

You can also control the actions that follow your instinctive response. What do you do with the adrenaline? Your body is primed for action; what actions will you take?

Some people respond to stress with anger, lashing out verbally or physically at those around them. But they cannot blame these actions on the stress. They are *choosing* to behave like this, even though their instinctive response is giving them the energy to do so. They should learn to rechannel that energy into something more productive.

The *recovery* is the next stage of response. After the energizing occurs, a person needs to cool down, get back to normal. Unfortunately, many find it hard to let go of their response to a stress event. They replay it in their minds, worrying about what might have happened if only . . .

If you've seen an action movie lately, you've seen some hero responding to a stress event. The adrenaline is pumping and the hero is doing what needs to be done. Chances are, the hero is cool about it, showing little emotion during or after the event. But that's not a good model for us. Especially in the recovery period, we need to let our emotions out. If we don't, it will only delay our return to normalcy.

But in our society it's bad form to cry or shout or shudder or take a day off. "Never let them see you sweat." We're supposed to grin and bear it, work through it, or "forget about it" (which we accomplish by stuffing ourselves with food, drugs, or alcohol). Many a Christian will mask his or her true emotions out of a desire to be a "victorious believer" who does not succumb to the trials of life.

All these denial tactics leave people in a vulnerable position. The bodily systems are not allowed to run their course and return to their balanced, pre-stress condition. And when you don't recover adequately from a stress event, you begin the next stress cycle off balance. That's when the real danger starts. That's when the unhealthy spiral begins.

Recovery from a stress event might include:

Emotional release. In the first moment of stress response, emotions may be pushed aside so you can deal with the matter at hand. But these emotions must eventually come out.

Physical rest. Especially if energy was expended during the crisis, you'll need to rest up. But even if all you did was slam on the brakes, your system has just run a marathon. Take it easy for a while.

Return to physical schedules of food, work, and rest. In the immediate crisis of a stress event, you might skip a meal or go without sleep. Afterward, your body is confused as to what it needs. It's something like a VCR blinking 12:00 after a power failure. Your system needs to be reset. As soon as you can, get back to your normal rhythms.

Talking about it with others. You need to process the event that just occurred. What happened? Why? Did you do the right thing? In the heat of the moment, you can tell yourself a lot of half-truths. Friends can help you see clearly.

Restoration of any damaged relationship. Often a stress event is an argument with a loved one, or even a violent confrontation. Or in the excitement of some other stress event, you might say hurtful words. As soon as you can, as much as you can, get these relationships back together. Don't let broken bonds hold you down.

Prayer and questioning of God. Many spiritual issues are raised in times of crisis. Don't run away from these. If you're wondering why God would allow something like this to happen, ask him. (Many biblical characters had similar questions.) Or perhaps you need to thank God for protecting you in the time of crisis.

Review of the issues involved. You can learn through crisis situations. You can get a better idea of who you are, how you act, what you're capable of. Sometimes a stress event can alert you to changes you need to make.

After the instinctive response and the recovery period, a person should return to a point of **equilibrium.** This should be a healthy way of life, involving proper diet and exercise, good relationships, emotional openness, and spiritual growth.

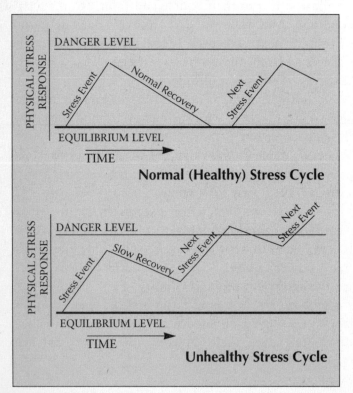

Normal (Healthy) Stress Cycle

Unhealthy Stress Cycle

The problem is that many people don't live at a healthy equilibrium. They don't care properly for their bodies, or they are burdened by emotional issues. So when stress events hit, they hit hard. The heart rate or blood pressure is already up, so the stress event pushes these to dangerous levels, and recovery is more difficult.

Stress Situations

The normal stress cycle gets complicated when there are repeated stress events with little time for recovery. Busy offices and factories can be like this, as well as schools and homes with many children. One crisis follows another, and your adrenaline is pumping all day.

We can call these *stress situations,* because they last longer than stress events. In fact, they may consist of strings of stress events. For people who live and work in stress situations, stress becomes a way of life. Their heart rate is high, their blood pressure up, their nerves on edge, their immunity down. Some people claim to find a sort of equilibrium in that—they're only happy when they're busy—but they can't keep it up for very long. Sooner or later they'll crash.

We will discuss more specific strategies later in the book, but for now let us suggest an easily remembered paradigm for management of stress situations: *accept, alter, avoid.*

Accept. Stress situations are often made worse because people are fighting their way through them. For instance, Julie hated her boss, Gwen. Julie resented the fact that Gwen was promoted and she wasn't. She found something wrong with every decision Gwen made. As a result, Julie's job was stressful. But what if Julie accepted Gwen as her boss and gave her the benefit of the doubt? The job would still be the same, the deadlines would still be there, but there wouldn't be this extra animosity. It wasn't easy for Julie to accept Gwen as her boss, but she tried it, and her job became a lot easier.

Melody and George didn't have a marriage; they had a world war. They fought over everything. He didn't dry dishes, preferring to let them air out, and she hated that. She didn't like to go out on weekends, preferring to stay home and watch TV, and he hated that. Their list of grievances was long and mostly petty. And the stress in their home could be cut with a knife. In counseling, they decided to try to accept each other's quirks. It wasn't easy, but ultimately they lessened the stress in their home.

Perhaps there are aspects of your job or your home life that you need to accept rather than fight.

Alter. Can you change certain aspects of your job or home life that cause you stress? Can you rearrange your schedule or take on fewer assignments?

You might find ways to lower the stakes of your responsibilities. Can you set false deadlines or extend your real deadlines? Can you revise your personal goals so you don't have to be vice president by next March? If you can make your performance less important in certain areas, you will reduce the stress level of your situation.

You could also try team building or delegation. Get others on board to share in your success or failure—at work or at home. This will help to ease the personal pressure.

You can also alter a stress situation by creating time for rest—and really resting. Proper rest should be as much of a priority as any deadline. You work better, in the long run, when you're rested. If you push yourself too hard, you will probably blow off steam by wasting time along the way. Set up rest time and don't waste it on other stressful pursuits. Really rest!

Avoid. Of course, you might just need to get out of that stressful situation. Let someone else be vice president. It's not worth it if it's going to kill you.

We would not advise avoidance in the case of a stressful marriage, but if there are other relationships that are too stressful for you, try withdrawing. If you have activities at church or in the neighborhood that are pressuring you, quit. Cut back. Ease your schedule. Avoid those stressful situations. And of course, it might be healthy to look for a job with less stress (though unemployment can be stressful, too).

Stress Catalysts

Some people make mountains out of molehills. They invent stress when it doesn't really exist, or they take a mildly stressful event and make it a major incident. There are several reasons for this.

Poor self-esteem. When people devalue themselves, they can begin to see each negative event as a personal put-down. This raises the stakes of these situations. These people are fighting for their own dignity. This can easily add stress to a mildly stressful situation.

Responsibility for others. Sometimes people feel overly responsible for other family members or close friends. They do not observe boundaries between their own fortunes and the fortunes of those around them. This can cause great anxiety, because other people, of course, don't always do what you want them to.

Antagonism. Some people just seem to have a sour attitude. They don't get along with others. In fact, they rub everyone the wrong way, whether or not they intend to. People like this can turn normal conversations into arguments, and mild disagreements into major fights.

Lack of faith. The Bible says, "Do not be anxious about anything" (Phil. 4:6), and yet many Christians worry constantly. They imagine the worst scenario possible and waste valuable energy fretting that it will turn out like that. They need to learn to trust God for these situations.

Ill health. If a person is already sick, he or she is less able to deal with the physical pressures of stressful situations. This makes those stressful situations even more critical than they would otherwise be.

Compulsive-addictive behavior. Many people try to "escape" from stress situations with compulsive-addictive behavior—getting drunk, getting high, smoking, gambling, shopping, and so forth. These actions may provide temporary diversion, but in the long run they worsen the stress.

MANAGING THE STRESS RESPONSES

Our instinctive response to a momentary stress event may be a rather simple thing, but the response to a stress situation can be complex. Good stress management requires attention to various aspects of the situation and our responses to it.

First, we need to clear away any stress catalysts, finding a sort of ground zero from which we can respond honestly to stress events. That is, we don't need to be worried about others, or making enemies, or taking personal offense at every little thing. Stress situations are bad enough without these factors adding to them.

Then we need to examine the stress situations to see if we can improve them by acceptance, alteration, or avoidance. At the very least, we need to establish "time-outs" along the way to allow for proper recovery.

But not only do we need *time* to recover, we need to learn *how* to recover—physically, mentally, emotionally, spiritually. And we need to establish good habits that will keep us at an equilibrium point, ready to face the next challenge.

YOUR TURN

1. Is there a particular stress event you have encountered recently? If so, what was it?

2. How would you describe your response to this stress event in
   - the instinctive stress response?

   - the recovery?

3. About how long did it take you to return to equilibrium (if you ever did return)?

4. Are you presently in a stress situation? If so, what?

5. What particular factors make this a stress situation?

6. Are there aspects of this situation that you need to accept? If so, what?

7. Are there aspects of this situation that you can alter? If so, what? What changes will you make?

8. Can you avoid the situation or aspects of it? How?

9. Are there stress catalysts involved in your life?

___ Poor self-esteem

___ Responsibility for others

___ Antagonism

___ Lack of faith

___ Ill health

___ Other:_____

10. How does this intensify your stress?

11. What can you do about these stress catalysts?

12. Of all the aspects of stress management that we mentioned, which is the one that you think you need most?

4

Irrational Fears

Anita worries. When her kids, who are now in their twenties, tell her what's going on in their lives, she worries about all the things that could go wrong for them. When they don't tell her anything, she worries about what they're not telling her.

In every situation she encounters, Anita imagines the worst possible outcome. In her church, she worries that there might be misunderstandings and division. At the office where she works, she fears that financial ruin is just around the corner. When her husband leaves on a business trip, she worries that the plane might crash and she will be left alone.

Her health worries her, too. She has high blood pressure, a weak heart, allergies, and was once diagnosed with cancer. Although it was detected and removed before much damage was done, the possibility always exists that cancer could return.

This woman is under stress, and she doesn't need to be. The external stresses she has to deal with are not very great, but she compounds them by her incessant worrying. So every minor problem becomes a major one. Every substantial problem becomes a disaster. She is stressed by a thousand imaginings that never take shape. In the battle with stress, she is her own worst enemy.

THE STRESS AGGRAVATORS

Let's consider that battle metaphor. Under normal circumstances, the battle with stress is usually just a skirmish. Stress-producing events occur, and our bodies are designed to meet these challenges. No problem.

But there are three major stress aggravators, which we'll deal with in this chapter and the next two. In our battlefield context, these are tendencies that either bolster the opposition or sabotage our own ability to fight it.

Compounded fears are the first of these stress aggravators. By worrying, we make Alps out of anthills. We imagine our stressors to be far worse than they really are. We're like the Midianites who were routed by Gideon's three hundred men—well, they were really routed by their own sudden terror at the sound and light that flooded their camp. Though they actually had the greater numbers, the Midianites feared that their foes far outnumbered them. Those unfounded fears helped a small force defeat a large army. Similarly, we can be routed by minor stresses when we imagine them to be major ones.

A second stress aggravator is the way we live *busy lives*. We take on too many commitments, and suddenly we're not making the decisions anymore—the decisions are making us (as we'll see in chapter 5).

> ## Stress Aggravators
>
> 1. Compounded fears—making mountains out of molehills
>
> 2. Busy lives that are spinning out of control
>
> 3. Unhealthy reactions to our stress that merely intensify our stress

The way we often resort to *unwise coping methods* is the third stress aggravator. We consume drugs or alcohol or resort to compulsive behavior, all of which sabotage our natural ability to deal with stress (more about this in chapter 6).

WHY PEOPLE FEAR

Anita is not alone. There are many whose lives are made needlessly difficult by worry. You might trace the symptom back to Jesus' day, when Martha was "worried and upset about many things." As a result, she was "distracted by all the preparations" that had to be made for Jesus and his disciples. You can sense the stress in her harried request, "Lord, don't you care that my sister has left me to do the work by myself? Tell her to help me!" (Luke 10:38–42).

Sometimes fear is a result of bad experiences in the past. Bob, for instance, will not swim underwater, because he was dunked as a child and held under until he nearly drowned. Though his adult fear is unnecessary, it is certainly understandable.

In our work with divorced people, we have found many fears about relationships, usually stemming from bad experiences—the pain of being deserted, the inevitable loss associated with divorce. People are usually shy about getting involved in significant relationships again, and rightly so! It takes time to deal with the issues of divorce, and that fear of relationships is a healthy way to give oneself the needed time for recovery.

Fear can be an honest appraisal of a dangerous situation. If a crazed terrorist is holding a gun to your head, you have a reason to be afraid. If a drunk driver swerves into the lane next to you, be afraid enough to move out of danger. No one would blame David for fearing Goliath. (He didn't—more on that in a moment—but no one would blame him if he did.)

Fear has a purpose: it gets us out of danger. The problem is, many of us get paralyzed by fear. Instead of running for safety, we stay put, our knees knocking, our jaws quivering. Just as our natural stress response is designed to help us meet temporary challenges, so our natural fear response is designed to help us run away. And just as we pile stress upon stress to the point of exhaustion, so we often pile fear upon fear to the point of paralysis.

While fear can be a reasonable response to situations in the past or present, all too often it's an unreasonable rejection of a good future. You can analyze it all you want, but at this level it boils down to a spiritual issue, a *lack of faith*. Are you trusting God to work all things together for your good, or are you worrying that some disaster will slip through his fingers?

It's hard to find a command more often repeated in Scripture than "Do not be afraid." The Bible makes it clear that spiritual wholeness involves trusting God for provision and protection.

THE FEARS OF THE FEARFUL

But still Anita worries. She's a fine Christian, well-versed in biblical teaching, but somehow this teaching has eluded her. There are thousands like her—people of faith who leave their faith in the umbrella stand when they go out to deal with everyday issues. As a result, they are stressed by phantom thoughts and minuscule possibilities.

Some fear that their daily needs will not be supplied. Ironically, this fear often surfaces among the affluent, who are insured up to their eyeballs and have more than enough socked away to provide for several lifetimes. Still, they worry that unemployment might strike, that the U.S. dollar might fail on the international markets, that they'll lose all in some IRS blunder.

Jesus was clear on this point: "Do not worry about your life, what you will eat or drink; or about your body, what you will wear. . . . But seek first [God's] kingdom and his righteousness, and all these things will be given to you as well" (Matt. 6:25, 33).

Others have a frequent fear of disastrous events. They watch a news report of a terrorist bombing, and it makes them afraid to go outside. They're afraid to fly or afraid to drive. Some fear that fire will devour their homes. Some will not set foot in California for fear of earthquakes.

Speaking to a people in a time of national turmoil, God said, "So do not fear, for I am with you; do not be dismayed, for I am your God. I will strengthen you and help you" (Isa. 41:10).

Some people add unnecessary stress to social interactions, because they fear rejection. Some feel extra pressure in taking on new projects, because they fear personal failure. Some keep a high stress level in relationships, because they are afraid of losing those they hold dear.

Probably ninety percent of what we worry about never happens.

"Do not be anxious about anything," Paul wrote, "but in everything, by prayer and petition, with thanksgiving, present your requests to God. And the peace of God, which transcends all understanding, will guard your hearts and your minds in Christ Jesus" (Phil. 4:6–7).

Many are afraid of injustice. They worry that others will take advantage of them. This, of course, results in a cynical attitude toward others, and a lack of trust all around. Increasingly we see Christians being afraid of persecution. Every court case that goes against a "Christian" cause is trumpeted as reason for alarm. Conspiracy theories are bandied about on Christian radio and in church lobbies. Most of this just adds unnecessary stress to our lives as we try to deal with the world.

As Peter wrote to persecuted believers, "But even if you should suffer for what is right, you are blessed. 'Do not fear what they fear; do not be frightened.' But in your hearts set apart Christ as Lord. Always be prepared to give an answer to everyone who asks you to give a reason for the hope that you have. But do this with gentleness and respect, keeping a clear conscience" (1 Peter 3:14–16).

In the middle of that passage, Peter quotes from Isaiah, where the frantic King Ahaz is advised not to react foolishly to conspiracy theories. (He did anyway.) For New Testament Christians, Peter advises that we adopt attitudes of "gentleness and respect," even in response to threats.

We have talked with some people who become afraid when things are going too well. Often suffering from poor self-esteem, they feel they don't deserve the good things that have happened to them. They worry that God is keeping some heavenly tally and will eventually even the score. In the same way, many Christians fear that God will punish them for various sins they struggle with. Overwhelmed by guilt, they have a hard time accepting God's free forgiveness. Though they claim to believe in God's grace, somehow they feel it doesn't apply to them.

The psalmist sings of the Lord's "benefits"—he "forgives all [your] sins and heals all [your] diseases" (Ps. 103:2, 3). Later he assures us that God "does not treat us as our sins deserve or repay us according to our iniquities" (Ps. 103:10). No heavenly scoreboard here. Our sins are removed "as far as the east is from the west." God understands when we slip up, because "he knows how we are formed, he remembers that we are dust" (Ps. 103:12, 14).

One of the most common, and strongest, fears we see is fear for one's children. This is a major part of Anita's daily litany of worries, and that of many other parents as well. It is very difficult *not* to worry about your children. Naturally, you love them and want what's best for them. But that love can easily turn into a desire to protect them from all pain. Since pain is a natural part of life and growth, this desire can turn into either an unhealthy control of your children's lives or a negative foreboding about the tribulations they inevitably face.

Parents must learn to let go of their children's lives. Though this is a very difficult process, it's absolutely necessary if the children are to develop into wise, mature adults. The process is gradual as teenagers take on more and more autonomy, reaching a certain amount of independence in adulthood.

Some parents try to maintain strict control of their children's lives well into adulthood, but many others maintain a pseudo control by worrying. They don't entirely trust their kids to make the best decisions. And they certainly don't trust the world to be kind to their kids. Therefore just as they tried to keep their five-year-olds from crossing the street without looking both ways, so they worry that their twenty-five-year-olds will enter into investments or marriages without looking both ways.

From a spiritual perspective, this again boils down to a lack of trust in God. It is one thing to love your kids. It is quite another to become obsessive about the many bad things that could befall them. We have scriptural examples of parents who loved their children but acknowledged that God was ultimately in control—from the extreme of Abraham nearly sacrificing his son, to Hannah giving up young Samuel, to David weeping over Absalom, to Eunice training Timothy in the faith and letting him join Paul's journeys.

> **Being overly worried about our kids boils down to a lack of faith in God.**

David marched out to face the giant Goliath. He wore no armor, just his faith in the power of God. The taunts of the Philistines did not daunt him. Was it a stressful situation? Certainly. Was his heart racing as he stooped to pick five smooth stones from the streambed? Probably. But God had rescued David in tight spots before, and he would empower the young shepherd against this titan. Whatever stress David felt at this momentous encounter, it was not compounded by fear. The stress was not pushed to the destructive point. David's adrenaline rush may have helped him take the right aim, whirl the sling with the proper force, and send the stone flying with its deadly aim. But fear was not binding him.

David's God is ours. We can count on his goodness and his power. We can meet the stresses of life, free from unfounded fears.

UNMASKING OUR PHANTOM FEARS

You remember how Dorothy was cowed by the Wizard of Oz—that is, until Toto pulled the curtain aside to reveal that the awesome wizard was really just a little man. Our fears can be like that—awesome images that mask little problems.

The way to deal with our unfounded fears is to unmask them, to remove the hype and get at the substance. What are we really afraid of?

As you evaluate the stress you are encountering, ask yourself, Is this stress being aggravated by my anxiety or fears about what might happen? Maybe not. There may be other stress aggravators at work in your situation. But look into this possibility.

Then ask, What specifically am I afraid of? Construct a complete worst-case scenario that you worry about. Since stress comes at us in many forms and many different situations, it might help to focus on a particular moment when you felt stress, or a particular activity in which you feel a high degree of anxiety. Don't let it be a vague feeling. Unmask your fears by getting to the specifics.

Ask, What are the chances that the scenario I fear will actually happen? Analyze the situation as best you can and come up with percentages of possibilities. Is there a ten-percent chance, a fifty-percent chance, or a one-percent chance? You don't have to do precise research, just make your best estimate. (Yet it might help to get someone else's estimate, too.)

Choose to live your life according to probabilities, not possibilities!

We often assume that negative things will probably happen, when actually the chances are slim. The chances of an airplane crashing, statistically, are tiny—smaller than your chance of being struck by lightning. Yet many people can only think about being in a hunk of metal thousands of feet in the air, and they remember news reports of the few planes that have crashed, and they worry that it will happen to them.

Then ask, Even if this scenario does take place, how bad will that be? What will I do? Construct a "stage-two" scenario. Maybe your worst-case scenario has you dying in some disaster. If you're a Christian, stage two puts you in heaven, enjoying fellowship with the Lord. That's not so bad. As people of faith, we know that even bad occurrences do not separate us from the love of God (Rom. 8:38–39).

Ask, Has God ever protected me from harm in the past? When? How? Be specific.

Ask, Has God helped me to endure difficult situations in the past? When? How? Again, be specific.

Now ask yourself, Can I count on God to protect me from the situation I fear? Or will he help me to endure this situation? Bad things sometimes happen to Christians, and even Christians have to endure hardship. But God gives us the strength we need to deal with these problems. The negative outcomes we fear, even if they do occur, need not be devastating for those who trust God.

Now it's time to take these questions back to real life. Ask, How will my trust in God affect my attitude—especially about the stress I face?

And ask, What will I do in my stress situations to show that I trust God? David walked out to face the giant, knowing that God walked with him. What steps of faith can you take?

YOUR TURN

1. Is my stress being aggravated by my anxiety or fears about what might happen?

2. What specifically am I afraid of?

3. What are the chances that the scenario I fear will actually happen?

4. Even if this scenario does take place, how bad will that be? What will I do?

5. Has God ever protected me from harm in the past? When? How?

6. Has God helped me to endure difficult situations in the past? When? How?

7. Can I count on God to protect me from the situation I fear? Or will he help me to endure this situation?

8. How will my trust in God affect my attitude—especially about the stress I face?

9. What will I do in my stress situations to show that I trust God?

5

Out of Control!

The most stressed-out beings on earth must be the lab rats, running mazes at the whim of the scientists who study them.

Think about it. They run all day and never get anywhere. And they have no control over their situation. They can't say, "Sorry, Doc, I've had enough of this. I'm moving in with my brother. He's got a tenement in the city." They can't go on strike, demanding more cheese and easier mazes. No, they have to take what's given them. The future is out of their paws.

Of course, the same is true of humans who have little control over their lives. Studying the experiences of hostages and prisoners of war, as well as incarcerated criminals, experts have found consistently high stress levels.

That might seem strange to some observers, who associate stress with nonstop activity. If people are sitting in prison cells, doing nothing, what do they have to be stressed about? Wouldn't that be somewhat relaxing?

Not at all. The lack of control over one's situation fuels anxiety, which sends stress sky high.

WHAT'S THE MATTER WITH KIDS TODAY?

Beverly has two children in their twenties. Her son has found the perfect woman, only he'll lose her if he doesn't propose soon. Her daughter, in the meantime, has strayed from the faith and resists Beverly's efforts to woo her back. Beverly feels considerable anxiety about her children, *because she has no control over them.* They must decide for themselves, and Beverly can only hope they make the right decisions. Meanwhile she has headaches; her doctor says they're stress related.

ON THE MOVE — BUT WHERE?

Jack has applied for a great job. Though he is well qualified and had a good interview, they are still interviewing other applicants. Meanwhile he has been told that his landlord is selling the house where he lives and he'll have to move. But where? If he gets that job, he'll be able to afford a nicer place, but if not—well, Jack doesn't know how to plan. He grows anxious as he waits, *but there's nothing he can do now.* Lately he's had trouble sleeping.

> **The lack of control over one's situation fuels anxiety, which sends stress sky high.**

CURRENT AFFAIRS

Mary Ellen knows her marriage is in trouble. She suspects that her husband, Ron, is having an affair. Though he adamantly denies it, he has been increasingly distant from her. She has tried everything—being loving, sexy, demanding, cryptic—but Ron isn't responding. *She doesn't know what else to do.* She fears her world is about to fall apart, but it's all up to Ron now.

EX-EMPLOYEE OF THE YEAR

Matt was laid off three months ago, shortly after being named "Employee of the Year." It was one of those economic decisions; the company was downsizing. Word was that the company might rehire some laid-off workers in the new fiscal year, so Matt hasn't tried too hard to find another job. Between his wife's secretarial salary and his unemployment checks, they can just scrape by. But the unemployment office has messed up on Matt's last two checks, which makes him mad—*but what can he do?* He feels he's at the mercy of his company, the government, the powers that be. He's been feeling stomach pain lately—an ulcer, maybe—but he's afraid to see a doctor. He fears that his health plan will find some way to withhold payment. That's just the way things are these days.

UNREWARDED EFFORT

All of these people are stressed by situations beyond their control. In fact, their lack of control is a significant factor intensifying their stress. It's all right to work hard at something, accomplish it, and tire yourself out in doing so. There is some stress in that, but you can handle it. Stress is magnified when you work hard *for no apparent reason.* When your company seems to put a ceiling above you—no more promotions—or when the government takes half your paycheck in taxes, or when your kids seem to resent the attention you give, there's no reward for your hard work.

If lack of rewards intensifies stress, the granting of rewards tends to reduce it. We're not talking primarily about financial rewards but about appreciation shown, compliments given. You have probably experienced this yourself. You're working hard at something, and you're getting stressed out—"Why am I doing this? No one cares. No one loves me. I'm just some drone doing the dirty work." But then someone comes by and says, "Hey, thanks for doing this. You're doing a great job." All of a sudden the work becomes easier, right? You're expending the same effort, but now you feel better about it.

Why? From a purely physical standpoint, the work is the same. A few appreciative words should have no effect on the physical stress of a particular job, you would think. But it goes back to the principle of wholeness. Our work is not just physical—there are emotional, mental, and spiritual components as well. We are not just drones, cogs in some machine. But when we do difficult, unrewarded work, we can often feel like spare parts. That knocks us off our equilibrium. It throws off our breathing, our posture, our muscle movement, our digestion.

But when someone shows appreciation, it reminds us of who we are—real people. It moves us back toward equilibrium. In the moment it takes to hear an encouraging word, our bodies "rest" a little. They begin to breathe, stand, move, and digest a little bit more healthily.

Some businesses have begun to realize that happy employees are good employees. It's part of that whole *Megatrends* and *Search for Excellence* thing. In *A Passion for Excellence,* Tom Peters and Nancy Austin talk about the value of "cheerleading" in business. It's vital to let employees know how important they are. "Cheerleading," they say, "is not merely legitimate; it's at the core of the most successful organizations."[1]

Cheerleading is just as important in homes and schools. With cheers in their ears, people work better, with less stress.

INVOLVEMENT

Ads for the Saturn car boast that every employee on the assembly line has a switch he or she can pull to stop the line if something doesn't look right. On one commercial, an employee proudly tells of the day he stopped the line.

Is that a good idea, giving that kind of control to every employee? Yes, it may slow production down a little, but it gives the employees a unique involvement in the process of making cars. Every employee is responsible for quality control. Every employee has power—in this case, the power to stop the assembly line when needed.

Stress is intensified by a lack of control and reduced when we gain control, or a share of control, in a situation. Some businesses (like Saturn) have recognized this, so there are now focus groups and employee polls and stock-option plans. Employees work better when they have a stake in the operation, when they have a say in how things are done.

Peters and Austin describe a scientific test ostensibly monitoring the effect of noise on production. Given mundane tasks, people were subjected to various distracting noises. Half of the subjects were given buttons that would suppress the noise; the others had no control over the noise. Those with the buttons performed considerably better than those without—despite the fact that *those buttons were never used.*[2]

So it was merely the *thought* of having control over this stressful situation that made half the group far more productive than the other half. Though the stress levels of these subjects were not tested, we would suggest that the group with control had less stress than the group without, and that allowed them to work more efficiently.

SURVIVAL TACTICS

So how will you succeed in business or at home or school when you feel totally out of control? Maybe your boss hasn't read any of those business books and runs your company like a nineteenth-century sweatshop. Or maybe the words of encouragement you get sound like lines from *1001 Sincere-Sounding Compliments to Tell Your Minions (and Thus Get Them to Work Harder)*.

Or maybe you're out of work. Or maybe your home is being wrecked by forces out of your control. Or maybe you have made commitments you can't get out of, and now you're stretched to the limit.

How do you regain control?

Reward Yourself

If you're not getting the rewards you need from others, give them to yourself. Periodically review what you have accomplished and congratulate yourself.

You may be able to work a "reward break" into your schedule. Take five minutes, or fifteen or twenty, to do something you really like doing, *as a reward for getting something done well*. Of course, you mustn't let these reward breaks get out of hand, but short breaks can pay off in better productivity. They're giving you rest that you need (and deserve).

If you're not getting the feedback you need from others, ask for it. Ask your boss how you're doing, or ask an opinion from a trusted coworker. At home, let the whole family talk together about their roles and needs.

Participate in Decision Making

Take any opportunity to join in the control of your situation. Do you have focus groups at work, or a suggestion box? Could you write a memo to the boss? The same ideas might apply to church or social commitments you have. And though the decision making may be a bit more complicated in your home situation, communication is still crucial.

Remember that your goal is *shared control*. You don't need to dictate how the company (or church or charity or home) is run. You're just offering suggestions, particularly regarding your own role. Be ready to have some ideas rejected—that's how it goes. But try to think like your boss. What are his or her priorities? What ideas would be accepted?

Take Control of Yourself

Sometimes you're not allowed to participate in the decision making. Or (even more frustrating) sometimes a company will give lip service to employee involvement but ignore all the employees' ideas. (The suggestion box empties into the trash can.)

In such situations, you are left to your own devices. You need to take control of *yourself*. You must not let your employer reduce you to the level of a machine part. Grab some self-respect.

Choose to stay or leave. If you are being taken advantage of, you may choose to leave your job and look elsewhere for work. If that creates other complications that you don't want to deal with, then you might choose to stay. But it's *your choice*. Weigh it carefully and then remind yourself from time to time that you have chosen to be where you are.

Choose to work hard or not. It is also your choice to push yourself an appropriate amount. Some employers demand far too much effort. You can choose to say no to that, working as hard as you can for eight hours but then leaving your work at the office. That may get you fired, and you need to weigh those options (work yourself to death or lose your job, hmmm), but it's still your choice.

Choose your attitude. You can work with a grudge, or you can choose to be cheerful. Veterans of prison camps have found that the one truly free choice they had was choosing to love their captors, choosing to keep their spirits up in spite of the hateful things going on. That was true victory. Now, your workplace may not be a prison camp, but you can make a similar choice. Assert your personal freedom by working with love and joy.

Choose your level of emotional involvement. This is a choice that has more to do with relationships than with the workplace. If you feel out of control in a relationship and are stressed by it, you need to take control of your emotional involvement. If a boyfriend or girlfriend, husband or wife, is toying with you emotionally, you need to set some boundaries. This may mean breaking off a nonmarital relationship. While we do not counsel people to seek divorce, if one spouse is acting irresponsibly and causing harmful stress, the other spouse needs to claim some level of emotional independence.[3]

Acknowledge God's Ultimate Control

We may do all these things and still feel that life is hurtling out of control. Events happen that change our lives drastically—a death, an accident, a fire, a theft—and there is no way we can control these things.

It helps to remember that God is in control. During a time of questioning, Israel needed to hear the Lord's assurance:

> Do you not know? Have you not heard? The LORD is the everlasting God, the Creator of the ends of the earth. . . . He gives strength to the weary and increases the power of the weak. Even youths grow tired and weary, and young men stumble and fall; but those who hope in the LORD will renew their strength. They will soar on wings like eagles; they will run and not grow weary, they will walk and not be faint.
>
> —Isaiah 40:28–31

There's a double truth here. First, our Lord is the powerful Creator. Second, he empowers *us*. We can make strong choices as we are strengthened and guided by God.

This does not mean that everything will always turn out as we hope. Like Job or Jeremiah, we may be disappointed with the things God allows to happen. But we still have a personal relationship with the King of the universe. As we grow in that relationship, we learn to trust his ways, even when we don't understand them.

YOUR TURN

1. Was there a time recently when you felt out of control? How did it feel? What aspects of your life were hurtling too fast?

2. Do you feel that you are rewarded enough for the work you do on the job or at home?

3. How does this make you feel?

4. Do you have a sense of ownership in your job or in other activities you're involved in? Do you have regular input into the decision making, or are you at the whims of others?

5. How does this make you feel?

6. What specific things could you do in the next week to

   • reward yourself?

   •participate in decision making?

   •take control of yourself?

   •acknowledge God's ultimate control?

6

Trying to Cope

The story is told of a man who took his young son out in a rowboat. In the middle of the lake, water began to seep through a crack in the bottom of the boat. "Look, Dad, a leak!" said the boy.

"We'll take care of that later," the father replied.

A few minutes later there was a thin layer of water at their feet. "Dad," the boy suggested, "maybe we could put something there to plug the leak."

"We can fix it later," the father answered. "I'll just row toward shore."

Soon the water was at their ankles. The boy was growing anxious. "Please, Dad, shouldn't we do something about the leak?"

The father was now rowing furiously toward shore, but the boat was moving slowly. "Later, Son," he snapped. "We can make it to shore. I know it."

The father kept rowing as the water rose. They were still thirty yards from land when the boat submerged. Both father and son swam safely to shore and lay there gasping for breath. "Wha—What happened?" the father groaned.

The son looked over at his stubborn father. "I guess it was later than you thought."

When stress seeps into our lives, like water into a rowboat, we often act like the father in that story. "Later. We'll deal with it later. Right now we have a job to do, a deadline to meet, a goal to achieve." But the stress accumulates, making it all the harder to get anywhere. If we allow the stress to build, refusing to deal with its causes, we will eventually sink. It will be later than we think.

But many of us have developed ways of coping with stress—or so we think. These methods help us get through the day, though we may have to pay for them tomorrow. These coping strategies allow us to keep rowing instead of plugging the leak in our boat. While they may seem effective at the time, in the long run they worsen our stress—or lead us into something more dangerous.

REPRESSIVE STRATEGIES

One of the most common ways of coping with stress is to pretend it's not there. We call these *repressive* strategies, because they hold back the awareness of stress from others or from oneself.

Denial

Believe it or not, denial is a healthy response to a stressful situation, part of that natural reaction to crisis. The adrenaline pumps, the heart races, and we conveniently "forget" how frightening the situation is. But denial becomes a problem when it lasts too long. God has given us a natural pattern in which we gradually become aware of our need to heal, so then we can seek the healing we need. But if we never reach that awareness, we never take the time to heal.

When Tom Whiteman (one of this book's authors) was a child, his family's house caught fire in the middle of winter. His father heroically carried the children from their beds to a neighbor's house, then went back and began furiously shoveling snow from the front porch into the living room to fight the fire.

In time, firefighters arrived to put out the flames. The house was damaged but not destroyed. Tom's father looked down and saw that his arms were black. The emergency squad offered to take him to the hospital, but he protested, "No, I'm fine, I'm fine." Fortunately, they insisted.

Halfway to the hospital, he began to feel the pain. His arms were, in fact, rather seriously burned.

His denial had helped to save the family's house. In the heat of the situation, he refused to think about the pain but worked to put out the fire. Although this was dangerous, it still might be considered "good" denial. He was able to put aside the pain *for a brief time,* to do what he had to do.

But minutes later denial nearly prevented him from being treated for his burns. This would be "bad" denial. Once the crisis is past, there is no need for denial. We need to come back to reality and get the help we need. (Fortunately, the emergency squad saw through his denial.)

People deny stress and its effects all the time. You have probably met people who are "rowing" through life as fast as they can, and you can see them falling apart. Their health is fading. They find it hard to concentrate. Yet they can't slow down—"No, I'm fine, I'm fine."

You may be one of those people.

Sometimes people deny the *magnitude* of a stress situation. Stress producers can pile up in our lives and we hardly notice. We take on new projects, agree to do certain things, and get extra assignments at work. Before we know it, we're working nonstop.

That can happen easily enough, and you can deal with it if you recognize the overload, rearrange your schedule as best you can, work hard in the short term, and plan a vacation for a month or two down the road.

But too often we deny the overload. We don't realize how many things are on the schedule. Or we don't recognize the stressful effects of a particular crisis.

One of the most common ways of coping with stress is to pretend it's not there.

We have seen people get divorced in the midst of their already stressful lives yet try to act as if nothing were different. Divorce is a huge stressor. Its impact on one's life is major. The same could be said for a death in the family or a job change. These are not punches you can roll with; you need to go down for the count and rest awhile before you come back swinging.

Sometimes people refuse to acknowledge certain *causes* of stress. A client came to Tom Whiteman's office seeking help for symptoms of stress. As they talked, Tom tried to zero in on the roots of her problem. Though she claimed to have a good marriage, the stories she told indicated otherwise. It was a highly manipulative, highly abusive relationship, but she had no clue that anything was wrong with that. No wonder she had stress symptoms! Yet the marriage seemed normal to her.

We see this often. There are many bad marriages causing great stress, and yet both parties are afraid to address the issues. Occasionally there is childhood abuse that has been denied or repressed all one's life. Or there may be hidden fears or phobias that a person refuses to deal with.

Sometimes people don't see their own symptoms and overestimate their own ability to handle stress. Men in high-stress situations often see stress as a personal opponent. If they acknowledge that they are stressed and need a rest, they are admitting defeat. They win by plowing through the situation and staying alive (and effective). But stress usually wins out in the end, wreaking havoc in their lives physically, mentally, emotionally, and spiritually. (Sometimes women feel this way, too, especially in high-powered work environments. But this attitude is far more prevalent among men.)

Such people become adept at explaining away the symptoms of stress when they appear. "An ulcer? No, it's just something I ate." "Shortness of breath? No, it's just a cold coming on."

And they continue to overload their schedules with high-stress activities, confident that they can handle it—"No problem."

But of course, denial is a problem. It blinds us to our true situation until it's too late.

Keeping Up Appearances

A second repressive coping strategy is closely related to denial. Where denial is refusing to admit the problem to *oneself,* "keeping up appearances" is a matter of hiding the problem from *others*. The person who uses this strategy becomes an expert at playacting, pretending that everything is fine.

We knew a businessman who played this game. His company was collapsing, and so was his marriage. Still, he kept up the pretense that everything was fine. He maintained all the trappings of the "good life"—limos, luxury, lavish spending—but he knew very well that it was all a sham.

This man's pretense took its toll on him physically. One day he woke up and could not move. Literally, he could not get out of bed. After several hours, he managed to struggle to a phone and call his doctor. After a slew of doctors failed to find out what the problem was, he came for counseling. His problem was clearly stress. Though he could hide it from everyone else, he could not fool his own body. Stress caught up with him.

After a few months in counseling, this man began to relax. He significantly downscaled his life and began to live more honestly.

Playacting, of course, adds extra pressure to every situation. The pretender is always looking over a shoulder to see what others are thinking. Though people like this may be well aware that they are fighting a losing battle with stress, the game must continue to be played. So stuff the problem, suck it in, gut it out.

This approach is actually a bit healthier than denial. At least the pretender is personally aware of the problem. This person is more likely to seek help from a counselor or from a book like this (though he might hide the book in order to keep up the appearance of an already well-managed life).

Isolation

Sometimes people in times of stress shut others out of their lives. This is most common among men, who tend to solve problems by themselves. If there is a lot of stress stemming from the person's relationships, this might be somewhat healthy in the short term. But it also closes a person off from the healing possibilities of human relationships.

If work is the main stressor, it may seem wise to lock yourself in the office until you get it done. But the work never gets done, you know that. There's always a new assignment when the current one is finished. And the isolated person has no one to offer feedback, to say when he or she is looking tired or acting irrationally.

COMPULSIVE COPING

People do the oddest things to relieve stress. One man we know plays computer games when he feels overwhelmed by work (actually, we know several who do this). Think about this. This man feels highly stressed, so he plays a game that *simulates warfare*. That can't be very calming, and when he finishes, his pile of work is still there.

There is something about stress that pushes us to crazy measures. Sometimes we try to numb ourselves—"drinking away our troubles," for instance. But in other cases—as with the computer game—it's as if we were seeking preoccupation, sending our energies in a different direction to take our minds off our stress. In some cases, we actually seek other, artificial stress producers to distract us from our real stress producers.

Numbing Substances

This is not so odd. It's dangerous but understandable. If your body is on red alert, you may seek some substance to calm it down. That may be a narcotic of some kind or alcohol or even the nicotine in a cigarette.

Many people eat when they're under stress, so food itself may have a numbing effect, although we also think there is a behavioral comfort involved in the act of feeding oneself.

In proper measure, numbing substances may be healthy. Doctors routinely prescribe medication that calms down their hyper patients. Some would argue that an occasional alcoholic drink serves to calm them down.

But when do these substances become dangerous? We would say that there's a problem of *dependence* and a problem of *distraction*.

The first question is, How long will you need this substance? As a temporary fix-it for a stress situation that gets out of hand, a numbing substance (in moderation and, in the case of drugs, properly prescribed) may be healthy. But if it remains a need, day in and day out for years, there's a problem. We have no worries about the woman who has a glass of wine every other Friday after a hard week of work. But we do worry about the man who needs to belt down two stiff drinks every night after work.

Some people seem to be addicted to stress.

The underlying problem has to do with the strategy of numbing. The whole purpose of taking one of these numbing substances is to "get rid of the pain," to distract ourselves from the things that are causing us stress. But sometimes distraction is the last thing we need. Sometimes there's a problem we need to solve. Sometimes there's a relationship out of whack, and we need to fix it. Sometimes our schedules need adjustment. If we regularly numb ourselves to these issues, they will never be dealt with.

Stress Substitutes

Stressed people often turn to compulsive behaviors to distract them from their stress. Ironically, these behaviors are often just as stressful as the rest of their lives.

While some deal with stress at the joystick of a computer game, others gamble, putting huge sums of money on the line and watching the roll of the dice. What could be more stressful? Yet there's probably some sort of inertia at work here. Once stressed, it's hard to get unstressed, so you gravitate to an alternate form of stress—far removed from the stressful details of your life but exciting enough to keep your interest.

In fact, some people seem to be addicted to stress. These are usually the workaholics, who stay with their stress producers day and night. Or they are constantly exercising, fanatical about jogging or working out. They don't know any other way to be. Just sitting and relaxing makes them more uncomfortable than sweating over some new project.

Other people indulge in pampering behaviors. Stress takes a toll on them, so they try to pay themselves back by eating, shopping, or pursuing sexual gratification. In the right contexts, each of these is a fine thing to do, but stress can push people into a sort of primal compulsion in these matters. People *cannot stop* eating; stress makes them do it. Or they *have to* go shopping, even if they have no money; it's the only way they know to "relax." Or people become sexually promiscuous or get caught up in pornography, because they feel these indulgences repay them for what their stressful situations take away. There is a passive-aggressive quality to these behaviors. People are trying to get back at all their stress producers, but they're really just punishing themselves.

And that's the problem with compulsive behaviors as coping mechanisms for stress. First, they do nothing to improve the original stress situations. Second, they often make things worse. You can go home from a hard day of work on Monday and consume a half gallon of Ben and Jerry's latest ice-cream sensation. But you still have to go to work on Tuesday, only you'll be five pounds heavier.

UNCONSCIOUS EXPRESSIONS

Tics and Habits

We're all familiar with nail-biters and foot-tappers. When they feel stressed, everyone knows it. It's as if the energy were just spilling out of them. They carry on their nervous tics and habits without thinking about them.

Most of these quirks are rather harmless, except in the extreme. Yet we've known people who would grind their teeth as they slept, resulting in substantial dental problems. This too was an unconscious response to stress.

The problem with unconscious habits is that they are largely uncontrollable. It's hard to tell a person to stop grinding her teeth at night when she doesn't know she's doing it. In some cases, behavior management techniques (like mittens for nail-biters) can break these habits, but often you just need to ease the stress.

Dreams

These can also signal high-stress situations. The unconscious mind breaks through to create frightful or tense scenarios. This is another way our minds cope with our daily stress, blowing off steam wherever they can.

Quick Temper

This is another way people unconsciously blow off steam. Even mild-mannered folks can be pushed to the edge by stress, responding with sudden anger. You may remember the old commercial where a young woman snaps, "Please, Mother, I'd rather do it myself!" This was an "Excedrin headache," clearly brought on by the stress this woman was facing.

"Blowing off steam" is an appropriate image in this case. Stress builds up within us, like steam in a boiling pot of water. If we do not turn down the heat (by easing our stress situations) or release steam in some productive way (exercising, working, solving the problem), our unconscious minds will find a way to vent all this pent-up tension—perhaps in a dream or a tic or an angry outburst.

Self-Destructive Behaviors

In some cases, the unconscious mind turns the tension inward, prompting some form of self-destructive behavior. This may be at the heart of heavy use of alcohol or drugs, or compulsive behavior such as gambling or overeating.

The behavior resulting from all these unconscious coping strategies may be complex. The symptoms may be difficult to correct. But the root of them is simple—stress.

The coping methods we use in dealing with stress are often ineffective, and more often they make things worse. Coping is not enough. We need to strike at the heart of the problem and ease our stress—both by reducing the magnitude of our stress producers and by learning healthier ways of responding to stress.

YOUR TURN

1. Which of the following coping methods have you used in dealing with stress?

   Repressive Strategies

   ___ Denial

   ___ Keeping up appearances

   ___ Isolation

   ___ Compulsive Coping

   Numbing Substances

   ___ Nicotine

   ___ Alcohol

   ___ Drugs

   ___ Food

   ___ Other: _____

   Stress Substitutes

   ___ Gambling

   ___ Spending

   ___ Workaholism

   ___ Sexual promiscuity

   ___ Pornography

   ___ Binge eating

   ___ Computer games

   ___ Other: _____

Unconscious Expressions

___ Tics and habits

___ Dreams

___ Quick temper

___ Self-destructive behaviors

2. Choose one of the coping methods you checked above (the one you use the most) and write it down here:_____

3. How have you used this method? Describe your behavior.

4. Why do you choose to do this? Do you know?

5. Are there particular times in the day or week when you do this sort of thing? When?

6. What effect does this behavior have on you? Does it make you less stressed? More stressed? Less stressed for a while and more stressed later?

7. If you think this behavior is unhealthy for you, what do you think you could do to stop it or at least control it? List three possible action steps.

    1.

    2.

    3.

8. Try to put at least one of these steps into action this week. When and how will you start?

7

Our Stress Environments

In the simplest terms, stress is an interaction. An outside agent—a deadline, a family fight, a sudden illness—exerts pressure, and we react to it. Stress production, stress reaction.

As we saw in the previous chapter, there are times when we hurt ourselves, on our side of the battle lines. We amplify a problem out of proportion, or we try some harmful coping method. But there are also times when those external pressures are too strong for us. One deadline follows another, or the fights occur every day.

Most of stress management has to do with *us*. Even when we can't control those outside stressors, we can control our own reactions. Most of this book will deal with personal habits, teaching you how to equip yourself for stress situations and how to react in a healthy manner to stress events.

But a stress management program would not be complete without some attention to your environment. Are you in a job or home or community where the stress is overwhelming? If so, what can you do about it?

THE A LIST

There's an ancient prayer that has been edited through the years and has found a home in the modern recovery movement.

> God grant me the serenity to accept the things I cannot change,
>   the courage to change the things I can,
>   and the wisdom to know the difference.

This can get us started on a helpful course of action. As we deal with a stressful environment, what can we do?

We can *accept* things.

We can try to change things (that is, *alter* or *avoid*).

And we need to *analyze* the situation to determine the wisest choice.

This is your "A List" of how to act in stressful environments. Let's flip it around and start with analysis. Is your environment truly stressful, or are you making the situation worse than it is? What aspects of your environment need to be changed or accepted? How can you accomplish this? When is it best to avoid rather than alter a situation? Some crisp analytical thinking will help focus your approach to your environment.

"Changing the things you can" may take different forms, which is why we're suggesting that you consider both alteration and avoidance. Sometimes you can change the things in your job or home that cause you stress. (It's more likely that you'll change only a few things, which will ease your overall stress level.)

Honest communication is crucial. Start by being honest with yourself.

Honest communication is crucial. Start by being honest with yourself. Have you taken on too many projects? Are you holding yourself to standards that are too high? It may be very difficult to admit to yourself that you can't do it all. It may be even harder to admit this to your boss or spouse—but you must. Explain your stress level in specific, even medical, terms. Even the worst Scrooge of a boss won't like the idea of losing an employee to a breakdown or heart attack. Search together for suitable solutions. Coworkers and family members can also help ease your burdens if you let them know about your plight.

But there are also stress producers at work or at home that you can avoid rather than try to change. Of course, if your job is full of stress that cannot be alleviated, you can quit. We don't recommend "quitting" your marriage, but you can learn to avoid the petty arguments that don't accomplish anything but raising your blood pressure.

Often there are people that get on your nerves. That guy in the next office. Your busybody aunt. The weird family across the street. Chances are, you won't change these people. But maybe, to keep your stress down, you can avoid them.

In the case of major issues, avoidance is a temporary measure at best. If these are not confronted at some point—and either altered or accepted—they will fester, and resentment will grow. But for minor issues that are somehow major stress producers, avoidance may be your best option. You can also use avoidance *temporarily* to choose your best time to deal with a serious conflict.

Acceptance is a decision, an intentional adjustment of the attitude. It does not mean that you like what's going on; it only means that you've decided not to fight it—externally or internally. Perhaps you have tried to change the situation and failed. Perhaps you have tried to avoid it but can't. But at this point, you decide that you will live with it, and you will not let it bother you.

Many people have never learned the art of acceptance. As a result, there are gripes and grudges gnawing at them constantly. The pseudo accepter may lose an argument but keep replaying the argument in her mind. Her boss may veto her proposal in favor of another course of action, and she secretly plots to sabotage her boss's plans. Such a person is a poor loser, perennially dissatisfied with things as they are.

True acceptance requires humility—somebody else may actually have a better idea. It also requires self-discipline. You have to steer your mind away from those rehashed arguments. The true accepter chooses to be free of the stress of dissatisfaction. This is never easy. You will have to rely on God's strength to get you to this point.

STRAIGHT A'S

The next couple of chapters will focus on the alter-avoid-accept strategy in the two most frequently stress-filled environments—job and family. But first we need to analyze. The following test should help you isolate your most serious environmental stress problems.

YOUR TURN

Read the following statements and indicate whether they apply to you, and to what degree. Note that the first seven questions deal with your "daily work." If you work at home or are self-employed, you may need to adapt these questions slightly, but try to understand the general sense of the question and answer it accordingly. Questions eight to fourteen deal with your home. If you live by yourself, you may need to expand the definition of "family" to include your family of origin or your closest friends.

Concise Index of Environmental Stress

Daily work

(If you work at home, are self-employed, or are unemployed, adapt the questions to your daily activity.)

1. In my daily work, I often face deadlines of major proportions.

1	2	3	4	5
Strongly Disagree	Disagree	Not Sure	Agree	Strongly Agree

2. My job is almost always on the line. If I don't perform well, I'm gone.

1	2	3	4	5
Strongly Disagree	Disagree	Not Sure	Agree	Strongly Agree

3. I find my coworkers difficult to work with.

1	2	3	4	5
Strongly Disagree	Disagree	Not Sure	Agree	Strongly Agree

4. I feel incapable of doing the work I'm paid to do.

1	2	3	4	5
Strongly Disagree	Disagree	Not Sure	Agree	Strongly Agree

5. I'm not sure what my boss wants from me.

1	2	3	4	5
Strongly Disagree	Disagree	Not Sure	Agree	Strongly Agree

6. When I get home from work, I'm so tired that I don't feel like doing anything.

1	2	3	4	5
Strongly Disagree	Disagree	Not Sure	Agree	Strongly Agree

7. It's difficult to drag myself to work.

1	2	3	4	5
Strongly Disagree	Disagree	Not Sure	Agree	Strongly Agree

Home

(If you live alone, let "family" include your family of origin or your closest friends.)

8. Members of my family are always attacking me verbally.

1	2	3	4	5
Strongly Disagree	Disagree	Not Sure	Agree	Strongly Agree

9. I would describe my home as spiteful and violent.

1	2	3	4	5
Strongly Disagree	Disagree	Not Sure	Agree	Strongly Agree

10. I would describe my home as cold and unfeeling.

1	2	3	4	5
Strongly Disagree	Disagree	Not Sure	Agree	Strongly Agree

11. It is difficult for my family to schedule all the things we need to do.

1	2	3	4	5
Strongly Disagree	Disagree	Not Sure	Agree	Strongly Agree

(For questions 12–14, if you're married, answer those marked "M." If you're single, answer those marked "S.")

12M. My marriage is in trouble.

1	2	3	4	5
Strongly Disagree	Disagree	Not Sure	Agree	Strongly Agree

12S. I tend to be involved in turbulent romances.

1	2	3	4	5
Strongly Disagree	Disagree	Not Sure	Agree	Strongly Agree

13M. My spouse knows just what to do to make me feel inadequate—and regularly does.

1	2	3	4	5
Strongly Disagree	Disagree	Not Sure	Agree	Strongly Agree

13S. I feel that I'm single because no one wants me.

1	2	3	4	5
Strongly Disagree	Disagree	Not Sure	Agree	Strongly Agree

14M. It is very tiring to keep my marriage going.

1	2	3	4	5
Strongly Disagree	Disagree	Not Sure	Agree	Strongly Agree

14S. I find single life very tiring.

1	2	3	4	5
Strongly Disagree	Disagree	Not Sure	Agree	Strongly Agree

General

15. Crime is a constant danger in my neighborhood.

1	2	3	4	5
Strongly Disagree	Disagree	Not Sure	Agree	Strongly Agree

16. I have few good friends in the area.

1	2	3	4	5
Strongly Disagree	Disagree	Not Sure	Agree	Strongly Agree

17. I am afraid to go out at night.

1	2	3	4	5
Strongly Disagree	Disagree	Not Sure	Agree	Strongly Agree

18. The things I own are constantly breaking down.

1	2	3	4	5
Strongly Disagree	Disagree	Not Sure	Agree	Strongly Agree

19. I regularly worry about paying my bills.

1	2	3	4	5
Strongly Disagree	Disagree	Not Sure	Agree	Strongly Agree

20. I regularly worry about my health.

1	2	3	4	5
Strongly Disagree	Disagree	Not Sure	Agree	Strongly Agree

21. I regularly worry about the well-being of people I love.

1	2	3	4	5
Strongly Disagree	Disagree	Not Sure	Agree	Strongly Agree

Now total the numbers you circled.

Questions 1–7: _____ (A)

Questions 8–14: _____ (B)

Questions 15–21: _____ (C)

Total of A, B, and C: _____

If your total score is 75 or more, you have a very stressful life at work and at home. You may need to find a new job, move to a new neighborhood, or put some serious effort into rebuilding your marriage or home life. You must look for ways to improve your environment.

If your total score is 50–74, you have some stress in your environment (work or home or both), but it is not overwhelming. It would make some sense to take moderate steps to lessen the stress of job or home, but you should be able to maintain a general equilibrium with the right stress management habits.

If your total score is less than 50, your work and home environments are not very stressful. There may be occasional danger zones, but you should be able to deal with these as you learn good techniques of regular stress management.

Look also at the balance of your A, B, and C totals. Your A total reflects your work situation; B is the home situation; and C is a collection of miscellaneous community and attitude items. If A is quite high (21 is average, 35 maximum), you may need to consider a job change or other major changes at work. If B is high, you need to concentrate on improving the spirit in your home.

The next two chapters will give you specific suggestions for altering, avoiding, or accepting stressful situations at work and at home.

8

On the Job

Joyce got a promotion last year, but it's like one of those good-news-bad-news jokes. Though she's getting a lot more money, she has no life. As an executive in a computer services company, she has an enviable position—or so you might think. But fourteen-hour days are common, and business trips take her away from her family every other week. She has had to drop out of several community and church involvements, just because she's never sure if she'll be at home or in Helsinki.

The job itself is OK, there's just too much of it. Joyce finds herself longing for the days when she was a few rungs down on the ladder, working hard but also enjoying weekends with her husband and kids. In her present position, she is nearly at a breaking point.

Whether you work in a factory or pharmacy, a school or salesroom, a business or boutique, your job is probably a major source of your stress.

Whether you work in a factory or pharmacy, a school or salesroom, a business or boutique, your job is probably a major source of your stress. You may hate your job and everything about it. Or you may love your job—except for this or that one little thing. Whatever your stress point is, you probably realize that work is a necessity of life. You just need to grin and bear it. Or scowl and bear it. Or just bear it.

ANALYSIS

If you're losing air in a bicycle tire, what do you do? You listen for the hiss, or you put it underwater and watch for bubbles. You need to find where the puncture is so you can patch it. Similarly, in a stressful job, you need to find out where the stress is. Is there a particular time of day when you have the most difficulty? Is there a coworker who bothers you? Is there a part of the job you can't stand?

- Phyllis works in an office shared by several doctors. While she generally enjoys her job and her coworkers, there is one doctor who regularly belittles her and the rest of the staff. Fortunately, he comes in only on Wednesdays. As you might expect, Wednesday is a high-stress day for Phyllis. Like one of Pavlov's dogs, she sees Wednesday on the calendar and begins tensing up. Sometimes the headaches begin Tuesday night.

- Linda is an editor for a professional newsletter. It's a fine job, except one of her duties is sizing photos—figuring out the percentages so the printer can fit the pictures in the right places. Somehow she never got the knack of sizing photos; she's insecure about it. With every issue, the time comes when she has to do this task. She'll put it off as long as she can, but then finally—greatly stressed—she has to do it.

- Gary, a writer, hates calling people on the phone. He always fears that he's intruding on the other person's life—especially if that person is busy or important. Though he loves writing articles based on library research, he dreads doing phone interviews—a task he postpones until the last possible moment, feeling terribly stressed about it.

- Wendy, a secretary in a small business, maintains the financial records of her company. She has never been trained in this; there's just no one else to do it. She dreads this task. "It's beyond my abilities," Wendy says.

It's easy for these people to forget—especially in the middle of their high-stress times—that they really like their jobs. It's just a certain part of the job that causes them stress, and that stress can sort of seep through the rest of their working days—and the rest of their lives.

STRESS CREEP

Tony is a young man, just out of high school, who's paying the bills with a part-time job at a local burger joint. After about a day and a half on the job, he realized that he hates it. One of his coworkers seems to be doing everything possible to put Tony down. The boss never explains anything well enough. And the whole job is gritty and grimy and greasy.

Since he works nights, Tony's stress begins around noon. Instead of enjoying his days, he anticipates the awful experiences of his night job. Though it's only a part-time job, it's dragging down his whole life. At first he thought it would get better, but he's been there three months now, and he still hates the place. He's looking around for another job, one that doesn't involve grease.

Tony—like Phyllis, Linda, Gary, and Wendy—is experiencing something we might call "stress creep." No, that's not a reference to his nasty coworker. It's the way a whole job can take on a sense of stress due to one of the job's components. From there it can begin to affect one's entire life.

While Tony's stress has crept through his idle afternoons, Phyllis's stress begins with her Tuesday night headaches. Every time Linda starts a new newsletter, or Gary maps out an article that requires a phone call, or Wendy picks up the ledger, they feel a general stress that has ballooned from their dread of one small activity.

The way to control stress creep is to keep monitoring your stress, tracing it back to its source, and dealing (as much as possible) with that source. Try to contain the stress in that particular time or with that particular person. Remind yourself that you really love your job—except for this or that. Try not to anticipate the stress ahead. That is, don't weigh down your present with fear of the future.

STRESS CONTAGION

We might look at stress as a kind of bacterial infection. It can grow, it's contagious, and though our bodies have natural defenses, it can overwhelm these defenses.

Just as the workplace can be a site for the transmission of the common cold or the flu, it often serves as a site for the transmission of stress. You may go to work relatively stress free, but then a coworker comes in furious from an argument at home. Your boss feels pressure from his or her boss and demands that you move your deadlines up a day or two. The photocopier breaks down, and everyone in the office is on edge.

If this is a regular occurrence in your workplace, you need to figure out who the carriers of stress are and how to deal with them. You would probably avoid a coworker who was sneezing all over the place, especially if you knew your resistance was low. It's the same with stress. You may have to avoid those that are spreading their stress to you. And if afflicted by a disease, you would slow down, take a break, allow yourself time to recover. You should do the same with stress.

GOING TO THE SOURCE

Where does your stress come from? That's a key question as you analyze your job-related stress. Like scientists for the Centers for Disease Control, you need to trace the infection back to its source. However, stress is not like a killer virus, which you would "contract" at a certain point. It's a substance that is harmless in small quantities. Problems occur when you *add* stress beyond your normal limits. So you'll be looking for several different sources of stress and looking for ways to reduce (but not necessarily eliminate) any or all of them.

Just as the workplace can be a site for the transmission of the common cold or the flu, it often serves as a site for the transmission of stress.

It would help to trace a timeline of your day. How stressed were you when you went to work? Was there a stressful commute—bad traffic, late trains? How did your day start?

Then "take your temperature" at different points of your working day. If you have a nine-to-five job (or thereabouts), you might want to consider your stress level at a midmorning break. Were you more stressed at this point than you were earlier? If so, why? Where did that stress come from? A person? A task? A deadline? Self-doubt?

Monitor your stress again at lunch, in midafternoon, at the end of your workday, and then back at home. (Adjust this pattern to fit your work schedule.) Find the points at which stress entered. Try to trace the sources.

YOUR TURN

Weekly Monitor

For every day of a five-day period at work, take seven "readings" of your stress level and plot them on the graph provided. For a nine-to-five schedule, we recommend these readings:

1. Just before you leave for work

2. Just after you arrive at work

3. Midmorning (one quarter through workday)

4. Lunch (halfway through)

5. Midafternoon (three quarters)

6. End of workday

7. At home after workday

(Adjust this schedule to fit your specific schedule.)

Note: This is a purely subjective reading—how "stressed" do you feel, on a scale of 0 to 100? It's possible to think back on your whole day and try to remember your stress levels at those different points. For better results, try to take a "time-out" at several points during the day to update this graph.

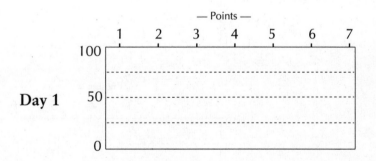

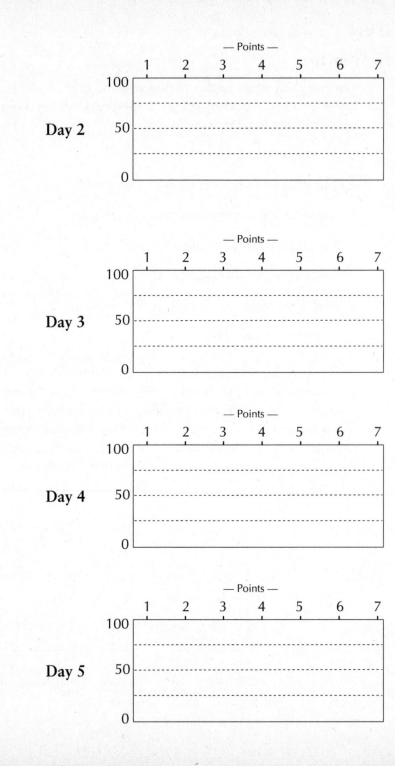

Analyzing the Graph

1. At the end of each day, evaluate your findings for that day. Look for sudden upturns of stress and try to explain them. Jot notes on the graph to help you remember people you saw, projects due, tasks involved in, news received, or sudden events.

2. When the week is up, look at the whole chart. Do you notice any patterns? Is there a time of day when you regularly feel great stress?

   My most stressful time of day is: _____

3. In explaining the upturns, did you jot down the same name or task or event more than once? Based on your analysis of your graph, list your five to ten most significant stress producers from this five-day period.

PEOPLE WHO GRIEVE PEOPLE

"Our marketing director thinks he knows everything," says Linda. "Whenever I suggest anything, he laughs at me. I have to edit his articles for our newsletter, and he's always giving me grief. I look things up two or three times, and if he's wrong, he's wrong—I have to fix it. But he'll never admit it."

Nearly every job has one: an "except for" person. As in, "This would be a great job *except for* Joe." Phyllis has that doctor who insists that she schedule a lot of patients and then scolds her for doing just that. She can't win. Tony has that fellow burger-burner who makes fun of him. Wendy has a business consultant who second-guesses everything she does in keeping financial records, an area she already feels insecure about.

In some companies, everyone knows that "Joe is just a jerk." It's as if he had that role in the company, with a nameplate on his desk—"JERK." Everyone expects him to cause problems.

But often there's just a person *you* have a conflict with. It's not the company jerk but someone who gets along fine with everyone else. Yet somehow you and this person have a conflict. Maybe you're vying for the same promotion, and this other person is always undercutting you. Maybe you just have different ideas about how the job should be done.

And sometimes stress is caused by someone you *like*. The boss you admire so much that you desperately want his or her approval. Or the disorganized worker who has a flurry of ideas but never follows through. Or the coworker you have a genuinely friendly competition with. Or the office busybody, who fills you in on all the latest gossip. Or the social butterfly who gabs and gabs and gets you further behind schedule.

Of course, there are also stress relievers, those wonderful people who get you back on track, who calm your fears and help organize your work. Find these people and hang on to them. They're valuable.

Besides analyzing our schedules, we should also analyze our interaction with our coworkers.

YOUR TURN

People Monitor

The people around us have a great effect on our stress levels. In the previous exercise, you sketched out a grid of your schedule, analyzing the stress factors. Now it's time to add people to that grid.

1. Start with the people you spend the most time with on the job, your inner circle. Choose three to five of your closest coworkers and list them here.

    _____

    _____

    _____

    _____

    _____

2. Then list your middle circle, people you deal with once or twice a day, if that. Try to find three to five people in this group as well.

_____

_____

_____

_____

_____

3. Finally, consider your outer circle, people you don't know all that well but see maybe once a week or less. List three to five of these.

_____

_____

_____

_____

_____

4. Now go back through all the people you've listed and give each one a score from +3 to -3. This score is based on *how they affect your stress level*. Those who give you the most stress should get a +3 score, while those who relieve the most stress should get a -3. Of course, you can use 2 or 1 on either side and 0 for those who have no effect on your stress level.

Extra Analysis

Try this. Go back to the graph of your weekly stress (p. 91). Take your highest-scoring stress-producing person and put an X wherever you had contact with that person. Take your lowest-scoring stress producer (-3, if you have one) and put an O on the schedule wherever you dealt with that person.

Now look at the graph. Is there a correlation? Did the stress producer cause upturns and the stress reliever cause downturns? (It doesn't always match up exactly, but it often does.)

OTHER JOB STRESSORS

There are a few general categories of stress producers that you may have missed as you perused your weekly schedule. They deserve mention here.

The Business World

Any business has its ups and downs, which cause a great deal of worry among those involved in that business. U.S. autoworkers worry about the balance of trade with Japan. Bank workers fret about the latest merger that may cost them their jobs. Factory workers fear the approach of automation. Book publishers wonder how long it will be before no one can read anymore. These social and business trends can bring great stress to individual workers.

Tim worked as a middle manager for a company that was in danger of going out of business. For a year he was in turmoil, not knowing whether his job was safe. It wasn't. The company downsized and let him go.

Ironically, he began a consulting business and was hired by his old company to advise them on a particular project. "I can't describe how great it was to walk out of that building after our first consulting session," Tim said. "I felt so free! For a year, I had been carrying the weight of that company with me wherever I went. But now I could walk out of that office and leave its problems behind. I hadn't realized how heavy those problems were."

In a fast-paced business world where mergers and acquisitions happen overnight, there are a lot of stressed employees.

Increasing Work Demands

Downsizing has its drawbacks, even for those who keep their jobs. They have a lot more to do. Increasingly, companies are giving three people the work of five. Deadlines come fast and furious. They're like buffalo in a stampede—you get trampled by one, and as you pick yourself up, you can hear the hoofbeats of the next one fast approaching.

In spite of all this fancy-schmancy analysis, you may be feeling stressed because you simply have too much work to do.

Project Cycles

You were already asked whether there was a particular time of day in which you felt the most stress. This is a related question. Is there a particular point *in a project* where you feel most stressed?

"We have to get a newsletter out to the printer every other week," says Linda. "And one of our writers is always late with her articles. We even give her false deadlines, and she still misses the real ones. So I just know that every other Thursday I will be frantically trying to put the newsletter together."

Linda's project is on a biweekly cycle. Yours may be every month or every week or every day and a half. It's fairly common to get stressed at "crunch time," right before a deadline, but some people feel more stress at the beginning of a project, when they're not sure yet what they're doing. Others reach a stress point somewhere in the middle, after they've procrastinated and before they've done much work.

"Project stress" tends to increase as the deadline approaches, but it decreases as parts of the project are completed. If you perform the project in a timely manner, your stress should stay pretty even. If you fall behind, of course, it will go up.

Conflicts

Inevitably, there are conflicts. When you work closely with people—even people you like—there will be times when you don't see eye to eye. These will tend to raise your stress level.

Working toward a common goal, you and your coworkers may disagree on how to get there. Or you may have different goals in view. Conflicts also result from differences in personality, background, assumptions, worldviews, ambitions, and values. Sometimes these problems are intensified by ambiguous lines of authority, scanty job descriptions, competition, and inadequate communication.

Conflict can be healthy, providing opportunities for personal growth and deepening relationships.

Insulting remarks, destructive rumors, factions, personality attacks, and smear campaigns can all make your life at work very unpleasant. You can find your own attitude caving in as you deal with this pressure.

But conflict itself is not all bad. Conflict can be healthy, providing opportunities for personal growth and deepening relationships. Conflict shows that people care about what's going on.

Certainly conflict will generate stress. But we can limit the damage of that stress by accepting the conflict, seeing its good aspects, and working through it.

Self-Image

For most of us, success at our daily work is interwoven with our self-esteem. If we aren't good at what we do, what good are we? This attitude raises the stakes of any work-related issue. Suddenly we're not just struggling with a particular project, we're battling for our own sense of personal adequacy. That in itself sends our stress soaring, and it often yields conflicts, which magnify the stress even more.

Linda's marketing director resisted any suggestion or constructive criticism, even though Linda had the task of editing his articles. That resistance is pretty common, and it usually boils down to a self-esteem problem. The person cannot set boundaries between himself and the paragraph he wrote for the company newsletter. It's all or nothing. Attack my writing and you attack me. If you say I misspelled a word, you are deeply demeaning my character.

We find this intertwining of self and work most often in men, who are culturally conditioned to identify with their work. In our society, men are what they do. (When you meet a man, what's the first question you ask? *What do you do?*) When a man fails at his job, he fails at life. At least, that's the way we think. Unemployment is distressing for anyone, but it hits men especially hard, we feel—not just in the practical questions involved ("How will we get the money we need?") but also in the personal affront ("What good am I?").

Women tend to draw their self-image from a broader range of sources. They see themselves as wives, mothers, friends, artists, and community leaders as well as executives or secretaries or managers or factory workers. But they also tend to have their self-esteem attacked on all these fronts. As a result, we have found general self-esteem issues more prevalent (at least more open) in women than in men, though *job-related* self-esteem issues are a smaller piece of their overall self-concept.

Still, self-esteem issues at work can be devastating for a woman, especially if she is feeling put down in other areas of life as well.

Women may also see, in their jobs, a variety of roles. That is, a female secretary may see herself as a sort of mom to the office staff, as the informal social leader for the company, as the morale booster, as the confidante, as the brains behind the boss, in addition to her typing and filing duties. She may also put pressure on herself to succeed in *all* these areas and feel inadequate if she "fails" in one or two.

"The Battle of the Sexes"

As long as we're discussing gender differences on the job, we should face up to the stress involved in male-female relations in the workplace. While the climate varies from company to company, the business world still tends to be male dominated, and many women feel a pressure to succeed by both male and female standards. High-ranking women may see themselves as representing their gender, trying to "prove" the ability of women and adding tremendous stress.

Some men were brought up to see women as inferior, at least in the workplace. Thus they feel an extra pressure to stay ahead of women who may be vying for their jobs. (We feel this is a misguided, unnecessary stress, but it exists, deeply imbedded, and it needs to be dealt with.) Other men want to be sensitive to women but aren't sure how. The rules keep changing, they feel. They try to be respectful but not patronizing, friendly but not harassing.

All of this adds a new dimension of stress to the workplace. And there's no magic elixir for it, except communication, acceptance, and re-examination of long-held biases.

YOUR TURN

Rating of Alternate Stressors

1. Is the following a source of stress for you? (Rate from 0 to 10, with 10 being the greatest source of stress.)

   ___ Fear of losing job

   ___ Fear that business realignment will leave you out in the cold

   ___ Too much work to do

   ___ Certain points in a "project cycle" are especially stressful

   ___ Conflicts with coworkers

   ___ Conflicts with boss

   ___ Doubts about self because of a job you failed at

___ Fears that others will think less of you if you fail at some task

___ The need to represent your gender as capable and effective

___ Sexual harassment or fear of being accused of it

2. Take your highest-rated stressor from the list above and think about a time when you felt that stress most acutely. What happened?

_____

_____

_____

3. What did you do to alter, avoid, or accept the situation, if anything?

_____

_____

_____

4. What could you have done better?

_____

_____

_____

9

Stress Strategies at Work

We have already presented the concept of altering, avoiding, or accepting the stress producers you face in different environments. After you have analyzed the stress producers in your work situation, you need to adopt at least one of these strategies.

It would be impossible for us to cover all the possible stressors you might face at work. But we do want to help you through the alter-avoid-accept process, and we'll do that by applying it to the three most common stressors in the workplace.

ALTER

Too Much to Do

How do you alter a situation in which you are overworked? It's not easy. There are usually reasons for the predicament—an unsympathetic boss, an inefficient system, a frugal company, an inability to say no—and these reasons are hard to change. Otherwise, you would have eased your workload long ago. But perhaps there are a few things that can be adjusted, which may help other things change, too.

Cry for help. Do this in your own way, at the appropriate decibel level, but somehow you have to let people know you're overworked. Some find it difficult admitting they can't do everything they're asked to do, but consider the alternative: a breakdown of some kind. Communicate your need.

Delegate responsibilities. If you have people working for you, let them do some of your work. Many executives get tangled up in the nuts and bolts of certain projects when they should merely be overseeing what others do. We knew a director of a Christian organization who insisted on doing a final edit of all the materials his ministry sent out, and he would often make minor changes in the wording. Since he was always overworked, he created a huge bottleneck in the whole company's schedule, and his editors resented his unnecessary involvement in the work they were hired to do. The point is, you can maintain a degree of control over a project even if you farm out some of the details. It's better for you and probably better for your company.

Altering stress on the job:

Cry for help.
Delegate responsibilities.
Rearrange duties.
Ease your expectations.
Learn to say no.
Set limits on overtime.

Rearrange duties. If you are part of a team, see if there are others who can take on some of your work in exchange for some of theirs. You want an even distribution of the workload, but you also want people working in areas where they're gifted. If Jill has vision and Jack sweats the details, give Jack the detail jobs and Jill the big-picture stuff. Find the specific tasks that weigh you down and see if there's someone else who could do them better.

Ease your expectations. It goes against the grain to say you should lower your standards, but you may have to. You may be your own worst enemy, pushing yourself way beyond your abilities. Identify where, exactly, your standards are. Pinpoint objective levels of what's "good enough." By all means, discuss this with your boss and coworkers. But you may be doing a lot of unnecessary work to reach standards that far exceed the standards of those you work with. It's nice to do good work, but don't kill yourself for it.

Learn to say no. Some people just take on too much. They underestimate the time and effort a project will take, and they want to be agreeable, so they say yes to everything. "Sure, I'll manage that project. No problem." But then it often becomes a problem. Draw the line early. Say no to a project at first and let yes come only after thorough examination.

Set limits on overtime. Whether you're a factory worker or chairman of the board, you need time off from work. Set limits. Talk with your family about this and write the limits down. "Maximum hours worked per week." "Maximum hours per month." Maybe you'll need to work sixty hours one week during crunch time, but then make it a point to ease up the next week. Set rules for yourself and be accountable to your family (or others). This is not easy to do, especially if your company depends on you or if you need the money from overtime hours. But how good will you be for your company or family if you run yourself ragged?

People You Can't Stand

If you try to alter the person you're dealing with, you'll probably fail. But if you try to alter the *relationship*, you have a chance. Relationships often sour due to lack of communication. People hold grudges and let resentments fester. People have assumptions about you that may be unfounded, but if you never address them, they will not be changed. Sometimes there are racial or sexual or religious stereotypes that enter the picture.

Or you may have done something wrong, knowingly or unknowingly. You may be in the job that the other person wants. He or she may have questions about how you got that job.

In most cases, communication is the first step in restoring (or establishing) a relationship. You may need to address a problem directly, and that may be difficult. "Why don't you like me? Why do you always try to hurt me?" These things aren't easy to say.

Of course, it's always best to enter such an encounter with humility. "Is there something I've done that I need to apologize for?" "What can I do to improve this relationship?"

In any confrontation, "I statements" are most effective. Instead of, "You make me feel bad," say, "I feel bad about the way we get along. Is there anything we can do to make things better?"

You may be met with denial ("Oh, nothing's wrong") or with anger ("Don't try to butter me up!"). Sometimes misunderstandings run deep.

Beware of the power factor. Some people see everything at work in terms of power—who has it, who doesn't. Some who have less power may resent you for having more and try to make you feel bad for the corporate power you have. Some who have more power may suspect your motives in trying to establish a relationship.

Of course, some people are just selfish or rude, and they may resist all your relationship-building efforts. Then you can only pray for healing. We are assuming that prayer is undergirding all your stress-reducing efforts. In the case of difficult coworkers, you'll find that you can't change them, but God can. And often he *does*.

Conflict

In marriage, the best couples know how to fight well. The same might be said of coworkers. Conflict will happen. The question is, Will it accomplish anything good, or will it just wound the people involved?

You will never alter the fact that conflicts happen at work. But you can change the *way* they happen. You can prevent them from destroying relationships, impeding the progress of your work, and causing you an unhealthy amount of stress. Some pointers:

See conflict as healthy. Welcome the exchange of views as a potential growth experience. Don't put up your personal defenses. Make up your mind to work together toward a common goal.

Look for a win-win solution. Your goal should not be to defeat the people you are in conflict with. You should try to find a way that their ideas can be heard and their needs met. Your own needs and ideas should be similarly affirmed.

Lose a fight once in a while. Yes, a win-win solution means a win for you as well, but you can't always find that. Don't be so intent on winning that you can't give in. Sometimes it's just not worth it to prolong the struggle. And if you willingly surrender on this round, you may ease the conflict in the next.

Focus on the issue, not the person. Our personalities usually take center stage in any conflict. But try to keep the conflict coming back to issues and directions. You may be able to get around the personal shields of defense that most people put up.

Use proper channels for conflict resolution. Many companies have systems set up for grievances and conflicts. Sometimes these are woefully inadequate, but sometimes they help. Acquaint yourself with these procedures.

Learn how to put conflicts behind you. Once the fight has been fought, you probably still have to face your combatant. Don't hold a grudge. Let bygones be bygones. Make peace—with a friendly gesture, a compliment, a talk—and move on.

AVOID

In Kenny Rogers's song, the gambler knows when to hold 'em and when to fold 'em. While the intricacies of poker playing may escape you, the rule still holds true in life. Sometimes it's simply best to fold 'em, to give up. The best warriors know when to run away, and live to fight another day.

Let's survey the avoidance tactic as it applies to our three major job stresses.

Too Much to Do

We have already discussed altering your situatiuon by avoiding some of the work in your pile of stuff to do. But so far we have skirted the main avoidance option—quitting.

It's a trend of the future, they say—individual downscaling. People are quitting their high-pressure, high-rise jobs in the city and moving to farms in Vermont to gaze at the mountains and raise goats. Trend tracker Faith Popcorn calls it "cashing out."

> **Lucrative jobs can be traps for people who literally kill themselves to earn that money.**

"The pace of life has quickened," she writes. "The ante has been upped. Traditional corporate success demands extraordinary, exhausting effort. We seem to be saying: 'Is all this stress really worth the reward?' 'Isn't this life I'm living shortening my life?' And the favorite refrain of our times, 'Is this all there is?'"[1]

Of course, life in Vermont (or Montana or the Virgin Islands) has stresses all its own. But if your job stress is endangering your health and if it can't be substantially decreased, you should seriously consider "cashing out." Revise your lifestyle. Live more simply.

And you don't have to move to the country. You could get a lower-pressure job in your current vicinity. Such jobs are usually lower-paying as well, so you will need to make some major lifestyle decisions. (Your whole family should be involved in this, of course, since it will affect them all.)

This sort of downscaling is not easily done. The Bible frequently speaks of the dangers of money, and we see it often in high-stress jobs. "People who want to get rich fall into temptation and a trap and into many foolish and harmful desires that plunge men into ruin and destruction," Paul warned Timothy (1 Tim. 6:9). Lucrative jobs can be traps for people who literally kill themselves to earn that money. They tell themselves they need that money to provide for their family's enjoyment and for their own. Ironically, these people seldom get to enjoy the fruits of their labors, and their families seldom get to enjoy *them*.

"Command those who are rich in this present world not to be arrogant nor to put their hope in wealth, which is so uncertain," Paul counsels his protégé a few verses later, "but to put their hope in God, who richly provides us with everything for our enjoyment" (1 Tim. 6:17).

There are certainly sacrifices involved in personal downscaling, but the well-ordered life that results is a rich reward.

Be careful, though, about jumping into unemployment too quickly. The job hunt can be extremely stressful, with the addition of self-esteem issues. In each interview, you are on trial—are you good enough to get this job? If your self-esteem is already shaky, you may need to build up your support systems before you take this plunge.

People You Can't Stand

This seems simple enough, doesn't it? If there are people you can't stand at work, *avoid them*. End of story.

Of course, it's not that easy. You *have* to work with some of these people, day in and day out. You can't get away from them.

But you can avoid talking about the issues that divide you. You can avoid doing the things that raise the hackles of the other person. You can avoid confrontations that will become shouting matches.

This may sound like denial, like sweeping problems under the rug. In fact, it is judicious management of a difficult relationship. By all means, confront a problem if it will do any good. (Alteration is your first option.) But if confrontation will do no good, save your energy. Choose not to be distracted in your work. Move ahead and avoid fireworks.

Conflict

As we have been saying, it is not necessary to avoid conflict. Conflict can be a healthy aspect of a workplace if it is sporadic, contained, and marked by good communication.

But needless conflicts can be avoided through good communication. People in a work situation need to know what their mutual goal is and what their individual roles are.

We authors are from the Philadelphia area, and we cheered our local baseball team, the Phillies, to the National League pennant in 1993. The amazing thing about that team, as with so many successful teams, was that each player knew his role and performed it cheerfully. Skilled players were sharing time in the field with others, right-handers platooning with left-handers, defensive replacements entering in the late innings, pinch hitters coming off the bench. Everyone knew what he had to do and did it. In the sweet glow of victory, there was little conflict.

But something happened in that strike-shortened season of 1994. The Phillies were losing, and conflict emerged. Suddenly players started mouthing off to the press. "Why am I not playing more? I want a different role on this team. I'm better than he is!"

There's nothing wrong with players wanting to play more. That's good. But when people start losing sight of the corporate objectives and start playing (or working) for themselves, there will be conflict. When people fail to see (or accept) their role in the big picture, there are big problems.

Good leadership will keep presenting the vision, the goals of the group. Capable leaders will also keep instructing employees about the value of each individual role. If you are in a leadership position, these simple points of communication will ease your stress considerably. If you find yourself "in the ranks," you can still exert that leadership from within, by clarifying your own role and the roles of those around you, honoring your coworkers for what they do, and reminding everybody of what you're all trying to accomplish.

Those basic on-the-job communication habits will prevent needless conflicts and pave the way for speedy recovery from conflicts that do occur.

ACCEPT

If things can't be changed or avoided, all that's left is acceptance. At heart here is a spiritual issue. Will you accept the goodness of God in leading you to this place? Will you trust in the power of God to get you through?

Too Much to Do

If you can't get out of it, the work is there in front of you. Acceptance means you buckle down and do it. Don't be distracted by anger about having all this work or by worry about how you're going to get it done. Don't daydream about how you're going to spend the money you make doing this job. Don't even count the hours till it will be finished. Just do it.

People You Can't Stand

This is one of the hardest things a person has to do, at work or in life. Sometimes you realize it's just a matter of personal style. You're conservative; the other person is liberal. You're type A; the other is type Z. You're jovial; she is dour. You may be able to look at these differences and shrug them away. "I know that's a good person. We're just different. We just don't get along."

But sometimes people are just evil. Sometimes they are intentionally obnoxious; they *try* to tick you off. Sometimes they are sour, sick people who want to spread gloom wherever they go. Sometimes they are so hateful, you wonder if there's any ray of light in their soul. Often they resist any attempt to make things better. What can you do with people like that?

See through God's eyes. God has been dealing with people like that for a long time. From the hard-hearted Pharaoh to the bloodthirsty Herod, God has encountered people who just would not open up to him. The Bible describes a "hardness of heart" that occurs. We'll sidestep the theology of that concept, but psychologically we see it often. People slam the doors of their hearts so hard, it's difficult to open them again.

But in a way, we can see the whole human race like that. We are rebellious, but God loves us anyway. Through God's eyes, the person you can't stand is still a created, beloved being—and God mourns over the rejection from that person.

Try to see your tormentor through God's eyes—eyes that are loving, mournful, hopeful.

Look for the wound. The "jerks" at work often thrive on intimidation. They try to make you feel inferior, and often succeed. There's a piece of folk wisdom that advises intimidated people to imagine the people they fear in their underwear. The idea is, we all are just people. See the person without the trappings of power.

Let's try a different idea: look for the person's wound. All human beings have been emotionally wounded in one way or another. Intentionally obnoxious people have probably been wounded deeply. The classic film *Citizen Kane* traces the dastardly behavior of the nation's most powerful man to a longing for his lost childhood, embodied in the sled named Rosebud. But every rascal has a "Rosebud." Every warrior has a wound.

You don't need to psychoanalyze the person you can't stand. You don't need to dig into that person's affairs. But be aware that this person is wounded. It will change your attitude, guaranteed.

If a parent denies ice cream to a three-year-old, the child may scream, "I hate you!" It's a terrible thing to say, but the parent is not devastated by it. Why? Because it's obvious that the child is speaking out of pain—at least a sense of deprivation. The child is wounded, in a way, and is not choosing words carefully. If you see your problem person in the same way, you will be able to let many hateful comments roll off you.

And if you display sensitivity to the person's wound, being willing to withstand the person's off-putting behavior, you may just break through the wall and find a person in there who's ready to find healing. That's unlikely, but it's possible.

Don't aim for this person's approval. If you're a people pleaser, you may be especially bothered by the thought that this person, for some reason, can't stand *you*. You try to be nice, but the person just hates you. You can do nothing right in his or her eyes.

Then let it be. You do not need that person's approval. Work your best for the company—and especially for God. As it says in Colossians 3:23, "Whatever you do, work at it with all your heart, *as working for the Lord, not for men*" (emphasis added).

Conflict

Once again we must emphasize that conflicts will happen and that's OK. Your acceptance of the potential value of conflict is crucial. If you are a people pleaser, this acceptance will not come easy. But you must learn to fight fairly and fight well—to listen, learn, and love in every conflict that arises.

Accept also the stress cycle that greets any conflict situation. Even if a conflict is healthy, it is still stressful. If you get into a heated argument during a staff meeting, your heart rate and blood pressure will rise, your stomach may churn, and your adrenaline will heat up your whole body. After that staff meeting, you may need a break. Let your system get back to normal. Go for a walk down to the mailroom or around the block. Take an early lunch or coffee break. Take five minutes to think of peaceful things before starting on your next project. This stress can be good for you, but you must allow time to recover.

You may also need to follow up conflict with some "conflict resolution." Don't let bridges burn behind you. If you felt that the staff meeting argument got out of hand, you may want to see the other party and patch things up. Agree to disagree, if need be, but reach out to affirm the other person. Do this as soon as possible, since unresolved conflicts get awkward. The scriptural principle is, "Do not let the sun go down while you are still angry" (Eph. 4:26). Accept conflicts but keep them short and to the point.

COMMUNICATION TIPS:
EASING THE STRESS OF RELATIONSHIPS

Listen hard.
Listen without drawing premature conclusions.
Show genuine interest in the other person.
Treat people fairly.
Discuss conflicts and concerns honestly and openly.
Keep confidences.
See things from the other person's point of view.
Understand the motive behind the conflict.
Ask questions to clarify.
Do not give commands.
Solicit ideas from the other person.
Show patience and love.
Overlook others' faults.
Forgive yourself and others.
Don't involve yourself in destructive gossip.

YOUR TURN

Assignment #1: AAA Action Plan

Look through your analysis from the previous chapter and select your five greatest issues or areas of job stress. List them in the numbered spaces below at the left.

In the spaces to the right, consider your alter-avoid-accept strategy. What can you do to alter, avoid, or accept these stressors?

1.

Alter: _____

_____

Avoid: _____

_____

Accept: _____

_____

2.

Alter: _____

_____

Avoid: _____

_____

Accept: _____

_____

3.

Alter: _____

_____

Avoid: _____

_____

Accept: _____

_____

4.

   Alter: _____

   _____

   Avoid: _____

   _____

   Accept: _____

   _____

5.

   Alter: _____

   _____

   Avoid: _____

   _____

   Accept: _____

   _____

Assignment #2: Stress Track

At the end of each day for a five-day period, review the major stresses you felt that day. In a few words, list each person, event, or situation that caused you stress. (For best results, do this at several points during the day.)

After listing the stressors, evaluate what you *did* to alter, avoid, or accept it. Write this down in a few words in the appropriate space. Then consider what you *could do,* that might be better, next time this occurs.

	ALTER		AVOID		ACCEPT	
	Did	*Could Do*	*Did*	*Could Do*	*Did*	*Could Do*
Day 1 Morning						
Noon						
Evening						
Night						
Day 2 Morning						
Noon						
Evening						
Night						

	ALTER		AVOID		ACCEPT	
	Did	*Could Do*	*Did*	*Could Do*	*Did*	*Could Do*
Day 3 Morning						
Noon						
Evening						
Night						
Day 4 Morning						
Noon						
Evening						
Night						

Day 5	ALTER		AVOID		ACCEPT	
	Did	*Could Do*	*Did*	*Could Do*	*Did*	*Could Do*
Morning						
Noon						
Evening						
Night						

10

Relaxing at Work

Apart from the alter-avoid-accept strategies of dealing with stress producers, you can help to ease your workday stress by *preparing* for it. Get into good physical habits—nutrition, exercise, rest, and maintaining a good working environment.

Later in this book, you'll find comprehensive plans for nutrition and exercise, but for now let's consider things you can do *at work* to maintain a stress-resistant equilibrium.

YOUR WORKSTATION

Where are you physically situated when you work? Do you sit at a desk? Do you stand at a counter? Do you have to walk around a lot? Do you drive?

It is important to make your work space as friendly as possible. It should be a home away from home. You should feel comfortable there as you do your work.

Within the guidelines of your company, personalize your workstation as much as possible. Include photos of loved ones, posters, mementos, plants.

If you sit most of the day, make sure your chair is comfortable but not too comfortable. You don't want to lean back and slouch. You need support for your back but proper padding as well. The chair should be the appropriate height relative to your desk, computer, and so on. Be careful about twisting arrangements, where you must regularly turn sideways to reach a file, phone, or keyboard.

If you have access to the thermostat, set the temperature at a comfortable level but not too warm. If you have to work at a less than optimal temperature, be sure you are dressed for it.

Make sure your workplace is as comfortable and relaxing as possible.

Adjust the phone ring to a level that won't jar you. Ordinary conversation is about sixty decibels, but phones are often set much higher. A loud phone will set you on edge at various points of the day.

Make certain the room is well lit. If the overhead lighting is inadequate, see if you can bring in a small lamp for your space. Be careful about your computer screen too. If you can adjust its brightness, find a medium level that won't make you squint but also won't shine too brightly.

Do what you can to limit excessive noise. If you work in a loud factory or store, consider using earplugs (at least during your break time). Many people prefer soft music to utter silence, but avoid raucous music and loud, distracting noise. As much as you might enjoy fast-paced rock music, we have found that it does not induce relaxation, even among its most avid fans.

YOUR CLOTHES

Many companies have dress codes, written or unwritten, so you may be rather limited in your options. But be sure your clothes fit properly, not too tight, especially at your stomach, chest, or neck.

Recently a doctor encountered several patients with stomach disorders—chronic indigestion. After a battery of tests proved inconclusive, this doctor realized that these patients—all middle-aged men of some girth—were merely wearing their pants too tight.

This is a common problem, actually. Many people gain weight as they age, and their wardrobes don't catch up. Men squeeze their bodies into suits that are too small, pants that are too tight, and shirt collars that choke them. Ties are constricting enough, but please make sure your collar is loose. Similarly, women constrict themselves in various ways. It's amazing how much more comfortable clothes can be when they fit right.

Be sure your clothes are warm enough for your environment but not too warm. They should allow you the proper range of movement you need in your job. Of course, you also want to look good. A lot of undue stress is caused by being the only one in the room without a suit, or having a spot on your tie that you try to hide, or realizing that your skirt is too short for the occasion. Take the time to plan appropriate dress for your various work situations.

Good shoes are also crucial, especially if you have to walk or stand on the job. Many businesswomen wear sneakers on the commute to work and change to heels when they get there. That's not a bad idea.

YOUR TIME

If you are a chronic latecomer, try to get to work early. Give yourself a nonwork project to do at your desk or workstation twenty minutes before the workday starts. That may make your commute less frantic, and even if you're running late for your prework project, you're still on time for work.

Take regular breaks of short duration. Many people go wrong by working for several hours straight and then "rewarding" themselves with a break that is far longer than they need. It would be much better to take a one-minute stand-up-and-breathe break every half hour than to work three hours solid and take an hour off.

YOUR BODY

Get in the habit of practicing good posture at work. Monitor your posture at various times of the day. If you sit, don't slouch. And don't arch your lower back. Bend forward from the hips. If you stand, adopt a straight but relaxed posture.

Don't sit in one position over a prolonged period of time. Stand up, move your feet up and down, and gently stretch. This will ensure better blood circulation. Remember to relax and breathe deeply a number of times during the day.

Be sure to eat properly at regular intervals. Avoid junk food at your desk, but you may want to have some fruit or whole-grain snacks available. You may have a coffee routine for yourself, but after the first cup or two, switch to water or unsweetened juice. Consider keeping a carafe or squeeze bottle at your workstation (or at least closer than the coffeepot).

A couple of times a day, take a five-minute break for *progressive relaxation*. This is a simple technique that stretches and relaxes various parts of your body. It will reenergize your body and get you well aligned for your next work period. (See the exercises at the end of this chapter for instructions on progressive relaxation.)

YOUR MIND

As work pressures mount, we can get into mental traps. We can focus only on the magnitude of our work or the difficulties involved in getting it done. We need to take *mental* breaks occasionally to keep our sanity.

One technique is the *key phrase*. When work is beginning to make you crazy, repeat to yourself, "I can do this. God is with me. This isn't the end of the world." Or something like that. Choose your own pithy statements and memorize them. Say them out loud if need be, but certainly in your conscious mind. Don't let the circumstances take control. With God's help, you can maintain a handle on the situation.

Another option is *calming visualization*. This is just a matter of using your imagination to "take a vacation" during one of those five-minute work breaks. Put yourself in the Bahamas or on a cool Colorado mountain, or perhaps with Jesus by the Sea of Galilee, and then come back to work refreshed. (Specific ideas for visualization are included in the exercises that follow.)

YOUR TURN

Checklist

___ My work space is friendly.
___ I have personalized my work space as much as I can.
___ My chair is comfortable (if applicable).
___ The temperature at work is comfortable.
___ The light at work is adequate.
___ My computer screen does not cause me eyestrain (if applicable).
___ The phone does not jar me when it rings.
___ My work space has a comfortable noise level.
___ My clothes are comfortable.

___ I am happy with how I look while I'm at work.
___ My clothes allow me the range of motion I need.
___ My shoes are comfortable.
___ I am usually on time for work and other meetings.
___ During my workday, I often take short breaks.
___ I eat properly so I am neither hungry nor stuffed at work.
___ I have good posture at work.
___ I take breaks for progressive relaxation.
___ I have key phrases that help me deal with pressure situations.
___ I practice calming visualization.

Review this checklist, paying attention to those items you haven't checked. Is there anything you want to do that will enable you to check any of those items? List one to three "action steps" you can take over the next few weeks.

Action steps

Week one: _____

_____

Week two: _____

_____

Week three: _____

_____

Progressive Relaxation

(It might be best to try this out by yourself at home before you practice it during your workday.)

As difficult as it might be, try to find a quiet place for this exercise. It's possible to do this at a desk if you don't have interruptions. Otherwise, look for a lunchroom, break room, or possibly a bathroom. You could even do this sitting in your car.

Assume a straight sitting position (or you could lie down or stand if need be). "Straight" does not mean rigid. Relax but don't cross your legs or slide down in the seat or bend forward. In this exercise, you will concentrate on your muscles, tightening and loosening each muscle group. (If you can already sense which muscles are tight, focus on those.)

Before you begin, take a few slow, deep breaths. Then start with your head. Work your face muscles by faking a yawn, then pouting, then making other faces.

Work your neck muscles by *slowly* turning your head right and then left and then in a gentle circular motion. Be extremely gentle with your neck stretches; any sudden movement could twist something that shouldn't be twisted.

Let your left arm tense up, beginning at the shoulder and moving down to your hand. Make a fist and clench it for ten seconds. Then relax it. Do the same with your right arm.

Shrug your shoulders. Slide them forward, then back. Then briefly tense your chest muscles, abdominal muscles, and hip muscles.

Lift your right knee, feeling a slight stretch in your upper leg, then extend your lower leg until your leg is straight. Point your toe, then stretch out your heel. Do the same with your left leg.

Calming Visualization

In your mind's eye, see a beautiful mountain scene. Now imagine . . .

The breeze begins to rise, making gentle waves over the green grasslands. The lightly fragranced breeze streams through your hair and over your face, making you feel chills up and down your body. As you walk along the side of the mountain, you see a small spring and hear its softly flowing sounds. You trace the stream's path and find yourself walking in a gorgeous pine forest. With pine needles beneath your feet, you feel that you are walking on nature's carpet. What a lovely world God has made!

The fragrance of the towering pines fills the air. The sun shines through the branches, warming your relaxed, calm body. As you contemplate, you feel at harmony within yourself, and you delight in being part of God's family. You can enjoy God's undisturbed, heavenly peace and tranquility in your body and spirit.

Smoothly and effortlessly, open your eyes and look around you with joy. God has made this part of your world, too. Enjoy it with a pleasant, peaceful mind.

Idea 1

Put the above description (or something you make up for yourself) on tape. During your relaxation breaks, put on some headphones and listen to the tape.

Idea 2

Find a painting or poster of a scene that relaxes you. Begin your visualization by looking at the painting and let your imagination carry you into it. Then, at various points during the day when you need to relax, you might look at the painting and imagine its serenity.

Note: Visualization may seem sort of "hocus-pocus" to some readers. But there's nothing sinister about it. Maybe others use similar techniques to "empty" their minds, but we Christians can use it to fill our minds with joy and appreciation for God's creation.

11

Home Stress

I want to wear my shorts!"

"It's too cold for shorts. Wear your jeans."

"They're dirty."

"Then wear your overalls."

"I don't like them."

The seven-year-old was going out to play, and the mother was making sure the girl would not catch cold. The fifteen-year-old son came bounding down the steps.

"Mom, do you still need those light bulbs?"

"Yes. You haven't gone to the store yet?"

"I was cleaning my room, like you said."

"Are you finished?"

"Not yet. Can I go to the store later?"

"No! I need those light bulbs."

"But I have to be at work at three. I can't clean my room and go to the store."

"Try."

A neighbor kid was at the door, looking for the ten-year-old daughter. The call rang through the house.

"Stephanie? Where's Stephanie?"

The father called from the living room, "I thought she was outside."

"Is she outside?"

"She's not outside."

"I saw her out there in the yard."

"She's not in the yard."

The seven-year-old was now begging the fifteen-year-old to watch her do a new step from dance class.

"I can't, Rachel. I have to go to the store."

"Please!"

"Mom! Tell Rachel I have to go."

"Rachel, he has to go. Find Stephanie. She'll watch you."

This is a genuine slice of life, sixty seconds of actual dialogue from an actual family. You may have played out scenes like this in your own home.

The point is, stress does not stop as you leave your workplace. It changes but it does not stop. For many, many people, the home holds even greater stresses. And if you are a single parent, a stay-at-home mom, or involved in a fairly dysfunctional family situation, the stress involved in dealing with your family day in and day out can be overwhelming.

> **Stress does not stop as you leave your workplace. It changes but it does not stop.**

The home has many of the same stressors that the workplace has—never enough time, the pressure to perform well, relationship problems. But there are usually emotional issues in the home that intensify the pressure. Home is where the hurt is. Our basic questions of identity often come from our home life. We learn who we are within our families of origin—our childhood homes—and we continue to play out our roles in the homes we create for ourselves as adults.

So the question of whether a child wears shorts or jeans is not just a fashion statement. In the home, things are never that easy. It's a power struggle between a child who's learning to dress herself and a mom who needs to feel appreciated for knowing what's best. The teenager is learning how to juggle his responsibilities—he is learning that there's never enough time—and his parents have to let him learn it. This slice of life is far more than the hustle and bustle of, say, a newsroom before deadline. It is the interweaving of each family member's growing and changing and hurting and healing.

The workplace is a *machine*. Each employee is a cog in the works—a semiconductor or fan belt or warning light. When one part feels stressed, the surrounding parts may share that stress to some extent. If one employee "breaks down," the whole machine will have to adjust while that "part" is replaced or repaired.

But the home is an *organism*, a living, breathing body with various parts. If one part feels pain, the whole body suffers along with it. It is not just an adjustment, as in the workplace, but a deep empathy, a symbiosis. In the home, one person's stress is everyone's stress.

In the home, one person's stress is everyone's stress.

Thus the home is the scene of the most traumatic events of our lives. A divorce rips up one's home life. A death in the immediate family is devastating. A lost job is a workplace trauma that comes home to roost with the family—there is disappointment, worry, frustration, and doubt all around. Though certain family members may try to shield themselves emotionally from such stress-inducing traumas, this is hard to do. These major events usually rock the whole family.

YOUR TURN

Stressors in the Home

Identify the stressful events that have occurred in the lives of your family members over the past year.

On the line at the left below, write the "point total" for each traumatic event. If the event happened twice, double it; three times, triple it; and so on.

Note: You may wish to define "home" and "family" in your own way, here and throughout this chapter. You may be single with roommates or just a group of friends you consider your "family." You may have extended family or blended family or split-custody arrangements. Adapt these items to apply to your situation.

Point Total	Event	Value
_____	Death in immediate family	4
_____	Separation or divorce	3
_____	Being jailed	3
_____	Pregnancy, new baby	2
_____	Loss of job or bankruptcy	2

____	Marriage in immediate family	2
____	Major change in financial situation	2
____	Injury or major illness in family	2
____	Extended conflict in marriage	2
____	Retirement	2
____	Sexual difficulties in marriage	2
____	Death of a close friend	1
____	New line of work	1
____	Financial concerns or major investment	1
____	Daughter or son leaving home	1
____	Moving to a new home	1
____	Major disciplinary problems with a child	1
____	TOTAL	

This is an adaptation of a detailed study that attempted to correlate specific stressful events with the likelihood of stress-related illness. It is remarkable how many of these major stressors are family related.

If you scored 12 or more, you can consider your home highly stressed.

If you scored 8–11, your home is moderately stressed.

If you scored 6–7, your home has minimal stress.

Below that, check your pulse. You may have stopped breathing.

FOUR GENERAL AREAS OF STRESS

Homes have many stressors, but the most serious (and most common) fall into these four areas: children, the marriage relationship, finances, and time constraints.

Children

The Bible calls children "arrows in the hands of a warrior," but sometimes they can feel like thorns in your side. They are the joy of your life, cute and innocent, and they say the darnedest things. They can also make your life crazy.

For the new parent, it is the constant attention, the messy diapers, the sleepless nights. For the parent with toddlers, there is the boundless energy—and the knowledge that they're always into something. Then they go off to school, and parents become chauffeurs until the kids take the keys and drive themselves. At some point, children realize that their

Examine your attitude toward money and make changes as needed.

Above all, you want to examine your attitude toward money, as a family, and try to alter this as needed. Money should never divide people, especially family members—it just isn't worth it. Money does not determine one's value or identity. It is a gift of God, to be used for God's glory. These attitudes should be taught and practiced within the home.

Avoid

It's hard to avoid money. Cold, hard cash is one of the necessities of life. But with a more Christlike attitude toward money, you can avoid a lot of money-induced stress. Jesus dealt specifically with people who worried about not having enough money. His message, loud and clear, was: "Don't worry. God will take care of you."

God takes care of flowers and birds, Jesus said, so of course he will provide for us. "Do not worry about your life, what you will eat or drink," Jesus taught. "Seek first [God's] kingdom" (Matt. 6:25–34).

The New Testament portrays the desire for money as "a root of all kinds of evil" (1 Tim. 6:10) and warns against giving it too high a priority. "People who want to get rich fall into temptation and a trap and into many foolish and harmful desires that plunge men into ruin and destruction" (1 Tim. 6:9).

We can avoid great stress in our homes by putting money in its place—as a necessity but not as a god. It's something we can use for many purposes, but we must not let it use us.

Accept

Finally, we need to accept what we have been given. Instead of reaching for more and more money, we should be thankful for what we have. The apostle Paul told Timothy, "Command those who are rich in this present world not to be arrogant nor to put their hope in wealth, which is so uncertain, but to put their hope in God, who richly provides us with everything for our enjoyment" (1 Tim. 6:17).

Whatever your current bank account looks like, you are rich. God gives you everything you need for your enjoyment. When an entire family adopts an attitude of thankfulness for the material things they have, their financial stress will be greatly curtailed.

TIME

In many homes, family members pass like minivans in the night, waving as they run off to choir practice, soccer games, business meetings, and church services. If this is Tuesday, these must be Belgian waffles we're having for dinner, zapped in the microwave by Dad or Junior or the babysitter. Teenagers have Day-timers these days, and preschoolers have to schedule their bedtime stories. How can families handle the time crunch?

Alter

You may need to make some major adjustments in your life or in your family's life. You may need to pull out of some commitments in order to spend time with your family. And your family may need to drop some activities to spend time with you. How important is your family life, and what sacrifices will you make to preserve it?

One family we know agreed that everyone would be home for dinner at six o'clock each evening. In rare circumstances, a family member might be excused, but in general this was a sacred time. The whole family scheduled its life around this time, and that wasn't easy with three teenagers in the house. All three were heavily involved in church and school activities, but they were home each night at six. That family's kids are now in their thirties, and they manage to get together every Christmas and for some summer vacations. Their togetherness has lasted.

However, you may need to alter your schedule merely by managing it better. If you arrange things well, you may be able to schedule family time together in the midst of a maze of other activities. The next three chapters give practical tips for time management. These may help you make the alterations you need in your family calendar.

Avoid

You can avoid some time stress by being careful about time wasters. One major culprit in most homes is the TV set. Children spend far too many hours watching mindless TV shows; then they complain that they don't have time to do their chores. They often learn the TV habit from their parents.

Parents need to model wise TV viewing for their children. Do not just sit and watch something because it's the next thing on. Decide as a family what shows are worth watching, and turn the set off in between those shows. Many families adopt a quota system for TV viewing. Children may watch only X number of hours per day or per week. When these regulations are strictly observed, it may bring on momentary stress ("Please, Mom, just one more show!"), but it will yield a better home life in the long run.

Increasingly, children (and many adults) are wasting time with video games and computer networking. Some of these activities can be instructive, but they can also be dangerously habit forming. Most video games are designed to be addictive, and computer chats can go on for hours. Kids are surfing the Internet late into the night and losing sleep. Parents should put restrictions on how much time is spent in these activities.

> **There is not enough time in the day to accomplish everything we have set our sights on. We need to accept that fact and revise our plans accordingly.**

Accept

Time stress can also be alleviated when we merely accept that we can't do everything. There is not enough time in the day to accomplish everything we have set our sights on. We need to accept that fact and revise our plans accordingly.

This attitude may also be taught to children. Yes, they should learn to honor commitments and abide by schedules, but there are often extenuating circumstances. And sometimes kids make bad choices, playing Myst for hours and leaving ten minutes to do homework. Adopt a wise but caring approach in such situations. Teach the children what they need to learn, but try to ease their panic.

Another point of acceptance is understanding time as a gift from God. When we see it that way, it makes sense to follow God's guidance in our use of time. God worked six days and then rested. In the Old Testament concept of the Sabbath, he has given us a pattern of work and rest.

Most Christians, of course, celebrate the "Sabbath" on Sunday, the Lord's Day. But Jesus taught that the Sabbath was intended for our benefit and that we shouldn't have to follow stringent rules about what we can and cannot do on that day. The purpose of the Sabbath is to *stop* what you normally do and rest! Unwind. Use the time to reflect on God . . . worship . . . go fishing . . . enjoy a ball game. We don't need to feel guilty for enjoying our Sabbath. That's what it was created for.

So accept this God-given principle—one day a week for restoration and rebuilding. Spend time with your family, have some fun, and put aside the normal pressures of life.

YOUR TURN

AAA Action Plan for the Home

What would you say are your four greatest stressors at home? Consider issues with children, family, money, and time, but don't limit yourself to these categories, and try to be more specific. (Don't write, "Children." Write, "Johnny always wants more attention.") List those four main stressors in the numbered spaces below.

Then, consider your alter-avoid-accept strategy. What can you do to alter, avoid, or accept these stressors?

1. _____

   Alter: _____

   _____

   Avoid: _____

   _____

   Accept: _____

2. _____

   Alter: _____

   _____

   Avoid: _____

   _____

   Accept: _____

3. _____

   Alter: _____

   _____

   Avoid: _____

   _____

   Accept: _____

4. _____

   Alter: _____

   _____

   Avoid: _____

   _____

   Accept: _____

13

Time Management: Priorities

When Tom Whiteman leads training seminars or workshops on communication skills, he often asks the participants to pair up and practice their listening skills. He asks one person in the pair to talk about the greatest stressors in his or her life, while the other person listens and empathizes. As he circulates through the room, listening, he finds a common theme to most of the conversations.

"I'm always rushing around and have no time to myself."

"I never seem to get caught up."

"I work all day but end the day even further behind than when I started."

"I just can't do all I have to do."

People just don't have enough time.

But Tom suspects that time is not really the problem. In fact, if we were to add five or six hours to every day, within a very short time we would be working at a hectic pace again, never really getting caught up.

When it comes to our stressful lifestyle, time is not the problem; the problem is how we manage our time.

No, it's *time management* that's to blame. And our stress will just get worse if we don't make gutsy changes in our time and lifestyle choices.

What are the results of ineffective time management?

1. We feel we are constantly rushing around.

2. We are never fully at peace, because there is always unfinished business that requires our attention.

3. We often force ourselves to make unpleasant choices, because we have overcommitted ourselves and don't know how to get out of obligations.

4. We are always rushing at last minute to finish projects, or we frequently miss deadlines.

5. We put off our own interests and hobbies, and other important activities, due to the "tyranny of the urgent."

6. Our family and loved ones suffer, because of our hectic pace.

7. We spend much of our time doing what we don't want to do, and very little time doing the things we wish we could.

YOUR TURN

1. How many of those seven things are true in your life?

___ I am constantly rushing around.

___ I am never fully at peace, because there is always unfinished business that requires my attention.

___ I often force myself to make unpleasant choices, because I have overcommitted myself and don't know how to get out of obligations.

___ I am always rushing at last minute to finish projects, or I frequently miss deadlines.

___ I put off my own interests and hobbies, and other important activities, due to the "tyranny of the urgent."

___ My family and loved ones suffer, because of my hectic pace.

___ I spend much of my time doing what I don't want to do, and very little time doing the things I wish I could.

2. Which is the most severe for you? _____

3. If you were to give yourself a letter grade on time management (A to F) what would it be? _____

PRIORITIES

Examining the literature on time management, we can reduce the suggestions into three basic categories.

1. Establish priorities in your life, set goals, and identify what is important to you.

2. Free up time by delaying or saying no to low-priority items.

3. Take items off your agenda by making effective decisions and delegating responsibility to others.

These actions will not be easy, especially if you have deeply ingrained time-wasting habits. It will take time to see significant changes, perhaps several weeks. And in the short term, a program of better time management may actually *increase* stress (as any lifestyle change will), but the long-term benefits are rich.

We have no desire to turn you into an automaton, rigidly following your date book down to each microsecond. Flexibility is a virtue—but so is sensibility. And there are some clear, workable steps you can take to make better use of the time you have.

LIFESTYLE CHANGE: DETERMINE YOUR PRIORITIES AND SET GOALS THAT WILL REFLECT THOSE PRIORITIES

Determining Your Priorities

Tom Landry of the Dallas Cowboys was one of the winningest coaches in pro football. Addressing a group of college students, he was asked about the secret of his success. At the beginning of his career, he replied, he determined his priorities for life—"God, family, and then football."

As you consider all of the jobs and responsibilities that you have, try to determine what your priorities will be. Probably your family, your spiritual life, your job, and yourself would be high on your priority list. But what other responsibilities do you now have that you find you just can't keep up with? Perhaps these include committee meetings, church and school organizations, family obligations, and so on. Even though all of these things are quite worthwhile, you may find that you just can't do them all. You may have to choose some of these activities to give up or at least to put on a back burner.

How do you determine which activities are most important? You need to consider how each matches up with your overall life goals and priorities.

Molly is a good example here. As the single mother of three children, Molly found she didn't have the time or energy for all of her obligations. She had a membership at the local YMCA, but with her new lifestyle, she found that she had little time to go there. She was about to cancel her membership, when she took the time to list her priorities. Her children and her own health were high on her priority list. So on second thought she decided to renew her membership and cut out some other activities that were keeping her out at night. She found the YMCA to be a great place for her to play together with her children, and found the aerobics classes to be beneficial to her state of mind.

This is a case where a seemingly unimportant activity actually became more important as a single mother thought about her priorities. It is critical that you not neglect yourself in this formula.

YOUR TURN

Priorities

Rate the following items in terms of their importance to you. Write H for high-priority items, M for middle-level priorities, and L for low-priority items. Be sure to fill in any high-priority items from your life that we may have missed.

_____ Spiritual life
_____ Career
_____ Home life
_____ Spouse (or other relationship)
_____ Children

____ School activities
     specifically:_____
____ Church activities
     specifically:_____
____ Yourself
____ Friendship
     specifically:_____
____ Social functions
     specifically:_____
____ Hobbies
     specifically:_____
____ Exercise
____ Reading
____ Sleep
____ Relaxation
Others:

_____
_____
_____

There's no need to come up with an exact sequence of priorities. But it does help to get a sense of your top four or five, then another handful in a middle echelon. You want to make sure there is enough time in your schedule for all of your high-priority areas, and some time in your week for midlevel items. Low-priority items can be put off until you have time to spare.

Setting Goals

Now that you have determined your priorities, it is important that your goals flow out of those priorities. What do you hope to accomplish in your life? Over the next five years? Over the next year? Tom tries to write these down each year for his work and his personal life. Each new year he reviews them, sees what he's accomplished and what he's neglected. His priorities rarely change, but each year several of his goals do change. Therefore even though you may have a five-year plan, you need to be willing to change these plans each year as things in your life change and as you grow and mature.

YOUR TURN

Family Goals

Lifetime

Example: Raise children who are independent but who love and honor God and other people.

_____

_____

_____

_____

_____

_____

Five years

Example: Have my children involved in a solid church and a good educational system.

_____

_____

_____

_____

_____

_____

One year

Examples: Start Bible memory plan with children.
Help Elizabeth with her homework.
Spend individual time with each child every week.

_____

_____

_____

_____

_____

_____

Now do the same kind of planning for other areas of your life. These areas should reflect your priorities, such as career, family, marriage, spiritual growth, and yourself. Some of these areas you may want to discuss with your spouse, your family, or your coworkers.

Work and Career Goals

Lifetime

_____
_____
_____
_____
_____
_____

Five years

_____
_____
_____
_____
_____
_____

One year

_____
_____
_____
_____
_____
_____

Spiritual Goals

Lifetime

_____
_____
_____
_____
_____
_____

Five years

_____
_____

_____
_____
_____
_____

One year

_____
_____
_____
_____
_____

_____**Goals**

Lifetime

_____
_____
_____
_____
_____

Five years

_____
_____
_____
_____

One year

_____
_____
_____
_____

_____Goals
Lifetime

_____
_____
_____
_____
_____

Five years

_____
_____
_____
_____
_____

One year

_____
_____
_____
_____
_____

ADJUSTING YOUR PERSONAL SCHEDULE

Good planning starts with good plotting. That is, to plan your future, you need to take a good look at the past and present. In order to develop a workable, priority-based schedule, start by plotting your activities over a seven-day period. Take a few minutes at several points of the day to list each thing you've done and how much time it took. Also record whether this is a high-, middle-, or low-priority activity. Don't neglect time when you did "nothing." Try to account for each fifteen-minute period.

Your log might look like this:

Lying in bed   Low priority   30 minutes

| Shower, shave, get ready for work | High priority | 45 minutes |
| Singing in shower | Low priority | 15 minutes |

. . . and so on.

It would probably help to use detachable worksheets that you can carry with you. You also might want to break your day into categories that fit your schedule. For Tom, it works best like this:

Before Work

	Activity	*Priority*	*Time*
Example:	Breakfast	H	20 min.
	_____	_____	_____
	_____	_____	_____
	_____	_____	_____
	_____	_____	_____
	_____	_____	_____

During Work

	Activity	*Priority*	*Time*
Example:	Returning phone calls	M	45 min.
	_____	_____	_____
	_____	_____	_____
	_____	_____	_____
	_____	_____	_____
	_____	_____	_____

After Work

	Activity	*Priority*	*Time*
Example:	Play with children	H	20 min.
	_____	_____	_____
	_____	_____	_____
	_____	_____	_____
	_____	_____	_____

After charting your daily activities for several days, write up a summary sheet on how you typically spend your time.

Summary Sheet

Total time spent on high-priority items:_____

Total time spent on midlevel items: _____

Total time spent on low-priority items: _____

Discernment

Now comes the work of discerning. You have probably reached the conclusion that you need to increase time spent on high-priority activities, find ways to do midlevel tasks more efficiently, and eliminate much of the wasted time on low-priority activities. Without adjustments to your schedule, you will probably not accomplish your goals, and this will keep you feeling as if you're spinning your wheels in life.

For example, when Tom examined his own schedule, he found that he spent much too much time watching TV, and even though he set his wife and children as priorities, they got less of his time. While he might find TV relaxing, he is not accomplishing what he needs to do, so ultimately it creates more stress in his life.

At work, Tom was wasting time thinking about whom to call or what to do next, so he concluded that a daily list of his priorities would help him to stay productive. Making a list may seem like more work to do, but again, Tom will feel more productive and less stressed if he can organize his day better.

You might find that you limit showers to five minutes, cut out a late-night TV show in order to rise early enough for prayer and Bible reading, or eliminate hot breakfasts except on Saturday mornings. Your discernment will have to determine what can be cut and what you can do differently in order to insure that your priorities and goals are accomplished.

Now go back over your schedule and write in where you need to make adjustments. Summarize your findings and write them here in the form of a goal. These goals are different from your long-term goals. These will be short-term goals, changes that should take place over the next couple of days, weeks, or (at the most) months. Therefore you need to make them as specific as you can.

YOUR TURN

Goals for Changing Your Schedule

Examples:

1. Watch only one hour of TV after work each day, except for two evening movies per week. (This requires that I get a *TV Guide* and plan my week ahead of time.)
2. Spend at least one hour playing with the kids each night and allow at least one hour to talk to my wife.

Personal schedule changes

_____

_____

_____

_____

_____

_____

Family schedule changes

_____

_____

_____

_____

_____

_____

Work schedule changes

_____

_____

_____

_____

_____

_____

Now all that's left is to put these into practice. Don't expect instant success but work slowly toward implementing these goals.

14

Limiting Time Involvements

During the fall term at college one year, Randy Petersen (one of this book's authors) quickly found himself overwhelmed. He was involved in theater, the school literary magazine, and leading a church youth group, besides trying to keep up with his studies. There just wasn't time for everything. One particular weekend, he felt harried by several specific responsibilities at church and school, and he knew that if he didn't get some more sleep, he'd get seriously sick. He was *almost* getting everything done but not quite. If he could have just one more hour . . .

Then he realized it was the weekend to come off daylight saving time. That night he got his extra hour. Gratefully he got the additional sleep he needed, but soon he was back in the same old grind.

Maybe you've experienced this sort of "found time" when an activity was canceled at the last minute. What a great feeling to have a couple hours—or a day or a week—with nothing scheduled!

But the fact is, we have the ability to "find" time whenever we want. If we really need time for something—for those high-priority parts of our lives—it's there. We just need to borrow it from some other activity.

LIFESTYLE CHANGE: FIND NEW TIME BY LEARNING TO LIMIT YOUR INVOLVEMENT

Learning to Say No

Tom Whiteman is still learning how to say no. If someone has a need and wants him to meet it, he has a terrible time turning that person down. But in order to stick to his priorities in life, sometimes he has to. He can't do it all.

Many others share his problem—perhaps you do, too. "People pleasing" is the culprit. We want to please others, even at the expense of our own well-being. The last thing we want to do is say no to someone. After all, they might think negatively of us if we do. We long for the approval of our children, our family, our church friends, or our coworkers. But no matter who they are, we still need to evaluate each request according to our stated priorities and goals.

> **We have the ability to "find" time whenever we want. If we really need time for something—it's there. We just need to borrow it from some other activity.**

One more person you might need to learn to say no to is yourself. Many stressed-out people make statements similar to this:

"I like a neat and orderly home. I like my children to be on a regular schedule, and I like to have everything in its place at the end of the day. But I just can't seem to do it all. I've had to learn to tolerate a little more chaos and to expect that at any given time, it is most likely that one room in the house is an absolute mess. But that's OK, because I've learned that my sanity is more important than order."

That's a priority statement. Did you catch it? "My sanity is more important than order." Many of us have similar compulsions. These may be seemingly positive, like cleanliness, seemingly trivial, like an "addiction" to video games or soap operas, or potentially harmful, like drinking too much or sleeping around.

In all of these cases, we must examine our choices in light of our priorities. If we have a limited amount of time, is it truly helpful to spend an afternoon in front of the TV or to lose a weekend on a drinking binge (not to mention the other harm that could do)? No. Nor is it very helpful to be frantic about cleaning every square inch of your home. Sometimes you must "just say no" to your own desires or compulsions in order to get on with what's really important.

YOUR TURN

Evaluating Time Requests

1. Look back over your list of priorities and see if there's anything you want to change. Are your priorities where you think they should be? Make any adjustments you think necessary.

2. Now see if you can remember five things you've recently been asked to do, regardless of whether you said yes or no. These may be simple things, like taking your kids to the zoo, or major things, like directing a school play. (If you have kids, try to include at least two requests that did not come from them.)

   1._____

   _____

   2._____

   _____

   3._____

   _____

   4._____

   _____

   5._____

   _____

3. Go back over these five requests and write yes or no in the left margin, to indicate how you responded to the request (or briefly note any compromise response you made).

4. Now consider how each of these tied in with your priorities. If one of these requests would help you accomplish one of the five priorities you listed earlier, write the number of that priority in the margin (next to the yes or no) and circle it.

5. Ideally, you should have numbers next to your yeses and not next to your noes. As you examine these requests in light of your priorities, are there yeses you should have said no to and noes you should have said yes to?

6. How can you use your priorities to make better decisions in the future?

_____

_____

_____

Getting Rid of Low-Priority Activities

If your higher-priority items are suffering from a lack of time, then one way you can gain time is to postpone or eliminate low-priority items. For example, Tom Whiteman identified TV as a big time-consumer of his but a low priority. Even when he has set the goal of only two movies a week, when he is falling behind and needs more time, then obviously he can cut out a week or two of TV.

On the other hand, TV might be a good way Tom can reduce stress, so he might choose to give up something else. Maybe he could stop going out for lunch for a few weeks. He could pack a lunch and work at his desk in order to get caught up, even if just for a limited time. Time management is a constant process of making decisions about our priorities and our needs, and protecting our mental health.

As you identify areas to eliminate, make sure they are not all things that you do for yourself. If you're a people pleaser and working on saying no, you might find it easier to give up your own needs in order to continue serving others. But your relaxation, quiet times, hobbies, or pleasure reading are important, perhaps more important than one more committee meeting, another family obligation, or a dinner with a client.

YOUR TURN

Ditching the Low Priorities

List two low-priority items you could give up for a period of time. Indicate how long you will try to live without these. (Try at least a week.)

_____Time period: _____

_____Time period: _____

Avoiding Time Traps

Before you can avoid wasting time, you must first identify where you are wasting it. You may need to look in some less obvious places. We typically think of sleeping in, long baths, sitting and staring into space, but many times these are just indications that we are overloaded and need to sit and regroup.

Some people are always busy. Every time you look at them, they're on the phone, writing, shuffling papers, or moving purposefully about the office. These are not people who get questioned about what they are doing all day. They are not lethargic, listless, or lazy. Yet even these people can be incredible time-wasters.

An employer had high praise for one of his middle managers, who left the company for another job. "Will was a terrific worker, always industrious, working late hours. I made it a point to warn the woman who replaced him that she would have difficulty keeping up with the job. Imagine my surprise when she was able to do the same job in half the time!"

As it turned out, Will had been very thorough but was very redundant and unorganized. He was constantly trying to keep up with the immediate demand and therefore didn't have time to plan ahead. His replacement did have some difficulty, the boss said, because Will had left a very disorganized filing system. Many important accounts were not keyed into the computer properly. The new manager had to retrieve the information from handwritten notes stuffed in drawers. For all of Will's hard work, it seems he wasn't getting a lot done.

Your work style, whether on the job or at home, can have a tremendous influence on how much time you waste. It is not the late mornings in bed or the sitting to watch a ball game that bothers Tom Whiteman the most. It is the unproductive time he spends on projects that turn out to be unneeded or redundant. Invariably he finds that if he had merely *planned his work* and then *worked his plan,* he would have saved himself much time and effort.

YOUR TURN

Suggestions

Look over the list of timesaving suggestions below. Check off the ideas that you think would be helpful to you. Now choose three that you could implement most easily, and begin to use them in your daily life. Once those are integrated into your work habits, come back to the list and choose three more.

____ Computerize your mailing lists and addresses.

____ Computerize your bill paying or pay by phone.

____ Each day, make a list of things you must do and then check them off as they are accomplished.

____ When you make a meal, make two and freeze one.

____ Write a list of things that can be done in five minutes or less and then do them when you have a free minute or two.

____ Get up a half hour earlier.

____ Reduce your get-ready time in the morning.

____ Learn to do two things at once: do nails while watching TV; dictate your "things to do" list while driving; plan your day while cleaning your room.

____ Organize your mail into an "immediate" pile, a "when you can" pile, and junk mail (to scan and toss).

____ Buy books on tape for those long drives in the car.

____ Organize your desk.

____ Schedule a time for meditation, relaxation, or planning your day.

____ Pray while you drive (but keep your eyes open).

____ Don't spend time worrying about things that may never happen.

____ Keep a list in the car of errands to run, so when you go out, you can do several at a time.

Rejecting Perfectionism

Being a perfectionist can cause you a great deal of unnecessary stress and anxiety. No one is perfect, and no project should be expected to be perfect. Some people rewrite the same letter a dozen times in order to make it just right. But for most people, the crunch of their workload does not afford them the luxury of doing everything the way they want it to be. Quality? Yes! But they may need to lower their expectations slightly in order to get the job done and move on to other business.

If you are a student, settle for B's. A's are nice if you can get them. But if they take too much time or energy, settle for B's or C's.

One of the best things that happened to Shelley was a D+ she got in college on her first exam in a freshman literature course. She had received straight A's in high school, graduating at the head of her class, and she assumed she would fare similarly well in college. But this literature course left Shelley clueless. The D+ was a shocker—she had never received a grade so low. Though she worked hard to get her final grade up to a B–, her straight-A record was broken, here in her first semester of college.

But looking back on it, Shelley sees that this helped her relax. She was able to enjoy college, getting involved in several extracurricular activities. Though she didn't get the 4.0 average she would have liked, she ended with a respectable 3.5—and many other great experiences.

It all goes back to your priorities. If you're headed for medical school, you need those A's. Work for the A's and cut out some of your other activities. But if you cannot maintain a healthy, well-rounded life and still do the work required for straight A's, stay healthy and get some B's. In the total scheme of life, it probably won't change your future very much.

If you are a parent, don't engage your children over every issue but instead pick your battles carefully, according to your priorities.

As a housekeeper, clean just one room at a time. That way, on any given day there is at least one room that is not clean. You can relax, knowing that one or two rooms are clean but that your house will never be perfect. It will still be, however, comfortable and livable.

Office workers, if being the best in your office means killing yourself and neglecting your family, then settle for being above average. Psychologist J. Clayton Lafferty studied more than nine thousand managers and professionals and reached this conclusion: "Striving for perfection is likely to harm employees and companies alike." Apart from the extra stress that perfectionists put on themselves, they regularly put themselves in time binds. "Because they equate their self-worth with flawless performance, perfectionists often get hung up on meaningless details and spend more time on projects than is necessary. Ultimately, productivity suffers."[1]

The thought life of a perfectionist is represented below. Which of these perfectionistic thoughts have you had?

1. I have a hard time determining what is realistically within my control. I take responsibility for things that are beyond my control (for example, my children's decisions, my spouse's behavior).
2. I'm afraid to try new things or to change, because I'm afraid I'll fail.
3. I try to take on too much or to control those around me.
4. I don't like the thought of being mediocre or average.
5. I'm not satisfied with less than one-hundred-percent effort in myself or others.
6. I'm too hard on myself. I continually do not achieve my own expectations.
7. I constantly compare myself to others and tend to come up lacking.
8. I have been accused of being too rigid or legalistic.
9. I have obsessional thoughts that plague me as I review over and over what I should have said or done differently.
10. I have a hard time enjoying social gatherings, especially if I am responsible for making sure everything runs smoothly.

If these thoughts sound familiar to you, then you are probably placing an undue burden or stress on yourself. You may in fact be your own worst enemy. You need to work on the following areas:

1. Learn to relax.
2. Give yourself permission to fail. (Send your next letter out with a spelling error.)
3. Let go of your need to control those around you. (If you are tempted to "play God," remember that even God allows his creatures to make free choices. You can do the same.)
4. Lower your standards and expectations.
5. Refuse to entertain thoughts about how it could have been or should have been. Remind yourself that you did what you did and that's fine. Now it's time to move on.
6. Learn to laugh at yourself and to enjoy life.

YOUR TURN

If you tend to be a perfectionist, choose one of the six recommendations above that you can begin to apply in your life. Think of a situation in the next week in which you could begin to put this into practice. How will you do this?

_____

_____

_____

_____

15

Decisions and Delegation

Meetings," Susan complained. "That's all we do at work anymore. We have meetings." She was on the management team for a financial services company.

"Like this morning," she went on. "We had this writer we hired to put together a training manual for this new area we're doing, and he brought us the copy. It was pretty good; we all liked it. Then George sees something on page twenty-seven that's not quite right, so we talk about it for five minutes, and of course everyone has an opinion. Tina has a problem with page thirty-five, which takes ten minutes."

Susan's smile was covering a deep frustration. "I'm all for group process and everything, but we had our five top executives in there this morning, and we wasted an hour trying to edit this manual *together*. I mean, can't we hire people and let them do that? I shudder to think of what that manual is costing us—if you were paying us by the hour, that's a pretty hefty sum. Why can't we just let the writer write?"

Susan's complaint is all too common. Especially in business but also in families and in general life, people waste precious time and face needless stress, because they can't make decisions or let others make them.

There is a value in the group process, to be sure. There are issues that executive teams need to review together. But efficient businesses know how to streamline the decision-making process, allowing adequate input but not time-wasting table tennis.

Wise executives know how to delegate responsibilities and let them go—perhaps with some review process but not with detailed involvement.

Time is also lost, however, when all the key decisions revert to one person. If that person has too much on his or her plate, there can be costly delays. Wise executives know how to delegate responsibilities and *let them go*—perhaps with some review process but not with detailed involvement.

LIFESTYLE CHANGE: LEARN TO MAKE DECISIONS AND TO DELEGATE

Learning to Make Decisions

For some people, just making a decision can be stressful. It can also be a time-wasting dilemma. A classic example is when Tom Whiteman moved himself and ten of his colleagues into new office space. They brought their furniture to the new location, where they had eleven private offices to choose from. Within a day, Tom picked his office and moved his things in, telling the others to decide among themselves who would get which office. Well, if you know any counselors, you know that the group process is very important. These counselors had to process how they felt about each office, how the sun hit it in the morning, how the ambience might change throughout all four seasons, how their furniture would fit and look, how the colors made the room feel, and a hundred other considerations. They ended up playing musical offices for the next four weeks.

Tom's colleagues would insist that he exaggerates the story, and they'd probably be right. But they do laugh about it whenever it comes up. What would Tom do differently the next time new space became available? He'd go in ahead of time and just assign office space. People might not like it as much, but it would sure save time.

If you're a person who has a hard time making a decision, then you are probably aware of the time and energy you expend in the process. Changing indecisiveness is a very difficult job, particularly if it is deeply ingrained into the fabric of your life. But indecisiveness is learned, and therefore it can be unlearned. It will, however, take tough choices and regular practice before decision making comes easily.

YOUR TURN

1. On a scale of 1 to 10, how decisive are you (10 is most)? _____

2. How long did it take you to answer that question? _____

3. What's the most major decision you've made in the last year?

   _____

   _____

4. List two decisions, major or minor, that you've made in the last week.

   _____

   _____

5. Do you think you would have decided differently on any of these matters if you had spent less time on the decision? _____

6. Would the outcome have been better or worse? _____

7. Major decisions still need major consideration. But wisdom lies in recognizing which decisions are minor and can be decided quickly.

Don't look back. Once a decision is made, you may still second-guess it. That's a problem for many, producing major anxiety. They live their lives in the land of "should haves" and "could haves." This is an incredible waste of time and energy, since most decisions cannot be undone. It's best to live with your decision—or learn from it and use that knowledge to make a better choice next time.

Practice telling yourself one or more of the following phrases.

1. "What's the worst that can happen?"

This is especially helpful for small decisions. When you're agonizing over whether you should go to the school conference tonight or stay home because you're feeling especially run-down, ask yourself, "What's the worst that will happen if I miss this conference tonight?" Here's how the conversation with the counselor in your brain should go:

Self: "Then the teacher won't give me feedback on my son."
Counselor: "So what's the worst that will happen if I don't get the feedback?"

Self:	"It might be very important."
Counselor:	"Well, if it's important, wouldn't the teacher call me or write me a note?"
Self:	"Yeah, you're right, but she's liable to think I'm a bad parent."
Counselor:	"Well, what's the worst that will happen if she thinks less of me?"
Self:	"Nothing will really happen. I can just send her a note tomorrow and tell her why I missed. If she is upset, then I guess that's on her. I can't be responsible for what she thinks."

2. *"I made the best decision I could with the information I had at the time. Whatever the outcome, I'll make the most of it."*

This applies to major decisions, which can be subject to major second-guessing. Practice this phrase for yourself. It really works! Whether the decision is big or small, we can only deal with the knowledge we have at the time. Hindsight might tell us more about what we might have done, but don't worry about hindsight. That's a no-win situation. We can't look back. We must learn and look forward.

Many have agonized over the decisions involved in buying a house. These choices can cost or save thousands of dollars. Should you lock in at a certain interest rate? Or should you wait in case the rates go down? Of course, the experts disagree on the direction of rates, so you can constantly agonize over this. But what's the worst that will happen? Well, a wrong choice would mean a higher mortgage payment each month. If that thought isn't very comforting, try the next phrase: "I made the best decision I could. Once the decision is made, there's no sense in looking back."

3. *"God is still in control, life still goes on, and I can adjust to whatever happens."*

This is another comforting phrase that we should practice often. God never wakes up and says, "Oh, no! Look at what happened while I wasn't paying attention!" As Christians, we can trust that God is in control of our lives. Yes, we make mistakes, but God is still in control. As long as our attitude is one of submission to him, there is really nothing for us to fear.

YOUR TURN

Take the gist of one of the phrases above and put it in your own words. Or make up a whole new pep talk, to keep yourself from wasteful second-guessing of decisions you've already made.

_____

_____

_____

_____

Learning to Delegate

You know what they say: "If you want something done right, you've got to do it yourself." This may be a common truism, but it's not really right. The truth is, you *can't* do it all yourself. We need to learn to ask for help and then to accept it graciously.

Once you've set your priorities and started saying no to any responsibilities that don't fit into your most urgent needs, there still remain those tasks that you would like to say no to but that must get done anyway—like cutting the grass or walking the dog or taking out the trash or maintaining the car—the list goes on and on. This is where the art of delegation comes in handy.

Look first to your spouse and children. Allow them to take on appropriate tasks that might ease your load. (Keep in mind, though, how busy *they* are.) There are other tasks for which you will need a support network of people you can count on. We suggest that you begin thinking now of people you would like to include in a list of trusted friends, counselors, and skilled professionals that you can call on for help.

YOUR TURN

1. What roles do you need help with? Put a check next to all that apply.

_____ Advisor	_____ Housekeeper
_____ Bill payer	_____ Investor
_____ Bookkeeper	_____ Landscaper
_____ Cook	_____ Launderer
_____ Counselor	_____ Decorator
_____ Mechanic	_____ Painter
_____ Gardener	_____ Provider

2. What other jobs do you need help with?

_____

_____

3. Now look back over the roles you checked or listed. Rather than take all of them on yourself, why not delegate? Try thinking of people who might help you accomplish those tasks. Next to all of the roles you've indicated, write the initials of the people whom you might ask to fill those roles or who are already filling them. (Remember that not all the roles need to be filled.)

_____ _____

_____ _____

_____ _____

_____ _____

_____ _____

4. In the space below, jot the names of your children and then list the tasks and roles they now have in the home. This is not what they *should* take on but the roles they are in fact assuming.

_____ _____

_____ _____

_____ _____

_____ _____

_____ _____

5. Now go back over this list. Are there any tasks or responsibilities that are just too great for them to take on? Are there any that are inappropriate for their age? If so, circle these.

6. Are there any that they *should* be able to handle, but they're just not doing them well enough? Put a box around these.

7. Are there other tasks that you need for them to take on (assuming that the tasks are appropriate to their age and abilities)? If so, write these in and underline them.

parents are not perfect, that they can make mistakes. Then comes the time when they are sure that their parents *always* make mistakes. Conflict is common in adolescence. And even if the kids go off to college, there are the financial obligations and constant worries about their welfare.

Is one age better than another? Most parents say NO. They typically describe headaches and joys of each developmental stage. As one parent advised us, "The problems are always there; they merely evolve."

> **It is important to remember that we don't want to remove stress from our lives; that would be impossible. Stress is normal and natural, especially with children.**

The Whiteman kids are at the toddler stage. Tom and his wife look forward to the day when they are a little more independent. (Tom wants to be reminded about this statement when they are teenagers.) They are glad to be out of the diaper stage, and at least they sleep through the night. And they thank God for the fact that they can actually take their eyes off them for a minute or so without worrying. There have been times when they thought this day would never come. Yet now that their kids are older, they find they are dealing with new stresses, such as peer pressure, schoolwork, and busy schedules. Those who are ahead of them in their parenting say, "Enjoy these good years with your kids, because it will all change."

Once again, it is important to remember that we don't want to *remove* stress from our lives; that would be impossible. Stress is normal and natural, especially for parents. There are several natural dynamics that enter the picture.

Growth. Growth brings stress. You can see this graphically when your seven-year-old pulls on last summer's T-shirt and it's two sizes too small. You can see the stress of that growing body pushing at the seams.

The same is true of emotional and intellectual growth. As children develop, they—and you as parents—encounter stress along the way. New ideas shatter the old assumptions. New loves and losses bring pain to innocent hearts.

Power struggles. Children are on a trajectory from the total dependency of the infant to the total independence of the adult. At every step of the way, there is a new negotiation to be made. Sometimes these happen easily, but usually there is struggle. Children often think they are further along that trajectory than they really are. Especially in adolescence, they reach for more independence than they can handle. Parents often try to hold children back, keeping them dependent, preventing them from moving forward on that trajectory.

These struggles can be violent and hurtful or sane and reasoned, but they are inevitable. There is a transfer of power going on, and it can be Civil war in Bosnia or free elections in South Africa. And even the easiest transfers cause stress.

Anxiety. Can there be anything more nervous than a parent giving a teenager the keys to the car and watching the kid drive away? Or watching the teenage daughter walk off arm in arm with her date, that mysterious boy with the nose ring?

Or sending the ten-year-old away on a weekend retreat? Or seeing the six-year-old off to school with his Power Rangers lunch box clanging at his side?

Parenting is a process of letting go. And it's never easy. It's natural to feel anxiety as children take each new, unsupervised step.

Special needs. We have great respect for single parents. How do they do it all? It's hard enough for a tag team of two parents, trading off the child-tending responsibilities when necessary. But what do you do when you're ready to scream but have no one else to help you? (That happens not only to single parents but also to married parents who feel they get no help from their spouses.)

And there are also stresses that arise from special needs of the children, or circumstances in the home:

- a handicapped child
- a rebellious teenager
- learning problems
- drug or alcohol abuse
- a teenage pregnancy
- a child-custody battle
- a heartbroken child

All of these scenarios can cause parents incredible heartache and stress. In the next chapter, we will give specific suggestions for altering, avoiding, and accepting these stresses. For now you need to remember that such stresses are natural, understandable. You are not necessarily odd, dysfunctional, or unspiritual if you have stress from your children. This stress will be there. The question is, How will you manage it?

YOUR TURN
Child-Related Stress

List the children in your home by name and age and consider the stresses they feel and the stresses they cause. (We offer space to list three children. If you have more, photocopy these pages before you fill them in.)

Child: _____ Age: _____

What stresses do you believe this child feels?

Growth (consider physical development, sexual development, learning, emotional experiences, etc.):

_____
_____
_____
_____

Activities and pressures (include school, sports, church groups, other organizations, and tasks):

_____
_____
_____
_____

Social involvement (include peer relationships, dating, best friends, etc.):

_____
_____
_____

Self-concept (what stresses does this child feel in his or her understanding of self?):

_____
_____
_____

Other stresses:

_____

_____

_____

How do any of these stresses affect the stress of the home?
In general:

_____

_____

_____

Power struggle (what issues of independence have been a matter of conflict?):

_____

_____

_____

Anxiety (what things do you worry most about?):

_____

_____

_____

....

Child: _____Age: _____

What stresses do you believe this child feels?

Growth (consider physical development, sexual development, learning, emotional experiences, etc.):

_____

_____

_____

Activities and pressures (include school, sports, church groups, other organizations, and tasks):

_____

_____

_____

Social involvement (include peer relationships, dating, best friends, etc.):

_____

_____

_____

Self-concept (what stresses does this child feel in his or her understanding of self?):

_____

_____

_____

Other stresses:

_____

_____

_____

How do any of these stresses affect the stress of the home?
In general:

_____

_____

_____

Power struggle (what issues of independence have been a matter of conflict?):

_____

_____

_____

Anxiety (what things do you worry most about?):

_____

_____

_____

• •

Child: _____ Age: _____

What stresses do you believe this child feels?

Growth (consider physical development, sexual development, learning, emotional experiences, etc.):

_____

_____

_____

_____

Activities and pressures (include school, sports, church groups, other organizations, and tasks):

_____

_____

_____

_____

Social involvement (include peer relationships, dating, best friends, etc.):

_____

_____

_____

_____

Self-concept (what stresses does this child feel in his or her understanding of self?):

_____

_____

_____

Other stresses:

_____

_____

_____

How do any of these stresses affect the stress of the home?
In general:

_____

_____

_____

Power struggle (what issues of independence have been a matter of conflict?):

_____

_____

_____

_____

Anxiety (what things do you worry most about?):

_____

_____

_____

The Marriage Relationship

Another key stressor in the home is the marriage relationship. (If you are not married, you can probably substitute a "significant other" in your life: a roommate, a romantic relationship, or a very close friendship.) Primary relationships in our lives can cause us significant stress when they're going well, and overwhelming stress when they're not.

The Bible describes marriage as "two becoming one." Two people with different minds, different wills, different backgrounds, and different dreams decide to merge their lives. Of course there will be stress!

There is something of a Trinitarian mystery here. As God is three and yet one, so a married couple is two and yet one. The partners do not totally give up their individuality, but they do enter this new corporation, this marriage. There is bound to be stress in this interaction. At some level, a married person is always dealing with "me" and "us."

> **Marriage can be your greatest source of joy, but it can also be your source of greatest stress.**

You might think of a marriage as a three-legged race. Remember that crazy activity from camp or Sunday school picnics? Two people are tied together at the leg and told to run across a field. Every other step is a joint effort. Every other step is an individual effort. Me. Us. Me. Us. Me. Us.

Some couples manage this very well, but even they experience stress. Where does marital stress come from?

Different backgrounds. We learn marriage from our parents, for good or ill. If a wife's father took out the trash, she will expect her husband to do it. If the husband's mother took out the trash, he will expect his wife to do it. They may sit around for weeks with the trash piling up, each resenting the other for not doing his or her job.

He may expect her to stay home and cook the meals, because that's what his mom did. She may expect to work outside the home, because that's what her mom did. She may look to him to provide spiritual leadership in the home, because her dad did. He may expect her to do so, because his dad wasn't a Christian.

She may be Baptist, he Presbyterian. He may be Republican, she Democrat. He may watch action movies, while she prefers love stories. She may want to spank the kids, while he finds that abhorrent. Each of these areas is a matter of conflicting assumptions. Couples must talk these issues through and decide where the compromises will be made.

Different styles. He may pick his nose. She may pick her teeth. He may snore. She may sneeze. Sometimes people have habits that their partners find disgusting.

But even more often it's a manner of speaking or thinking that causes conflict in marriages. The Myers-Briggs Type Indicator is one of several tests that delineate different personality types.[1] Some people, they say, are perceivers, while others are judgers. These two types may work well together, but there is bound to be conflict. The perceiver never makes up his mind, while the judger decides things quickly. There are also feelers and thinkers, introverts and extroverts.

These are not insurmountable differences, but they will cause stress. Husbands and wives need to understand each other's styles and allow for those.

Of course, there are also major differences in just being male or female. A growing body of research indicates that there are clear differences in brain structure between men and women. Not that one is better than the other—they're just different. Men and women think differently. Surprise! (The brain differences combine with cultural differences in our upbringing to make us operate in very different ways.) So there are reasons that men don't ask for directions, and that women talk about feelings before facts. There are reasons for men to withdraw from conversation and for women to feel threatened by that.

As we understand our gender differences, we can alleviate some of the stress this causes.[2]

Different dreams. What if one partner dreams of buying a comfortable split-level in the suburbs, while the other dreams of getting involved in an inner-city ministry? What if one dreams of corporate success, while the other wants to chuck it all and be a freelance writer? What if one wants to retire to Florida and the other to Vermont?

We invest a lot of mental and emotional energy in our dreams. It's tough to adjust them and, in some cases, scrap them to accommodate the dreams of our partners. This is yet another edge of conflict in marriage.

Disappointment. We marry our partners and then they change. Sometimes those changes delight us, but often they disappoint us.

Part of this is the natural change from wooing to working. Before a marriage, the partners try to show each other their best sides. Men bring flowers and open doors. Women dress their best and try hard to seem interested in the minutiae of the man's life. But once the commitment is made, people get back to their real selves. This can be a disappointment for both.

We also age. Many people are, frankly, disappointed that their partners have grown fat or bald or gray or sickly or just plain old. Our cultural obsession with youth and looks does nothing to help this situation.

Marital stress is eased as we come to accept and even appreciate the aging process and learn to accept our partners for who they are.

Power struggle. Who really calls the shots? If the two marriage partners want separate things, what do they do? Who wins?

This power struggle occurs even when a couple agrees on the husband being the "head of the home." In this arrangement, wives often find ways to influence the husbands' decisions. The struggle goes on under the surface, in hurt feelings and innuendoes. In homes that practice "mutual submission," the struggle may be more obvious. And many Christian couples struggle because both partners want to give in to the other.

These struggles are not always bad—they are the natural exchange of different opinions. You want to dine at Houlihan's, but I want to go to the Olive Garden. Let's decide. You want to buy new drapes, but I want a power mower. Let's decide.

Whether the exchange is congenial or nasty, there is potential for stress. The best relationships are not those without conflict but those that manage their conflicts well.

Great expectations, and needs not met. Many people enter marriage expecting it to solve all their problems. They soon learn that for every problem marriage solves, it creates two new problems. This goes beyond the disappointment mentioned earlier. This is a matter of needs.

A woman may need her self-esteem regularly bolstered, but that flattering lady-killer she married is now tearing her down at every opportunity. A man may need a wife to support him in his profession, but that fawning beauty he married is now complaining that he spends too much time at work.

Needs also change as we grow. In many homes in the past few decades, wives have "grown" from homemakers to career women. Whether that's a good move to make or not, many husbands have found it hard to deal with. They "needed" the house cleaned, meals cooked, and so on, and they stopped getting those needs met. Meanwhile the wives "needed" the challenge of employment, or the self-esteem of their own jobs, and they felt that their husbands were holding them back.

> **People enter marriage expecting it to solve their problems. They soon learn that for every problem marriage solves, it creates two new problems.**

We often counsel men and women who feel they have "grown beyond" their spouses—they have new needs that are not being met—and they wonder if they need to find someone new. Many times this is just a smoke screen for a midlife crisis or a seven-year itch, but sometimes people's needs do change. Couples have to learn how to deal with this, and that can bring great stress.

Fear of losing one's spouse. Especially in this age of rampant divorce, people are often afraid that their spouses will leave them. This fear can create a very tense cat-and-mouse game.

Say a woman feels her husband is withdrawing from her. She panics and clings desperately to him, which makes him want to withdraw more, which makes her panic more, and so forth.

Or say a man fears that his wife might leave him. Fearing the emotional pain he might suffer, he holds back from investing himself in the relationship. Sensing that he is not investing in the relationship, she holds back, too.

This is the sort of stress that is usually held inside. Most of the time, it does not come out in arguments and fights, but it churns in the heart of each marriage partner. "What should I say? What should I do? I can't do that or that. What will my spouse think?"

As with so many aspects of interpersonal stress, communication is crucial.

YOUR TURN

Marital Stress

Background

1. Describe ways in which your background and your spouse's are similar.

   _____

   _____

   _____

   _____

2. Describe ways in which your background and your spouse's are different.

   _____

   _____

   _____

   _____

3. Circle any of those differences that cause stress in your home.

Style

1. Describe any of your spouse's habits or quirks that get on your nerves.

   _____

   _____

   _____

   _____

2. Have you and your spouse taken any personality tests, such as the Myers-Briggs Type Indicator? If so, what have you learned about the compatibility or incompatibility of your personalities? If not, what can you say about the difference in your personality styles?

_____

_____

_____

_____

3. What "typically male" or "typically female" behaviors does your spouse exhibit? What are the most bothersome for you?

_____

_____

_____

_____

Style (for the spouse)

Now ask your spouse these same questions about you.

1. Describe any of your spouse's habits or quirks that get on your nerves.

_____

_____

_____

_____

2. Have you and your spouse taken any personality tests, such as the Myers-Briggs Type Indicator? If so, what have you learned about the compatibility or incompatibility of your personalities? If not, what can you say about the difference in your personality styles?

_____

_____

_____

_____

3. What "typically male" or "typically female" behaviors does your spouse exhibit? What are the most bothersome for you?

_____

_____

_____

_____

Dreams

1. How would you describe your dreams for yourself and your marriage? (Where would you like to be ten, twenty, or thirty years from now?)

   _____
   _____
   _____
   _____

2. How would you describe your spouse's dreams for himself or herself and for the marriage?

   _____
   _____
   _____
   _____

3. Are there any differences here that cause stress? How?

   _____
   _____
   _____
   _____

Disappointment

Note: This can be deep, personal stuff, and it might be best to keep it private. If you don't feel comfortable writing these answers down, that's fine, but take time to think them through.

1. In what ways has your spouse disappointed you since you got married?

   Appearance:_____
   _____

   Attitude:_____
   _____

   Spiritual Life:_____
   _____

   Health: _____
   _____

Ability and Talent: _____

_____

"Sex Appeal": _____

_____

Other:_____

_____

_____

_____

2. Looking over these same categories, are there ways in which you think you've disappointed your spouse?

_____

_____

_____

3. How has this caused stress in your relationship?

_____

_____

_____

_____

Power struggle

1. If you disagree about something you need to do together, what happens? Who "wins"? Or is there a compromise?

_____

_____

2. Give a specific example of this happening.

_____

_____

_____

_____

3. How did you feel afterward?

_____

_____

4. How do you think your spouse felt afterward?

    _____

    _____

5. Do you use power or manipulation or some other technique to get your way? Or do you submit pretty easily?

    _____

    _____

6. How frequently do you and your spouse engage in power struggles? Daily? Weekly? Several times a day? Hardly ever?

7. How stressful are these power struggles usually? Give them a rating from "highly stressful" to "hardly stressful at all."

8. How would you describe your attitude toward disagreements with your spouse? Do you hate them, avoid them, welcome them, use them to blow off steam, etc.?

    _____

    _____

    _____

Great expectations, and needs not met

1. On the scale of one to ten below, rate how fully you have expected your marriage to meet your needs. On the adjacent scale, rate how fully your marriage is meeting your needs.

    10   10

    9   9

```
8        8

7        7

6        6

5        5

4        4

3        3

2        2

1        1
```

2. What needs of yours do you wish your spouse would meet?

   _____

   _____

   _____

3. What needs of your spouse do you think you're not meeting?

   _____

   _____

   _____

4. In the last year, which of the following statements have you said (mark with your initials) or heard your spouse say (mark with spouse's initials).

   "You're never here for me."

   "I don't feel as if you REALLY love me."

   "You care more for your job than you do for me."

   "You don't care at all about MY day."

   "Why don't we ever _____ anymore?"

   "Don't you find me attractive anymore?"

   "I don't feel as if you respect me."

   "Even when you're here, you're not really paying attention to me."

5. How do great expectations and unmet needs cause stress in your home?

_____

_____

_____

_____

Fear

1. Do you have any fear that your spouse might leave you, that death might separate you, or that you may be losing the love you once had?

2. Does your spouse have any such fear?

3. If so, how does this add stress to your relationship?

_____

_____

_____

Finances

Money—getting it, keeping it, spending it—is an area of major stress in our individual lives and in our families. Whether you're in a situation of wealth or want, problems come up.

Many families are torn apart by having *too much* money—they struggle with values and limits. Others only wish they had such problems. They never seem to have enough. The bills need to be paid, the children need new clothes, and you're fighting about who wrote the last check. When different family members tussle over limited funds, there can be significant emotional stress.

From time to time, surveys will be released on the major causes of marital discord. What do husbands and wives fight about most often? Money is regularly at, or near, the top of the list. Why? Because the handling of money brings out some very personal issues. It's interesting that Jesus talked more about money than about anything else, except "the kingdom of God." He knew that our finances reflect the basic decisions we make about who we are and what's most important to us.

Spending vs. saving. There are two basic philosophies about money: one is that prudent people save their money; the other is that money exists to be spent.

Generally, we see the savings principle held by those who have come out of situations of great need or who have suffered a major financial loss. The depression generation in the U.S. is deeply savings oriented. When you have lost it all, you want to sock away some emergency funds to get you through the next disaster. Such people are usually well insured, with savings accounts and CDs and retirement plans.

Others see a certain folly in saving too much money. What good is it if you never enjoy what it can buy? Some people live frugally and stow away huge amounts that just sit in their bank accounts until they die— does that make any sense? It's far better, the spenders say, to buy what you want with the money you have. Enjoy it while you can.

> **If you want to see what's most important to people, look at their checkbooks. People pay for what they care about.**

Of course, there are variations on both these themes. Most people are somewhere in between, saving some and spending some. But often there are conflicts in a marriage because one partner is a saver and the other a spender. These philosophies are so deeply rooted, it's hard to make compromises.

"How can you be so irresponsible?"

"How can you be so cheap?"

These disagreements, unless they're confronted and (to some extent) accepted, will cause significant stress in the home.

Priorities. If you want to see what's most important to people, look at their checkbooks. People pay for what they care about.

If a neighbor came to you and said he was raising money to build some memorial to the town's founder and would you chip in a hundred bucks, you'd probably say, "I'd love to, but I can't afford it." But if your child became ill and you needed to pay a hospital bill of a *thousand* dollars, you'd find a way to pay it. We "afford" what's important.

So if you really wanted to give more to church or a charity, you could move to a cheaper home, trade in for a cheaper car, and cancel your cable TV. But you've made certain decisions along the way about how much you could spend for this or that. Those decisions have reflected your priorities.

So in any home, there will be conflicts about what's most important. Say you get a thousand-dollar bonus at work. Ask each family member how to spend it. You'll probably get a different answer from each one. College fund. Roller blades. Summer vacation. New carpeting. Car detailing. Basketball camp. Therefore when a decision is finally made, there will be sharp disagreement from some family members.

One friend of ours still remembers that her father claimed he didn't have enough money to send her to her first-choice college. But after she enrolled at a less desirable school, he bought a luxury car. As she figured it, the car could have helped pay for at least the first two years of the top-rate college. Apparently, as he figured it, he "needed" that car. It was a priority for him, more important than his daughter's preferred school. She was hurt by that decision, but it was his money.

In cases where family expenditures are clearly for this spouse or that one, for this child or that, the money management can send messages about who's more important—whether you intend to send those messages or not. For that reason, it's best to try to keep things fairly even.

Still, there will be conflict as family members say, "I can't believe you bought that, when we could have had this!"

Identity. Unfortunately, our society often judges one's personal worth on the basis of money. People with high-paying jobs tend to be more respected than those in low-paying jobs. This is foolishness, of course, but it can create problems of identity and resentment in a family.

If a man sees his role as breadwinner for his family, he will feel worthless if he loses his job. If his wife gets a better-paying job, he may feel threatened. He will tend to compare himself to the fathers of other children on the block and gauge his personal value accordingly. Both mother and father may feel ashamed that they are unable to provide more for their children.

Children don't always understand financial limits, especially in the early years. If Johnny next door has a complete collection of Pogs, your little Suzy will want some, too. If Gina down the street has a new bike, your Robby will want one. If all the other kids playing hoops after school have three-hundred-dollar sneakers, your resident athlete will feel poorly shod. If all the other seniors are getting new cars for graduation, your family scholar will feel disappointed if she doesn't get one, too.

If children understand that they are "poor" or "middle class" or "not able to afford all the neat things everyone else has," they may accept that, but there may also be some resentment at times. Through no fault of their own, they share the financial lot of their family. If kids at school look down on your kids because they don't dress as well or have as much stuff as others, your kids may resent you for that.

So you have to talk about these things, get them out in the open. Let your kids know how unimportant money is in the great scheme of things, that money is not a proper judge of character or personal value. Both kids and adults need to learn that.

Mine and yours. In family finances, there can also be some confusion about whose money is whose. If one partner earns forty thousand dollars a year and the other earns twenty thousand, does the higher-paid person get to make two thirds of the financial decisions? Or does all the money belong to everybody? These things need to be figured out.

If children get an allowance, do they have any limits on how to spend that money? Is that money all theirs? Again, these matters should be discussed and clearly understood.

The notions of "mine" and "yours" can cause some bickering in a family. Naturally, we would like to encourage sharing. But at the same time, "good fences make good neighbors." Clear delineation of possessions can save a few family fights.

YOUR TURN

Financial Stress in the Home

1. On the line below, the far left is the "frugal saver," living cheaply and saving nearly everything earned. The far right is the "spendthrift," spending everything and saving nothing. Put an X on the line to indicate your own position. Put an O on the line to indicate your spouse's.

Frugal Saver   Spendthrift

_____

2. Are you two far apart? Does this cause stress in your home? Give an example.

   _____

3. If you had a thousand-dollar bonus, what would you do with the money?

   _____
   _____
   _____

4. What would your spouse do with the money?

   _____
   _____
   _____

5. If you have kids old enough to make such decisions, what would they do with the money?

   _____
   _____
   _____

6. If there's anyone else in your household (and you might include your own parents or in-laws if they visit often), what would they do with the money?

   _____
   _____
   _____

7. Look through your checkbook for the last few months. How do your expenses reflect your priorities?

   _____
   _____
   _____

8. Do you tend to gauge your personal value by the money you make?

   _____

   Does your spouse?_____

Do your kids?_____

9. Do you think your family has more, less, or about the same amount of money as most of the people you deal with on a regular basis (neighborhood, work, church, school, etc.)? _____

10. Does this make you feel more important or less important, or does it have no effect? _____

11. List ten things in your life that are more important than money.

_____
_____
_____
_____
_____
_____
_____
_____
_____
_____

12. Have you ever fought in your home over whose money belonged to whom? If so, describe the disagreement.

_____
_____
_____
_____
_____

13. If you have children, do they get allowances? _____

Why or why not? _____
_____

14. Do you and your spouse have any "personal money" that you can spend without consulting the other person? _____ Why or why not? _____
_____
_____

15. Would you consider money a major stressor in your home, a moderate stressor, a minor stressor, or no stressor at all? _____

Time

There's never enough time in the day. For most of us, that's true at work and at home. Time is money, they say, and what we've just been saying about money is true of time as well. It's just another kind of currency. It's a valuable commodity that we have in limited supply. How we spend it tells a lot about who we are.

Here again the question of "affordability" comes up. Friends invite you over to see slides of their vacation in the Ozarks, and you politely say, "Sorry, I don't have time." But if your kid makes it to the state Little League finals, you'll make time to be there. You'd better.

We spend time on what's important to us. Every day, we make decisions along these lines. In a family, there can be demands for time that go unmet, and some hurt feelings along the way.

Providing vs. being there. Joe works ten to twelve hours a day. When he comes home, his wife scolds him for missing their daughter's band concert. Joe is understandably perplexed. He is spending long hours at work in order to provide for his family, and he doesn't have much time left to spend with them.

Becky is a single mom who works hard at two different jobs to support her ten-year-old son. One day he complains that she never spends any time with him.

In both these cases and many more, family decisions need to be made. The children and spouses need to understand that a breadwinner's time at work is a gift to them. But they may all need to rearrange their lives— maybe these families can get by with less money in order to have more time to spend together.

Cave time vs. group time. Many people, especially men, need to spend a good deal of time by themselves. One author calls this "going into his cave," when a man retreats from group activities to figure things out on his own.[3] In many family situations, this is difficult. It can also be misunderstood.

If one family member frequently goes off alone, others can feel rejected. Yet if that family member is forced to participate in family activities—and given no time alone—that person can grow cranky and nervous. Some people are introverts, drawing energy from being alone and then expending that energy in public. Others are extroverts, who draw energy from public interaction and expend it when they are by themselves. Most families include both types and must allow for both types.

Decisions should be made about which family activities are compulsory and which are optional. A certain amount of cave time can be allowed and honored, but then the person can be drawn out into the family again. This is true of children or parents. We know one woman who asked her children and husband to give her a half hour of quiet when she got home from work. No questions, no problems, no noise. After that half hour, she was up and ready to spend quality time with them.

Learning time responsibility. In the dialogue that started this chapter, a teenager was upset because he didn't have time to finish cleaning his room *and* go to the store *and* go to his part-time job. This is typical. Children are learning how to manage their time, and they don't always get it right. This too can be a source of some stress in the home.

For children and adults, there are time-consuming chores to do. Sometimes other people in the home depend on you to do your chores on time. The person who dries the dishes has to wait for the person who washes the dishes. Sometimes there is some complex orchestration to be done.

For the most part, children should be held to their commitments and expected to do chores on time, even if that means giving up some other activity. The child who put off doing homework until the last minute should not be excused from sweeping the kitchen floor. In this way, kids will learn to schedule their time better. But parents should be reasonable, allowing some slack if it seems appropriate.

Everyone in the family should understand his or her responsibility to the rest of the family, the responsibility to be with the family at certain times and to do certain tasks on time. This will not eliminate time stress in the family, but it will prevent some misunderstandings that can intensify the stress.

YOUR TURN

Time Stress in the Home

1. Check off any of the following difficulties that apply to you.

   I have trouble

   ___ balancing time commitments between home and work

   ___ trying to spend time with my kids, while still getting the work done around the house

   ___ keeping my house or apartment in good condition

   ___ running errands for the kids (car pools, etc.)

   ___ spending "quality time" with my spouse and children

   ___ doing things that I enjoy without feeling stress or guilt

   ___ having any time to myself

2. What family activities have you participated in during the last month?

   _____

   _____

   _____

   _____

   _____

3. How often does everyone in your household come together? Most of the time? Every meal? Every dinner? Once a week?

   _____

   _____

4. Does your family understand and accept the time you spend earning money to provide for them? _____

5. If not, what can you do to help them understand this better? Or do you need to cut back on your money earning?

   _____

   _____

   _____

   _____

6. If you were independently wealthy and no longer had to work for a living, how would you spend your time?

_____

_____

_____

_____

_____

7. Are you more of an introvert or extrovert?

_____

8. List the other people in your household and whether you think they are more introverted or extroverted.

_____

_____

_____

_____

_____

9. Are allowances made for the introverts to spend time alone? _____

_____

10. How well do you think your children are learning time responsibility?

_____

_____

_____

11. Are you and your spouse good models for them in this area?

_____

_____

12

Stress Strategies for the Home

A single mother came to Tom Whiteman's office recently to talk about difficulties she was having with one of her teenagers. The latest issue: ear piercing for her thirteen-year-old. Tom didn't quite understand her concern at first. The problem was, she explained, this was her thirteen-year-old *son*.

Sure, it's in fashion for kids of both sexes to get their ears drilled, but this mom didn't understand it. She reacted in anger and frustration, scolding her son vehemently about his values, styles, and generally liberal attitudes. During the session, she unloaded her frustration on Tom. What had she done wrong?

Then Tom talked with her son. As the boy saw it, his mom was just using this issue as an opportunity to do what she enjoyed most—lecturing him. "She goes on and on. I get the point, but she turns it into a big issue over my clothes, my friends, everything about me. I just tune her out, because I've heard it all before."

There is stress in this home. The mom feels it and the son feels it. But what can they do about it? And what can you do when you encounter your own inevitable home stress?

As we saw in chapter 10, we have three good choices for dealing with stress: alter, avoid, accept. These strategies can work not only in the workplace but also in the home. In the last chapter, we focused on four main home stressors: children, marriage, finances, and time. Here we'll see how the alter-avoid-accept strategy can apply to each of those areas.

CHILDREN

How should Mom respond when her son wants an earring? How can the stress in this home be reduced?

Alter

First, the mother might attempt to alter her parenting style. In this example, Mom used the classic lecture. It obviously wasn't working, yet she pressed on with it. It's a common mistake.

It's a lot more effective, and *much* less stressful, to make a decision and merely state the rules. Arguing about it is counterproductive, especially if you launch into personal attacks and extraneous issues.

In fact, there are three broad parenting styles: the authoritative style, which is rigid and highly structured; the laissez-faire style, which is unstructured and permissive; and a balanced style, which combines a loving, supportive atmosphere with flexible yet firm limits. Most would agree that the balanced style is the goal, yet we often get out of balance to one degree or the other.

Avoid

In parenting, the key avoidance strategy is to pick your battles. When things get tense with kids, every interaction becomes a major power play. I've known parents who would fight with their youngsters about a last carrot or pea left uneaten on the plate. Now, maybe there's a bit of rebellion involved there, but parents need to be wise in choosing where they will expend their energy.

Avoid battles that are not worth fighting.

Part of this is preparation. You need to anticipate the issues you'll face with your kids and be ready for them. In the earring example, Mom needs to decide ahead of time how she is going to deal with all the cultural issues her son will face: music, makeup, dress, friends, styles, and so forth. She needs to decide where to lay down the law on these things—and decide which of these issues is not worth fighting over. Ideally, she could talk with her son in advance about some of these things so she can get his input before it becomes a federal case.

If you have a spouse, discuss with him or her beforehand about the issues you will take a stand on and the issues you would prefer to let go of. It is important that you present a united front and that you avoid battles that are not worth fighting.

Finally, you will want to accept the fact that your children are different from you. They may like different kinds of music and different styles. This is to be expected and accepted as part of growing up. Let your kids talk to you about the things in their lives—the temptations they face as well as the inspiring things they encounter. You may be surprised at how morally responsible they are.

It's true that children often rebel. Many ordinary parts of our lives become power plays as children seek to gain the upper hand. But sometimes children are just learning to think for themselves, in a healthy way. Sometimes they are just going through an identity crisis of sorts. They need to make some independent decisions to know who they are. You may avoid some unnecessary conflict if you support your kids in some of their decisions. Trust them. Give them some leeway.

Accept

Your child also has a unique personality, with specific gifts and interests and a specific "bent." In Proverbs we are told to "train a child in the way he should go." Scholars have interpreted this as "train a child according to his bent." That is, seek to understand your child's uniqueness, affirming and encouraging those qualities. Each child is different and needs to be raised differently. Accepting these differences and making allowances for them will go a long way toward making the job of parenting less stressful.

MARRIAGE

Marriage is the site of our highest expectations, deepest hurts, and broadest needs. Many people intensely love and hate their mates at the same time. For many relationships, stress is a given.

Alter

In stressful marriages, there are many areas that could be altered—too many to mention here. But change is an essential ingredient of healthy marriages. We cannot do what we want day after day, but we must be willing to change for the good of the relationship. This attitude of servanthood does not come naturally to us. It is something we have to work at daily.

Even communication demands a servant attitude. Good communication in a marriage requires that you listen even when you are not interested, that you talk when you don't feel like talking, and that you apologize when your pride resists it. Even though the skills come hard, using them in your relationship will surely reduce stress.

> **Good communication in a marriage requires that you listen even when you are not interested, that you talk when you don't feel like talking, and that you apologize when your pride resists it.**

Couples develop patterns of interacting. Sometimes these are very healthy, but often they can become hurtful and damaging. Marriages become less stressful as partners change their patterns of interaction, revising their interpersonal habits—listening, sharing, supporting, sacrificing.

Avoid

When a child scrapes his elbow, it bleeds, he cries, a bandage is applied, and eventually a scab develops. Then what does he do? He keeps picking at the scab. It hurts a little, but he has this morbid fascination with his wound.

Couples do this in relationships all the time—except they're picking *each other's* scabs, emotionally speaking. The wife knows exactly what galls the husband, so she does it and says it whenever she can. The husband knows how to needle his wife, and he *can't stop doing it*. She makes him feel jealous. He makes her feel inadequate. Both bring up old wounds, arguments from last year, last month, last week, issues that have never been resolved.

Healthy couples know how to let it rest. They avoid those old scabs. They stay off the touchy subjects.

This is not the same thing as denial or "stuffing" our problems. If issues need to be resolved, for goodness' sake, resolve them! But if an issue has been laid to rest, let it rest. Don't keep bringing old baggage into the relationship.

Stress management in relationships also requires that partners limit their arguments to issues and stay away from personal attacks. Take the time to ask, "What are we fighting about?" Define the issue and have a good argument, but do not demean the other person.

Avoid statements like

"You always . . ."

"You never . . ."

"How can you be so . . .?"

"There you go again!"

Healthy couples also schedule their fights. This sounds a bit crazy, but it can go a long way toward alleviating stress. In order for an issue to be truly resolved, you want both parties at their top form. George Foreman doesn't want to fight Mike Tyson when Tyson has the flu. (Well, maybe he does.) To have a fair fight, you need to find a time when you're both ready to deal with the issue.

> **Healthy couples know how to resolve issues. They avoid old wounds and do not use touchy subjects to gain the upper hand.**

You can say, "Could we talk about this some other time?" But if you say that, *be sure to find another time to resolve this issue.* One gem of wisdom Scripture gives us is this: "Do not let the sun go down while you are still angry" (Eph. 4:26). Some couples have observed this as a rule in their relationship, and it has spared them many problems. Avoid late-night squabbles that will seem silly in the morning. Even if you can't resolve an issue before bedtime, go to bed in peace, agreeing that you will revisit the issue later.

Accept

Much of the stress in a relationship is unavoidable, a natural part of intimacy. But a great deal of what we quarrel about *can* be avoided through learning to accept each other. Stop trying to remake your spouse in *your* image.

Ray was complaining about his wife. She didn't keep the house the way he liked, she didn't have the same interests, and her personality was very different from his. In frustration, Ray related how for years he had tried to get her to change, to appreciate his perspective, even just to sit and watch an entire baseball game with him. But to no avail. He couldn't get her to be the wife he wanted her to be.

Finally, Ray concluded that he was going to give up on her and give up on his marriage. He decided to stop caring about how she cleaned the house or what she did in her free time. He watched his games by himself and let her watch what she wanted in another room. This created a distance between them, but in time he noticed that they were also getting along a lot better, and he felt a lot less stressed.

Today, almost six months later, Ray reports that his marriage is quite improved and the power struggles are almost gone. Now that he has learned the value of accepting his wife, he doesn't try to change her as much.

When we enter marriage with ultrahigh expectations, we can become very disappointed in our mates. We're trying as hard as we can to have the perfect marriage, but our spouses are messing it all up. Or so we think. Of course, they may be thinking similar things. We may be ruining their ideas of the ideal marriage.

> **We're trying as hard as we can to have the perfect marriage, but our spouses keep messing up our plans.**

Acceptance may involve some distance, as Ray discovered. It may mean letting the marriage find its own level, not forcing it. We need to accept our spouses as the wonderful people they are and let the marriage grow—not into some prescribed ideal but into a unique and marvelous relationship between two unique and marvelous people.

FINANCES

We've examined the stresses that finances can bring. Financial bickering has torpedoed many a relationship. But this too can be brought under control with the alter-avoid-accept strategy.

Alter

First, wherever you can, try to make changes that will improve your overall situation. Many people think all they need is to earn a little more money in order to manage better, but they actually would do better to learn how to live within their means. Somehow people who live beyond their means when they're making twenty thousand dollars a year are still living beyond their means when they're pulling down forty thousand. Setting a budget and learning the discipline of living within that budget would be a lot better than any raise.

How do you make financial decisions in your home? Perhaps you could ease stress by altering this method, giving more or maybe less input to other family members. Perhaps you could start or stop giving allowances to children. You could also make some difficult decisions together about simplifying your lifestyle—home, car, clothes, vacations, and so on.

Action Point

Have a family meeting about the division of responsibilities in your home. You might use this opportunity to hear your kids' perspectives on the roles they are filling. (Make sure you have talked through this with your spouse ahead of time and that you support each other through the meeting.)

Be sure to do the following:

1. Go through the circled items on your list and explain that you do not expect them to do these things anymore. Be sure that this does not come across as a put-down but that your concern and love shows through.

2. Go through the boxed items on your list and talk about how your children could do these things better. You may need to give instructions or explain your expectations.

3. Introduce your children to the underlined items on your list. Ask them if they'd like to help you out in these ways. Explain what a great help it would be to you. Make sure they know how to do these things and what is expected of them.

Time management is a critical issue for all of us. Therefore you must determine your goals and priorities, say no to obligations that don't fit into those priorities, and build a support network that can help you manage some specific tasks.

16

Self-Talk

Imagine yourself in a crowded airport. Your plane is already forty minutes late. You're going to miss your connecting flight, and the first day of your vacation is going to be ruined. As you look around the waiting area, you notice two people in particular. One man is pacing back and forth, intermittently stopping to verbally abuse the woman behind the counter. He's so agitated that he won't even speak to his wife, who is obviously embarrassed by his behavior.

Another man is sitting with his wife and children. He's using the time to play with his young children, while his wife is reading a novel. If he weren't in an airport, you would guess he was already on vacation.

What's the difference between these two men? Their *self-talk*. One is obviously stressed, his mind racing with thoughts: "This no-good airline ... That stupid lady ... My vacation is ruined ... My wife just sits there ... Who's going to pay for this?..."

The other man is probably thinking, "Well, there's nothing I can do, so I might as well make the most of it ... This is a good time to connect with my kids ... At least I'm not at work ... I've been looking for a time when I could talk with my wife ..."

Of the two examples, which one is more like you? Put yourself in the scene. You're waiting for your plane and now faced with missing your connection. This is truly a stressful event for even the calmest of us. So the question is, What is your self-talk in this situation?

Having been there himself, Tom Whiteman knows that for him there is the initial anxiety: "What am I going to do? Is there another flight I can take? Can I still make my connection?"

This anxiety is a normal part of being human. But once Tom determines that he's going to miss his connection and there's no other flight, then he usually begins the process of changing his self-talk. He forces himself to do this, actually rehearsing his self-talk as follows: "There's nothing I can do. I'll just relax and make the most of the time. Things could be much worse; at least I'm safe."

> **The difference between a really good day and a really awful day is not found in what happened but in what you tell yourself about that day.**

Tom hasn't always been good at this. God taught him a powerful lesson one weekend when he was traveling. He had missed a flight, was rerouted through two other cities, and spent all night trying to get home—normally it would have been just a two-hour flight. He arrived home about six o'clock Sunday morning in the foulest of moods. He had told off three flight attendants, had several very nasty conversations with God, and when he walked in the door of his home, he proclaimed to his wife, "Don't expect me to go to church with you this morning!" (as if this were all her fault).

He was just dozing off when the phone rang. It was about seven o'clock in the morning. You can probably imagine his reaction: "Who in the world is calling at this time in the morning! Why can't I get some sleep around here! @#%^&**!!!"

The man on the phone was the Sunday school teacher for the couples class Tom and his wife attended. He was calling to ask Tom to teach the class for him that morning. Tom immediately thought, "He's got a lot of nerve. He doesn't have any idea what kind of night I've had!"

But before Tom could respond, the man continued, giving the reason for his request. "Our son was killed last night by a drunk driver."

Suddenly everything changed. After agreeing to do whatever he could to help, Tom hung up the phone and had a whole new conversation with God. "Be with this family . . . and thank you for getting me home safely."

That night was several years ago, and yet its impact has changed every trip and inconvenience Tom has had since then. He's changed his self-talk.

He's redefined "a bad night," and he's tried to stop worrying about things that really are not that bad.

THE INTERVENING VARIABLE

What determines how a person responds to a difficult experience? An event itself can be serious, but different people respond in different ways. Some greet new challenges with determination, even a kind of joy. Others are defeated by hard times, lashing out in anger or withdrawing into sullenness. Scientifically, it doesn't add up. This equation needs another variable.

Self-talk is that variable. It's what separates the go-getters from the dead ducks. It's what makes one person greet a stress event with panic and another with calm assurance. It is the filter through which we deal with the events of our lives.

The importance of your self-talk is obvious. It's not the event itself that causes stress, fears, or anxiety. *It's what we tell ourselves about the event.* Our feelings and behaviors are not determined by other people or events but by our own minds. This brings the responsibility back to us. A sad event does not make us depressed. No, we understand this event in a way that depresses us. A hateful action does not make us feel angry. We choose to see it as a wrong, an injustice, and we respond with the anger appropriate to our perception.

When Tom answered the phone at seven in the morning, he was angry at the rudeness of the early caller. What "made" him angry? The phone? The caller? The crazy night he had just experienced? No, all of those factors were filtered together in his mind. He processed them and decided that he had a right to feel angry for this unwelcome wake-up call.

But his attitude changed considerably during the course of the call. He wasn't angry anymore. What changed? He had still been awakened early after a terrible night. None of the events had changed; it was merely *the*

THE INTERVENING VARIABLE		
Event	Self-talk	Reaction: Feeling or Behavior
Neutral	Positive or Negative	Positive or Negative

way he interpreted them. In his inner monologue, he suddenly put his sufferings in perspective. With the intervening variable of his self-talk, newly revised when he heard of his caller's tragedy, he changed his response to this stressful situation.

One key for managing stress is monitoring our own self-talk. Other people or events do not actually cause our stress; rather, our stress comes from what we tell ourselves.

It's much easier to blame others for our problems. "God isn't fair . . . The airlines are run by incompetent people . . . If only my wife would do what I ask . . . My boss drives me crazy." These are all reasons that our clients give for the anxiety in their lives. The hard work of counseling is to help them understand that they cannot do anything about those events or those other people. But they can decide how to think about those events or people.

LISTENING TO LIES

There are several problems with the self-talk we normally engage in. First, it is often *distorted.* Like the serpent in the Garden, we tend to seize on half-truths, which are the most dangerous lies. Our self-talk tends to be *negative,* magnifying bad situations, discounting good elements, and putting down our own abilities.

Our self-talk is often *self-centered,* but this does not mean we're proud of ourselves. We may focus on our own failure, our own unworthiness, or our own needs, but we do tend to focus on ourselves. Certainly, Tom's self-talk as he tried to make flight connections was rather selfish. He saw only his own needs until he was jolted out of his myopia by the early morning call.

Ironically, much self-talk is also *self-defeating.* The self-focus does not stem from self-exaltation but the opposite. We focus on our own inability. We tell ourselves, "I'm no good . . . I really messed up . . . People think that I'm stupid . . . I could never do that . . . God must be mad at me."

In the throes of such a self-defeating attitude, we can interpret everything that happens as (a) brought on by our own foolishness, (b) intentionally done by someone else to hurt us, or (c) a test from God. Self-centered self-defeaters are magnets for suffering. Or so they see themselves. They often bring needless stress on themselves, because they personalize every external event.

Some Observations about Negative Self-Talk

Our negative self-talk is usually automatic. It is not something we consciously think about, but it just "kicks in" whenever there is a triggering event.

Negative messages and stories tend to be on a "tape." In other words, once an event or a word triggers our reaction, the tape begins to play. It can go on and on, repeating the same negative message in our minds, sending us into a tailspin that can last for hours, days, or months. For example, you may have a tape called "My Mother Predicted That I'd Never Amount to Anything." At times, someone can use just one negative word in referring to you or something you did, and the whole tape begins to play again. It will play over and over if you let it.

Negative thinking is usually irrational, but to you it sounds like the truth. You have deceived yourself into believing a lie, and sometimes only a close friend or a counselor can point out the deceptiveness of the message you are listening to. "What if" statements fall into this category. (What if my spouse leaves me? What if my kids are run over by a truck?) We can beat ourselves up with the what ifs, but in truth these are usually irrational.

Negative tapes can lead to panic attacks, obsessive thinking, and phobic reactions. Just like bad physical habits, sometimes our mental habits cause us to become sick or out of control. Negative self-talk can also lead to serious problems when it remains unchecked.

YOUR TURN

1. What is some of your negative self-talk? What things, untrue or half true, do you tell yourself regularly? (Check any that apply, and add others specific to your case.)

    ___ I am no good.

    ___ If anything can go wrong, it will.

    ___ When I do something wrong, God plays hard to get.

    ___ I'll never live up to the expectations of my parents.

    ___ My parents never expected much of me, and they were right.

___ I'm not really good at anything.

___ I'll never be as good a person as _____.

__ _____

__ _____

__ _____

__ _____

2. Many of us have negative "tapes" that we replay in our minds. These may be comments that have come from relatives or friends or others over the years. As you evaluate those negative messages, where do they seem to have come from?

____ Parents (Message: _____)
____ Siblings (Message: _____)
____ Other relatives (Message: _____)
____ School friends (Message:_____)
___ Boyfriend or girlfriend of the past (Message:_____)
____ Teachers (Message: _____)
____ Church leaders (Message:_____)
____ Spouse (Message:_____)
____ Children (Message: _____)
____ Coworkers (Message: _____)
____ Other (Message:_____)

3. What are some areas in your life in which your self-talk has caused you undue stress?

_____ Your job　　　　_____ Concern for the future
_____ Your family　　　_____ Fear of what others think
_____ Your marriage　　_____ The way you look
_____ Finances　　　　_____ A past trauma
_____ Church　　　　　_____ Personal insecurities
_____ The pace you set　_____ The friends you keep

Types of Negative Self-Talk

The Anxiety and Phobia Workbook identifies four types of self-talk. We might consider these as four different "characters" that could live within our minds: the worrier, the critic, the victim, and the perfectionist.[1]

The worrier. This type tends to suffer from irrational fears. In an extreme, this attitude can lead to obsessive thoughts and panic attacks. Often statements begin with "What if" or "If only." The worrier will take a situation and immediately imagine the worst-case scenario, in spite of logic that would indicate that the chances of such an outcome are slim. When they fly, they think about crashing. When they have chest pain, they think heart attack. And when they hear reports of a new kind of flesh-eating bacteria, they assume they will get it. They anticipate the worst, they overestimate the odds of something bad happening, and they imagine tremendous failure, embarrassment, or catastrophe.

Your best defense? Choose to live your life by *probabilities,* not *possibilities*!

The critic. The critic is the voice inside you that is always ready to judge you and will jump on you for even the slightest flaw. It loves to put you down, to humiliate you and remind you that you're no good. The critic lowers your self-image. The voice may mimic your mother or father and remind you that "You'll never amount to anything" or "You could have done it better." This self-talk compares you with others and always has you coming up short.

Your best defense? Discover your God-given strengths. Drown out the critic's voice by constantly reminding yourself what these strengths are.

The victim. The victim is that part of you that keeps you feeling hopeless and helpless. It feeds depression and makes you powerless. "No one really appreciates me," it cries. "Everyone takes advantage of me." This voice bemoans where you are today and convinces you that you'll never be able to change it because there will always be others out there who will hold you back or victimize you some more. You become convinced that you'll never succeed, so why try?

Your best defense? Stop pointing fingers of blame toward others and take full responsibility for your future.

The perfectionist. The perfectionist is similar to the critic, but instead of putting you down, the perfectionist constantly reminds you that you could have done better. Nothing is ever good enough for the perfectionist. This voice will keep you in constant stress and at the edge of burnout. No matter how hard you try, there is always that little bit more that you could have done or that slight imperfection that should have been fixed. "I should have ..." or "If only I had ..." are common expressions.

Your best defense? Only God is perfect, so give yourself some slack!

YOUR TURN

Which of the four negative self-talk types is a problem for you? On a scale of 1 to 10 (1 being "not a problem" and 10 being "a serious problem") rate the negative self-talk in your life. Then begin your work on changing your self-talk, by writing a positive response or a "counter-statement" to each negative message.

The worrier

1   2   3   4   5   6   7   8   9   10

Negative statements that you say to yourself	Counterbalancing statement
Example: If I get a checkup, they'll probably find cancer.	I need to take care of myself by getting a checkup. I'll leave the results up to God.

The critic

1   2   3   4   5   6   7   8   9   10

Negative statements that you say to yourself	Counterbalancing statement
Examples: You're stupid and can't do anything right	You've got a good head on your shoulders. You just made a bad decision this time.

The victim

	1	2	3	4	5	6	7	8	9	10

Negative statements that   *Counterbalancing statement*
you say to yourself

Example: I can't get a good grade in this class,   If I put my mind to it, I can
because the teacher doesn't like me.   earn a good grade.

The perfectionist

	1	2	3	4	5	6	7	8	9	10

Negative statements that   *Counterbalancing statement*
you say to yourself

Example: The meal was OK, but the   Everyone had a good time,
rolls were a little overcooked.   and the meal was fine.

TELLING YOURSELF THE TRUTH

As you think about what you tell yourself, sometimes the most important issue becomes a search for what is true. For example, to a very disturbed mind, the truth might be presented as, "I'm a total failure and deserve to die." A more subtle distortion might lead one to conclude, "The whole evening was ruined, because of my bumbled presentation." So how do we determine what is truth?

As Christians, we know that we must search the Scriptures to determine the truth about ourselves and how we interact with others. Christ told us that "the truth will set you free" (John 8:32). But free from what?

We believe that Christ was speaking primarily of the truth about who he was. But this truth goes beyond a statement of Christ's deity. Knowing who Christ is *and knowing who we are in Christ* is what truly sets us free. As his children, we are unconditionally loved, eternally secure, and therefore free from worries of death, free to live a victorious life, and free to fail. Most of us go through life worrying about failing, *but Christ has already paid for those failures.*

From the very beginning of this book, we have acknowledged God's sovereignty and the fact that if we trust completely in him, we will never need to worry. Yet as human beings, it is natural for us to worry from time to time. We must conclude that the process of becoming more Christlike is a process by which we renew our minds, constantly seeking to view ourselves the way he views us.

> **Knowing who Christ is and knowing who we are in Christ is what truly sets us free.**

We're not just saying, "Don't worry, be happy." We're saying that we all must learn to accept God's opinion of us. We are sinners, yes. We are incapable of earning God's love, yes. But apparently, in our Lord's eyes, we are also worth loving and worth dying for.

YOUR TURN

1. In a typical day, what is the balance between negative self-talk and positive? Take a guess.

   _____% Negative   _____% Positive

2. Now keep track for a twenty-four-hour period. Carry a tally sheet with you. Every time you make a negative self-statement, put a mark on the negative side, and then also mark the positive self-statements. After a day of this, mark your tally here.

   _____% Negative   _____% Positive

3. How close are you to being balanced? How close was your guess?

4. If you are out of balance on the negative side, or even if you are fairly balanced in your percentages, then you may want to begin to "transform your mind" according to Philippians 4:8. Ask God to show you how important you are to him.

Changing Your Self-Talk

Scripture tells us to "renew our minds" (Rom. 12:2). Change your self-talk from the negative ways you view yourself to the truth. To renew your mind, you may want to follow the following steps.

Recognize the self-statements that are negative. Identify them immediately and acknowledge them as lies.

Stop saying these lies to yourself. Once you've identified your negative self-talk and conclude that it is contributing to the stress in your life, you want to make a conscious effort to stop this self-talk.

Take a breather. Stop for a minute—relax—take a few deep breaths, and think about where these "tapes" came from. Usually they are deep-seated. They are deeply rooted in our personality and may be very tough to stop. Think back. Where have you heard these messages before? From a parent, an old teacher, a spouse, or a friend? (Sometimes we make them up all by ourselves, a natural part of our sinful nature.) It sometimes helps to identify who made these tapes. It is up to us to rerecord these tapes with new, more truthful information.

Spell out the negative self-statement. Don't let it lurk there in your mind as some vague certainty. Write it down so you can examine it. Identify which of the four types it is.

Write out a counterbalancing statement. Once again, you want to bring these transactions out into the open. Find the errors in the negative self-statement and substitute a positive statement, carefully worded to reveal the truth of who you are.

Practice saying this new, positive statement to yourself. Renewing your mind takes time, but with some practice, you'll get used to your new, positive approach.

YOUR TURN

Keep a daily log of your self-talk. Try this for at least a week.

Situations that affected my self-talk: My response:

_____   _____
_____   _____
_____   _____
_____   _____

Compliments received: My reaction:

_____   _____
_____   _____
_____   _____
_____   _____
_____   _____

Insults received or inferred: My reaction:

_____   _____
_____   _____
_____   _____
_____   _____
_____   _____

Thoughts I want to get rid of:

_____
_____
_____
_____

Things I want to keep telling myself:

_____
_____
_____
_____
_____

Photocopy this page for as many days as you want to keep this log.

17

Asserting Yourself in Nonstressful Ways

When one of Tom Whiteman's employees mentioned that she was taking a course on assertiveness, he thought, "Oh, no! She's going to come back to work with a list of unreasonable demands and ultimatums." He was already stressed enough. He didn't need some newly assertive colleague telling him what to do.

But that's not what happened. Instead, he saw a gradual, healthy change in her. She began to speak up more in staff meetings, saying valuable things she had previously held back. When she didn't understand something, she would go directly to someone and ask for clarification. Her assertiveness training was a very good experience for her, and a tremendous stress reducer!

If you are under stress, you may be afraid to assert yourself. Assertiveness means confrontation, and confrontation can be stressful. You might think it's better to go with the flow, to let your life go on as it always does. But using that strategy, you'd also be letting the stressful patterns of your life go on. Instead of taking control of the situation and trying to improve it, you'd be putting yourself in the *more* stressful position of "powerless victim" (see chapter 5).

You may also have a faulty picture of assertiveness. Assertive people are not necessarily obnoxious, rude, or selfish, though you may know people who take assertiveness to this level. Assertive people can be winsome and caring. They can actually be quite skilled at maintaining good relationships.

> **As people accept their unique position as human beings created and loved by God, they can love themselves in a healthy way and give of themselves to others.**

In order to be assertive, you must first know what you want and then learn how to ask for that. It's that "learning to ask for it" that the obnoxious ones don't get. They may know what they want, but they alienate people so much that they often *don't* attain their goals. People who are properly assertive know how to work with others to accomplish mutual objectives.

A THEOLOGY OF ASSERTIVENESS

Assertiveness grows out of the belief that you have the *right* to express yourself. It goes to the core of your self-image and also to the heart of your theology. Some Christians have a hard time being assertive, because they believe that we have no rights. They demand nothing, ask for nothing, and maybe even expect nothing.

There is a germ of truth in their thinking, but overall it's a distorted perspective, and one reason some Christians are so hung up and stressed out. That germ of truth is servanthood. We are clearly instructed to look out for the best interests of others, to give ourselves freely, following the example of Jesus. But even Jesus expressed his own needs. After a long day of healing, he took the time for rest and prayer. He invited himself to Zacchaeus's house for dinner. He sent his disciples to find a beast for the Triumphal Entry by saying merely, "The Lord needs him." Even on the cross, Jesus said, "I am thirsty."

We see a big difference between selfishness and expression of one's opinions and needs. Of course, you must not "think of yourself more highly than you ought" (Rom. 12:3), but isn't there a parallel problem in thinking too little of yourself? Jesus said, "Love your neighbor *as yourself*" (Matt. 22:39, emphasis added), indicating an equilibrium that should exist in our relationships.

In counseling sessions, we have discovered time and again that relationship problems arise from a lack of healthy self-respect. It's hard to have an honest give-and-take with a doormat. While we appreciate the servant attitude held by those who adopt a "doormat theology," we feel they are misguided. As people accept their unique position as human beings created and loved by God, they can love themselves in a healthy way and give of themselves to others.

In that context, assertiveness is a way of *honoring a relationship*. By taking the risk of expressing yourself, you enter into a relationship and strengthen it. If you never say what you really feel or need, you are not really entering into a relationship as a full participant. In that case, a relationship cannot grow.

For those who are stressed out, especially those who live with unreasonable fears or phobias, there is usually a downward spiral of negative self-talk, bottled-up emotions, and unexpressed fears. These worsen, accumulate, and may even cause physical problems or emotional disorders.

Other times, our stress is less global and more specific. For example, people who lead a fairly normal life may go into a tailspin whenever they have to make a presentation in front of a group or whenever they're around a certain person. Sometimes this is because that person or event is a trigger for some unresolved issue or conflict. You may experience this yourself—certain situations and encounters that you try to avoid but can't. Yet by learning to be more assertive, you can express emotions as they come up, you can ask for what you want or need, and you can learn to say no when you need to. These three skills can reduce your stress, increase your self-esteem, and improve your relationships.

Balancing Two Extremes

Learning to be assertive is usually a matter of balancing two extremes—the tendency to be a "wimp" and the tendency to be too aggressive. Christians are rarely rewarded for being too aggressive. As we have seen, this is generally non-Christlike behavior. On the other hand, however, Christians are often revered for being submissive, conforming, subservient. To some extent, this is Christian love in action. But when does it cross the line? When does meekness become weakness? When does the servant become a wimp?

(If we were writing for, say, an association of salespeople, we would be asking an opposite question: When does healthy assertiveness become selfish aggression? In that context, aggressive behavior is rewarded, but Christians tend to lean the other way. We all need to find a proper balance.)

Servanthood. Christian servanthood does not mean telling people what they want to hear, just so you'll be liked. Nor does it mean cowering in fear before others. The Bible says that "perfect love drives out fear" (1 John 4:18). Christian love is strong. While it may be sacrificial and self-giving, it is consistently honest and brave.

That's a challenge we seldom take. We are too concerned with being polite and nice and not rocking the boat. We deny or repress our feelings for the sake of others, feeling guilty about doing anything for ourselves. While we help others to the point of our own burnout, we deny our own valid needs, not wanting to be a burden on anyone else.

> **We may be so concerned with being polite and nice that we deny or repress our feelings for the sake of others, feeling guilty about doing anything for ourselves.**

This is a way of life that's out of balance. Ultimately this lifestyle will stress you out, burn you out, and destroy your ability to minister to others. Self-sacrifice is good, but there's a simple matter of *stewardship* involved. Even Jesus put boundaries on his ministry, taking time for rest. If you give until there's nothing left, there will be nothing left. Trust God to give you guidance on healthy limits to your servanthood.

The fact is that we do have needs—not only physical needs of food and rest but emotional needs of encouragement and satisfaction. When we ignore those needs, we repress some pretty strong emotions—anger, pain, disappointment. These emotions can simmer into resentment and perhaps explode into an emotional meltdown, a physical breakdown, or inappropriate behavior.

Inappropriate behavior can be overt wrongdoing or secret indulgence in pain-numbing addictions. It can also come in the form of "sabotage" or noncooperation. This is *passive-aggressive behavior,* a fairly common psychological phenomenon involving a surface response of passivity and a hidden cache of aggression that ultimately leaks out. Passive-aggressive people don't get mad, they get even.

For instance, you might say yes to something you really don't want to do—leading a Bible study at church because they couldn't find anyone else to do it. But then you come late each week or don't prepare well. You may not even admit it to yourself, but under the surface, you are getting even for being pressured into taking on this task.

Or say a person at church needs to talk and pray with someone about her emotional problems. Always willing to help, you say you'd love to meet with this person, though you really don't want to. Somehow you never get around to scheduling a meeting. (You might even find yourself screening your phone calls to avoid the person.)

Passive-aggressive people don't get mad, they get even.

You find yourself with a bad attitude toward someone in your church or family. When they ask what's wrong, you say, "Nothing." Yet your body language and tone betray you.

Your spouse does something wrong and then asks forgiveness. You *say*, "I forgive you" and seem to patch things up, but then you do subtle things to make your partner pay for the offense.

We human beings have natural tally sheets inside our heads. We regularly keep score in our interactions with others, whether or not we realize consciously that we're doing this. Often a submissive attitude out front is countered by a vengeful subconscious. If we give up our valid rights and concerns in our external dealings with people, we may be internally plotting to get even.

Overaggressiveness. The other extreme is being *too aggressive*. This might include a selfish attitude and abrasive language. You don't just express your needs, you *demand* them. In the process, you show no concern for other people's rights and needs.

Overaggressive people get their needs met by controlling and manipulating others—usually the nonassertive people. An overaggressive person thrives on confrontation, wanting to win in most aspects of life. The nonassertive person most likely fears confrontation and thus allows the aggressor to win without a fight.

In many cases, this is merely turning the other cheek. Christians are taught to return good for evil. The problem comes when a whole relationship is built on such an imbalance. We have counseled numerous couples in which one partner is overaggressive and the other is nonassertive. This makes for major tension in the home. On the surface, the aggressive one gets his or her way, but there are usually many hurt feelings and frustrations underneath the surface. We try to encourage the nonassertive partner to begin talking about his or her feelings and needs, and we encourage the aggressive partner to appreciate the value of the other person's desires. If both partners make the necessary changes, the relationship can be greatly improved.

Defining Assertiveness

Assertive behavior involves three levels of interaction:[1]

Communicating your feelings to others in a way that is honest and respectful. The best way to describe this is found in Ephesians 4:15— "speaking the truth in love." Keeping your mouth shut will cause you stress. It is irresponsible to cover over something that needs to be addressed for the good of a relationship. You may think you are being unselfish, but actually you may be letting your fear of confrontation damage the relationship. You need to "speak the truth." But you also must do this in a loving way. Don't be too aggressive. Focus on the other person's needs as well as your own.

Learning to ask for what you want or need. This category includes asking for help when you need it, taking things back when they're not the right size, and expressing your physical and emotional needs in a relationship without apologizing or feeling guilty. You learn to ask for what is right, without obnoxiously demanding your rights. We've known people who will never return something they've purchased, even if it is obviously defective. They get sick but will not take a break from working or caring for their family. They would feel guilty for expressing what they need. They don't want to be a bother to anyone.

Do you ever hear your car's brakes begin to squeak? This is a signal that you need new brakes—the brake pads have worn down, and metal is scraping metal. Now, wouldn't it be great if someone invented a "squeakless" brake so you wouldn't have to be bothered by that nasty sound? No! Without the squeak, you wouldn't realize there was anything wrong. You'd grind your brake drums to the point where they'd be ineffective. The squeak is valuable, because it tells you what you need to do to keep the car in good working order.

The same is true of us as people. We need to squeak once in a while when there's something wrong. We need to express our needs so something can be done.

Imagine your brakes saying, "You know, we really aren't very important in this car. There are so many more important parts—the carburetor, the battery, the muffler. If we squeak when we get run down, it will just draw attention away from those more important parts, so we'll just suffer silently." That would be disastrous. The brakes are important—not all-important but a key piece of the whole machine—and you need to know when there's a problem with them.

ASSERTIVE RESPONSES

1. Communicating your feelings to others in a way that is honest and respectful

2. Learning to ask for what you want or need

3. Learning how to say no

If our marriages, our families, our companies, our churches, and our communities are going to stay in good working order, we need to understand that we are important components in those operations—not all-important but part of the whole—and we need to remain effective, so we need to get our needs met. We need to learn to squeak.

Learning how to say no. People pleasers are those who say yes to just about everything because their self-image is based on what others think of them. They reason, "If I say no to this, So-and-so is going to think less of me, and I can't afford to let that happen." All their yeses catch up to them when they find themselves helping everyone but themselves (and often they neglect their own families too). People in ministry are particularly prone to this problem, as verified by the high incidence of ministry stress and burnout.

Balance

A properly assertive person learns to live with a sense of *balance*—balance between one's own needs and the needs of others, and balance between submissive, aggressive, and assertive behavior. There are times for all three of these styles of behavior, and much of that determination depends on a proper weighing of one's own needs in relation to those of others. A healthily assertive style—being a sort of middle ground—will be the most helpful in most cases. But there are also times when we just need to submit. For the good of a relationship, we may choose to sacrifice our needs for the needs of the other person. That can be, of course, a noble and loving thing to do.

> **A properly assertive person has learned the art of balance—balancing the need to take care of self, while being willing to sacrifice for the needs of others.**

There are also times when we need to be aggressive. We may need to *demand* our rights at times. Such situations are rare, but they do exist, particularly in situations with other aggressive people. We need wisdom to determine whether an aggressive approach is called for or whether a mere assertion will suffice.

YOUR TURN

Styles of Response

Do you tend to be submissive, aggressive, or assertive in your daily interactions? In the hypothetical situations below, indicate which response is closest to the way you would normally respond.

1. You order a meal that is not to your liking. You would

Submissive	Assertive	Aggressive
just eat it	kindly ask for something else	ask to see the manager

2. You're in a relationship (with a boyfriend or girlfriend or perhaps a business partner) that is causing you significant stress. You would

Submissive	Assertive	Aggressive
hang in there and say little or nothing	address the issues that are bothering you	break it off

3. You're at a show, and the people behind you are making noise. You would

Submissive	Assertive	Aggressive
sit quietly	turn around and ask them kindly to stop	tell them to "Shut up!"

4. You need your spouse or friend to pick you up at the airport after a trip. You would

Submissive	*Assertive*	*Aggressive*
ask but feel guilty	politely ask for what you need	tell them when and where to pick you up

5. You're in a group conversation and have something to say that you think is important, but there are no breaks in the conversation that would allow you to jump in. You would

Submissive	*Assertive*	*Aggressive*
keep it to yourself	jump in after waiting patiently	interrupt and say what you think

6. You watch as your neighbor is digging up a garden that he begins to extend into your yard. You would

Submissive	*Assertive*	*Aggressive*
continue to watch and wonder what's going on	walk out and ask what he's doing	march out and demand an explanation

7. You're sitting in a "no smoking" area, when someone near you starts to smoke. You would

Submissive	*Assertive*	*Aggressive*
let it go	ask them kindly to refrain from smoking	insist that they put out their cigarette, or report them to an authority

8. Your friend or spouse says something sarcastic about you at a dinner party in order to get a laugh, but it hurts your feelings. On the way home that night, you would

Submissive	*Assertive*	*Aggressive*
try to forget it, even if it's bothering you	tell the person in a loving way how you feel	let them have it!

9. You need ten dollars for gas, and you notice that your friend or spouse has cash in their wallet. You would

Submissive	*Assertive*	*Aggressive*
try to get by on the gas you have	ask to borrow ten dollars	insist that they lend (or give) you the money

10. Your spouse or friend calls you unexpectedly and asks you to run out and do something. But you've already made plans to do something else, and their request will make it impossible to do both. You would

Submissive	*Assertive*	*Aggressive*
cancel your plans and do as they ask	tell them that you are sorry but have other plans	tell them no and make them feel bad for asking

Evaluating Your Responses

As you look over your responses, do you see a tendency toward one extreme or the other?

Are there circumstances in which the submissive or aggressive response would be best? Look back over the cases mentioned and imagine the circumstances that might change your response.

Does your response vary depending on the other people involved? Are there some people you need to be more submissive toward and others with whom you should be more aggressive? Are you more assertive with a spouse (or boyfriend or girlfriend)? When it is a stranger or just an acquaintance, do you change?

Also, review the hypothetical situations and try to determine the spiritual implications. Can we be loving and giving and also find that middle ground of healthy assertiveness? What is the "Christian" response when people are gabbing behind you at a concert? (Demanding quiet from the talkers might reflect your love for the performer or the rest of the audience.)

HEALTHY ASSERTIVENESS

Assertiveness requires the learning of habits. Most of us have been brought up to be submissive. That is, as children we are taught to "be seen and not heard," to do what adults tell us to do. Certainly, many of us chafe under this way of life and find various ways to rebel, but we all grow up as smaller, weaker, more dependent people. In the context of growing up, submissive habits can become ingrained.

Some families, however, teach a parallel track of aggressiveness. As children watch their elders, they learn that they can get what they want by demanding it, fighting for it, or manipulating others. It might be argued that the baby who cries for a bottle is actually learning aggressive (or at least assertive) behavior. "I need this! Waaaaaa!" And suddenly the bottle appears.

> **You may need to learn new habits. You may need to train yourself to turn around at the concert and shush those behind you. Or you may need to teach yourself not to lash out in anger at those who are bothering you.**

Whatever your background, you may need to work at learning new habits of healthy assertiveness. You may need to train yourself to turn around at the concert and shush those behind you, if your natural tendency is to let it ride. Or you may need to teach yourself *not* to lash out in anger at those who are bothering you. (If anger is a problem for you, there are probably larger issues involved. There are several fine books available on controlling anger.[2] Or you may want to consult a counselor. Our discussion here will focus on those who are naturally submissive and need to assert themselves more.)

As you seek to develop habits of healthy assertiveness, there are four steps you need to take:

1. Understand what balanced assertiveness looks like.

2. Practice assertive responses.

3. Develop positive body language.

4. Learn to say no.

Understand What Balanced Assertiveness Looks Like

We have already touched on the definitions and descriptions of assertiveness. It's important to remember, though, that the goal is not to "be more selfish." That point can easily be forgotten if you read too many self-help books and popular magazines. *Looking Out for Number One* was a best-selling book that baldly stated a certain frame of mind: you have to put yourself first. That is *not* our message in this chapter. You can surely see that it does not square with biblical teaching.

Healthy assertiveness is primarily *stewardship* of who you are, what you can do, and the relationships you're in.

Jesus told a story of a man who went on a journey. Before the man left, he gave three servants different sums of money to manage in his absence. Two of the servants invested the funds and reaped great returns. The third, afraid that he might lose this venture capital, buried it in the ground. When the master returned, he scolded this fearful servant for not even getting interest on this sum.

The servant did not use what he had. Afraid of squandering this fortune, he squandered an opportunity instead.

Christian teachers routinely use this parable to talk about our talents— that is, our skills and abilities. This is a valid application (in fact, the English word "talent" comes to us from this parable, in which it originally referred to an amount of money). But we'd like to expand the idea even more—to include not just your skill at playing clarinet or growing marigolds but your ability to enter into a conversation, your well-thought-out political opinions, even your opportunities to enjoy the beautiful sounds of a concert. These are all gifts that you are given. Will you use them or bury them in the ground?

> **Healthy assertiveness is primarily *stewardship* of who you are, what you can do, and the relationships you're in.**

Too many Christians, in the name of Christian submission, keep quiet when they should be voicing their valuable opinions. They are trying to be humble, and that's admirable. They think they have nothing important to say—but wait a second! God gave them the ability to think. God gave them the ability to analyze a situation. God even gave them the ability to determine whether something is worth saying or not. If we stay mum when God has given us something good to say, are we not making the same mistake of the bashful servant?

And speaking of stress, maybe we should add to the parable in another way. When we bury our feelings and needs inside us, it's like burying toxic waste in the ground. It can eat away at us, causing stress and making other stress situations worse. So not only are we squandering opportunities to use what God has given us, we are also polluting the bodies God has given us!

Stewardship also occurs in relationships. Marriages, close friendships, working relationships, and business partnerships all need regular maintenance, from both parties. It's hard work to keep a relationship in good health, and both partners must pitch in.

But often a relationship will grow lopsided. One partner stops working at it, and the other has to pick up the slack. In our work with married people, the question often comes up, "As a Christian, should I just accept this? My spouse has been repeatedly unfaithful [or keeps moving out and back in or is abusive]. Do I have to submit to this?"

While we do not advise divorce, we do urge people to assert themselves—and to "assert the marriage." That is, they need to say, "*You* (wayward spouse) are not playing by the rules of this marriage. You made promises that need to be kept." Some Christians (especially women) fear that this would not be following God's ideal of submission—but it *is* submission to God's ideal of marriage. The person is calling the errant partner to enter into a healthy relationship.

The same principle applies in less volatile situations. If a wife feels her husband is ignoring her, she can say to herself, "There's something wrong with this relationship. As a joint steward of this relationship, I need to call this to my husband's attention." There is nothing selfish about it; it's a matter of upholding a certain *quality of relationship*.

If a friend of yours regularly puts you down, it is not selfish to complain about it. You can say, "You're not treating me as a friend should. Is there a problem here?"

In our era, everyone seems to be clamoring for their rights. It's true, there's a lot of selfishness there. We wish people would start talking about their *responsibilities*. The Bible doesn't talk a lot about our rights, but it does say we should put others ahead of ourselves. Yet there's a phrase it uses repeatedly in describing relationships within the church—"one another." We are to love, honor, speak truth to, submit to, encourage, and pray for *one another*. That's mutuality. Back and forth. We give and receive. God doesn't want lopsided relationships. He wants us to work at maintaining "one another" relationships, in which we have responsibilities *and* rights.

Practice Assertive Responses

In preparation for a conversation or event in which you think you might be intimidated, practice some assertive responses in advance. If you know your friend is going to call and ask you to do something you don't want to do, rehearse in advance what you want to say, so you're not caught speechless when the moment comes. (When we don't know what to say, we usually revert to old habits, so you'll probably end up agreeing unless you practice saying no.)

Role play may also help. One employer had a hard time telling employees they were not working up to par, and as a result, some unsatisfactory situations dragged on. In counseling, he played out certain scenarios in which he would confront an employee before the situation became an even bigger problem. You can do the same thing with a good friend, acting out potentially difficult scenes.

As you plan your assertive responses, keep several strategies in mind:

Use "I language." This may be difficult if you're not used to talking about your own needs, but it will smooth the way for your message. Don't go into this confrontation with guns blazing, saying, "*You* are so inconsiderate, incompetent, and ignorant!" Plan to describe your own feelings:

"*I* can't hear when you're talking like that."

"*I* feel uncomfortable when you tell jokes like that."

"*I* need you to work harder, and I get the feeling you've been sloughing off lately."

Chances are, the person will react less defensively this way. Also, you are talking about what you know (your feelings) as opposed to what you don't know (you can only make assumptions about their motives). They may be able to deny your assumptions, but they can't deny your feelings. They may say, "Oh, those jokes are harmless! Can't you take a joke?" But you can stand by your feelings: "I still feel uncomfortable. I wish you wouldn't tell them when I'm around."

Personal Bill of Rights

1. I have the right to ask for what I want.
2. I have the right to say no to requests or demands that I can't meet.
3. I have a right to my feelings, and the right to express them.
4. I have the right to stand by my convictions and values.
5. I have the right to make mistakes and to not be perfect.
6. I have the right to be treated with dignity and respect.
7. I have the right to change my mind.
8. I have the right to my own personal time and space.[3]

It's OK if they disagree. You don't have to make the other person agree with you. You are merely asserting your feelings. Many of us (people pleasers) want to see eye to eye with everyone, but that will never happen. As you practice your assertive responses, do not imagine situations in which you "convert" the other to your point of view. Practice saying, "Well, maybe we can just agree to disagree," or something along those lines.

The point is, you are achieving a victory by merely stating your views. You don't have to win anyone over.

Uphold the relationship. This may not apply to those ignorant loudmouths sitting behind you at the concert, but if you are asserting yourself *in a relationship,* try to affirm the relationship. Whether you're dealing with a spouse, friend, or business colleague, you may want to establish your common ground before entering into the confrontation. A spouse may begin by saying, "I love you. You know that. But when you do this, it really bugs me." A boss may say to the scuffling employee, "It's my job to ensure that everything gets done properly and efficiently in this office. And I've noticed that you're holding us back in certain areas." With a friend, you might say, "Your friendship means a lot to me, but ..." You get the idea.

Remember, you're not just saying, "You have to please me by doing such-and-such differently." No, you're calling them to a better relationship.

> **In preparation for a conversation or event in which you think you might be intimidated, practice some assertive responses in advance.**

YOUR TURN

1. List some situations in which you need to practice assertive responses.

   Spouse (or girlfriend or boyfriend)?

Your boss, employee, or colleague at work?

Other friends?

Other family—parents or kids?

2. Now choose one of the relationships listed and try to write down a "practice" assertive response. What do you need to say to this person?

_____

_____

_____

_____

_____

3. Now try acting out this scene, saying these lines as if you were actually confronting the person. Do this by yourself or with a trusted friend.

Develop Positive Body Language

Positive body language sends a message of confidence to all those around us. Suggestions for sending this kind of message include:

1. Maintain good eye contact while speaking with others. Don't look down or away.
2. Sit or stand with good posture—not slouched or turned away from the person.
3. Keep an open posture—not with arms or legs crossed tightly.
4. Stand firm in your convictions and speak assertively but without getting angry or hostile.

Learn to Say No

Have you been getting those phone calls lately? Salespeople are always calling you, trying to interest you in a new product, service, or credit card. And it's hard to be polite to these people, isn't it?

You say, "No, I'm sorry, I'm not interested."

You *want* them to say, "Oh, all right. Have a nice day. Bye." But of course they never say that. Somewhere in some textbook of telephone sales, it says: DON'T TAKE NO FOR AN ANSWER.

So they say, "Yes, but have you considered our four-point option plan?" Or "I understand your concern, Mr. So-and-so, but our system is far superior." Or "Here's a number you can call if you have any questions." (You're trying to hang up! Why would you want a number to call?)

Maybe a true test of assertiveness is how long it takes you to hang up on unwanted sales calls.

An important part of your assertiveness training is learning to say no when you really need to. It's about setting limits on those who will make demands on your time and energies.

> **An important part of your assertiveness training is learning to say no when you really need to. It's about setting limits on those who will make demands on your time and energies.**

For most of us, demands on our day keep us moving at a feverish pitch, always feeling that we're falling further and further behind. Then someone comes along and asks you to do one more thing. You know you can't do one more thing, but you see the request as an opportunity to build a new relationship or to endear yourself to the person making the request. What do you do? Many times, we just agree but then later regret the decision.

Does that sound like you? Maybe you just need to learn how to say no! It's a simple word, but it can be very hard to say. This too may take some practice.

Granted, we don't want to seem selfish. We want to help out when we can. But once again, it's a matter of stewardship. If we are already stretched to our limit, we will do no one any good by agreeing to do one more thing. If we are not gifted in a certain area, it makes no sense to agree to take on a project in that area. Saying no in these cases is not selfish—it's using what God has given us.

In these "no-saying" situations, we recommend the following steps.

Make sure you listen to the entire request and clarify what they are asking you to do. You may want to repeat back to the person, "So what you are asking me to do is . . ." You want to make sure the other person knows that you have heard and understood the request.

Thank the person for asking. This will solidify your relationship and make you feel better, even though you have to turn it down.

Regretfully decline. (Assuming that you are regretful.) Say no in a firm but loving way. Don't say "maybe," don't say "if you really need me," don't say "next year"—unless that's what you really mean. Say no.

Give an honest reason. This may be the hardest part. Essentially, you're saying, "Other things I do are more important than this." You don't need to give a detailed reason, however. You might just say, "I'm too busy."

Stick to your guns. If they do not take no for an answer, then you need to state it again, but this time more simply and succinctly. "Thank you again, but my answer will have to be no!"

Some people make it a point never to agree to do something right away. Their answer is always, "I'll let you know tomorrow." Then, with some time to weigh the decision, it's easier to say no. If you are a people pleaser, this might be a good idea. It also gives you time to examine a decision and pray about it. It's hard for even the most zealous church recruiter to argue with an answer like, "I've prayed about it, and I don't feel God wants me to do this."

YOUR TURN

The situations below are designed to help you practice your newfound assertiveness skills. Fill in the blanks with an assertive response to each case.

1. A friend stops by at about five o'clock in the evening and starts chatting with you. But at six o'clock your family is having dinner—and discussing some important family business. As dinnertime approaches, your friend shows no signs of leaving. What do you say?

   _____

   _____

   _____

   _____

2. You hire a contractor to do some work in your kitchen, refacing cabinets and replacing countertops. But you get a bill that's fifty percent higher than the estimate, and it includes some work you didn't ask for. What do you say?

   _____

   _____

   _____

   _____

   _____

3. You're in the express lane at the grocery store with just a few items in hand. But while you're looking at the latest issue of *TV Guide,* somebody with a full cart (and far more than "ten items or less") squeezes in front of you, saying, "I'm in a hurry. I'm sure you don't mind." What do you say?

   _____

   _____

   _____

   _____

   _____

4. You're out driving with a friend who keeps telling you when to slow down, advises which lane to get into, and warns of potential obstacles in the road. All of this unsought driving instruction annoys you. What do you say?

   _____

   _____

   _____

   _____

5. You've planned a quiet night at home, your first free night in a month. But then a friend calls and wants you to come over and talk. There's no crisis. This person just feels a bit lonely. What do you say?

   _____

   _____

   _____

   _____

6. At church, the hospitality chairperson tells you, "Kathy said you wouldn't mind bringing cookies for fellowship hour, so I signed you up for next week. They need to be here half an hour before the service so we can set them out." Of course, you have a terribly busy weekend coming up, and you're not sure when you'll have time to make (or even buy) cookies. What do you say?

_____

_____

_____

_____

_____

7. A decision was made at work that affects your department greatly, but you had little input. You learn that the other employees on your level were consulted, but somehow you were left out of the loop. You wonder if it was an oversight or an intentional slap in the face. In any case, it deeply bothers you. What do you say?

_____

_____

_____

_____

_____

8. The Sunday school superintendent at church calls you and says, "We're desperate for a teacher for the fourth-grade boys. We really need you to do this." You had a previous experience with fourth-grade boys that went badly, nearly ending in a significant loss of sanity. It is clear that you do not have the spiritual gift of teaching fourth grade. What do you say?

_____

_____

_____

_____

_____

18

Breathing Correctly for Better Health

Nancy, a thirty-three-year-old TV producer, faced stressors dozens of times during any given working day. As a day progressed, so did her anxiety and fatigue. She would catch herself holding her breath or notice that her breathing was fast and shallow. On certain hectic days, she felt dizzy and experienced chest pain. By seven o'clock in the evening, she often felt light-headed, weak, and completely drained.

Jack, a forty-year-old emergency room physician, suffered from muscle tension, migraines, and neck and shoulder pain—but only on the days he was on duty. Assuming that certain foods might trigger his headaches, he stayed away from caffeine, red wine, smoked meats, ripened cheese, and foods containing MSG. But he still experienced the same symptoms. Finally, he came to Samuel Verghese. Samuel first asked him to monitor his breathing and posture while he was under pressure. For Jack, most of the pressure came when he was sewing a severed leg back onto an accident victim or frantically pumping a heart that had stopped beating. Yet he decided he would try to keep a record of his breathing.

To his great surprise, Jack discovered that he began to breathe rapidly during high-stress times, and his chest, neck, and throat felt tight. Also, he realized that he was frequently bent over while working on a patient, making it difficult for his diaphragm and lungs to function freely.

What did Nancy and Jack have in common? Shallow, rapid breathing and, as a result, an oxygen-starved brain and body. In this short chapter, we'll examine the process of inspiration and expiration, and the problem of incorrect breathing.

THE BREATHING PROCESS

The primary function of the respiratory system is to supply the body cells with oxygen and to remove the carbon dioxide. In order for body cells to oxidize nutrients and release energy, cells must be supplied with oxygen. As we inhale, the diaphragm, that dome-shaped muscle that separates the lungs from the abdomen, contracts and moves downward. When the diaphragm lowers, the abdominal organs beneath it are compressed. These activities ensure sufficient room for the lungs to expand. As these things occur, air is channeled into our lungs by atmospheric pressure, and the lungs expand. If we need a deeper breath, the diaphragm and intercostal muscles may be contracted further and for a longer period.

When we exhale, the diaphragm and the external intercostal muscles return to their original positions. The abdominal

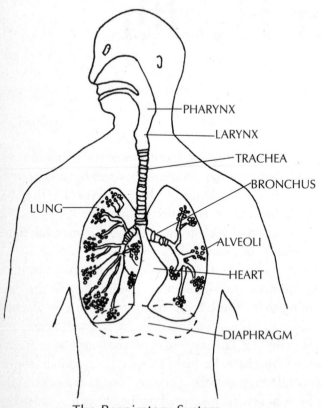

The Respiratory System

organs also return to their previous locations, pushing the diaphragm upward. These activities push the lungs up and force out the air that is inside them.

INCORRECT BREATHING

Incorrect breathing is a natural response to stress. As we have already seen, the body mobilizes for action when it encounters a stressful situation. It grabs the air it needs for a short spurt of activity. As we've been saying about the whole stress response, it's fine if it occurs for a short time and if there is time allowed for recovery. The same thing is true of our breathing. The short, fast breaths taken during a moment of stress can be very good if you need to run somewhere quickly or fend off an attacker. But if you *stay* in a stress situation, those short, fast breaths will rob you of oxygen.

This shallow breathing limits the full function of the diaphragm and the external intercostal muscles. This causes the body to eliminate too much carbon dioxide. Low levels of carbon dioxide disturb the blood's alkaline balance and induce hyperventilation, which can cause dizziness or fainting. Shallow breathing (also called "chest" or "shoulder" breathing) does not get enough air to the lower part of the lungs. It has been suggested that this can bring about anxiety, momentary memory loss, and panic attacks. Other results of poor breathing include exhaustion, cold hands or feet, chest pains, headaches, gulping, sighing, and frequent yawning.

YOUR TURN

Check Your Breathing

1. While sitting or standing straight, breathe normally. Count your breaths per minute. About ten to twelve breaths per minute should be fine.
2. Stand in front of a mirror. Place one hand on the upper part of your chest, the other on the lower edge of your ribcage. Inhale. If your stomach (and lower ribcage) expands more than your chest does, you are breathing correctly. If your chest rises more than your abdomen, your breathing is faulty.

Breathing Correctly

The following exercises can help uncoil your tense, aching body and help you breathe in a healthy manner.

1. Inhale slowly through the nose and fill your lungs with fresh air (inhale for four to six seconds). Then breathe out slowly and smoothly, drawing your abdomen in and back toward your spine.

2. Consciously inhale and concentrate on your rising stomach. While exhaling, focus on your stomach pulling in comfortably and force the air out.

3. As you breathe, visualize the process. Imagine, just below your ribcage, a deflated balloon. While inhaling, feel the balloon slowly inflating. While exhaling, feel it deflating.

4. Imagine the air-exchange that goes on when you breathe. As you inhale, sense the oxygen-rich air pouring into your body. Imagine the molecules of oxygen being carried in the blood to the various parts of your body. Even your fingertips should feel full and energized. As you exhale, sense the elimination of the carbon dioxide you don't need. Every breath can clean your mind and energize your body and help you manage your stress better. Breathing correctly of course, may not fully solve your stress-related symptoms; you need to combine all options discussed in this book—absolute faith and love in God, eating right, correct exercise, sufficient rest, relaxation, healthy habits, and stress management skill.

19

Exercise for Body and Mind

A reliable body of scientific evidence supports the immeasurable value of exercise and relaxation, and affirms both as critical to total health and well-being. A longitudinal study published in the *Journal of the American Medical Association* showed that the least-fit individuals had greater risk of premature death. The study of 10,224 men and 3,120 women was conducted to determine if regular physical exercise helped people live longer.[1]

Even after all risk factors such as high blood pressure, smoking, and cancer were included in the results, men and women with low levels of physical fitness were more than twice as likely to die early as people who exercised moderately. The study defined "exercise" as planned workout time rather than normal, everyday-life-related activities.

For doctors and researchers, debate about physical and mental exercise and relaxation is a nonissue. It is widely recognized among health professionals that cardiovascular improvement through exercise is a life and brain extender. An effective exercise program can reduce your brain stress and body stress, improve health, firm muscles, and help you lose weight.

Remember, one of the most effective ways to manage stress is through developing your own style of exercise to fit your needs. So adapt or design a program that is most useful for you.

NO AGE LIMIT ON BODY AND BRAIN EXERCISE

Do you remember the fun you had as a child—running, chasing, jumping, and biking?

Sure you do! Well, you can experience those exhilarating feelings again. Who knows, you may feel like a kid again!

> **An effective exercise program can reduce your brain stress and body stress, improve health, firm muscles, and help you lose weight.**

At any age, walking, stretching, low-impact aerobics, physical yoga exercises, slow body movements, and deep breathing can improve overall wellness, including mental functions. Even inactive elderly people can enjoy better physical and mental health with regular exercise, according to a report in *Geriatrics*. Seventy-five patients ranging in age from sixty-five to ninety-eight participated in a slow exercise routine for six weeks in a program called SMILE (So Much Improvement with Little Exercise). They attempted a variety of exercises: gentle neck and shoulder rolls; slow back twists; side bends; feet and arm extensions, rotations, and flexes; and slow, deep breathing. After six weeks, most of the elderly reported more flexibility, less stiffness, and more energy.[2]

Getting Started

Here are some tips for staying strong, relaxing, and having fun with exercise!

Get medical tests and assessments. Ask your physician to check your urine, blood pressure, lungs, and heart functions to rule out any conditions such as hypertension, irregular heartbeats (arrhythmias), or diabetes. If you are a healthy thirty-or-younger athlete, expensive exercise stress tests are unnecessary. In fact, they frequently result in false positives (meaning that the test may show problems that are not present) according to Victor Frollicher, M.D., chief of cardiology at Veterans Administration Medical Center, Long Beach, California. Request tests that confirm your levels of cholesterol, protein, vitamins, minerals, and hormones if needed. This is especially important if you are over forty, have not exercised for a number of years, and have risk factors for heart disease or stroke.

Assess your body type and pick correct exercise. There are usually three body types:

1. People who are lean

2. People who are heavy

3. People who are in the middle

Jogging may be fine for the lean, light person. If you are a heavy person, walking or other low- or non-impact exercise is safer.

Set reasonable exercise goals. Don't conquer the world your first time out. Consult your doctor or fitness professionals to establish good goals and limits for your program.

Slowly ease in by pacing your fitness activities. The first few times out will be the hardest. So take it easy! Don't rush to meet your goals. Take your time getting used to your exercise regimen.

Schedule your exercise time when you are not extremely tired but alert. If your mind slacks off during exercise, you may not do the exercises properly, resulting in harm to your body, or at least decreased benefit. Also, you may fail to notice warning signs of overexertion.

A good rule: After exercising, rest for five minutes and count your pulse. If the count is above 120 beats per minute, you're doing too much.

Make exercise convenient and pleasant. The key thing to an exercise program is that you *do* it. If you join a health club, find one close enough that you can visit a few times a week. Don't push yourself so hard that it stops being fun.

Don't overstrain your body. Overdoing can increase the chances of injury and internal infections. Be sensitive to warning signs: chronic fatigue, unexplained weight loss, persistent aches and pains after exercise, appetite loss, excessive thirst, disturbed sleep, serious hormonal changes, and severe gasping for breath while exercising.

If you exercise in a hot environment, quench your thirst before starting. Then continue to drink a small amount of fluids *during* exercise if you're thirsty. Spray water on yourself to keep cool. If you are taking aspirin, keep in mind that hot weather can cause dehydration through excessive sweating and urination, especially if you are involved in long-distance running.

Finish strenuous exercise gradually. This eases the effect of your falling blood pressure and heart rate. If these drop too quickly, you may feel dizziness or cramps or something worse. Do a light exercise after a heavy exercise, to wind down.

Use deep, regular breathing. (See chapter 18.)

Avoid harmful exercise. This would include bouncing on a hard surface, serious back bends, deep knee bends and push-ups, jumping jacks with rapidly swinging arms, hanging upside down, high-impact aerobic dancing, running on hard surfaces, heavy wrist and ankle weights, and touching the toes while standing with the knees in locked position (which places abnormal pressure on the lumbar vertebrae; slightly bend your knees to avoid back problems).

Consider setting up a home gym. If you don't like the outdoors or the social aspects of working out in a club, a setup in your home can be ideal. Arrange an open space for running and walking in place and floor exercise. Look into an exercise bike or stair climber. But do take precautions: have a phone or alarm system nearby for emergency health needs.

Wear good walking or jogging shoes. The proper foot support can prevent injury and maximize the value of your exercise.

Avoid exercising outdoors during peak traffic hours, to avoid toxic pollutants. Try not to run along the road during rush hour.

Swing your arms as you walk. This can increase the intensity of your walk. Don't hold your arms straight and stiff. Bend your elbows and swing loosely. Slow down if you tire.[3]

Take stairs rather than elevators and escalators. Walk on the golf course and carry your own clubs. Park your car far enough (during the daytime) from the store, the office, or the train station to give you the pleasure of extra walking. In short, find the value of exercise in everyday movements.

Buy good fitness books or videos for inspiration. To prevent you from getting bored with your preferred exercises, learn more about total fitness. There are plenty of good helps on the market.

Try exercising with a friend. If the going gets tough, you may need some encouragement. Make your exercise time a social time by joining up with a companion.

Engage in "complete" physical activities. Certain sports and pastimes such as cross-country skiing, rowing, swimming, low-impact aerobic dancing, skating, or biking can give you complete body conditioning, burn off calories, and enhance shaping and cardiovascular fitness. And they're fun too.

Give yourself rewards. For example, buy a plant for your bedroom or get a massage or facial. Set certain goals for your program and give yourself a trophy of some sort when you reach them.

Wipe your mental slate clean of negative thoughts by thinking positive thoughts. "Oh, I hate this. I'm really out of shape. Only one more lap and I'm free from this dungeon. I'm so fat." Have you heard any of those comments in your head lately? Replace those thoughts with brighter ones. Celebrate the joy of movement. God has given us our bodies, and we can praise him for them, whatever shape they're in.

Get Used to Timing Heart Rates

Fitness experts generally agree that there are three heart rates we need to become accustomed to: the resting heart rate, the maximum heart rate, and the recovery heart rate.

The resting heart rate. This is the number of pulse beats per minute *when you are at rest*. The resting rate of those in good physical shape is usually lower than those who are out of shape, because the healthy heart pumps a sufficient volume of blood for every contraction; it doesn't have to drudge as hard as a weak heart.

The maximum heart rate. This is the safe range at which your heart should beat *while you exercise*. It serves as an internal guide to keep us away from working too hard or not hard enough. You can estimate your maximum heart rate by subtracting your age from 220. If you are 40 years old, your maximum heart rate is 180 beats per minute (220 minus 40).

Depending on your health and fitness level, you can decide whether you should be exercising below or near this rate. The American College of Sports Medicine (ACSM) recommends that you maintain a heart rate of sixty to ninety percent of your maximum safe heart rate during exercise. Beginners should work at the lower end of this range, and only competitive athletes should work as high as eighty-five to ninety percent. Take your pulse and note how you feel within your range.

You can estimate your maximum heart rate by subtracting your age from 220.

If you are overweight, you should exercise at the low end of the training heart rate range or even slightly lower than the range, because of the added stress on your body.

Therefore if you are 40 years old and not overweight, your target heart rate during exercise should be between 108 and 162 beats per minute (60–90% of 180). When you exercise, therefore, test your pulse to ensure it is within the proper range.

The recovery heart rate. This is your pulse rate taken five minutes *after you have stopped exercising*. It shows how quickly you recover. If the pulse rate is higher than 120 beats per minute, you need to reduce your exercise intensity or its duration. As you slowly build up, your heart will become stronger and you'll see your recovery heart rate drop.

Measuring Your Heart Rate

Each heartbeat is a pulse or stroke. The pulse is a manifestation of the expansion of the arteries that occurs when the heart contracts and forces blood into the circulatory system. Pulse can be measured almost anywhere an artery lies near the skin surface; the wrist is one such location.

Press lightly with the first two or three fingers on the inside of the wrist near the bone, about an inch below the base of the thumb. If you are going to measure the pulse for the first time, it is best to count all the beats for sixty seconds. Later, you may count for fifteen seconds and multiply by four. Or count for ten and multiply by six to get the heart rate for one minute.

Reminder: If you are over forty and have not been exercising regularly, you should consult your personal health care provider before starting an exercise program. People with preexisting cardiac or respiratory disease or with any other medical or physical condition need to consult their personal health care provider prior to embarking on an exercise program.

Your heath care provider may assist you in determining your training zone, based on your needs and current condition.

SAMPLE EXERCISES FOR A FIT BODY AND MIND

Until recently, many (including the American College of Sports Medicine) promoted the idea of a thirty-minute aerobic exercise program. Today most sports medicine specialists, exercise physiologists, and other researchers acknowledge that *any* physical activity is beneficial for overall fitness. (This does not apply for those interested in advanced weight and strength training.)

A recent study conducted at Stanford University determined that ten minutes of aerobic exercise three times a day is as beneficial to heart and lungs as thirty continuous minutes.

Indeed, you too can design your exercise program and enjoy a fit body and mind.

What Is Fitness?

Body and brain fitness means a well-conditioned, well-nourished muscular and brain system. Your brain, heart, muscles, and other vital organs need regular exercise to stay fit. Your body fitness is important for a healthy brain. You are fit if you can

- carry out daily mental tasks and challenges without feeling fatigue or being irritable, impatient, or upset
- climb one or two flights of stairs without gasping for air or feeling fatigue in your legs
- carry out daily tasks with little or no struggle and have energy to spare

Warm-Up

Before beginning any exercise program, for safety's sake make specific stretching a habit. First, warm up for five minutes with low-intensity, low-impact aerobics such as walking around or marching in place. Follow with five minutes of stretching the arms, shoulders, neck, trunk, and legs. Stretching is like flexibility training; it prevents injury and increases your range of motion.

Before beginning any exercise program, for safety's sake make specific stretching a habit.

Low-Impact Movement Exercises

These exercises flow from one to another. Do about ten to fifteen repetitions of each exercise or spend fifteen to twenty seconds on each exercise. Choose your own intensity for ten minutes of warm-up or for regular exercises. If you are a beginner, your body may not maintain the advanced stretch position with good form; if you shake and feel intolerable muscle and joint pain, go slowly. Avoid quick, vigorous stretching, which may tear muscle fibers and tissue. If you have back or other physical problems, consult your physician.

Low step kicks. Stand and kick your left leg forward while swinging your right arm. Then plant your left leg and kick your right leg while swinging your left arm. Continue alternating.

Low Step Kicks

Multiple Knee Lifts

Multiple knee lifts. Stand with legs shoulder width apart, knees slightly bent, and hands on your shoulders. Lift one knee as you push both arms straight overhead. Drop knee and arms and repeat with the other side. Keep alternating.

Straddle lift. Start with arms at your sides and feet a little more than shoulder width apart. Then stand on your toes while lifting both arms overhead. Return to starting position and repeat.

Straddle Lift

Alternating knee lifts. Stand with knees slightly bent, feet a little more than shoulder width apart. With your arms, grab your right leg at the thigh and lift it up and to the right. Return to starting position and repeat with the left leg.

Alternating Knee Lifts

Marching. Stand straight, knees and arms relaxed. Raise right knee toward your stomach until your thigh is parallel to the floor, while swinging left arm forward. Repeat opposite side. Continue in a marching motion.

Marching

Power lunges. Stand with your feet shoulder width apart and arms slightly bent at your sides. Lift your right leg and lunge forward, shifting your weight onto that leg. At the same time, lift your right arm straight overhead. It's a karate move. Switch sides and continue.

Power Lunges

Hip, groin, and thigh flexors

Hip, groin, and thigh flexors. Kneel on one knee. Bring the front (raised) knee back to the other knee, then bring the other knee forward. Continue. You may need to place your fingers on the floor to keep your balance.

Gluteus and hamstring stretch. While lying on your back on a padded carpet or exercise mat, lift one leg and grasp the back of your upper thigh with both hands and pull your leg gently toward your chest, keeping the leg straight up in the air. Hips and buttocks should remain on the floor. Opposite leg may bend slightly. Return to starting position and repeat with other leg.

Gluteus and Hamstring Stretch

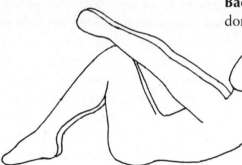

Back-knee sit-up. This exercise strengthens the abdominal muscles. Lie on your back on the floor, mat, or carpet with your knees bent and feet flat on the floor about a foot apart. Slowly move your chin up toward your chest while lifting your shoulders up and reaching your palms toward your knees. Stop at the point of struggle, hold for about five seconds, then return to starting position.

Back-knee Sit-up

Start with a manageable number in the beginning and increase as needed in the future. Caution: don't place your hands behind your head and lift your upper body.

Lower Back Exercise

Lower back exercise. Stack two pillows on the floor and lie face down on your stomach with your lower abdomen on the pillows. With arms to the side or forward, push up so your midsection is three to five inches off the pillows, hold for five to ten seconds, then slowly lower your body. Repeat.

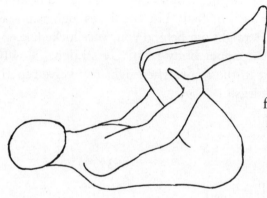

Lower back stretch. Lie on your back on a floor mat and bend knees toward chest. Place hands on the back of thighs and draw legs tighter toward chest. Hold for a moment, then slowly lower your legs. Repeat eight to twelve times, if possible.

Lower Back Stretch

If you are a beginner, start with the lighter weights and the fewest sets and repetitions. Follow your program for one day, and the next day take a break.

If you are at the intermediate or advanced level and able to stretch to the limits of each position while maintaining correct form and good stretching sensation, then go for it. If you are interested in strength training, even with light ankle weights and dumbbells, you can improve your strength and endurance and feel even better about yourself. You can alternate weight-bearing activities with non-weight-bearing activities. This can make your workout more fun.

Twenty-Five-Minute Weight Training Program

You will need:
      Ankle weights—as you can handle
      Dumbbells—as you can handle
      A firm, armless chair with a back support

   Begin at a level that is right for you.

Standing hamstring curl, hip extension, and knee flexion. This strengthens calves, back of hamstrings, and buttocks muscles. With the weights around the ankles, stand holding on to back of chair. Lift one leg as high as possible, straight out behind you, knee locked, keeping the upper body relatively straight. Slowly lower leg to the floor. After eight to twelve repetitions, switch legs.

Standing Hamstring Curl, Hip Extension, and Knee Flexion

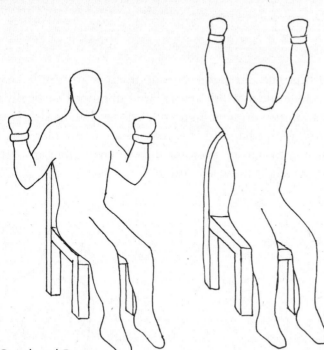

Overhead press. This strengthens the upper back and upper chest. Sit on the chair with your back straight and feet flat on the floor. Hold dumbbells in each hand at shoulder level and push the weights directly up above the shoulders. Don't lock the elbows. Slowly lower weights to shoulder level and repeat up to eight to twelve times.

Overhead Press

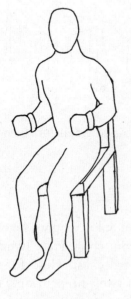

Side shoulder raise. Strengthens shoulder, chest, and upper back muscles. While relaxed, sit on chair with your back in a straight position, feet shoulder width apart and toes pointing forward. Holding dumbbells vertically with palms inward, bend elbows to ninety degrees and hold them close to your sides. Now slowly raise your arms straight out to the side (not unbending your elbows), just above shoulder level. Lower slowly to starting position and repeat up to eight to twelve times.

Side Shoulder Raise

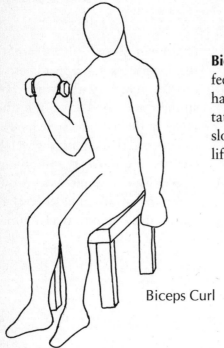

Biceps curl. Strengthens front of upper arm. Sit in chair, feet shoulder width apart. Hold dumbbell vertically in hand, then draw palm up to chest level while slowly rotating your hand to face toward your shoulder. Lower slowly to starting position and switch to other arm after lifting eight to twelve times.

Biceps Curl

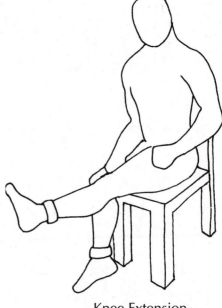

Knee Extension

Knee extension. Strengthens front of thigh. Sit straight and relaxed in chair, with feet flat, toes forward, and weights around your ankles. Hold side of chair if you need support, and slowly extend one leg out in front until knee is straight but not locked. Slowly lower your leg. Do the same with the other leg. Repeat eight to twelve times on each side.

Lower back stretch. Strengthens lower back. Without ankle weights, lie on your back on a floor mat and bend knees toward your chest. Place hands on the back of thighs and draw legs tighter toward chest. Hold for a moment, then slowly lower your legs. Do eight to twelve repetitions, if possible.

At Tufts University a group of adults of various ages participated in a one-year strength-training exercise program that included a similar routine. The participants acquired many benefits from the exercise, including gain in muscle mass as well as muscle strength. "After one year of strength training," the researchers found, "they emerged physiologically younger by fifteen to twenty years than when they began. Even their psychological profiles were much more youthful." One does not have to buy expensive exercise equipment or even join a health club. With simple homemade or store-bought dumbbells and ankle weights, one can replicate the Tufts exercise program at home.[4]

If you are a beginner, start with light weights (2–5 pounds) and only two or three sets of ten repetitions each. Follow your program for one day, and the next day take a break. Strength training two days in a row is not recommended. If you need outside help, many local fitness and health organizations such as the YMCA—or individuals certified by the American College of Sports Medicine, a college or university, or a physical education or sports medicine center—may offer classes at a reasonable cost.

Using high resistance and a low number of repetitions is the quickest way to increase muscle strength and achieve ideal muscle conditioning. While the above exercises can improve your health, if you are interested in a more vigorous workout program, you may also use good exercise videos and books, such as those listed below.

- *The Stanford Health & Exercise Program,* Crocus Entertainment Inc., 120 minutes, $19.95. A video with three levels of excellent, well-planned aerobic workouts.
- *Jane Fonda's Workout—Light Aerobics and Stress Reduction Program,* Warner Home Video, 55 minutes, $29.98. A video with a unique stress reduction component.
- *Step and Slide,* Club Cardio Video, 62 minutes, $24.95 (to order, call 1-800-433-6769). A video designed to enhance cardiovascular endurance while forming all muscles of the lower body. The two major pieces of equipment necessary are the slide and the step. Exercise veteran Linda McHugh, a dynamic choreographer, does a nice job.
- Donna Richardson's *Back to Basics,* Video Treasures, 65 minutes, $19.95 (to order, call 1-800-745-1145). A video that is funky, fun, always stresses safety and good form, and is definitely worth the effort. Donna, a familiar face on ESPN, really gets the viewer motivated.

- *Steppin' Out*, New and Unique Videos, 60 minutes, $19.95 (to order, call 1-800-365-8433). Carrie Weiland challenges exercisers to work harder, better, and stronger, with advanced step aerobics and weight training featuring lunges, squats, and propulsions, in which safety and form are stressed.
- *Ken Levy's Fighting Trim Workout*, Ken Levy, 60 minutes, $29.00. A video with interesting, motivating self-defense moves with aerobics for intermediate and advanced exercisers.

SUMMARY

Although a sedentary life is one of the worst things for our body and brain, most of us spend a great deal of our time sitting. The benefits of regular exercise reduce overall risk of death from all causes, including cardiovascular disease and cancer, by about seventy percent. Some studies show that exercise promotes development of new coronary arteries if existing arteries are blocked due to blood fats. Regular exercisers are also less likely to suffer from stroke, high blood pressure, and other circulatory disorders. Some studies have shown that if you have non-insulin-dependent diabetes, exercise can reduce the level of your blood sugar. It may even prevent diabetes. Exercise can also increase blood flow to the brain, improving mental ability.

20

Nutrition

Donna, age forty-eight, was a successful mother and teacher going through a divorce. She felt emotionally and physically exhausted in the morning, early afternoon, and sometimes throughout the day. When she felt her energy level getting low, she was anxious and irritable and she reached for sugar-rich snacks or caffeine, only to experience short-lived energy boosts.

Michael was plagued by fatigue and exhaustion. At thirty-nine, he owned a company that had more than sixty-five employees. Frequently he became irritable, tense, and moody due to low energy levels. He also had difficulty concentrating on his work. Since his yearly physical examinations, including blood tests, had satisfactory outcomes (ruling out diabetes, hypoglycemia, and thyroid problems), his complaints seemed to have a nutritional basis. Was he eating right?

The simple fact is this: You can enhance your body's ability to deal with stress, if you eat well. Your body will be prepared for its natural stress responses.

Nine-year-old Christine and eighteen-year-old Todd were both experiencing a roller-coaster effect in their energy levels. Their roller coaster ascended strongly but bottomed out by midmorning. Sometimes they did not eat breakfast or skipped lunch, and they usually ate poorly. The typical sugar-laden breakfast foods and fatty lunches (made with hydrogenated oils and processed flours) can make anyone feel fatigued, sleepy, and sluggish within about two hours.

Jerry, forty-two, was a healthy insurance executive who had a physical exam and came out with flying colors. Nobody expected him to suffer a sudden cardiac death (SCD) without a history of heart disease; the autopsy showed no evidence of atherosclerosis. He had not experienced any arrhythmia or ischemia. But his wife indicated that work-related stress, along with a stressful family situation and poor eating, had been taking a severe toll on him.

Donna, Michael, Christine, Todd, and Jerry share a common problem with millions of others—chemical imbalances in the brain and body, caused by incorrect foods and nutrients. Mental and physical stress caused by poor nutrition is a great threat to our immune system.

The simple fact is this: You can enhance your body's ability to deal with stress, if you eat well. Stressful events will still occur, but you can take them in stride. That is, your body will be prepared for its natural stress responses.

On the other hand, you can hurt your body's ability to deal with stress, if you eat poorly. Your body's natural stress reactions can cause you *greater* stress, resulting in a snowball effect.

BRAIN AND BODY, AND STRESS REACTION

Stress in the body usually accompanies heightened physical, neural, chemical, and emotional stimulation. Earlier we discussed the way the body gears up for a stress event, in a fight-or-flight response. A series of events occurs in the brain, mainly through two closely connected systems—the *hormonal* (endocrine) system and the *autonomic nervous* system.

In the hormonal route, when the brain experiences a stressful thought or event, neurons (cells of the brain or nervous system) communicate through chemicals called neurotransmitters. These chemical molecules seep (travel) out of one neuron to another, then send dangerous electrical triggers, causing the hypothalamus region of the brain to activate the *sympathetic* nervous system.

The sympathetic nervous system is the half of the autonomic nervous system that is *active* while experiencing stress. Via this system, commands received from your brain travel down your spine and branch out to almost every organ, muscle, artery, and vein throughout your body. This system is chiefly responsible for activating the pituitary, adrenal, and thyroid glands to secrete a number of hormones into the bloodstream. These in turn trigger a chain reaction of hormonal and autonomic responses that affect the total person.

During the fight-or-flight process, the sympathetic nervous system is hyperactive and increases the adrenal gland's secretions of hormones, especially the *stress hormones*—corticotropin (CRF) and glucocorticoid along with epinephrine and norepinephrine. At the initial stage of response, adrenaline levels are at the highest, to help confront the challenges. But noradrenaline is released later as the stressful exertion continues. (Adrenaline and nor- adrenaline are British terms for the American designations epinephrine and norepinephrine.) The effects of these hormonal secretions include increased heart rate, constricted abdominal arteries, dilated pupils, increased release of glucose from the liver, additional hydrochloric acid in the stomach, increased blood cholesterol, and elevated blood pressure, to mention a few.

In short, your brain and body is made to believe that you are in danger, hormones electrify your system for action, and blood rushes to the vital organs to help you face the challenge. When this happens, you vasoconstrict in other parts of your body. This means that the blood vessels tighten up in the extremities of your body, causing the heart to pump harder to push blood to the feet and the fingers. This state of alertness causes the hormones and nervous system to ignore other important bodily functions.

When we don't care for our bodies, it affects us physically, emotionally, and even spiritually.

The body can afford to do this temporarily, while a short-term danger exists. But if this process does not stop after the emergency situation, it can result in numerous neurophysiological damages.

The sympathetic nervous system not only triggers the negative effects, it also suppresses the activities in the *parasympathetic* nervous system, the other half of the autonomic nervous system.

The parasympathetic nervous system controls many crucial mind-brain-body functions such as sleep, relaxation, and internal calmness—and is involved in quiet mediation and prayer. It is active in bodily recovery and healing processes. It also promotes growth, energy, storage, blood pressure control, correct heart rhythms, maintenance of essential minerals, and positive cognition. Parasympathetic activity is also associated with controlling many of our emotions, including anger, rage, and irrational fears. But this half of our autonomic nervous system is generally *inactive* during a stress response.

Chronic Stress and Risks

A prolonged fight-or-flight response overstimulates the sympathetic nervous system, triggering hypersecretions of the stress hormones, "turning off" the parasympathetic nervous system, and thus seriously threatening our immune system. Immunologists are not always absolutely able to predict the subtle interrelation of stress, immune function, and disease, because the process is an intricate web, involving factors such as diet, nutrition, mind, social interaction, spiritual issues, risk factors, and other nonlinear components. Yet many valid scientific studies clearly show the immunological consequences of stress.

At the National Institutes of Health Conference in Bethesda, Maryland, one doctor reported the results of a study indicating that stress robs a person's energy, increasing susceptibility to infection with rhinoviruses. The study also discovered that with each virus, the patients' assessments of their own level of stress correlated with their likelihood of being infected. And people with a higher degree of stress contracted colds twice as frequently as people with less stress.[1]

We have learned from AIDS-related research that stress can suppress or impair our immune system. The immune system's primary function is to protect our bodies against infection from bacteria, fungi, parasites, and viruses. But chronic secretions of the stress hormones impede our immune system, weakening our defense from within. This means that the lymphatic system—including the thymus gland, spleen, lymph nodes, lymphatic vessels, tonsils, white blood cells, and other hormonal and blood components—is severely inhibited, making us susceptible to numerous disorders.

Also, when the immune system is weak, invading microorganisms may not be destroyed effectively and may enter our body and make us sick. Tremendously accelerated demand placed on our vital organs, immune system, and especially the master gland—the thymus—can weaken them prematurely. In fact, immunologists have discovered that the chronic oversecretion of stress hormones can cause the thymus to shrink prematurely. Normally, thymic levels are low in the elderly and people exposed to chronic infectious immune disorders.

Increased secretions of the stress hormones can also accelerate our metabolic rate, placing a greater demand on the pancreas to produce more glucose to keep the blood sugar level stable. This can prematurely weaken or even impair the pancreas.

Continued high production of stress hormones can accelerate the breakdown of proteins and muscles, a process known as *catabolism*. This chemical interaction, under prolonged stress, can disturb the balance of specific amino acids. Depletion of certain amino acids can result in neurobiochemical disturbances, causing depression, mood swings, sleeplessness, and other behavioral and physical disorders. These imbalances can disturb or deplete the balance of vitamins, minerals, enzymes, and other nutrients.

It is also well known that the cardiovascular system is weakened with each succeeding stressor experience, making the system progressively vulnerable to sudden cardiac death. In his research at NASA, Robert S. Eliot, M.D., discovered that healthy aerospace engineers and scientists between the ages of twenty-eight and thirty-five were dropping dead—not because of any apparent heart disorder but due to mysterious microscopic lesions that appeared in the fibers of their heart muscles *(contraction band lesions).*

About half of all heart attacks happen within forty-eight hours of a major stress event.

Experts confirm that frequent large doses of adrenaline-like chemicals released during stressful experiences could cause such lesions! For those at high risk, daily excessive levels of stress may imply silent heart problems lurking within.[2]

Noting that about half of all heart attacks happen within forty-eight hours of a major stress event, Sandra McLanahan, M.D., director of stress management training at the Preventative Research Institute in Sausalito, California, urges people to develop heart-healthy habits in their diet and their life. "Since about half of Americans develop some sort of heart disease, we all need to consider eating a lower-fat diet and learning how to manage *stress.*"[3]

Clearly, stress is hazardous to your health. But there are ways to prepare your body nutritionally for the onslaught of stress. Proper food will boost your immune system and help your bodily systems get back to normal after a sudden stressor.

The kind of food you eat affects measurably your mind, brain, body, emotions, and consequently your Christian walk. So learn to eat foods that help you view stressors positively. Learn to avoid or reduce the intake of harmful foods. And learn what supplements will minimize your health risks.

USING FOOD POWER TO MANAGE STRESS

The food we eat has power—power to reduce the negative impact of stress, to produce a healthy immune system, to boost energy, to prevent fatigue, to make us feel good, to heal, to prevent diseases, perhaps even to slow down premature aging and to allow us to experience a hundred other wonders. To make those miracles happen, we need to gain a wealth of knowledge about the foods God has given us.

At the University of Illinois in Chicago, scientists are storing data about edible and nonedible plants. The database, called NAPRALERT, contains over 110,000 entries. In recent years, scientists have been able to isolate and test the efficacy of minute quantities of bioactive plant and food compounds on disease and healing processes. Also, research scientists have conducted intervention studies in which people with a certain disorder are placed on specific foods, and records are kept on who improves, deteriorates, or remains stable during a course of two, three, or more years. Numerous such tests, along with population and epidemiological research, have given us the knowledge to confirm that foods do have specific medicine-like properties to be used as immune protectors, cancer fighters, antihypertensives, antidepressants, sedatives, tranquilizers, analgesics, antibiotics, and anti-inflammatory agents, to name a few important uses.

Of course, you are free to put this food power to use without any prescription. But if you are going to substitute foods for medications, you need to consult your doctor first.

On the Stress-Fighting Front

In recent years, a vast body of physicians and scientists from around the world have focused on a number of nutrients—vitamin C, beta-carotene, and vitamin E—as capable of fighting cancer, heart disease, and other diseases. But in April 1994, when results of the Alpha-Tocopherol (vitamin E) and Beta-Carotene Cancer Prevention Study (ATBC) were published in the *New England Journal of Medicine*, it dampened the enthusiasm of some researchers. Yet the now famous Finnish clinical trial administered only small daily doses of vitamin E and beta-carotene (50mg and 20mg respectively), amounts far less than the several hundred milligrams found in most commercially available supplements. Another shortcoming is that participants (Finnish smokers) were monitored for an average of only six years, a relatively short duration.[4]

You are free to put healthy foods to use without any prescription. But if you are going to substitute foods for medications, you need to consult your doctor first.

In the same issue of *NEJM*, three leading epidemiologists advised that the results of the ATBC trial should not be viewed as showing these vitamins to be ineffective or hazardous.[5]

In fact, a study from China published in the *Journal of the National Cancer Institute* revealed that vitamin E and selenium given in combination with beta-carotene appeared to reduce the risk of stomach cancer.[6]

Preliminary research presented in the *American Journal of Clinical Nutrition* suggests that a multivitamin a day boosted the immunity in people over age sixty.[7] Since scientists have been unable to precisely target antioxidant vitamins or foods to specific cancers, heart disease, or other diseases, the best thing is to eat plenty of vegetables—especially green, leafy kinds—and fruits. These can boost our immune defenses against bacterial and viral infections and destroy carcinogens. Vegetables and fruits are rich in thousands of compounds such as the lesser-known indoles, lutein, cryptoxanthin, zeaxanthin, lycopene, quarcotin, selenium, glutathione, and the well-known vitamins C and E.

The Oxygen War

Imagine two opposing forces in our bodies, engaged in battle. The valiant defenders of health and vitality are the *antioxidants,* and the deficient defectors are the *oxidants.*

It may surprise you, but oxygen is the bad guy here. It's actually a two-edged sword. Though it sustains life, oxygen can also damage our cells the same way it can rust iron. A combination of environmental pollutants, poor nutrition, smoking, and normal cellular metabolic processes (such as breathing and immune functions) can rob normal oxygen atoms of crucial electrons. This produces unstable oxygen molecules with an insufficient number of electrons *(free radicals)*. These are simply waste products, but they possess fierce destructive potency.

When our bodies are exposed to chronic stress, free radicals gain strength and attack our immune system. Antioxidants strive to protect our bodies by fending off these destructive oxidants.

The free radicals take various forms. Since the molecules of the free radical atoms lack one of the electrons that is required to keep them stable, they furiously travel throughout the body in search of the missing electron. In the process, they steal electrons from good but weak cells and create more free radical renegades. Then they continue their savage journey. This robbing and pairing of electrons creates a damaging free radical chain reaction in our bodies that erodes our cell membranes and can alter the many cells that encode genetic information in the DNA, these cells to mutate. This is the first step on the path to cancer and other illnesses.

Only the free radical *scavengers* that occur naturally in our body can neutralize the radicals. This neutralization process is accomplished chiefly by antioxidant substances such as vitamin A and beta-carotene, vitamins C and E, glutathione, coenzyme Q_{10}, selenium, lycopene, and other nutrients. You can get a sufficient supply of antioxidants by eating lots of fruits and vegetables. This will help maintain tissue concentrations of these vital nutrients.

ANTIOXIDANT FOOD AND SUPPLEMENT GUIDE
Disease-Fighting Antioxidant Foods

almonds	ginger	peppermint
apricots	grapes	peppers
asparagus	grapefruit (pink)	pumpkin
basil leaf	guava	sage
berries	kale	sago palm
broccoli	lettuce (dark green)	salmon
Brussels sprouts	mackerel	sardines
cabbage	mustard greens	sesame seeds
cantaloupe	nutmeg	spinach
carrots	oats	sweet potato
chili pepper	onions (red or yellow)	Swiss chard
collard greens	low)	tangerines
cumin	oranges	tomato
fish	papaya	watermelon
garlic	peanuts	

As a rule, shop for the darkest-green, leafy vegetables and colorful fruits. Fresh and frozen vegetables and fruits have more antioxidants than canned or cooked.

Vitamin A and carotenoids. Vitamin A helps your body's immune system by keeping the microbe-catching membranes of the mouth, respiratory passages, and skin intact. Also, it is essential for healthy eyes, bones, and organs. Vitamin A deficiency is not very common in the United States, so do not overdose. You can get natural and synthetic forms of vitamin A. Synthetic forms of vitamin A are generally water-soluble supplements, making it more absorbable than the fat-soluble form of vitamin A derived from fish liver oils or other animal fats. Retinol is the vitamin A in animal foods. This also helps to produce healthy mucous cells and manufacture germ-killing enzymes. Remarkably, foods rich in beta-carotene and vitamin A appear to reduce your risk of stroke dramatically. A Harvard study that tracked about ninety thousand female nurses for eight years revealed that eating carrots five times a week or more reduced stroke a surprising sixty-eight percent, compared with eating carrots just once a month or less.[8]

Major food sources of vitamin A are: carrots, spinach, apricots, dried peaches, dark green, leafy vegetables, sweet potatoes, pumpkins, beets, and mangoes. Daily dose is 25,000mg combined. Note: cooking does not destroy these vitamins.

Scientists have discovered forty or so carotenoids in foods that protect our body from various diseases, including cancer.

Vitamin C. Essential for collagen formation, vitamin C combats stress and muscular weakness, and stimulates immune systems. Numerous scientific studies indicate that the energy function of your immune system is strengthened by vitamin C. It assists in activation of folacin, in iron absorption, and in other brain functions. It aids in tissue repair, increases appetite, heals wounds and bleeding gums, and serves as a powerful antioxidant to protect against asthma, bronchitis, cataracts, angina, and male infertility. It is useful for fatigue, depression, headaches, and loss of appetite.

Major food sources of vitamin C: all fruits, especially citrus fruits, tomatoes, papaya, berries, greens, sago palm, cabbage, peppers, barley greens, and cabbage. Daily dosage is 500–1,000mg or more. Take natural sources of vitamin C, like rose hips, cherries, alma fruit, guava, and

Carotenoid Food Guide[9]

Alpha-carotene: fresh or canned pumpkin, carrots

Beta-carotene: sweet potatoes, carrots, apricots, spinach, collard greens, canned pumpkin, cantaloupe

Beta-cryptoxanthin: papaya, oranges, tangerines, mangoes

Lutein and Zeaxanthin: kale, collard greens, spinach, Swiss chard, mustard greens, red pepper, okra, romaine lettuce

Lycopene: tomato juice, watermelon, guava, pink grapefruit, tomatoes

This is only a partial list, since many tropical fruits and vegetables that contain carotenoids are not readily available in all grocery stores.

mango. If it upsets your stomach, try sustained or time-released vitamins. Bioflavanoids enhance the function of vitamin C.

Vitamin E. Vitamin E is a powerful antioxidant that protects the heart and arteries. It keeps brain cells healthy with a good supply of oxygen, which detoxifies the body. When topically applied, it speeds healing. People with higher blood levels of vitamin E are less likely to suffer angina, arrhythmia, and heart attacks. During chronic stress, vitamin E can reduce or stop the free radical destruction. Vitamin E also helps increase circulation. The *New England Journal of Medicine* published two studies, one involving 87,245 nurses who took 100 IU of vitamin E daily for more than two years. The participants had a 41% lower risk of heart disease compared to nonvitamin E users.[10] In the second study, 39,910 male health care professionals took over 30 IU of a vitamin E supplement and had a 37% lower risk of heart disease.[11]

Major food sources of vitamin E: wheat germ oil, almonds, whole wheat, vegetable oils, green, leafy vegetables, whole-grain cereals, meat, and eggs. Daily dose: 400–1,000 IU. Take D-alpha tocopheryl acetate is a good vitamin E supplement. Consult your doctor for appropriate dosage.

Glutathione. This is another powerful antioxidant and anticancer agent. By preventing lipid peroxidation and acting as an enzyme to disarm free radicals, glutathione lends protection against cataracts, heart disease, asthma, and cancer. It protects against damage caused by cigarette smoke, chemotherapy, and radiation. It also protects our bodies from indoor and outdoor toxic pollutants.

Major food sources of glutathione: avocados, watermelon, asparagus, oranges, grapefruit, peaches, cauliflower, broccoli, and okra. Cooking and processing destroys some glutathione. If you take a glutathione supplement, consult your doctor for appropriate dosage.

Coenzyme Q_{10} (ubiquinol$_{10}$). This is one of the strongest antioxidants to support the effectiveness of the immune system. CoQ_{10} is routinely used in Japan in the treatment of heart disease, asthma, allergies, and high blood pressure. It protects the stomach lining and seems to help heal duodenal ulcers in some. It is also useful to improve blood circulation.

Major food sources of coenzyme Q_{10}: sardines, salmon, mackerel, pistachio nuts, garlic, sesame seeds, soybeans, and certain meats. Daily dose: 10–30mg.

Selenium. This powerful mineral antioxidant helps to combat numerous bacterial and viral infections. It has shown to improve gastrointestinal functions, appetite, memory, and mood. Selenium works synergistically with vitamin E, zinc, and glutathione. A controlled study conducted at University College in Swansea, Wales, revealed that people who ate the least selenium foods were the most anxious, depressed, and tired. These subjects improved drastically after increasing their intake of selenium.[12] Some researchers think that selenium biochemistry may be one of the major factors in understanding the life cycle of the human immunodeficiency virus (HIV) and the pathology of AIDS. These scientists have discovered that HIV, which can develop into AIDS, gradually depletes the body of selenium.

Major food sources of selenium: tuna fish, Brazil nuts, garlic, wholegrain flour, and most organ meats. Daily dose: 50–100mg or as directed by your doctor.

Lycopene. This is a well-known, inexpensive source of nature's strongest antioxidant, linked to preventing various types of cancers. At the University of Illinois in Chicago, researchers have discovered low blood levels of lycopene in women who were candidates for a precancerous condition called cervical intra-epithelial neoplasia. Also, researchers at Johns Hopkins University detected low blood levels of lycopene in people with pancreatic cancer. Lycopene's antioxidant ability, many experts think, helps keep LDL cholesterol from becoming oxidized. Lycopene works somewhat like vitamin C and works synergistically with vitamin E.

Major food sources of lycopene: watermelons and tomatoes. Lycopene is the ingredient that gives them their red color (but not all red fruits have lycopene). A small amount is also found in apricots and certain tropical wild berries found in the Amazon forests. Lycopene is not destroyed by cooking or processing.

Are Supplements for Me?

Since the discovery of antioxidants, many physicians and scientists who never before believed in the effectiveness of nutrient supplements are increasingly and in overwhelming numbers using supplements personally, while learning how they work to prevent and heal diseases.

There are at least five major reasons why one may need to add supplements to regular meals. In the first place, every person differs from others biochemically, genetically, and psychologically. Two people of the same age, sex, weight, and ethnic background can have vastly different hormone levels. Their brain chemicals, moods, state of mind, and quality of health can also vary a great deal. What is adequate for one may be inadequate for another.

Second, for many of us our usual diet does not contain enough necessary nutrition, due to the amount of processed foods we consume.

Third, the ways we prepare our foods may also decrease nutritional levels.

Fourth, the immediate environment we live in, the kind of air we breathe, the water we drink, and our place of work may require that we take supplements to maintain good health.

Finally, special groups of people such as heavy smokers, problem drinkers, poor eaters, women on oral contraceptives, expectant mothers, the elderly, those taking certain medications, strenuous exercisers, people suffering from chronic disorders, and patients recovering from fractures or surgery may need supplements to enjoy a well-nourished mind and good health.

As discussed earlier, the food we eat influences our thinking and behavior. This applies to nutritional and herbal supplements as well. If we consume too much or too little, the influence may be negative. The key is to maintain overall mental and physical *balance*. Imbalances aggravate illnesses. We can restore the balance from time to time by consuming specific nutrients. The right nutrients can alter the biochemistry and function of the brain and body and help us defend against the negative impact of stress.

Numerous studies have clearly demonstrated that people who are deficient in certain nutrients suffer from psychological, behavioral, and physical symptoms. Yet it's crucial to determine your *personal* need. Obviously, the degree of supplemental need and toleration is different for each person. Here is a simple checklist of common complaints that might be remedied through better nutrition or vitamin supplements. For specific guidance, consult a nutrition-oriented doctor who can help guide you in developing a program that is just right for your needs.

YOUR TURN

Evaluating Your Supplemental Need

Indicate which of the following most clearly correspond to you in the past three to six months.

_____ Under chronic stress
_____ Tense and anxious
_____ Irritable
_____ Tire easily
_____ Restless sleep
_____ Trouble falling asleep
_____ Frequent headaches
_____ Can't relax
_____ Smoker
_____ Negative feelings
_____ Heavy smoker
_____ Constant stomach problems
_____ Can't make decisions
_____ Depressed
_____ Poor eating habits
_____ Teeth grinding
_____ Family history of cancer
_____ Feel like a social outcast
_____ Need coffee, alcohol, etc. to function
_____ Suffer premenstrual symptoms
_____ Prone to colds and infections
_____ Recovering from surgery
_____ Suffer "sugar blues"
_____ Cravings for sweets
_____ Family history of high blood pressure
_____ Family history of heart disease
_____ Family history of diabetes
_____ Sweaty palms

_____ Hostile
_____ Constant conflicts at work
_____ Frequently late to work or appointments
_____ Worry
_____ Chest tightness
_____ Moody
_____ Lack of concentration
_____ Exposed to toxic substances
_____ Elderly
_____ Feel helpless
_____ Chronic fatigue
_____ Family problems interfering with work
_____ Tempted to use drugs or alcohol as an escape
_____ Poor attention and concentration skills
_____ Nonassertive
_____ Low self-esteem

21

Delicious Eating to Transform Stress

E ating is enjoyable. Yet many find it stressful. Nowadays, the process of planning meals, preparing them, and consuming them is fraught with "shoulds" and "oughts" and "bewares." Even this book, with its detailed discussions of the nutrients found in common foods, might be daunting for some.

For those who struggle with their weight, every meal is a conflict. "Should I have this delicious thing or this healthy thing?" "Should I have a second helping or not?" "Will I show self-discipline, or will I give up and pig out?"

Others have special diets, reducing salt, sugar, fat, or cholesterol. Similar issues enter the picture. Food loses its fun.

In some cases, the stress involved in making these food decisions can sabotage a diet plan. You can get so worked up about saying no to certain foods that you might try to salve your stress by eating *more*. Feeling guilty about eating is unhealthy and counterproductive. Guilt sounds the stress

For those who struggle with their weight, every meal is a conflict.

alarm, which makes you angry, and in the end you're robbed of the joy of eating.

The secret, we feel, is to keep a positive outlook on the whole process. Substitute positive thoughts for your negative thoughts about food. Instead of concentrating on what you're choosing *not* to eat, celebrate the goodness of what you *are* eating.

In this way, you can adopt an exciting eating style that will pave the way for you to reduce health risks and to meet the stresses of your life in a healthy manner.

POSITIVE SUBSTITUTION

Much has been written about having a "positive mental outlook" and so on. It can be ridiculous in the extreme, as it overlooks the solid realities of life in favor of some rose-colored image. That's not what we're talking about.

Positive substitution is a decision to focus on the good instead of the bad. We might find the principle in Philippians 4:8, where Paul urges his readers to "think about" (dwell on, ponder) things that are "true ... noble ... right ... pure ... lovely ... admirable ... excellent ... praiseworthy." You don't close your eyes to negative realities but you choose to dwell on positive aspects. You look at the future instead of the past, the possibility instead of the failure.

Later we'll talk more about the "self-talk" messages we send ourselves. But in this discussion of healthy eating, it's an important consideration.

YOUR TURN

Positive Substitution

Here are a few examples of positive messages. Look them over and decide whether you can claim any of them as your own. But don't look only at the present or past, look at the future too. In the space at the left, write "now" (if it's something that is true of you already) or "soon" or "someday" (depending on when you think this will be true of you). Then write in a few more positive messages that pertain to your specific food situation—present or future.

_____ I love the feeling of being in good shape and being attractive and thin.

_____   I find it easy to lose weight gradually and safely.

_____   I deserve to be healthy.

_____   My body is healthier, attractive, and stronger.

_____   I am confident in myself and about losing weight.

_____   I am in control of my attitude and behavior toward eating.

_____   I don't eat because I am angry and/or frustrated and upset.

_____   I keep a food diary until I get used to eating nutritiously.

_____   I drink a glass of water or diluted juice twenty minutes before eating.

_____   My desire for salt, sugar, fat, and junk food decreases.

_____   I munch on veggies for snacks.

_____   I am satisfied with smaller portions and stop eating before feeling stuffed.

_____   I like staying on a low-fat diet.

_____   I visualize myself as a disciplined eater and shopper.

_____   I read labels on food and buy only healthy food.

_____   My investment in my well-being is profitable.

_____   I eat about four hours before going to sleep.

_____   I brush my teeth after every meal.

_____   I like the feeling of being in control of my body and my eating habits.

_____   I am very happy that I am losing weight permanently.

_____   _____

_____   _____

_____   _____

BUYING AND EATING

The most important second step to practice is to buy and eat smart. Every time you shop for food, you are making decisions about what foods will be available to you (and your family) at home. If you do the shopping for your family, you know it's not easy to account for everyone's tastes and differing nutritional needs. Planning is crucial *before* you go shopping. Prepare to choose foods that are both healthy and delicious.

Then, of course, there are decisions to be made in the preparing and eating of the food. As with other stress issues (see chapter 5), it's important that you maintain control of these decisions. *You* decide what you eat and how much. In a family situation, those decisions may be shared, but you

Planning is crucial before you go shopping. Prepare to choose foods that are both healthy and delicious.

should have some input. You don't need to eat just to be nice or to be sociable—you have a free choice.

With that in mind, consider the following suggestions for your food decisions.

Eat a well-balanced nutritional variety. According to nutrition scientists, the human body requires over forty nutrients to maintain food health. These are classified as vitamins, minerals, amino acids, essential fatty acids, carbohydrates, enzymes, and water. Only a few of us will be able to keep an accurate track of these requirements. The wise advice is to eat a well-balanced and vast variety of foods that contain these nutrients, to meet the demands of our body.

What is a well-balanced, nutritional variety plan? Most health and nutritional experts agree that a balanced variety contains the following proportions.

- Protein: 15 to 20 percent of total calories
- Carbohydrates: 55 to 60 percent of total calories
- Fat: 20 to 30 percent of total calories (mostly monounsaturated fat)
- Fiber: 40 to 50 grams per day
- Water: 6 to 8 eight-ounce glasses per day

Such a plan includes the six basic food groups:

1. Vegetables: all types, especially dark green, leafy vegetables.

2. Fruits: all kinds, including berries, melons, and citrus fruits.

3. Whole grains: rice, cereals, legumes (peas and beans), nuts, seeds, and added fiber.

4. Dairy products: nonfat or low-fat milk, including natural cheese and nonfat yogurt. Soy milk is a good substitute for some.

5. Meats: fish, lean meats, poultry (skin and fat removed), and vegetable protein.

6. Liquids: clear water, unsweetened and diluted juices (pulped), and drinks that are caffeine free, fat free, and artificial-sugar free.

Eat every meal. More than fifty-five percent of Americans now eat their breakfast, lunch, and dinner regularly. Breakfast is the most important meal of the day, because calories consumed early in the day are given more opportunity to be converted into energy. If you also eat a well-balanced lunch, you won't feel tired and irritable in the afternoon. Your body will enjoy a steady source of fuel for energy from the food eaten throughout the day. Furthermore, your blood sugar will not plunge. Heavy, sweet breakfasts eaten on the run, meager lunches, and bingeing for dinner can only increase chances of becoming overweight.

Watch out for hidden sweets and artificial, low-calorie sweeteners. Most food we eat contains sugar. Cereals, cookies, candy bars, breads, soft drinks, canned fruits, vegetable soups, salad dressings, yogurt, sauces, ketchup, and canned vegetables all contain sugar. When you read the labels on some products, you'll notice more than one form of sugar listed, though they don't always sound like sugar—fructose, maltose, lactose, sucrose, sorghum. In order to avoid sugars, therefore, keep a watch out for any of these names.

> **"Why is it that everyone I see drinking diet sodas seems to be overweight?"**
>
> **—Jay Leno**

Strong evidence from at least three recent studies suggests that artificial sugar substitutes like aspartame (sold under the brand names "NutraSweet" and "Equal") and saccharin have *no benefit at all* in weight control. For example, the American Cancer Society's study of seventy-eight thousand women showed that users of artificial sweeteners were more likely to put on pounds than nonusers. Sadly, women who used artificial sweeteners gained weight faster.[1]

A team of researchers at Leeds University in England discovered that aspartame increased hunger feelings, while sugar reduced hunger and created a feeling of fullness in the participants.[2]

What does this mean to you? *Be cautious about using artificial sweeteners!* They could be counterproductive. Use less-refined sugars in moderation.

Fight saturated fats and LDL cholesterol. According to the surgeon general's report on nutrition, the U.S. populace eats too much fat. We need only the equivalent of one tablespoon per day.

The risk of heart attack triples when blood cholesterol rises from 150–250mg per 100 g of blood, and increases even faster after that. Levels above 240 LDL are a primary cause of the atherosclerotic plaque that clogs coronary arteries. Fat is the most concentrated source of energy. It provides nine calories per gram, while carbohydrates and protein provide only four. However, a high-fat diet is simply counterproductive to weight loss and good health and lowering serum cholesterol. In fact, fatty foods elevate blood cholesterol and triglycerides.

FACTS ABOUT DIETARY FATS

Saturated fats: Usually those that remain solid at room temperature. Examples: meat fats, butter, fats from chicken and other poultry and fowl. These contribute most to a buildup of LDL ("bad" cholesterol).

Hydrogenated fats: Vegetable oils that have been artificially hardened, making them into saturated fats.

Subtle saturated fats: Usually fats that remain liquid at room temperature. These oils include palm oil, palm kernel oil, and coconut oil. These oils are just as artery-clogging as the animal fats.

Unsaturated fats: Primarily those that remain liquid at room temperature, including most vegetable fats. They are divided into two categories:

Monounsaturated fats: These are the least-unsaturated fats, including olive, canola, and peanut oil. Olive oil has demonstrated to be better for lowering LDL than once thought.

Polyunsaturated fats: Among the most-unsaturated fats are safflower, sunflower, corn, cottonseed, and soybean oils.

By adhering to the following tips, you will reduce fat in your diet.

- When cooking poultry, remove the skin and all visible fat. Choose white meat, because it has less fat. The skin adds a hefty one hundred calories per serving, and dark meat another thirty to fifty calories.
- When you cook meat, drain off fat before eating. Eliminate butter or hard margarine made with hydrogenated oil or olive oil and use soft margarine made of unhydrogenated oil.
- Avoid eating commercially cooked and baked foods if they contain animal fat, coconut oil, palm oil, and a great deal of sugar. Cook with the following oils: soybean, sunflower, cottonseed, or canola. Better yet, steam as much as possible.
- Reduce salad dressings containing saturated fats.
- Cut back on fatty dairy foods. Use skim milk, low-fat cheeses, and nonfat yogurt.

- Eat more seafood, fish, tofu, beans, and peas for protein. Reduce animal dairy products. When you eat meat, eat only the leaner cuts. Grill or broil meat so the fat drips off.
- Cut down the intake of cocoa, coconut palm products, and nuts.
- Eat no more than two eggs per week.
- Eat plenty of fruits and vegetables.

If your cholesterol level is slightly elevated, discuss with your doctor the possibility of taking niacin, L-carnitine, chromium picolinate, and vanadium sulfate supplements.

Increase complex carbohydrates and fiber in your food. A low-saturated-fat, high-fiber diet can keep you healthy and regular. Numerous studies have shown that the thermic effect (production of heat by the body) of carbohydrate food is much higher than thermic effects of fat. Whole-grain foods, breakfast cereals, oatmeal, oat bran, rye, pumpernickel, corn kernels, whole-wheat pasta, starchy vegetables, brown rice, and beans are rich in complex carbohydrates, fiber, minerals, protein, vitamins, and oils. A diet high in fiber will be low in fat. Your hunger is satisfied by bulk and not calories. Fiber is an essential ingredient needed for proper function of the digestive tract.

In addition to the above fibers, add fruits and vegetables to your diet, such as apples, most berries, strawberries, avocado, carrots, broccoli, okra, parsnips, peas, cabbage, green beans, potatoes, summer squash, and zucchini. Leave the skins on fruits, vegetables (if they are not contaminated with insecticides and pesticides), and legumes to enhance their fiber content.

Buy only necessary foods. Make a shopping list of things you need and stick to it. Don't buy empty-calorie foods (most snack foods and sugary treats).

Cook with a variety of spices for palate-pleasing flavors. See the tasty recipes that follow.

Watch your salt intake. Our bodies need only 200mg of salt daily, but the average daily intake per person is 4,500mg. A high intake of table salt (sodium chloride) in the American populace has been attributed to causing high blood pressure and associated disorders. Salt also retains water, causing swelling, especially in women. Unfortunately, food manufacturers are using more and more salt in prepared foods. Rinsing certain canned foods for two to three minutes reduces the salt content by almost half in most cases, and more in other foods.

Like sweets, salts also come under different names, such as sodium chloride, monosodium glutamate (MSG), baking powder, and baking soda. To reduce salt, rather than adding a large quantity while cooking, sprinkle a limited amount of salt on top of foods after preparation.

Also limit salt-cured, smoked, and nitrite-cured foods. These foods are impregnated with tars from the smoke. Smoke, tar, and nitrates are capable of causing cancer.

If you must prepare fatty, salty foods, give leftovers away. Occasionally you may have to prepare some fatty, salty food for a social occasion. All right, if you must. But don't hang on to the leftovers. Give them away (or toss them).

> **Rapid weight-loss or weight-gain schemes are harsh on the body's organs.**

Avoid crash diets and dangerous weight loss programs. Rapid weight-loss or weight-gain schemes are harsh on the body's organs. These programs can lead to disorders like high blood pressure, diabetes, and kidney disease.

Don't use PPA but use guar fiber or "natural" diet aids. Fifteen to twenty million Americans, mostly women, buy over-the-counter diet aids. Two popular diet aids approved by a government review panel are phenylpropanolamine (PPA, the active ingredient in Dexatrim) and benzocaine.

PPA is used in about 150 prescription and over-the-counter medications. PPA primarily works on the hypothalamus (the appetite center in the brain) by convincing the body to reduce the desire to eat. It's chemically linked to amphetamines. The concern originates from the potential for abuse and resultant side effects, which are similar to the effects of amphetamines: dizziness, heart palpitations, rising blood pressure, and addiction.

Some physicians believe that the 75mg found in diet aids is safe. However, isolated incidents of negative side effects are steadily reported to emergency rooms and poison-control centers around the country. Peter Nash, assistant clinical professor of medicine at the University of California in Los Angeles, warns that PPA can cause blood pressure to rise, resulting in cerebral hemorrhaging and strokes. It should not be used by children.[3] It has also been suggested that diet drugs can cause glaucoma.[4]

Benzocaine is widely used in prescription and over-the-counter drugs, including cough lozenges that numb sore throats. It is also sold as a gum.

It works on the tongue by anesthetizing the taste buds on the tongue, which suppresses the appetite.

Stop binge eating. You need to deal honestly with your anxieties, fears, hopes, and goals in life. It's fine to allow small eating binges if you usually eat well. However, don't try to compensate for boredom, poor self-esteem, depression, or disappointment in life by going on food binges. Use positive substitution to program useful images and get rid of negative habits that trigger the urge to eat when you should not be eating.

Don't fast without consulting a doctor. Prolonged periods of fasting do result in weight loss. But you may gain it all back. If you plan to fast more than twenty-four hours, drink fluids to avoid dehydration. Intake of pulped juices is a good way to supply the body and brain with a minimal amount of glucose. Lack of glucose can cause *ketosis,* a chemical imbalance in the body that can result in dehydration and nausea. Take small doses of vitamin and mineral supplements and avoid strenuous activities.

Assess your eating style. If you have no control over your eating, to experience a health breakthrough, you may analyze your eating style and specific needs. For example, until you have control over your eating, keep a simple weekly food chart of the following things:

- Everything you eat
- Calories
- Place of eating
- Time of day or night
- Duration of meal
- Physical and mental condition while eating

Try to avoid drinking or cooking with chlorinated water. Drink filtered water. Make sure that your drinking and cooking water is not contaminated with insecticides, pesticides, fertilizers, and other chemicals such as alum, carson, chloride, lime, phosphate, soda, ash, sodium, aluminates, cyanides, asbestos, and arsenic. These chemicals in various combinations are believed to cause cancer.

Avoid unhealthy buffets. Many restaurants have sumptuous buffets filled with rich foods. With a fixed price, you'll be tempted to eat a lot to get the most for your money.

QUICK AND DELICIOUS POWER FOOD PLAN

If you are exposed to daily stress and could use some extra brainpower and body energy, here are some great antistress menus for the whole week. You may combine, mix, match, and alter as you desire. ENJOY!

Monday

Breakfast:	It's the most essential need of the day. So don't skip! Eat cereals containing oats, oat bran, brown rice, millet, and fruits. Granola, half-ripe bananas, peaches, apples, or other fruits. Add nonfat yogurt, nonfat milk, or orange juice. If you have special nutritional needs, take your supplements.
Midmorning snack:	Herbal tea or diluted fruit juices. An apple or a peach or a nectarine.
Lunch:	Eat a fresh garden salad containing lettuce, cabbage, carrots, beans, sprouts, tomatoes, and beets, etc. Use low-fat or nonfat salad dressing. If you like turkey, add one ounce turkey breast, chopped.
Afternoon snack:	Carrots or apples or some other fruit. A healthy natural beverage.
Dinner:	Steamed or boiled white or brown rice or whole-grain vegetable pasta (without eggs). One skinned and baked chicken breast. One cup nonfat milk. Fruits for dessert (fresh if possible).
Bedtime snack:	One cup chamomile tea or warm nonfat milk.
Throughout the day:	Drink steam-distilled or filtered water (6–8 glasses).

Tuesday

Breakfast:	One glass of orange juice. One slice of whole-wheat toast. -1/2 cup Cream-of-Wheat or granola cereal.
Midmorning snack:	Fresh apple and carrots or similar substitutes.

Lunch:	Mixed vegetable soup with saltless whole-grain crackers. Unsweetened canned peaches or a fresh peach.
Afternoon snack:	Fresh peach or nectarine or sliced pineapple.
Dinner:	Asian combination (steamed or boiled brown rice, beans, cabbage, and sprouts, mildly seasoned with Japanese teriyaki or tamari sauce; add watercress, tomatoes, celery, and peppers as you like). One serving of fish or turkey breast. Fresh fruit dessert or fruit salad.
Bedtime snack:	1/2 or 1 cup warm low-fat or nonfat milk.

Wednesday

Breakfast:	1/2 grapefruit or an orange. Multigrain or buck-wheat pancakes.
	Unsweetened fruit or jelly spread or topping. One glass low-fat or nonfat milk.
Midmorning snack:	Herbal tea and an apple.
Lunch:	Lentil vegetarian soup. Mixed salad.
Afternoon snack:	Any fruit and herbal tea.
Dinner:	1/4 skinned and baked chicken. -1/2 cup steamed or boiled rice. Fresh, diversified salad.
Bedtime snack:	One cup low-fat or nonfat milk or chamomile tea.

Thursday

Breakfast:	Granola or multigrain hot or cold cereal mixed with apples, bananas, or peaches. Nonfat or low-fat milk or yogurt.
Midmorning snack:	Fresh apple or carrots. Herbal tea.
Lunch:	Pita pocket (whole-grain) stuffed with cooked vegetables, including pepper and stone-ground mustard. Slide a slice of nonfat cheese into the pocket if you'd like. Vegetable juice.
Afternoon snack:	Fresh fruits and whole-grain crackers or yogurt.

Dinner:	Fish or chicken or turkey, skinned and broiled or fried in thin olive oil. Fresh, diversified salad. Fresh fruit or a slice of natural carrot cake.

Friday

Breakfast:	Pulped juice. Oatmeal or granola cereal (add fruits). Nonfat milk.
Midmorning snack:	Herbal tea. Bran muffin.
Lunch:	Multi-bean soup with a variety of vegetables, including ginger, garlic, onion, tomato, and other spices. Baked fish or skinned and baked chicken.
Afternoon snack:	Fresh apple or yogurt.
Dinner:	Brown rice. Vegetable-bean soup cooked in garlic, onion, and other spices.
	Fresh mixed garden salad. Fresh fruit salad for dessert.
Bedtime snack:	Nonfat milk or chamomile tea.

Saturday

Breakfast:	Multigrain pancakes or Belgian waffles made with egg whites and "Pam" for oil. Fruit juice.
Midmorning snack:	Popcorn cake with peanut or almond butter.
Lunch:	Kale soup (with onions, garlic, potatoes, green pepper, ginger root, and cabbage). Diversified, fresh salad with dandelion and nonfat dressing. Fruit for dessert.
Afternoon snack:	Whole-grain blueberry muffin.
Dinner:	Brown or white rice, boiled or steamed. A diversified, fresh salad. 1-1/2 cup whole-wheat and vegetable spaghetti with marinara sauce. Water or diluted juice.
Bedtime snack:	Nonfat warm milk or chamomile tea.

Sunday

Breakfast:	Make your own cereal for breakfast if you like: 3/4 cup raw rolled quick oats 2 tbsp. wheat germ 1 tbsp. wheat bran 1 cup puffed rice or millet 1 tbsp. chopped almonds 1/2 ripe banana, chopped (sprinkle on a bit of cinnamon powder) Combine all in a mixing bowl, pour nonfat milk or juice or soy milk and enjoy.
Midmorning snack:	One large apple. Ten or fifteen unsalted almonds.
Lunch:	Stir-fry veggie plate: 2 cups mixed veggies 2 tsp. olive oil (add garlic, onions, ginger root, or other spices) 1 cup boiled rice One cup or more of lentil soup
Afternoon snack:	One large apple and carrots or one cup nonfat yogurt with fruit.
Dinner:	Cook salmon, tuna, or mako shark in your favorite spicy sauce with garlic, ginger root, and chopped onions if you like. Diversified, fresh garden salad. Steamed mixed veggies. Fruits and frozen yogurt for dessert.
Bedtime snack:	Chamomile or mint tea.

22

Medication and Nature's Resources to Reduce Stress

In the movie *Outbreak,* a deadly virus is unleashed on a small American town. Amazingly (perhaps too amazingly), scientists find the "host" animal that carried the virus to the U.S. Inside this animal's system are the antibodies needed to fight the fatal disease. Soon a serum is produced. Happy ending, fade to credits.

It's only a movie, but it reminds us of some important realities. Researchers believe that outbreaks of diseases more resistant to antibiotics is inevitable. Scientists acknowledge that it is just a matter of time before some superdeadly strain mutates again, killing millions of people.

But it is also true that the human body has built-in defenses against disease. God has given us *immune systems* that, when properly maintained, fight against the many germs and diseases that cross our paths. As we enter the crowded twenty-first century of our shrinking planet, our immune systems may be pushed to the limit.

Consider the jetliner, where air is recirculated in the cabin. A passenger who carries a virus and, say, sneezes will introduce that virus to all the other passengers. The recirculating air will keep bringing the virus back to those who missed it earlier. Those whose immune systems are strong will fight off the intrusion, but those who have been weakened—by other diseases, by lack of sleep or food, or by stress—are very susceptible. Unfortunately, jets are usually filled with harried business travelers, sleep-deprived students, and snack-happy vacationers.

In a way, our world is a jetliner, recirculating disease-filled air and water. And as the stresses of our world increase, people will be more susceptible to germs and viruses.

In the face of such frightening reality, what should we do? Worry? No, that will only make things worse. We can trust God in all situations. That doesn't mean we won't ever come down with some dread disease. Many Christians have become seriously ill, but they can still rely on God's comfort and strength.

When we're healthy, we should be thanking God for the built-in disease-fighters he has given us. And we should do everything we can to be sure our immune systems are ready for the challenge.

The more you study the way God has made us, the more you realize how everything is connected—body, mind, emotions, soul. Doctors who treat the body as if it were merely a machine do us a great disservice. The physical aspects of healing are important, of course, but there's much more to it. We see this especially in the area of immunity to disease. Studies have shown that immunity is greatly affected by one's mood and one's thought. As Christians, we might suggest that even one's relationship with God affects a person's response to disease.

As we have seen, stress weakens us at every level, stripping our immune systems of strength at every level. We need, then, to strengthen ourselves at every level. An *integrated* treatment plan can help us to participate in life fully and with joy. Since we are complex physical, chemical, psychological, and metaphysical units and not mere parts put together, we need to consider the brain, mind, and the body as one unit.

The medical community is just beginning to understand this. For years, it has needlessly separated the brain, mind, spirit, soul, and body. Only now are doctors beginning to see that there may be alternate ways to achieve healing or to alleviate stress, ways that may focus as much on the mind or soul as on the body. Future hospitals may have a battery of new methods at their disposal that would integrate the mind (psycho), the brain (neuro), and the bodily processes (physio) to assist us in dealing with stress. For example, in the immediate future, treatment based on neurochemicals, hormones, and genetic changes underlying specific diseases may become a part of the standard treatment plan for stress.

We realize that some Christians are concerned about the "New Age" overtones of such a new approach to medicine. It is true that Eastern religions emphasize the unity of body and spirit (in fact, the unity of all things). But this is a Christian principle, too. We are "fearfully and wonderfully made" by a God who wants us to love him with all our heart, soul, mind, and might. Yes, we must be careful that health care professionals don't lead us into a false religion, but we should applaud the medical community for generally moving in the right direction as they understand the interrelatedness of the physical and nonphysical. And we should continue to urge them to understand the full breadth of how God has created us.

When we talk about immune systems, we're talking about *prevention*. We're talking about closing the barn door *before* the animals get out (or, more properly, before the intruders get in). The chief medical component of a stress management program is a healthy lifestyle of body, mind, emotions, spirit, relationships, and so on. Such a lifestyle can prevent stress-related diseases from taking hold.

MEDICATIONS AND NATURE'S HEALERS

The nature of our complex biochemistry requires an integration of traditional medicine and natural means of treatment in order to achieve the best possible results. From conception, our brain chemistry shapes our behavior, and as we progress, our behavior affects the structure of our brains. The brain is affected by numerous factors, including changes in the body. Therefore to achieve correct neurochemical balance between brain and body—as well as healthy behavior—any effective treatment plan should consider vitamins, minerals, proteins, essential oils, amino acids, enzymes, natural healing substances, a healthy diet plan, exercises, relaxation, medication, and surgery, if needed. Many problems can be prevented and treated through natural means. However, medication may be required for those suffering from disturbed brain metabolism, chronic hypertension, and a host of other disorders.

A moderate dose of prescription medications combined with nutritional treatment can bring comfort and best results in many disorders. The goal is to benefit from all valid sources for a healthy mind, brain, body, and spirit. The key is to achieve a successful delicate balance.

Nutritionally-oriented treatment offers an amazingly effective, safe, and long-term healing approach to emotional and stress-related disorders. Nutritional therapy is unique because it can be tailored specifically to heal each individual's condition. Due to high-tech health research and testing capabilities, nutritional diagnosis and treatment modality is no longer a leap in the dark. Specific causes can be identified, and appropriate nutritional therapy can be tailored according to each individual's condition. Nutritional supplements and specific foods along with modern medicine can do wonders in preventing, improving, and even curing many common mental and physical disorders. An integrated treatment approach is the best choice in treating all ailments, including the idiopathic (no known cause) illnesses such as fatigue, hypertension, sleep disorders, anxieties, and allergies.

Stress Medications

Medications are not usually prescribed for stress per se but for stress-related *disorders* such as high blood pressure, anxiety disorders, digestive disorders, insomnia, headaches, sleep disorders, arrhythmias, and fatigue, to mention just a few.

Since approximately sixty million American adults have high blood pressure, which is often attributed to internal and external stressors, let us look first at antihypertensive medication therapy and then natural healing therapy.

Antihypertensive Medications

Blood pressure-lowering medications are most commonly used when an individual's diastolic pressure (the bottom number in the blood pressure equation, representing resting pressure) is above 94 millimeters of mercury (mmHg) or above 90 in smokers. Some people are able to control high blood pressure with diet, exercise, stress management training, biofeedback, and other modifications of related factors. Others still require a combination of home remedies and medication to achieve and maintain normal readings. Without the use of medication, the risk of fatal stroke or heart attack is high. It is good to keep in mind that unless your blood pressure is consistently, say, 150 over 95 or unless you have certain specific risk factors for heart disease, medication may not be imminently warranted. Check with your physician.

Types of Medications

Once it is determined that you need medications, you need to find out from your physician which will work best for you. The options are numerous, and this chapter can only discuss a few in brief. Those interested in a detailed study may need to read *Physician's Desk Reference*[1] (or *The Pill Book*[2] by Harold M. Silverman, which is less expensive, written for the general public, and probably all you will need). These medications fall into eight categories. Here is a short introduction:

Diuretics. Thiazide diuretics are the most commonly used. These drugs help increase the removal of sodium and water by acting on the kidneys to stimulate the production of large amounts of urine. This results in a reduced volume of blood in the arteries and veins, making it possible to lower blood pressure. Long-term use of thiazide medicines may deplete potassium and magnesium along with excess water from your body. Thiazide diuretics may also raise blood sugar.

Calcium channel blockers. By blocking the penetration of calcium into blood vessel walls, these medications allow blood vessels to relax and blood to flow unrestricted. They also decrease muscle spasms in those blood vessels. According to recent research, calcium channel blockers such as diltiazem, nicardipine, and verapamil do not interfere with patients' sex lives, sleep, emotions, and work habits as propranolol, a beta-blocker, does. Also, it seems that beta-blockers increase LDL (bad) cholesterol and lower HDL (the good kind). Nicardipine should not be used if you have advanced hardening of the arteries, especially the aorta.

Beta-blockers. Drugs such as acebutolol, atenonlol and nadolol, known as beta-adrenergic blocking agents, block the spontaneous responses of beta-nerve receptors to reduce the amount of blood pumped with each heartbeat. They block the action of naturally occurring substances, like epinephrine (adrenaline), that increases the heart rate. This helps to lower blood pressure. Often they are prescribed with a diuretic. These drugs do interfere with patients' sex lives, sleep, emotions and work habits and may cause depression. Combining them with one a day multi-mineral vitamins may reduce the bad effects. These are good medications for people with diabetes and high blood pressure.

Angiotensin-converting enzyme (ACE) inhibitors. This class of drugs primarily works by suppressing angiotensin. Angiotensin II is a powerful blood vessel constrictor, and it also causes salt and water retention. This group of drugs is effective alone or in combination with other antihypertensive agents, especially thiazide-type diuretics. Vasotec is a commonly prescribed ACE-inhibiting medication. People with kidney disorders or collagen disease need to be closely monitored while taking this type of medication. Pregnant women should not take ACE inhibitors.

Vasodilators. By relaxing and dilating the arteries of the heart and smooth muscles, these drugs allow increased blood flow. They are prescribed along with a beta-blocker, a diuretic, or a nerve inhibitor. These drugs, in normal doses, have minimal actions on the central nervous system. Hydralazine and Minoxidil are commonly prescribed vasodilators.

Alpha-blocking agents. These drugs block alpha receptors in the blood vessel walls, causing arteries to dilate. Alpha-blockers are used only when other medications have proven inadequate. Prazosin and terazosin, two common alpha-blockers, can cause dizziness or fainting.

Peripheral adrenergic antagonists. Although most of these drugs are usually alpha-blocking agents, some block the release of (adrenaline) norepinephrine caused as a result of stress. Given in combination with a diuretic, these drugs act in various ways on the sympathetic nerve endings to dilate blood vessels, and are used to treat severe hypertension. Examples: dotazosin, quanadrel and prazosin. These can cause low blood pressure and a loss of balance when one stands up quickly.

Centrally acting drugs. These medications dilate peripheral arteries, lowering arterial pressure. But they do not have a direct effect on the amount of blood pumped out of the heart. They are not used as an initial medication. Some of these drugs are made from the roots of the rauwolfia plant of India. They can cause dry mouth, drowsiness, depression, diarrhea, and excessive dreaming.

Combination drugs. Different types of drugs are sometimes prescribed to have the greatest efficacy. Examples: bendroflunethiazide and nadolol; chlorthalidone and clonidine.

There are also the coronary vasodilators that dilate the heart vessels to help blood pump with less restriction.

Initially, patients are usually given one of the medications based on their specific need. For example, age, medical history, mental illness, risk factors, race, pregnancy, interaction with other drugs, and even genetic factors are considered.

Natural Ways to Reduce Blood Pressure

Controlling high blood pressure without medications is usually not easy for most people. However, if you work with your doctor, a natural approach to reducing high blood pressure can be rewarding without the medicinal side effects such as fatigue, depression, and impotence. If you don't have high blood pressure and you're interested in keeping it that way, you also can benefit from the following proven tips.

Exercise. Walk, bike, run, or get into a training program. The role of exercise in reducing high blood pressure is well documented in the medical literature. Exercise may be as effective as medication in lowering blood pressure. As indicated earlier in the exercise section of this book, discuss with your doctor before starting a vigorous exercise program. Keep in mind the acronym FIT: Frequency, Intensity, and Time (duration). Your workout should have these three components:

1. Warm-up

2. Steady exercise at your target heart rate

3. Cool-down

Eat less fat and more fiber. Watch out for saturated fats (see discussion on nutrition in chapter 21). *Trans fats* in margarines, and hydrogenated oils and animal fats, raise heart disease risk. Total fat should not exceed twenty to thirty percent of daily calories. Some believe that thirty to forty percent is high. You can find fiber in psyllium, barley, bulgar, bran buds, whole wheat, oat bran, and certain fruits and vegetables, like asparagus.

Eat plenty of fish. Fish such as tuna, mackerel, and salmon contain omega–3 fatty acids, which appear to help reduce hypertension. Eat fish at least twice a week.

Lose weight. Shoot for an optimal body weight. Studies show dramatic drops in blood pressure after men get rid of their potbellies. Some did not even require medication after they lost weight. Eat plenty of high-fiber foods. They are high in complex carbohydrates and low in fats. Fiber can fill you up without adding too many calories. (To reduce the chances of gas or diarrhea from fiber, add yogurt to your diet. You can also buy anti-gas enzymes at your health food store.)

Don't smoke or drink coffee. Limit coffee intake to one or two cups a day. If you don't drink coffee, don't start. Those who don't drink coffee at all may experience elevated blood pressure if they begin to drink coffee.

Get enough calcium, potassium, and magnesium. Many studies have shown that lack of calcium (less than 600mg a day) can increase the risk of high blood pressure. Calcium appears to help control blood pressure by decreasing contraction of muscles in the walls of blood vessels or by affecting certain hormones.

How much calcium is enough?

1,200mg a day if you are eleven to twenty-five
1,500mg a day if you are over fifty and not taking estrogen
1,000mg a day for other adults

Calcium sources: a supplement or dark green, leafy vegetables, skim milk, nonfat yogurt, tofu, fortified cereals, or orange juice.

Lack of magnesium is closely linked to high blood pressure, abnormal heart rhythm, and heart attack.

Magnesium sources: green, leafy vegetables (raw), plus barley greens, nuts, cereals, seafood, and whole grains.

Potassium, combined with calcium, magnesium, and sodium, plays a vital role in the contraction, nerve impulse response, and other functions of the heart. Evidence suggests that a high-potassium diet may reduce hypertension.

Potassium sources: potatoes, pumpkins, fruits, vegetables, grains, nuts, seeds, and chicken breast.

Avoid black licorice. Licorice causes your body to retain sodium and lose potassium, which can raise blood pressure. If you do not have high blood pressure or heart disease, licorice in moderation can help, especially to reduce a cough.

Reduce salt. Excess salt in the blood absorbs additional fluid into the blood, increasing the volume of fluid in the body. This means that the kidneys are required to work harder to remove the extra salt and fluid. If the kidneys are unable to function at optimum capacity, the demand is placed on the heart to pump this excess fluid. This process also affects numerous other functions of our body, because various hormones are involved in the salt-wasting system. (See sidebar.)

Eat hawthorn berries. These appear to mildly dilate coronary blood vessels to allow unrestricted blood flow. You may buy them from a health food store. Health food stores also carry combination natural high-blood-pressure-lowering tablets, capsules, or liquids.

Take a complete multivitamin and mineral supplement. Take a time-released tablet with meals in the morning or at noon.

Try coenzyme Q_{10} (coQ_{10}). CoQ_{10} is a vitamin-like compound that occurs naturally in our bodies. However, our bodies may not synthesize enough to promote sufficient healing. Increased amounts of coQ_{10} promote healing of heart muscles and lower blood pressure. At dosages lower than 10mg per day of coQ_{10}, no side effects have been reported. The usual preventive dosage of coQ_{10} is 10–30mg per day. Larger amounts are used to treat various disorders. Read more about coQ_{10} and discuss with your nutritionally oriented doctor.

Reduce on-the-job stress. Employees ranging from stockbrokers to sanitation workers were asked to carry portable monitors at work to measure their blood pressure. This study showed that those who reported high job-stress were three times as likely to have high blood pressure as those who did not report a great deal of stress. To reduce job stress, take a five-minute job-stress break every two or three hours and do

Ways to Reduce Salt

1. Reduce salt intake to about half a teaspoon (1,000mg) or less per day.

2. Read food labels and avoid foods with high salt content, such as (canned) baked beans, luncheon meats, (canned) tuna fish, corned beef, and chips.

3. Stop adding salt at the table.

4. At home, add a very small amount of salt to foods after they are cooked.

5. In place of salt, use herbs, lemon juice, and spices to enhance flavor and taste.

6. Avoid carbonated drinks, club soda, powdered milk, reconstituted instant milk, and other drinks containing sodium.

7. Add potassium-rich foods to your diet and add potassium supplement when needed.

some simple exercises in deep breathing, complete-body relaxation, and stretching (see chapter 10).

More Tips to Reduce Stress Naturally

Today it is widely agreed that many disorders that result from stress and aging are often the result of nutrient deficiencies in the brain and body. When faced with a high degree of stress, our bodies do not handle nutrients well. Thus you can fight stress and related disorders by feeding your body enough of the right vitamins, minerals, and other nutrients. What you eat is brain and body fuel. A high-nutrient supply is the key to improve your immunity, and a strong immune system means more power to fight stress. Here are some nutrients we need most. In addition to eating well, take supplements as needed.

The B-complex vitamins. They play a key role in helping our nervous system. Vitamin B_6 in particular is a powerful immune booster. It protects against formation of kidney stones and helps promote better sleep. People with depleted vitamin B_6 reserves have shown fewer antibodies to fight disease.

Brewer's yeast. Brewer's yeast or bio-strath (a tonic), when used as directed on the label, can provide the B vitamins needed along with your foods.

Chlorophyll and spirulina. Chlorophyll (found in all green foods) and spirulina (an algae) are recognized around the world as the most promising of all microalgae, containing concentrations of nutrients unlike any other single plant, grain, or herb. Spirulina is a powerful, naturally digestible food used to protect against the ravaging effects of chronic stress.

Phytotherapy. Some use plants to help reduce high blood pressure. You might want to investigate how specific herbs can affect your immune function. You can choose from a variety of standardized herbal preparations that provide consistent, active ingredient levels to reduce blood pressure and boost your immune system. Among the herbs that have been shown to reduce blood pressure: garlic, gingko leaf, hawthorn, passion flower, catnip, valerian, parsley seeds and leaf, hibiscus flowers, and saw palmetto. Caution: do not overuse or abuse. Consult your doctor.

Vitamin C. Vitamin C is important for adrenal functions. Stress depletes the adrenal hormones.

CONCLUSION

In this chapter, we have given you examples of how medications and certain natural treatments can affect various stress-related disorders. Some disorders can be fully and completely treated with natural means. Others need medication. Consult your prescribing doctor to discuss if you could combine natural means with medication. If your doctor is unfamiliar with natural treatments, he or she may refer you to another doctor who can help you. *Do not discontinue any medication abruptly.* At your local library, you can read about medications in the *Physician's Desk Reference.* Many other books on nutritional prescriptions are available.

In order to make the stresses in your life work for you, you need to be aware of the stresses that you experience. You need to know yourself, your physical, nutritional, psychological, spiritual, and social needs. Eat balanced meals, be involved in regular exercise, be humorous, and practice positive substitution in your thinking. Indeed you can, with God's help, overcome stress and benefit from those experiences for a healthy and joyous life.

23

Putting It Together

If you're already trying to put into practice every suggestion we've made, you're probably under more stress than when you started. It can be pretty overwhelming, all this talk about diet and exercise and healthy habits. You can go crazy trying to do it all.

But you can do some of it.

Maybe there's only one thing that you can change about your stressful lifestyle in the next month. But that's one thing that will make you a bit healthier than you were before. And if you do another thing the next month and another the next, in a year you'll have made ten or twelve positive changes in your life. You will not be as susceptible to stress. You'll have broken the stress spiral.

So don't let yourself be overwhelmed. We're giving you the "complete" picture of a healthy, stress-managing life. You don't need to adopt it all instantly, but you can take a step in that direction.

This final chapter will guide you in creating your own plan to combat stress. In essence, you get to write your own self-help book now. How will you change your life?

STRESS EVENTS

Way back at the start, we talked about stress events and stress situations. Stress events happen to us regularly, and our bodies respond naturally with heightened energy, which slowly dissipates as the danger passes. Major problems occur when we live or work in stress situations and our bodily responses stay at a heightened level and never subside.

Therefore your personal battle strategy against stress has to operate on both fronts—dealing with short-term events and long-term situations. Let's start with those events.

If you're a football quarterback, you call a play in the huddle and everyone knows where to run. The play has been carefully designed by the coach, with X's and O's on a chalkboard. You're confident that it will get big yardage for you. But then you line up for the snap and see that the huge middle linebacker is perched in front of your center and that your primary receiver is double-covered. The play will never work now!

What do you do? You call an "audible." It's a backup play that has been previously arranged. Everyone on your team knows that "A5" is a pitchout to the fullback. When you shout that signal, your teammates forget the play called in the huddle and go with this new play.

You need to have some audibles ready in your life. You need to have a course of action that you prepare in advance to use in stress events. You need to design this play and practice it.

What elements will this course of action include?

Body prep. Your body is going to go on high alert. You may need this energy if, say, you're facing a physical threat. But if the stress producer is not a physical threat, your high-tension response will not help you. And even if you are facing a physical threat—that truck that cuts you off on the highway—you need to restore your body to a calmer status as soon as the threat is gone.

We recommend that you breathe deeply. Try taking ten breaths, holding each one a little longer, and "sending" the breath deeper. Remember what we said about diaphragmatic breathing? Don't let your shoulders do the breathing, and don't keep the air in your upper lungs. Fill your abdomen with air, and let your diaphragm muscles move naturally.

To aid in your breathing, you will need to sit or stand straight. This will also help your muscles to avoid some unhealthy tension. Take a moment to check your body alignment. Sometimes people hunch forward or twist their bodies when they're tense. If you do that, don't. Make it a point to straighten out in moments of stress.

Fighting fears. Often stress will bring on irrational fears, which fly like crazy through our brains, and we can't capture them. We wind up worrying about little things. Even the big things should not overwhelm our faith, but often they do.

When you feel those fears flying around, pray. Ask God for comfort. Trust the Spirit to sort through the muddle and help you think straight.

It might also be helpful to have some Bible verses memorized, ready to use in moments of stress. "Do not fear, for I am with you" (Isa. 41:10). "I will fear no evil, for you are with me" (Ps. 23:4). "In all things God works for the good of those who love him" (Rom. 8:28). And there are many others. Be prepared with verses of comfort, and if memory fails you, have these verses written on business cards in your wallet.

Control your coping. If stress pushes you toward some unhealthy coping mechanism—such as alcohol, drugs, tobacco, overeating, gambling, or sex—you need to face this head-on. Those coping methods promise to alleviate your stress, but they just make it worse. There may be a momentary escape, but you need long-term freedom.

How will you counter these tendencies? Again, you can pray. Again, you can consult Bible verses. You may also want to give yourself a clear picture of the consequences of your indulgence. (Those people who put a picture of a fat person or skinny person on their refrigerators have the right idea.) Your self-talk at this moment might be something like, "This may seem like something I need right now, but if I do it, here's what will happen. . . . I'll be worse off, and the stress producer will still be here."

Taking control. If, in your moment of stress, you feel as if life is spinning out of control, take a moment to evaluate what exactly is still in your control. You always have the power of your responses. No one can *make* you angry. They can give you reason to choose to be angry, but it's still your choice. If control is frequently an issue in your stress events, pause to ask yourself, "What do I still control? And how will I responsibly use the control I have?"

Talking to yourself. Often our stress moments make us doubt our own value. We enter a self-esteem crisis, and we lash back defensively, intensifying the stress of the moment. You may need to develop a personal patter of self-affirmation.

Again, prayer and appropriate Bible verses will be valuable. Remember that God loves you. God even *likes* you. He enjoys spending time with you. And if God is for you, who can be against you (Rom. 8:31)?

Withdrawal. In sudden moments of overwhelming stress, it is often helpful to withdraw. Yes, sometimes you're at work and you have to get a job done, or you're in some other inescapable situation. But often you can withdraw in some way—leave the room, stop arguing, stay quiet for a while, go for a walk.

YOUR TURN

Your Personal Plan for Stress Events

Write out what you will do, think, and/or say in moments of stress. Keep your self-talk and prayers short and pithy. You want to create an audible here that you can memorize and practice. Ideally, you should be able to rewrite this plan on an index card that you can carry with you for stressful moments.

Body prep (breathe, stretch, straighten) _____

_____

_____

Fighting fears (a quick prayer, Bible verses) _____

_____

_____

_____

_____

_____

Control your coping (if applicable, a strategy against unhealthy coping mechanisms, a plan to fight temptation at vulnerable moments, a self-talk message, an image to consider) _____

_____

_____

_____

_____

_____

Taking control (self-talk)_____

_____

_____

_____

_____

Self-esteem (self-talk)_____

_____

_____

_____

_____

_____

Withdrawal (an action to take) _____

_____

_____

Now practice this. Think back to your last stress event and pretend you're going through it again—only now you're using this personal stress plan. Does it work? Make adjustments as you practice, but get used to following this plan. Then memorize it for use when you need it.

STRESS SITUATIONS

Much of this book has dealt with ways of easing your general stress level. Many of us live in what we might call "stress situations." A long time ago, stress stopped being an event here and an event there—now it's a steady pattern. Everything gets us stressed out. Our bodies don't know what normal is.

The stress event plan you just worked out will not do much to ease those general stress situations—although it may help keep things from getting any worse.

Imagine that your house is flooded with water because there's a hole in the roof. Every time it rains, your house fills up with water. You used to be able to bail it out (let's pretend there are no electric pumps) after each rain, but then the storm season hit, and you've been flooded ever since.

That stress event plan is like patching the roof. If you practice it faithfully, it will keep you from adding new stress to your flooded life. But you still have a house full of water, and there's only one way to get rid of it—one bucket at a time.

As we have seen, stress wreaks havoc on your body, emotions, mind, and spirit. It affects your diet, your exercise, your relationships, your schedule, your daily work, and your prayer life—and it is affected by all those areas. Round and round it goes. Stress makes you stressed, and your stressedness adds new stress to your life.

Let's tackle an area or two and try to make some positive changes. One bucket at a time, with God's help, we can bail ourselves out.

YOUR TURN

Making Progress Toward Healthy Stress Management

Diet

As you look back over the material on diet and nutrition in this book, list three to five changes you would like to make in your diet to become healthier.

_____
_____
_____
_____
_____

Exercise and other health factors

Looking back over the material on exercise in this book, list three to five changes you would like to make in this area. Include exercise habits you'd like to begin as well as other health factors, such as cutting back on alcohol or tobacco, or getting more sleep.

_____
_____
_____
_____
_____

Job situation

List up to three specific things you could do to improve your job situation, making it less stressful for you.

_____
_____
_____

Home situation

List up to five specific things you could do to improve your home situation, making it less stressful for you.

_____
_____
_____
_____
_____

Time management

List up to three things you could do to improve your time management (be better organized, say no, delegate, etc.).

_____
_____
_____

Self-talk

List three short messages that you need to hear on a regular basis (regarding self-esteem, fighting fears, taking control, etc.).

_____
_____
_____

People

List up to three relationships you have that are more stressful than they should be. For each one, list one thing you could do to improve that relationship.

Person:_____
To do: _____

Person:_____
To do: _____

Person:_____
To do: _____

Spiritual life

List three to five things you could do to improve your relationship with God.

_____

_____

_____

_____

_____

Next Step

Now you should have a list of fifteen to thirty possible improvements to make. If you did all of these, think how much better your life would be! Now the bad news: you can't. Well, maybe in time you could make all these changes, but this is far too many to start with. We want to narrow it down to three.

Review what you listed for the first two categories—"Diet" and "Exercise and other health factors." Choose one of those changes to concentrate on over the next month. List it here.

Change #1 (Health) _____

_____

Then review the next three categories: "Job situation," "Home situation," and "Time management." Choose one of those changes to concentrate on over the next month. List it here.

Change #2 (Environment and Schedule)_____

_____

Now review the last three categories: "Self-talk," "People," and "Spiritual life." Choose one of those changes to concentrate on over the next month. List it here.

Change #3 (Relationships) _____

_____

At the risk of making this seem like a tax form, we ask you to write these three proposed changes on the appropriate lines on the following pages. Also, fill in the dates that correspond to one week from now, two weeks from now, and so on.

Try to make these three changes in your life. Chart your progress each week on these pages. At the end of the month, evaluate your progress in each area. Have you made the change you desired? Is it firmly ingrained as a good habit (or thoroughly left behind as a bad habit)? Do you need another month to work on it? Or can you choose another change from your master list of possible changes? Make your choice and continue.

We've given you progress charts for three months, but feel free to photocopy these pages if you want more.

May God's grace go with you as you continue to move toward healthy stress management.

PROGRESS CHARTS
Month One

WEEK 1 DATE_____

Change #1 _____

How successful was I this week in adopting this change?

Were there factors that made it more difficult than I expected? How will I overcome these?

Do I need to revise my goals?

What strategies will help me do better in the next week?

Change #2 _____

How successful was I this week in adopting this change?

Were there factors that made it more difficult than I expected? How will I overcome these?

Do I need to revise my goals?

What strategies will help me do better in the next week?

Change #3 _____

How successful was I this week in adopting this change?

Were there factors that made it more difficult than I expected? How will I overcome these?

Do I need to revise my goals?

What strategies will help me do better in the next week?

....

WEEK 2 DATE_____

Change #1 _____

How successful was I this week in adopting this change?

Were there factors that made it more difficult than I expected? How will I overcome these?

Do I need to revise my goals?

What strategies will help me do better in the next week?

Change #2 _____

How successful was I this week in adopting this change?

Were there factors that made it more difficult than I expected? How will I overcome these?

Do I need to revise my goals?

What strategies will help me do better in the next week?

Change #3 _____
How successful was I this week in adopting this change?

Were there factors that made it more difficult than I expected? How will I overcome these?

Do I need to revise my goals?

What strategies will help me do better in the next week?

•••

WEEK 3 DATE_____

Change #1 _____
How successful was I this week in adopting this change?

Were there factors that made it more difficult than I expected? How will I overcome these?

Do I need to revise my goals?

What strategies will help me do better in the next week?

Change #2 _____
How successful was I this week in adopting this change?

Were there factors that made it more difficult than I expected? How will I overcome these?

Do I need to revise my goals?

What strategies will help me do better in the next week?

Change #3 _____

How successful was I this week in adopting this change?

Were there factors that made it more difficult than I expected? How will I overcome these?

Do I need to revise my goals?

What strategies will help me do better in the next week?

....

WEEK 4 DATE_____

Change #1 _____

How successful was I this week in adopting this change?

Were there factors that made it more difficult than I expected? How will I overcome these?

Do I need to revise my goals?

What strategies will help me do better in the few days remaining in this month?

Change #2 _____

How successful was I this week in adopting this change?

Were there factors that made it more difficult than I expected? How will I overcome these?

Do I need to revise my goals?

What strategies will help me do better in the few days remaining in this month?

Change #3 _____

How successful was I this week in adopting this change?

Were there factors that made it more difficult than I expected? How will I overcome these?

Do I need to revise my goals?

What strategies will help me do better in the few days remaining in this month?

· ·

MONTH-END DATE _____

Change #1 _____

How successful have I been in adopting this change?

What have I learned about myself, others, or God as I attempted to make this change?

How has this life change affected the stress in my life?

Do I need to keep working on this for another month? (If so, fill this same change in as "Change #4" on the following pages.)

Change #2 _____

How successful have I been in adopting this change?

What have I learned about myself, others, or God as I attempted to make this change?

How has this life change affected the stress in my life?

Do I need to keep working on this for another month? (If so, fill this same change in as "Change #4" or "Change #5" on the following pages.)

Change #3 _____

How successful have I been in adopting this change?

What have I learned about myself, others, or God as I attempted to make this change?

How has this life change affected the stress in my life?

Do I need to keep working on this for another month? (If so, fill this same change in as "Change #4" or "Change #5" or "Change #6" on the following pages.)

If you do not need to keep working on these changes, go back to your master list and choose other changes to focus on during the next month. Label these as "Change #4" or "Change #5" or "Change #6" and fill them in on the following pages.

Month Two

WEEK 1 DATE_____

Change #4 _____

How successful was I this week in adopting this change?

Were there factors that made it more difficult than I expected? How will I overcome these?

Do I need to revise my goals?

What strategies will help me do better in the next week?

Change #5 _____

How successful was I this week in adopting this change?

Were there factors that made it more difficult than I expected? How will I overcome these?

Do I need to revise my goals?

What strategies will help me do better in the next week?

Change #6 _____

How successful was I this week in adopting this change?

Were there factors that made it more difficult than I expected? How will I overcome these?

Do I need to revise my goals?

What strategies will help me do better in the next week?

. . . .

WEEK 2 DATE_____

Change #4 _____
How successful was I this week in adopting this change?

Were there factors that made it more difficult than I expected? How will I overcome these?

Do I need to revise my goals?

What strategies will help me do better in the next week?

Change #5 _____
How successful was I this week in adopting this change?

Were there factors that made it more difficult than I expected? How will I overcome these?

Do I need to revise my goals?

What strategies will help me do better in the next week?

Change #6 _____
How successful was I this week in adopting this change?

Were there factors that made it more difficult than I expected? How will I overcome these?

Do I need to revise my goals?

What strategies will help me do better in the next week?

....

WEEK 3 DATE_____

Change #4 _____

How successful was I this week in adopting this change?

Were there factors that made it more difficult than I expected? How will I overcome these?

Do I need to revise my goals?

What strategies will help me do better in the next week?

Change #5 _____

How successful was I this week in adopting this change?

Were there factors that made it more difficult than I expected? How will I overcome these?

Do I need to revise my goals?

What strategies will help me do better in the next week?

Change #6 _____

How successful was I this week in adopting this change?

Were there factors that made it more difficult than I expected? How will I overcome these?

Do I need to revise my goals?

What strategies will help me do better in the next week?

....

WEEK 4 DATE_____

Change #4 _____

How successful was I this week in adopting this change?

Were there factors that made it more difficult than I expected? How will I overcome these?

Do I need to revise my goals?

What strategies will help me do better in the few days remaining in this month?

Change #5 _____

How successful was I this week in adopting this change?

Were there factors that made it more difficult than I expected? How will I overcome these?

Do I need to revise my goals?

What strategies will help me do better in the few days remaining in this month?

Change #6 _____

How successful was I this week in adopting this change?

Were there factors that made it more difficult than I expected? How will I overcome these?

Do I need to revise my goals?

What strategies will help me do better in the few days remaining in this month?

....

MONTH-END DATE _____

Change #4 _____

How successful have I been in adopting this change?

What have I learned about myself, others, or God as I attempted to make this change?

How has this life change affected the stress in my life?

Do I need to keep working on this for another month? (If so, fill this same change in as "Change #7" on the following pages.)

Change #5 _____

How successful have I been in adopting this change?

What have I learned about myself, others, or God as I attempted to make this change?

How has this life change affected the stress in my life?

Do I need to keep working on this for another month? (If so, fill this same change in as "Change #7" or "Change #8" on the following pages.)

Change #6 _____

How successful have I been in adopting this change?

What have I learned about myself, others, or God as I attempted to make this change?

How has this life change affected the stress in my life?

Do I need to keep working on this for another month? (If so, fill this same change in as "Change #7" or "Change #8" or "Change #9" on the following pages.)

If you do not need to keep working on these changes, go back to your master list and choose other changes to focus on during the next month. Label these as "Change #7" or "Change #8" or "Change #9" and fill them in on the following pages.

Month Three

WEEK 1 DATE_____

Change #7 _____

How successful was I this week in adopting this change?

Were there factors that made it more difficult than I expected? How will I overcome these?

Do I need to revise my goals?

What strategies will help me do better in the next week?

Change #8 _____

How successful was I this week in adopting this change?

Were there factors that made it more difficult than I expected? How will I overcome these?

Do I need to revise my goals?

What strategies will help me do better in the next week?

Change #9 _____

How successful was I this week in adopting this change?

Were there factors that made it more difficult than I expected? How will I overcome these?

Do I need to revise my goals?

What strategies will help me do better in the next week?

....

WEEK 2 DATE_____

Change #7 _____

How successful was I this week in adopting this change?

Were there factors that made it more difficult than I expected? How will I overcome these?

Do I need to revise my goals?

What strategies will help me do better in the next week?

Change #8 _____

How successful was I this week in adopting this change?

Were there factors that made it more difficult than I expected? How will I overcome these?

Do I need to revise my goals?

What strategies will help me do better in the next week?

Change #9 _____

How successful was I this week in adopting this change?

Were there factors that made it more difficult than I expected? How will I overcome these?

Do I need to revise my goals?

What strategies will help me do better in the next week?

....

WEEK 3 DATE_____

Change #7 _____

How successful was I this week in adopting this change?

Were there factors that made it more difficult than I expected? How will I overcome these?

Do I need to revise my goals?

What strategies will help me do better in the next week?

Change #8 _____

How successful was I this week in adopting this change?

Were there factors that made it more difficult than I expected? How will I overcome these?

Do I need to revise my goals?

What strategies will help me do better in the next week?

Change #9 _____

How successful was I this week in adopting this change?

Were there factors that made it more difficult than I expected? How will I overcome these?

Do I need to revise my goals?

What strategies will help me do better in the next week?

• •

WEEK 4 DATE _____

Change #7 _____

How successful was I this week in adopting this change?

Were there factors that made it more difficult than I expected? How will I overcome these?

Do I need to revise my goals?

What strategies will help me do better in the few days remaining in this month?

Change #8 _____

How successful was I this week in adopting this change?

Were there factors that made it more difficult than I expected? How will I overcome these?

Do I need to revise my goals?

What strategies will help me do better in the few days remaining in this month?

Change #9 _____

How successful was I this week in adopting this change?

Were there factors that made it more difficult than I expected? How will I overcome these?

Do I need to revise my goals?

What strategies will help me do better in the few days remaining in this month?

. . . .

MONTH-END DATE _____

Change #7 _____

How successful have I been in adopting this change?

What have I learned about myself, others, or God as I attempted to make this change?

How has this life change affected the stress in my life?

Do I need to keep working on this for another month? (If so, fill this same change in on your photocopies of the progress chart.)

Change #8 _____

How successful have I been in adopting this change?

What have I learned about myself, others, or God as I attempted to make this change?

How has this life change affected the stress in my life?

Do I need to keep working on this for another month? (If so, fill this same change in on your photocopies of the progress chart.)

Change #9 _____

How successful have I been in adopting this change?

What have I learned about myself, others, or God as I attempted to make this change?

How has this life change affected the stress in my life?

Do I need to keep working on this for another month? (If so, fill this same change in on your photocopies of the progress chart.)

....

If you plan to continue this process, make photocopies of the following progress chart.

Progress chart (to photocopy)

WEEK _____

Change #__ _____

How successful was I this week in adopting this change?

Were there factors that made it more difficult than I expected? How will I overcome these?

Do I need to revise my goals?

What strategies will help me do better in the next week?

Change #__ _____

How successful was I this week in adopting this change?

Were there factors that made it more difficult than I expected? How will I overcome these?

Do I need to revise my goals?

What strategies will help me do better in the next week?

Change #__ _____

How successful was I this week in adopting this change?

Were there factors that made it more difficult than I expected? How will I overcome these?

Do I need to revise my goals?

What strategies will help me do better in the next week?

Notes

Chapter 5: Out of Control!

1. Tom Peters and Nancy Austin, *A Passion for Excellence* (New York: Random House, 1985), 258.
2. Ibid., 216–17.
3. Authors Whiteman and Petersen discuss this at length in their book *Love Gone Wrong* (Nashville: Nelson, 1993).

Chapter 9: Stress Strategies at Work

1. Faith Popcorn, *The Popcorn Report* (New York: HarperCollins, 1991), 51.

Chapter 11: Home Stress

1. The Myers-Briggs Type Indicator by Peter B. Myers and Katharine D. Myers is available from Consulting Psychologists Press, Inc., 3803 E. Bayshore Rd., Palo Alto, CA 94303.
2. On male-female differences, we recommend John Gray's *Men Are from Mars, Women Are from Venus* (New York: HarperCollins, 1992) as well as our own *Men Who Love Too Little,* by Thomas Whiteman and Randy Petersen (Nashville: Nelson, 1994).
3. Gray, *Men Are from Mars,* 29–41.

Chapter 14: Limiting Time Involvements

1. "Impossible Dream," *Psychology Today* (May-June 1995), 8.

Chapter 16: Self-Talk

1. Edmond J. Bourne, *The Anxiety and Phobia Workbook* (Oakland, Calif.: New Harbinger, 1990), 153–54.

Chapter 17: Asserting Yourself in Nonstressful Ways

1. Bourne, *The Anxiety and Phobia Workbook*, 238. We would also recommend Robert Alberti and Michael Emmons, *Your Perfect Right* (San Luis Obispo, Calif.: Impact Press, 1974). This will give you a better understanding of assertive responses.

2. Recommended books on anger include Les Carter and Frank Minirth, *The Anger Workbook* (Nashville: Nelson, 1993) and *Those Who Need to Control* (Nashville: Nelson, 1993).

3. Adapted from Bourne, *The Anxiety and Phobia Workbook*.

Chapter 19: Exercise for Body and Mind

1. *Journal of the American Medical Association* (November 3, 1989).

2. *Geriatrics* (Vol. 44, No. 6), 13.

3. For a pamphlet on walking, write to the President's Council on Physical Fitness and Sports, Washington, DC 20001.

4. *Tufts University Diet and Nutrition Letter* 13, no. 1 (March 1995).

Chapter 20: Nutrition

1. Sheldon Cohen, M.D., "Stress May Raise Viral Susceptibility," *Medical Tribune* (February 10, 1994).

2. Robert S. Eliot, M.D., *From Stress to Strength* (New York: Bantam, 1994), 10–11.

3. Sandra McLanahan, M.D., "Preventive Medicine Through Stress Management," *Macrocosum Magazine* (Fall 1994), 6–7.

4. *New England Journal of Medicine* 328 (April 1994), 1,029–35.

5. Ibid., 1,040 ff.

6. *Journal of the National Cancer Institute* 85 (1993), 1,483.

7. *American Journal of Clinical Nutrition* (September 1994).

8. Jean Carper, *Food, Your Miracle Medicine* (New York: HarperCollins, 1993), 98–99.

9. This list comes primarily from the *Journal of American Dietetic Association* 93 (1993), 284.

10. *New England Journal of Medicine* 328 (1993), 1,444–49.

11. Ibid., 1,450 ff.

12. David Benton, Ph.D., "The Impact of Selenium Supplementation on Mood," *Biological Psychiatry* 29 (1991), 1,092–98.

Chapter 21: Delicious Eating to Transform Stress

1. James Balch, *Prescription for Nutritional Healing* (Garden City Park, N.Y.: Avery Publishign Grove, 1990), 133, 169, 196.

2. Samuel Verghese, *The Working People's Guide to Stress Management* (Philadelphia: Continental Press, 1989), 126.

3. Jay Stein, ed., *Internal Medicine* (4th ed.) (St. Louis: Mosby Yearbook, 1994), 315, 1160, 506–07, 284.

4. Note to editor: This note was heard on the radio. No details known.

Chapter 22: Medication and Nature's Resources to Reduce Stress

1. *Physician's Desk Reference* (PDR) is the only compendium of official, FDA-approved prescription drug labeling. It is published annually by Medical Economics Data Production Company at Montvale, N.J. You may buy a PDR from your local book store. Suggested price about $60.00.

2. *The Pill Book* answers most questions in a style so that the general public can easily understand the medication that their doctors prescribe. It describes everything you may need to know about more than 1500 prescription drugs, including generic and brand names, usual doses, side effects and much more. It is published by Bantam Books and may be purchased from your local book store. Suggested price is $8.00.